369 0246385

Physician
Assistant
Review

ON

Physician Assistant Review

4TH EDITION

EDITOR

Patrick C. Auth, PhD, MS, PA-C

Chair and Program Director
Physician Assistant Department
Hahnemann Physician Assistant Program
Drexel University
Philadelphia, Pennsylvania

ASSOCIATE EDITOR

Morris D. Kerstein, MD, FACS

Professor of Surgery
Jefferson Medical College of Thomas Jefferson University
Philadelphia, Pennsylvania

Wolters Kluwer | Lippincott Williams & Wilkins
Health

Philadelphia • Baltimore • New York • London
Buenos Aires • Hong Kong • Sydney • Tokyo

Senior Acquisitions Editor: Sonya Seigafuse
Senior Product Manager: Kerry Barrett
Vendor Manager: Alicia Jackson
Senior Manufacturing Manager: Benjamin Rivera
Senior Marketing Manager: Kim Schonberger
Design Coordinator: Terry Mallon
Production Service: S4 Carlisle

Printed in China

Library of Congress Cataloging-in-Publication Data

Physician assistant review/editor, Patrick C. Auth; associate editor, Morris D. Kerstein.—4th ed.
     p. ; cm.
   Includes bibliographical references and index.
   ISBN 978-1-4511-4409-3 (alk. paper)
   I. Auth, Patrick C. II. Kerstein, Morris D.
   [DNLM: 1.   Clinical Medicine—Examination Questions. 2.   Clinical Medicine—Outlines.
3.   Physician Assistants—Examination Questions. 4.   Physician Assistants—Outlines. WB 18.2]

610.76—dc23

2012008078

Care has been taken to confirm the accuracy of the information presented and to describe generally accepted practices. However, the authors, editors, and publisher are not responsible for errors or omissions or for any consequences from application of the information in this book and make no warranty, expressed or implied, with respect to the currency, completeness, or accuracy of the contents of the publication. Application of the information in a particular situation remains the professional responsibility of the practitioner.

The authors, editors, and publisher have exerted every effort to ensure that drug selection and dosage set forth in this text are in accordance with current recommendations and practice at the time of publication. However, in view of ongoing research, changes in government regulations, and the constant flow of information relating to drug therapy and drug reactions, the reader is urged to check the package insert for each drug for any change in indications and dosage and for added warnings and precautions. This is particularly important when the recommended agent is a new or infrequently employed drug.

Some drugs and medical devices presented in the publication have Food and Drug Administration (FDA) clearance for limited use in restricted research settings. It is the responsibility of the health care provider to ascertain the FDA status of each drug or device planned for use in their clinical practice.

To my parents, Patricia and Clifford,
PATRICK C. AUTH

To Margaret and Lars for your love and understanding.
MORRIS D. KERSTEIN

PREFACE AND ACKNOWLEDGMENTS

This fourth edition of *Physician Assistant Review* includes an expanded online, updated test bank with rationales for the correct and incorrect answers, and a new chapter, Preventive Medicine. Each chapter has been updated to reflect the latest standards of care and revisions based on our readers' feedback. The online material allows readers to take a simulated certification examination on their computer to test their knowledge. Readers will receive a complete assessment of their score, which will allow them to discover areas of weakness and better focus their studying. In addition, a team of test-item reviewers have reviewed the test questions.

Physician Assistant Review was written to prepare certified physician assistants for the recertification examination, and recent physician assistant graduates for their first certification examination. The goal of the book is to provide a review of the required primary care medical knowledge for physician assistants. The book is organized into 22 chapters. Chapters 1 through 13 detail body systems, Chapters 14 through 18 are organized into subspecialties, Chapter 19 provides a review of ethical and legal issues related to physician assistant practice, Chapter 20 discusses environmental emergencies, Chapter 21 provides a review of preventive medicine topics such as family violence,

unintentional household injuries, and falls prevention in older adults and lead levels in children and adults. Chapter 22 provides test taking and study strategies. Chapters 1 through 18 are subdivided into sections. Each disorder is presented using the following categories: etiology, pathology, clinical features, diagnostic studies, and management. The book has been prepared using an outline format to allow the reader to review a segment of material quickly. The online test questions will help guide the reader toward mastery of the material.

Physician Assistant Review has found itself the standard for comparison. This is a direct result of the contributors from the first, second, third, and fourth editions who are leaders in their field. I would like to offer a very special thank you to Kerry Barrett of Lippincott Williams & Wilkins for her patience, dedication, and editorial assistance. In addition, I would like to extend a thank you to the founding parents of the physician assistant profession, the physician assistants who volunteer their time at the local, state, and national level, and the physician assistant educators dedicated to our students. Without your commitment to the physician assistant profession this book would not be possible.

Patrick C. Auth

CONTRIBUTORS

Naveed Ahmed, MD, MPAS, PA-C
Academic Coordinator
Physician Assistant Program in the Kingdom of Saudi Arabia
George Washington Medical Faculty Associates
Department of Emergency Medicine
Kingdom of Saudi Arabia
Chapter 8

Michael R. Arnold, MCMs, PA-C
Adjunct Faculty
Physician Assistant Program
Center for Community Health and Minority Medicine
Barry University
Miami Shores, Florida
Chapter 16

Patrick C. Auth, PhD, MS, PA-C
Chair, and Program Director
Physician Assistant Department
Hahnemann Physician Assistant Program
Drexel University
Philadelphia, Pennsylvania
Chapters 7, 11, 21, and Test Review Committee

Matt Dane Baker, DHSc, PA-C
Dean, School of Science and Health, Professor
Philadelphia University
Philadelphia, Pennsylvania
Chapters 3 and 17

Jose "Pepe" E. Barcega, MHS, BS, PA-C
Director of Clinical Education, Clinical
   Assistant Professor
Hahnemann Physician Assistant Program
Drexel University
Philadelphia, Pennsylvania
Chapter 11

Adrian S. Banning, MMS, PA-C
Clinical Instructor
Hahnemann Physician Assistant Program
Drexel University
Philadelphia, Pennsylvania
Chapter 6

Kathryn T. Beishline, MSPAS, PA-C
Chair, Department of Physician Assistant Studies
Jefferson School of Health Professions
Thomas Jefferson University
Philadelphia, Pennsylvania
Test Review Committee

Reamer L. Bushardt, Pharm. D. PA-C
Chair and Professor
Department of Physician Assistant Studies
Wake Forest School of Medicine
Winston-Salem, North Carolina
Chapter 18

Jeffrey Bonfield, BS
Director, Center for Student
Academic Resources
Drexel University
Philadelphia, Pennsylvania
Chapter 22

George S. Bottomley, DVM, PA-C
Associate Professor and Program Director
Physician Assistant Program
University of New England
Portland, Maine
Chapter 6

M. Rebecca Buckley, MHS, PA-C
Associate Director of Clinical Education,
   Clinical Assistant Professor
Hahnemann Physician Assistant Program
Drexel University
Philadelphia, Pennsylvania
Chapter 5

Jill M. Calvalet, MHS, PA-C
Clinical Associate Professor
Department of Physician Assistant Studies
Saint Francis University
Loretto, Pennsylvania
Chapter 12

Lawrence Carey, Pharm. D.
Program Director, Associate Professor
Philadelphia University
Philadelphia, Pennsylvania
Chapter 18

Torry Grantham Cobb, PA-C, MPH, MHS, DHSc
Dartmouth Medical School/Dartmouth-Hitchcock Medical Center
Department of Surgery
One Medical Center Drive
Lebanon, New Hampshire
Chapter 2

Randi Beth Cooperman, DHSc, MCMSc, PA-C
Assistant Professor of Medical Education
Associate of Clinical Education
Physician Assistant Program
Center for Community Health and Minority Medicine
Barry University
Miami Shores, Florida
Chapter 16

Rosalie G. Coppola, MHS, PA-C
Assistant Clinical Professor
Hahnemann Physician Assistant Program
Drexel University
Philadelphia, Pennsylvania
Chapter 4 and Test Review Committee

Eric W. Cucchi, MS, PA-C
Adjunct Professor – School of Physician Assistant Studies
Massachusetts College of Pharmacy and Health Science
Faculty – UMass Memorial Physician Assistant Critical Care
    Residency
University of Massachusetts Memorial Hospital
Worcester, Massachusetts
Chapter 10

William Demshok, MS, PA-C
Assistant Professor Medical Education
Associate Director of Didactic Education
Physician Assistant Program
Center for Community Health and
    Minority Medicine
Barry University
Miami Shores, Florida
Chapter 16

G. John DiGregorio, MD, PhD
Medical Director
Hahnemann Physician Assistant Program
Professor, Pharmacology
Drexel University
Philadelphia, Pennsylvania
Chapter 18 and Test Review Committee

Diane Abercrombie, PA-C, MA, MMSc, PhD
Assistant Professor, Interim Chair
Department of Physician Assistant Studies
University of South Alabama
Mobile, Alabama
Chapter 2

Susan M. Dubendorfer, MPA, PA-C
Clinical Assistant Professor
Hahnemann Physician Assistant Program
Drexel University
Philadelphia, Pennsylvania
Chapter 15 and Test Review Committee

Ellen D. Feld, MD
Associate Clinical Professor
Hahnemann Physician Assistant Program
Drexel University
Philadelphia, Pennsylvania
Chapter 9

Richard Fien, MD, MPH, FACC
Associate Professor of Medical Education
Director of Didactic Education
Physician Assistant Program
Center for Community Health and
    Minority Medicine
Barry University
Miami Shores, Florida
Chapter 16

F. J. (Gino) Gianola, PA, DFAAPA
MEDEX Northwest Division of Physician
    Assistant Studies
Physician Assistant Training Program
Seattle, Washington
Chapter 19

Chandak Ghosh, MD, MPH
Senior Medical Consultant for Federal Policy
U.S. Department of Health and Human Services
Health Resources and Services Administration
New York, New York
Chapter 21

Lee Dresden Goldberg, MD, FACP, FACE
Adjunct Professor
Physician Assistant Program
Center for Community Health and Minority Medicine
Barry University
Miami Shores, Florida
Chapter 16

Debbie Hanson, MCMSC, PA-C
Assistant Professor of Medical Education
Associate Director of Medical Education
Physician Assistant Program
Center for Community Health and Minority Medicine
Barry University
Miami Shores, Florida
Chapter 16

Kelly Harrison, MSPAS, PA-C
Clinical Instructor
Hahnemann Physician Assistant Progam
Drexel University
Philadelphia, Pennsylvania
Test Review Committee

Michelle L. Heinan, EdD, MS, PA-C
Chair/Program Director
Physician Assistant Program
Concordia University
Mequon, Wisconsin
Chapter 1 and Test Review Committee

Jennifer Hixon, DHSc, PA-C
Program Director and Professor
Physician Assistant Progam
Bay Path College
Longmeadow, Massachusetts
Chapter 7

Robert D. Howard, MD, MSPT
Clinical Assistant Professor
Emergency Medicine Department
School of Medicine
Drexel University
Philadelphia, Pennsylvania
Chapter 7

Melissa M. Kagarise, DHSc, MMS, PA-C
Assistant Professor,
Department of Physician Assistant Studies
Saint Francis University
Loretto, Pennsylvania
Chapter 12

Morris D. Kerstein, MD, FACS
Professor of Surgery
Jefferson Medical College of Thomas Jefferson University
Philadelphia, Pennsylvania
Co-Editor

Julie J. Kinzel, MEd, PA-C
Clinical Instructor
Hahnemann Physician Assistant Program
Drexel University
Philadelphia, Pennsylvania
Chapter 4 and Test Review Committee

Joseph C. Krolikowski, MHS, PA-C
Adjunct Faculty
Hahnemann Physician Assistant Program
Drexel University
Philadelphia, Pennsylvania
Chapter 20

Vicki D. Lachman, PhD, MBE, APRN, FAAN
Clinical Professor
Drexel University
Philadelphia, Pennsylvania
Chapter 19

Grace P. Landel, MEd, PA-C
Program Director, Joint MSPAS/MPH Program
Associate Professor
College of Education and Health Sciences
Touro University California
Mare Island
Vallejo, California
Chapter 11

Clara LaBoy, MS, PAC, CAQ
Assistant Professor
Psychiatry School of Physician Assistant
    Studies-Worcester/Manchester
Massachusetts College of Pharmacy and Health Sciences
Worcester, Massachusetts
Test Review Committee

Daniela Cheles-Livingston, PA-C, MD
Clinical Instructor
Hahnemann Physician Assistant Program
Drexel University
Philadelphia, Pennsylvania
Chapter 9

Joseph Mileto, Jr., MHSc, PA-C
Associate Director of Clinical Education and
Clinical Assistant Professor
Hahnemann Physician Assistant Program
Drexel University
Philadelphia, Pennsylvania
Chapter 15

Keith Moore, PA-C, JD
Associate Professor of Medical Education
Associate Program Director
Center for Community Health and Minority Medicine
Physician Assistant Program
Barry University
Miami Shores, Florida
Chapter 16

Nina L. Multak, PA-C, MPAS
Clinical Assistant Professor
Hahnemann Physician Assistant Program
Drexel University
Philadelphia, Pennsylvania
Test Review Committee

Judy Nunes, PA-C
Lead Physician Associate in Neurosurgery
Yale-New Haven Hospital
New Haven, Connecticut
Chapter 6

Doreen Parkhurst, MD, FACEP
Associate Dean and Program Director
Physician Assistant Program
Center for Community Health and Minority Medicine
Barry University
Miami Shores, Florida
Chapter 16

Elizabeth Quinlan-Bohn, MS, RPA-C
Clinical Coordinator, Clinical Instructor
Physician Assistant Program
D'Youville College
Buffalo, New York
Chapter 13

Scott Richards, PhD, PA-C, DFAAPA
Assistant Professor of Physician Assistant Studies
School of Physician Assistant Studies-Worcester/Manchester
Massachusetts College of Pharmacy and Health Sciences
Manchester, New Hampshire
Test Review Committee

Theresa J. Riethle, MS, PA-C
Assistant Program Director
Associate Professor
Physician Assistant Program
Bay Path College
Longmeadow, Massachusetts
Chapter 10

Parmjeet S. Saini, PA-C, MPA, DHSc
Senior Public Health Analyst
Health Resources and Services Administration
Bureau of Clinician Recruitment & Services
New York, New York
Chapter 21

Margaret Schwedler, MD
Associate Professor of Anesthesiology
Thomas Jefferson University and Health Science Center
Medical Director
Jefferson Surgical Center
Philadelphia, Pennsylvania
Chapter 11

Todd Philip Smith, PA-C, MT (ASCP)
Assistant Professor
Department of Physician Assistant Studies
University of South Alabama
Mobile, Alabama
Chapter 2

Gloria M. Stewart, EdD, PA-C
Director and Professor
Physician Assistant Studies
Marietta College
Marietta, Ohio
Test Review Committee

Rebecca Lovell Scott, PhD, PA-C
Associate Clinical Professor and Academic Coordinator
Bouve College of Health Sciences
Physician Assistant Program
Northeastern University
Boston, Massachusetts
Chapter 14

Charles Stream, MPH, PA-C
Director of Critical Analysis, Clinical Instructor
Hahnemann Physician Assistant Program
Drexel University
Philadelphia, Pennsylvania
Chapter 20

Robin Wempe, PA-C
Joint MSPAS/MPH Program
Assistant Professor
College of Education and Health Sciences
Touro University California
Mare Island
Vallejo, California
Chapter 11

Anthony S. Zaza, PhD
Adjunct Assistant Professor
Department of Pyschiatry
School of Osteopathic Medicine
University of Medicine and Dentistry of New Jersey
Chief of Mental Health
VA Medical Center
Beckley, West Virginia
Chapter 5

CONTENTS

16 Surgery Disorders 383

William Demshok • Richard Fien • Debbie Hanson • Randi Beth Cooperman • Michael R. Arnold • Doreen Parkhurst • Keith Moore • Lee Dresden Goldberg

17 Geriatric Disorders. 416

Matt Dane Baker • Florida Olivieri

18 Pharmacology 430

G. John DiGregorio • Reamer L. Bushardt • Lawrence Carey

19 Ethical and Legal Considerations 455

Vicki D. Lachman • F. J. Gino Gianola

20 Environmental Emergencies. 474

Joseph C. Krolikowski • Charles Stream

21 Preventive Medicine 482

Parmjeet S. Saini • Patrick C. Auth

22 Study and Test-Taking Strategies 494

Jeffrey Bonfield

Head, Ears, Eyes, Nose, Throat Disorders

1

Michelle L. Heinan • Aaron L. Shapiro

I. Eye

THE EYELIDS/CONJUNCTIVA/LACRIMAL GLAND

A. Hordeolum (Figure 1-1)

1. **Definition**
   - Acute localized swelling of upper or lower eyelid.
2. **Etiology**
   - Caused by staphylococcal organism.
   - Internal hordeolum is a meibomian gland abscess.
   - External hordeolum is smaller and on the margin of the lid.
3. **Clinical Features**
   - May occur on the upper or lower eyelid.
   - Tender to touch, painful.
   - Red, swollen.
   - Vision acuity is normal.
4. **Diagnostic Studies**
   - None.
5. **Management**
   - May resolve spontaneously.
   - Topical antibiotic solution or ointment may assist in the acute phase.
   - Warm compresses three to four times per day.
   - May need incision and drainage (I & D) if no improvement within 48 hours.

B. Entropion

1. **Definition**
   - Inward turning of the lower eyelid.
2. **Etiology/Pathology**
   - Older population.

FIGURE 1-1. **Hordeolum (sty).** (From Weber J, Kelley J. *Health Assessment in Nursing.* 2nd ed. Philadelphia, PA: Lippincott Williams & Wilkins; 2003, with permission.)

- Extensive scarring of the conjunctiva and tarsus.
- Scarring, infection, or spastic conditions.
- May be congenital.
- Caused by weakness of the muscle surrounding the lower part of the eye.
3. **Clinical Features**
   - Redness.
   - Light sensitivity.
   - Dryness.
   - Increased lacrimation.
   - Foreign-body sensation.
   - Scratching of the cornea by lashes.
   - Eye irritation.
4. **Diagnostic Studies**
   - None.
5. **Management**
   - Artificial tears; ocular ointment at bedtime for lubrication.
   - Surgical tightening of muscles if lashes rubbing against cornea.
   - Cool compresses to decrease swelling.
   - Epilation of the eyelashes.

C. Ectropion

1. **Definition**
   - Outward turning of the eyelid exposing palpebral conjunctiva.
2. **Etiology**
   - Common in elderly individuals.
   - Following a seventh nerve palsy.
   - Orbicularis oculi muscle relaxation.
   - Can be congenital or have cicatricial causes.
3. **Clinical Features**
   - Excessive lacrimation.
   - Drooping of the eyelid.
   - Exposure keratitis.
   - Cosmetic deformity.
   - Redness.
   - Light sensitivity.
   - Dryness.
   - Foreign-body sensation.
4. **Diagnostic Studies**
   - None.
5. **Management**
   - Artificial tears.
   - Surgery (lid tightening).

1

FIGURE 1-2.   **Blepharitis.** (From Weber J, Kelley J. *Health Assessment in Nursing.* 2nd ed. Philadelphia, PA: Lippincott Williams & Wilkins; 2003, with permission.)

D. Blepharitis (Figure 1-2)

1. **Definition**
   - Bilateral eyelid margin inflammation.
   - Anterior or posterior; can coexist.
   - **Anterior:** *Staphylococcus* or seborrheic.
   - **Posterior:** Meibomian gland dysfunction (MGD).
2. **Etiology**
   - May be caused by a *Staphylococcus aureus* infection (usually ulcerative).
   - May be caused by *Staphylococcus epidermidis* or coagulase-negative staphylococci.
   - Seborrheic is associated with brows, ears, and/or scalp seborrhea and is nonulcerative. Pityrosporum ovale is involved but is not a causative agent. Seborrheic has no ulcers, scales are greasy, lid margins are less red than the ulcerative.
   - Possibly caused by type IV hypersensitivity reaction.
   - Associated with dry eye syndrome.
   - More common in women than in men.
   - Caused by excessive secretions from eyelid glands, poor eyelid hygiene, bacterial infection, viral or fungal infection, Gram-negative organisms, *Streptococcus,* herpes simplex, herpes zoster, or mites.
3. **Clinical Features**
   - **Anterior blepharitis:** Granulations or scales are attached to the eyelashes; eyes are red and swollen (red rimmed).
   - **Posterior blepharitis:** MGD that causes inflammation of the eyelid; bacterial infection.
   - With *Staphylococcus,* a primary glandular dysfunction with a strong association to acne rosacea; telangiectasis.
   - Orifices are plugged; glands are dilated; abnormal secretions (cheesy secretions).
   - Epithelial keratitis.
   - Cornea develops peripheral vascularization and thinning.
   - Meibomian glands are inflamed.
   - Mild entropion with tears of an abnormal greasy or frothy consistency.

- Burning, itching, and irritation of eyes.
- Complications include chalazion, hordeolum, recurrent conjunctivitis, epithelial keratitis, corneal infiltrates, abnormal lid or lash positioning, and inferior corneal thinning.
4. **Diagnostic Studies**
   - Cultures in severe cases.
5. **Management**
   - **Anterior:** Keep scalp, eyelids, and eyebrows clean.
   - Warm compresses followed by scrubbing the lids.
   - Remove scales with damp cotton applicator and baby shampoo, rinse with clean water.
   - Apply bacitracin or erythromycin eye ointment every day to lid margins.
   - **Posterior:** Eyelid massage and expression of the meibomian gland on a regular basis; management of face and scalp dermatology problem.
   - To control MGD, need to add an oral antibiotic (tetracyclines, doxycycline, minocycline, or erythromycin). Prednisolone may be used.
   - Artificial tears should be used on a daily basis.

E. Chalazion (Figure 1-3)

1. **Definition**
   - A localized swelling on the upper or lower eyelid.
2. **Etiology**
   - Most are caused by blockage of the meibomian gland duct by an accumulation of secretion.
   - Other factors may be the presence of seborrhea, viral infection, immunodeficiency, or acne rosacea.
3. **Clinical Features**
   - Hard, nontender swelling of the upper or lower eyelid.
   - Conjunctiva is usually red and elevated in the area of the lesion.
   - Lesion usually points inward.
   - If large enough, may cause astigmatism or distort vision from pushing on the cornea.
   - May have a history of blepharitis.

FIGURE 1-3.   **Chalazion.** (From Tasman W, Jaeger E. *The Wills Eye Hospital Atlas of Clinical Ophthalmology.* 2nd ed. Philadelphia, PA: Lippincott Williams & Wilkins; 2001, with permission.)

4. **Diagnostic Studies**
   • None.
5. **Management**
   • Visual field and visual acuity testing.
   • Warm compresses three to four times per day.
   • Referral to ophthalmologist if no improvement on its own.
   • Injection of a corticosteroid or I & D may be necessary.

F. **Conjunctivitis**
   1. **Definition**
      • Inflammation of the conjunctiva.
   2. **Etiology/Pathology**
      • **Viral:** Usually caused by an adenovirus type 3.
      • **Bacterial:** Chlamydiae, gonococci, *S. aureus, Streptococcus pneumoniae, Haemophilus* species, *Pseudomonas, Moraxella.*
      • Allergic.
      • Chemical.
      • Direct contact via fingers, towels, or other contaminated objects or surfaces.
      • *Staphylococcus* species found more in adults.

      GONOCOCCAL
      • Contact from genitalia-infected secretions.
      • Consider other sexually transmitted diseases or HIV.
   3. **Clinical Features**

      BACTERIAL
      • Eyelashes stick together in the morning.
      • Purulent discharge.
      • Very contagious.
      • Vision does not blur.

      GONOCOCCAL
      • Lid edema.
      • Purulent discharge.
      • Tender to palpation.
      • Redness.
      • Preauricular lymphadenopathy.
      • Urethritis is probably present.

      VIRAL
      • Associated with malaise, fever, pharyngitis, and preauricular lymphadenopathy.
      • Burning or gritty sensation.
      • Watery discharge, injected conjunctiva.
      • Watery eyes; second eye usually becomes infected within 1 to 2 days.
      • Eyelashes stick together in the morning.

      ALLERGIC
      • Watery discharge, injected conjunctiva.
      • Eyelashes stick together in morning.
      • Both eyes are affected.
      • Scratchy, erythema.
      • Burning sensation.
   4. **Diagnostic Studies**
      • Scrapings and cultures to be done in serious cases.
   5. **Management**

      IN ALL CASES
      • Avoid rubbing eyes.
      • Wash hands frequently; avoid using same towels as everyone else.
      • Contact lens wearers should dispose of the lens case, disinfect contact lens, and not use contacts until treatment is completed.

      VIRAL
      • Usually will heal itself within 2 weeks.
      • Possible topical decongestant/antihistamine.

      BACTERIAL
      • Topical antibiotic drops or ointment such as erythromycin ophthalmic ointment (mainly used for children) or sulfa ophthalmic drops for 5 to 7 days.
      • If no improvement in 48 to 72 hours despite treatment, refer to ophthalmologist.
      • Gonococci: Gram stain confirmed by Gram-negative diplococci, refer immediately to ophthalmologist, hospitalization for intravenous (IV) and topical antibiotic therapy. Considered emergency due to corneal involvement.

      ALLERGIC
      • Remove allergen if known.
      • Possible treatment options are use of lodoxamine tromethamine, cromolyn Na, olopatadine, ketorolac tromethamine, levocabastine HCl, naphzoline HCl, or pheniramine maleate.
      • Systemic antihistamines.

G. **Dacryocystitis (Figure 1-4)**
   1. **Definition**
      • Nasolacrimal system obstruction resulting in a lacrimal sac infection.
      • Reason for obstruction is unknown.
   2. **Etiology/Pathology**
      • Usually present in people over 40; peaks at ages 60 to 70; postmenopausal women; and infants.
      • Congenital: Both sexes are at equal risk. In acute cases, *S. aureus* and *β*-hemolytic strep.

FIGURE 1-4. **Acute dacryocystitis.** (From Tasman W, Jaeger E. *The Wills Eye Hospital Atlas of Clinical Ophthalmology.* 2nd ed. Philadelphia, PA: Lippincott Williams & Wilkins; 2001, with permission.)

- Usually unilateral.
- In chronic cases, *S. epidermidis,* anaerobic strep, *Candida albicans.*
- Results from chronic mucosal degeneration, ductile stenosis, stagnation of tears, and bacterial overgrowth.
- *Haemophilus influenzae* in children.
- Cause is usually unknown, but can be the result of trauma, nasal diseases, or a dacryolith.
- Congenital, may be due to infection or an incomplete canalization of the duct.

3. **Clinical Features**
   - Sudden onset of pain, redness of tear sac region, tenderness, and swelling.
   - Purulent material may be expressed from the sac.
   - Must remove obstruction or recurrences are common.
   - In chronic cases associated with obstruction of the nasolacrimal duct, pus or mucus may be expressed in these cases.
   - In some cases, may cause orbital cellulitis.
   - Discharge and tearing is present in chronic cases (tear film may decrease visual acuity).

4. **Diagnostic Studies**
   - Usually none; consider computed tomography (CT) scan or magnetic resonance imaging (MRI) when the etiology is in question.
   - Staining of smear taken from expressed tear sac secretions.
   - Complete blood count (CBC) to check for leukocytosis.
   - Antinuclear antibody to rule out lupus.
   - Antineutrophil cytoplasmin antibody testing to rule out Wegener granulomatosis.

5. **Management**
   - **Children:** Oral Augmentin, Unasyn, or Levaquin along with topical antibiotic drops/ointment, warm compresses, and acetaminophen. Aggressive treatment in children needed to avoid orbital cellulitis.
   - **Adults:** Augmentin, Unasyn, or Levaquin along with topical antibiotic drops/ointment, warm compresses, and ibuprofen. Usually dacryocystorhinostomy is needed.
   - **Acutely ill patients:** Should be hospitalized and treated with IV antibiotic (nafcillin or cloxacillin), blood and secretion cultures, warm compresses, and ibuprofen.
   - Imaging studies.
   - Removal of obstruction.
   - Probing of the nasolacriminal system.
   - Laser-assisted endoscopic dacryocystorhinostomy and balloon dilation.
   - **Congenital:** Warm compresses, lacrimal sac massage, antibiotics (topical and/or oral). Usually resolves spontaneously. Probing of the nasolacriminal system can be done.

H. Conjunctival Foreign Bodies
1. **Etiology**
   - Results from trauma to the conjunctiva by a foreign body.
2. **Pathology**
   - Foreign body sets off inflammatory reaction.
3. **Clinical Features**
   - Acute pain.
   - Foreign-body sensation.
   - Redness.
   - Excessive tearing.
   - Visual acuity may or may not be affected.
4. **Diagnostic Studies**
   - Check visual acuity and visual fields.
   - Slit lamp and/or funduscopic examination.
   - Fluorescein staining.
   - Evert the eyelids to check for foreign body and abrasions.
5. **Management**
   - Instillation of a local anesthetic.
   - Normal saline flush and removal of the foreign body using a sterile cotton-tipped applicator.
   - Reassessment in 24 hours by fluorescein staining.
   - Antibiotic ophthalmic ointment.
   - Referral to ophthalmologist if corneal epithelium is not healing properly within 24 hours or if unable to remove the foreign body completely.

I. Orbital Cellulitis
1. **Definition**
   - Severe infection of the eye tissue.
   - May cause intracranial infection, vision loss, or potential death.
2. **Etiology/Pathology**
   - Occurs in children, immunocompromised and geriatric populations.
   - Bacteremia.
   - Complications from eye surgery.
   - Paranasal sinusitis (most common).
   - Dental infection.
   - Orbital trauma.
   - *S. aureus, Streptococcus pyogenes, S. pneumoniae, H. influenzae* are most common in children under the age of 5.
   - Erosion of the orbital bone is possible, resulting in a brain abscess or meningitis.
3. **Clinical Features**
   - Decreased vision, double vision, proptosis, and pain and warmth around the eyes.
   - Purulent drainage may be present in case of infection.
   - Diffuse unilateral lid swelling, fever, and conjunctival hyperemia.
   - Limitation to extraocular movements.

4. Diagnostic Studies
- Check visual acuity.
- Cultures/smears to determine organism (nasal, blood, conjunctiva).
- Consult otolaryngologist.
- Consult neurologist if suspected meningitis.
- CT of orbit to check for foreign body, abscess, or sinusitis.

5. Management
- Requires prompt treatment and hospitalization.
- Refer to ophthalmologist.
- Immediate treatment with IV antibiotics.
- Local sprays to reduce sinus decongestion, oral or nasal decongestants, or antihistamines can be administered.
- Monitor body temperature, visual acuity, degree of proptosis, and ocular motility to determine progress.
- Examine patient on outpatient basis (after switching to oral antibiotics) every 2 to 4 days until resolved.
- Surgical drainage may be needed if an abscess has formed.

J. Pterygium
1. Definition
- A thickening of the conjunctiva in the shape of a triangle usually on the nasal side growing inward toward the cornea.

2. Etiology/Pathology
- Male.
- Comes from the limbus and grows toward or onto the cornea.
- Genetic.
- Linked to those in tropical climates, exposed to the sun, working outside, HPV infections, tumor suppressor gene p53 has an abnormal conjunctival expression, and abnormal HLA antigen expression.

3. Clinical Features
- Eye is usually red.
- Irritation.
- Sight can be affected if the pterygium grows into the region of the cornea.
- Causes difficulty for those who want to wear contacts due to irritation.

4. Diagnostic Studies
- Photographs or video keratography that shows progression.

5. Management
- Over-the-counter topical ointment, drops, or gels.
- Surgery.
- Refer to ophthalmologist.

THE CORNEA

A. Corneal Abrasion (Figure 1-5)
1. Definition
- An irregularity of the cornea, superficial in nature.

2. Etiology/Pathology
- Results from trauma to cornea by a foreign body, contact lens, fingernail.

FIGURE 1-5. **Corneal abrasion.** (From Tasman W, Jaeger E. *The Wills Eye Hospital Atlas of Clinical Ophthalmology.* 2nd ed. Philadelphia, PA: Lippincott Williams & Wilkins; 2001, with permission.)

3. Clinical Features
- Acute pain.
- Redness.
- Photophobia.
- Excessive tearing.
- Foreign-body sensation.
- Blurred vision.
- History of recent trauma.
- Usually presents with the eye closed.

4. Diagnostic Studies
- Check visual acuity and visual fields.
- Slit lamp and/or funduscopic examination.
- Fluorescein staining: defect will appear as a bright green area with black light.
- Evert the eyelids to check for foreign body or abrasions.

5. Management
- Remove foreign body, if present. Depending on how embedded the object is into the cornea, use a moistened, cotton-tipped applicator, sterile 22G needle, or Alger brush.
- Antibiotic ophthalmic ointment.
- Application of eye patch with firm pressure.
- Oral pain medication.
- Reassessment in 24 hours by fluorescein staining.
- Referral to ophthalmologist if corneal epithelium is not healing properly within 24 hours or if unable to remove the foreign body completely (if present).

B. Corneal Ulcer
1. Definition
- Corneal tissue necrosis.

2. Etiology/Pathology
- Most commonly caused by an infection of bacteria, fungi, amoeba, or virus.
- Noninfectious causes can be from inflammatory disorders, dry or allergic eyes, or neurotrophic keratitis.

- Caused most commonly by *Pseudomonas, S. pneumoniae, Staphylococcus, Chlamydia,* and *Acanthamoeba.*
- Usually with corneal trauma, corneal foreign body, inadequate contact lens sterilization, or sleeping in contact lenses.
- Can occur as a result of complications from chronic blepharitis, conjunctivitis, herpes simplex keratitis, trachoma.
- Can result from a vitamin A or protein deficiency.
- Can result from eyelid abnormalities where the cornea is exposed due to lack of complete eyelid closure.

3. **Clinical Features**
   - Photophobia, foreign-body sensation, ache, increased tearing initially (minimal).
   - Begins as a gray, circumscribed opacity that eventually necroses, forming an excavation of the cornea.
   - Eye is red, injection circumcorneal.
   - If fluorescein is applied, this area will stain green showing the defect.
   - In chronic cases, corneal neovascularization and pus in the anterior chamber may be present.
   - There may be purulent or watery discharge.
   - Decrease in visual acuity.
   - Perforation can occur causing leakage of aqueous humor.

4. **Diagnostic Studies**
   - Fluorescein staining.
   - Giemsa and Gram staining.
   - Culture.

5. **Management**
   - Immediate referral to ophthalmologist for treatment.

C. **Corneal Foreign Body (Figure 1-6)**
1. **Etiology**
   - Results from trauma to the cornea by a foreign body on the surface of, or embedded into, the cornea.

FIGURE 1-6. **Corneal foreign body.** (From Tasman W, Jaeger E. *The Wills Eye Hospital Atlas of Clinical Ophthalmology.* 2nd ed. Philadelphia, PA: Lippincott Williams & Wilkins; 2001, with permission.)

2. **Pathology**
   - Foreign body sets off inflammatory reaction.
   - If foreign body is not removed, can cause infection, tissue necrosis, or both.

3. **Clinical Features**
   - Acute pain.
   - Redness.
   - Photophobia, excessive tearing.
   - Foreign-body sensation.
   - Blurred vision.
   - History of recent trauma.
   - Usually presents with the eye closed.
   - May see a ring infiltrate surrounding the site of the foreign body if embedded for >24 hours.

4. **Diagnostic Studies**
   - Check visual acuity.
   - Slit lamp.
   - Visual fields.
   - Tetanus immunization status.
   - Fluorescein staining: the foreign body will be dark with an area of green surrounding it under the black light.
   - Evert the eyelids to check for foreign body or abrasions.

5. **Management**
   - Instill topical anesthetic.
   - Depending on how embedded the object is into the cornea, use a moistened cotton-tipped applicator, a sterile 22G needle, or an Alger brush.
   - Antibiotic ophthalmic drops should be applied such as Polytrim, Sulamyd, or Tobrex.
   - Application of eye patch with firm pressure.
   - Oral pain medication, if needed.
   - Reassessment in 24 hours by fluorescein staining.
   - Referral to ophthalmologist if corneal epithelium is not healing properly within 24 hours or if unable to completely remove the foreign body.

THE GLOBE

A. **Optic Neuritis**
1. **Definition**
   - Inflammation of the optic nerve.

2. **Etiology/Pathology**
   - Associated with demyelinative disease (i.e., multiple sclerosis).
   - May occur in association with viral infections (mumps, measles, influenza, and those caused by the *Varicella zoster* virus).
   - May occur with systemic lupus erythematosus.
   - Toxic substance exposure (e.g., methanol, tobacco).
   - Metabolic or nutritional issues.
   - Vascular insufficiency.

3. **Clinical Features**
   - Unilateral vision loss that develops suddenly.
   - Vision varies from 20/30 to no light perception.
   - Patient has pain particularly with any type of eye movement.

- Monocular field defects are possible.
- Color vision loss.
- Afferent pupillary defect (Marcus Gunn pupil).
- Disc margin blurring.
- In acute phase, the optic nerve appears normal and then becomes swollen.
- Occasional flame-shaped peripapillary hemorrhages are present.
- Optic atrophy occurs if enough optic nerve fibers are destroyed.
- Visual acuity usually improves within 2 to 3 weeks and frequently returns to normal.

4. **Diagnostic Studies**
   - Referral to ophthalmologist.
5. **Management**
   - Referral to ophthalmologist.
   - Referral to a neurologist if demyelinating disease.

B. Retinopathy

1. **Definition**
   - Progressive damage to the eye's retina.
   - One of the leading causes of blindness.
2. **Etiology/Pathology**
   - Can be caused by long-term uncontrolled diabetes or hypertension.
   - Can result in vision loss.

   DIABETIC RETINOPATHY
   - **Nonproliferative (Figure 1-7A, B)**
     - Capillary microaneurysms develop.
     - Tortuous and dilated veins.
     - Flame-shaped hemorrhages.
   - **Maculopathy**
     - Increasing ischemia.
     - Cotton-wool patches.
     - Retinal vein beading.
     - Closure of retinal capillaries.
   - **Proliferative**
     - Ischemia stimulates vessels that leak serum proteins.
     - Neovascularization can result.
     - Massive vitreous hemorrhage can result, causing sudden loss of vision.
     - Adhesions can develop.
     - Bands form and contract on the vitreous, causing retinal detachment or retinal tear.
     - Hemorrhage and swelling, leaking of fluid into the retina.
     - New growth of blood vessels within the eye.

   HYPERTENSIVE RETINOPATHY
   - Accumulation of the development of atherosclerosis from long-standing hypertension.
   - Acute elevation of blood pressure results in loss of autoregulation in the retinal circulation, causing vasoconstriction and ischemia.
3. **Clinical Features**

   DIABETIC RETINOPATHY
   - Decreased visual acuity and color vision.

FIGURE 1-7. A: Fundus with diabetic retinopathy and neovascularization of the optic disc. B: Hypertensive retinopathy. (From Tasman W, Jaeger E. *The Wills Eye Hospital Atlas of Clinical Ophthalmology.* 2nd ed. Philadelphia, PA: Lippincott Williams & Wilkins; 2001, with permission.)

- Retinal hemorrhage, retinal edema, hard exudate, neovascularization, macular exudate, retinal detachment.

  HYPERTENSIVE RETINOPATHY
  - Decreased visual acuity.
  - Retinal hemorrhage, retinal edema, cotton-wool exudates, copper/silver wiring, arteriovenous nicking, optic disc swelling, retinal detachment.
4. **Diagnostic Studies**
   - Referral to ophthalmologist.
5. **Management**
   - For patient with type 1 diabetes: Referral to ophthalmologist 3 years after onset and then annually.
   - For patients with type 2 diabetes: Referral to ophthalmologist at the time of diagnosis and annually.
   - Control blood glucose levels and lipid levels.
   - Women wishing to conceive should be referred to an ophthalmologist for evaluation.
   - For pregnant patients: Should be seen by ophthalmologist in the first trimester, then every 3 months until delivery.
   - Removal of vitreous hemorrhage.
   - Treatment may include argon laser panretinal photocoagulation, vitreoretinal surgery, treatment of systemic disease.

C. Retinal Detachment (Figure 1-8)

1. **Etiology**

   THREE TYPES
   - Rhegmatogenous retinal detachment (RRD)—the most common.
   - Exudative or serous retinal detachment (ERD).
   - Tractional retinal detachment (TRD).

2. **Pathology**
   - RRD—a break in the retina allows the vitreous fluid to leak, causing the detachment. Caused by spontaneous, penetrating, or blunt trauma.
   - ERD—accumulation of subretinal fluid causes the detachment. This detachment usually results from inflammation or a tumor.
   - TRD—adhesions form, causing a traction on the retina, which forces it to separate or tear. This type of detachment occurs with sickle-cell disease, trauma, or proliferative diabetic retinopathy.
   - Bilateral detachments are possible for patients who have had bilateral cataract extractions.
   - More common in patients with myopia >6 diopters.
   - Young people can sustain traumatic detachments.
   - Occurs between 40 and 70 years of age.
   - Cataract extraction and myopia are possible causes.
   - Can result in blindness or loss of light perception.
   - Leukemia, diabetes, angiomatosis, eclampsia, breast cancer, melanoma, and sickle-cell disease all increase the risk of retinal detachment.

3. **Clinical Features**
   - Photopsia.
   - Shower of floaters.

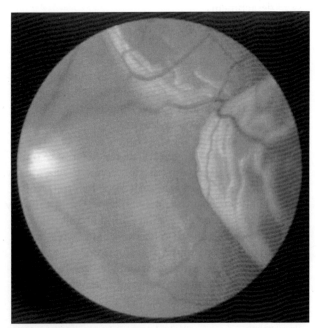

FIGURE 1-8. Retinal detachment. (From Moore KL, Dalley AF II. *Clinical Oriented Anatomy.* 4th ed. Baltimore, MD: Lippincott Williams & Wilkins; 1999, with permission.)

- Decreased visual acuity.
- Objects appear to have a wavy type of distortion.
- Visual field defects show as a late symptom.
- Flashing lights occur when the posterior vitreous separates.
- Asymptomatic until the inferior detachment progresses and reaches the fovea.
- Intraocular pressure (IOP) is >4 to 5 mm Hg in comparison with the unaffected eye.
- On examination, multiple tears may be present.
- Usually asymptomatic unless central vision is threatened, in which case the patient can suffer severe and abrupt vision loss.
- Appears as a concave, smooth-surfaced detachment with marginal fibrovascular bands extending into the vitreous body.

4. **Diagnostic Studies**
   - Referral to ophthalmologist.
   - Slit lamp.
   - No laboratory tests are usually needed unless a cause for the detachment is unknown. CT or MRI is used only if a tumor or foreign body is suspected.

5. **Management**
   - Emergent referral to ophthalmologist.
   - Choice of treatment depends on the size, location, and type of detachment. In some cases, the detachment can be handled medically.
   - Possible treatment methods include surgery, laser therapy, pneumatic retinopexy, and cryotherapy, scleral buckling, reattachment, and intraocular gas.

D. Retinal Vascular Occlusion

1. **Definition**
   - Occlusion of the central retinal artery or vein by an embolus, causing profound vision loss.

2. **Etiology/Pathology**
   - Artery: Usually occurs in patients between the ages of 50 and 80 who often have concurrent hypertension, hyperlipidemia, cardiac arrhythmia, diabetes, or atherosclerosis.
   - Artery: May be secondary to giant cell arteritis.
   - Artery: Systemic vasculitis, thrombophilia (congenital or acquired), hyperhomocysteinemia, oral contraceptives, or migraine in younger patients.
   - Vein: Most common on awakening. Screen for systolic hypertension, diabetes, hyperlipidemia, and glaucoma.

3. **Clinical Features**
   - Sudden, painless, unilateral loss of vision, visual field, or both, lasting from minutes (amaurosis fugax) to permanent.
   - Vein: Retinal venous dilatation, retinal cotton-wool spots, optic disk swelling, retinal hemorrhages, and dilation and tortuosity of the retinal veins.

- Vein: Possible neovascular glaucoma can develop in the first 3 months.
- Artery: A cherry red spot is seen at the fovea.
- Artery: Blood in the veins has a "box car" appearance.
- Occasionally an embolus can be visualized.
- Artery: Visual acuity is restricted to the temporal areas or by counting fingers.
- Artery: Swelling of the retina (lasts 4 to 6 weeks).
- Artery: After 4 to 6 weeks, retina appears normal, but the optic nerve is pale and arterioles attenuated.
- Artery: Cotton-wool spots are limited to the region affected.
- Artery: If head and neck pain are associated, consider internal carotid artery dissection.

4. **Diagnostic Studies**
- In addition, order electrocardiogram, fasting blood sugar, lipid profile, partial thromboplastin time, erythrocyte sedimentation rate, antiphospholipid antibiotics, plasma homocysteine, lupus anticoagulant, and C-reactive protein in younger patients, labs to rule out associated conditions, duplex ultrasound of the carotid.

5. **Management**
- Cause must be determined to prevent stroke.
- Emergency referral to ophthalmologist.
- Vein: Panretinal laser photocoagulation for those at risk for neovascular glaucoma.
- Intravitreal injections.
- Vein: Vitrectomy with radical optic neurotomy.
- Vein: Branch vein occlusion may benefit from injection of tissue plasminogen activator.
- Artery: Patient must lie flat with high levels of inhaled oxygen.
- Artery: IV acetazolamide.
- Thrombolysis may improve outcome.
- Artery: If giant cell arteritis is suspected, give high dose of corticosteroids and biopsy the temporal artery, possible involvement of the other eye.
- Low-dose aspirin.
- Check for sources of emboli including carotids or cardiac.
- Artery: Inhaled oxygen.
- Artery: Reduction of IOP and vascular resistance to flow (digital globe massage, paracentesis, and carbonic anhydrase inhibitors).
- Referral to cardiologist to rule out arrhythmia.

E. **Cataract**
1. **Definition**
- Opacities of the lens.
2. **Etiology/Pathology**
- Usually bilateral (but asymmetric).
- Due to injury, age, systemic disease, congenital, or inhaled corticosteroid treatments.
- Common loss of vision, particularly in elderly people.
- Usually occurs at >60 years of age.
- Cigarette smoking increases risk.
- Exposure to ultraviolet (UV) light.
- Malnutrition.
3. **Clinical Features**
- Can be visualized with ophthalmoscope or slit lamp.
- Shadows or black spots in red reflex.
- Hazy, blurred, or distorted vision.
- Loss of color vision.
- Double vision.
- Difficulty visualizing the retina due to opaque lens; fundus reflection is absent and the pupil becomes white.
4. **Diagnostic Studies**
- Thorough eye examination by ophthalmologist or optometrist.
5. **Management**
- Surgery indicated when there is visual impairment.

F. **Glaucoma**
1. **Definition**
- Disease of the optic nerve related to abnormal drainage of aqueous from the trabecular meshwork, which may cause increased ocular pressure resulting in decreased peripheral fields and possible blindness.
2. **Etiology**
- Populations at risk for open-angle glaucoma include people of African American origin; Asian and Inuits heritage for angle closure; people with vascular diseases such as hypertension; those with migraines, diabetes, or cardiovascular disease; older adults; those with high myopia; and people with a family history of glaucoma.
3. **Pathology**
   OPEN-ANGLE GLAUCOMA
- Lack of proper drainage of the aqueous through the trabecular meshwork, causing damage to the optic nerve and resulting in vision loss.
- May be associated with increased ocular pressure.
- Occurs in 90% to 95% of glaucoma cases.

   ACUTE (ANGLE CLOSURE) GLAUCOMA
- Primary can occur only with the closure of a preexisting narrow anterior chamber angle.
- Secondary to long-standing anterior uveitis or dislocation of the lens.
4. **Clinical Features**
   OPEN-ANGLE GLAUCOMA
- Asymptomatic until late in the disease.
- Chronic, slow, and progressive visual field loss.
- Increased cup:disc ratio on funduscopic examination.

   ACUTE GLAUCOMA
- Ocular pain and decreased vision.
- Halos around lights.
- Conjunctiva is injected; cornea is cloudy.

- Reduced visual acuity.
- Pupil is mildly reactive in a mid-dilated state.
- Nausea and abdominal pain may occur.
- IOP is >50.
- Physical examination: Visual field defects.
- Enlarged or excavated optic disk with pallor.

5. **Diagnostic Studies**
   - Thorough eye examination by ophthalmologist including tonometry.
   - Central field testing.
   - Pachymetry.

6. **Management**

   OPEN-ANGLE GLAUCOMA
   - Adrenergic blocking eye drops (timolol, levobunolol, betaxolol), epinephrine eye drops, β_2-agonist eye drops, prostaglandin analogs, or carbonic anhydrase inhibitors.
   - Laser surgery (trabeculoplasty).
   - Surgery (trabeculectomy).
   - Cyclophotocoagulation.

   ACUTE-ANGLE CLOSURE GLAUCOMA
   - Decrease of IOP by laser (argon or yttrium aluminum garnet).
   - Systemic acetazolamide, with or without osmotic agents.
   - Laser peripheral iridotomy, iridoplasty, or iridectomy.
   - Pilocarpine after IOP begins to drop.
   - Prophylactic iridotomy on uninvolved eye.
   - Refer to ophthalmologist.

G. Strabismus

1. **Etiology**
   - Basically unknown, but can be hereditary.
   - Can be the result of stroke, thyroid disease, tumor, nerve conditions, or trauma.
   - Can present at birth or shortly thereafter.
   - Also can develop from 6 months to 7 years of age.

2. **Pathology**
   - Poor development of one eye with decreased visual acuity, which can lead to amblyopia and blindness if not corrected.

3. **Clinical Features**
   - Most common presentation is esotropia (crosseyed) or exotropia (wall-eyed).
   - Both eyes are not able to align simultaneously on an object.
   - Presentation at birth is a congenital esotropia.
   - Development between 6 months and 7 years has some accommodative component.
   - One eye wanders out when patient is ill, tired, or compromised in some way (intermittent exotropia).
   - Eye wanders longer and more frequently with time. Eventually leads to eye turning outward all the time (constant exotropia).

4. **Diagnostic Studies**
   - Hirschberg light reflex test.
   - Cover/uncover test.
   - Referral to ophthalmologist or optometrist.

5. **Management**
   - Check visual acuity; if amblyopia is present, patch good eye.
   - Make sure that there is no regression of the good eye during the time it is patched.
   - Surgery may be necessary to straighten eyes.
   - Late onset cases usually cause diplopia.
   - May be treated with eyeglasses, prisms, or a vision therapy program called orthoptics.
   - Eye patch or surgery may be necessary.
   - Referral to a neurologist if underlying disease is suspected.

H. Nystagmus

1. **Definition**
   - Unilateral or bilateral oscillation of the eye that is dependent on gaze with one eye more pronounced.

2. **Etiology/Pathology**
   - May occur with ocular lesion, esotropia, or hypoplastic visual pathways.
   - Likely ocular, but may have central nervous system (CNS) or inner ear involvement.

3. **Clinical Features**
   - Must occur in normal fields of vision.
   - Occurs in one or more planes.
   - Refer to pediatric ophthalmologist to do an iris transillumination.

4. **Diagnostic Studies**
   - When testing eyes, material to occlude the eye should be held 12 in away from the eye not being tested. Placing the material close to the eye worsens the condition of nystagmus and does not give a good read on acuity.
   - Electroretinogram to rule out retinal pathology.
   - Referral to ophthalmologist.

5. **Management**
   - Referral to ophthalmologist.
   - Possible surgery or treatment with prisms.

I. Macular Degeneration

1. **Definition**
   - Unilateral progressive vision loss.

2. **Etiology/Pathology**
   - Over the age of 55.
   - Family history.
   - Smoker (current or previous).
   - Light colored iris.
   - Lack of physical activity.
   - Possibly due to low intake of essential vitamins.
   - Cardiovascular disease.
   - Red or blond hair.
   - Female.
   - Caucasian.

3. **Clinical Features**
   - Hard and soft drusen on ophthalmoscopic examination.
   - **Neovascular type:** Confluent, large soft drusen.
   - **Neovascular type:** More rapid loss of vision.
   - **Atrophic type:** Bilateral gradual and progressive vision loss.
   - Central vision loss, periphery remains intact.
4. **Diagnostic Studies**
   - Biomicroscopic fundoscopic exam.
   - Fluorescein angiography to confirm wet age-related macular degeneration.
   - Optical coherence tomography to assess treatment response.
5. **Management**
   - Stop smoking and increase physical activity.
   - Eat dark green leafy vegetables and foods high in omega 3 fatty acids.
   - Avoid excessive sunlight.
   - Consult retina specialist.

J. Papilledema
1. **Definition**
   - Increased intracranial pressure that causes swelling of the optic disk.
2. **Etiology/Pathology**
   - Causes can be meningitis, encephalitis, pseudotumor cerebri, cerebral trauma or hemorrhage, brain tumor or abscess.
3. **Clinical Features**
   - Most of the time is bilateral.
   - No warning symptoms except for a couple of seconds of diminished vision.
   - Headache, nausea, vomiting if increased intracranial pressure.
   - Tortuous retinal veins, optic disk retinal hemorrhages, swollen and hyperemic optic disk.
   - Pupillary response and visual acuity are abnormal in advanced conditions.
4. **Diagnostic Studies**
   - Thorough ophthalmoscopic examination.
   - Possible neuroimaging to search for cause.
5. **Management**
   - Determine the cause.
   - Treat the underlying condition.
   - Reduce intracranial pressure.

K. Blowout Fracture
1. **Definition**
   - Fracture of the floor of the orbit resulting in an increase in IOP.
2. **Etiology/Pathology**
   - Blunt force trauma against the eye.
3. **Clinical Features**
   - Intraocular muscles and fat pads may be caught in fracture.
   - Enophthalmos.
   - Possible infraorbital rim, upper lip, and cheek anesthesia.
   - Upward gaze diplopia signifying inferior rectus muscle entrapment.
   - Step off of infraorbital rim.
   - Look for retinal detachment, lens dislocation, ruptured globe, hyphema.
4. **Diagnostic Studies**
   - Orbital CT.
5. **Management**
   - Tetanus.
   - Pain control.
   - Possible prophylactic antibiotics.
   - Educate patient on avoidance of nose blowing and valsalva.
   - Consult with ophthalmologist and maxillofacial surgeon.

L. Hyphema
1. **Definition**
   - Anterior chamber bleeding.
2. **Etiology/Pathology**
   - Usually blunt trauma.
   - Nontraumatic: newborn after stressful birth, blood dyscrasias, juvenile xanthogranuloma.
3. **Clinical Features**
   - May be associated with other ocular injury such as retinal detachment or edema, glaucoma, subluxation of the lens, or iritis. Those patients with sickle cell trait or anemia who have an elevated intraoculation pressure.
4. **Diagnostic Studies**
   - Refer to ophthalmologist.
5. **Management**
   - Refer to ophthalmologist.
   - Shield over eye, head elevated.

II. Ear
THE EXTERNAL EAR
A. Otitis Externa
1. **Etiology**
   - A bacterial infection of the external auditory canal.
   - Fungal infection.
   - Swimming or use of cotton-tipped applicators removes the protective layer of cerumen, resulting in maceration.
   - Trauma, eczema, foreign body, otorrhea, and contact dermatitis are contributing factors.
2. **Pathology**
   - *Pseudomonas aeruginosa.*
   - *S. aureus.*
   - *Streptococcus.*
   - *Moraxella catarrhalis.*
   - *H. influenzae.*
   - *Proteus.*
   - Chronic cases are fungal—*Candida, Aspergillus.*

3. Clinical Features
- Localized infection sometimes forming a boil, called furunculosis, which causes pain on pushing on the tragus.
- Generalized, painful.
- May note drainage at the opening of the external auditory canal.
- Hearing not affected, or minimal.
- Swelling of the canal.
- Discharge noted in the canal.
- Facial nerve function should be normal.
- Severe infection may show signs of auricular or postauricular cellulitis, which may resemble a mastoid abscess.
- Malignant external otitis is a separate entity caused by *P. aeruginosa* in patients with diabetes, which results in erosion of tissue and bone and needs immediate attention by an otolaryngologist.
- Discharge noted in the canal.

4. Diagnostic Studies
- Cultures in cases of treatment failures or refractory.

5. Management
- Cortisporin otic (if tympanic membrane [TM] is intact). Ofloxacin otic or Cipro HC Otic can be used. Ofloxacin otic is the drug of choice when a perforated TM cannot be ruled out.
- Systemic antibiotics in case of cellulitis, or possible system involvement.
- Refer resistant cases to an ENT specialist.
- Oral analgesics if needed for pain.
- Educate patient on not getting water in ear.
- No swimming until completion of antibiotics.
- Recommend baths instead of showers.
- Educate patient on not storing medications in the refrigerator.

B. Foreign Body
1. Etiology
- Most often seen in children.

2. Pathology
- Foreign body of metallic origin.
- Foreign body of plant or organic matter.

3. Clinical Features
- May have conductive hearing loss.
- May have otalgia or discharge if secondarily infected.
- Bleeding is possible if the object is sharp.

4. Diagnostic Studies
- None.

5. Management
- For solid material, a loop, or a hook, or an alligator forceps may be used. Be careful not to rupture TM; may irrigate if it is a rounded object, such as a bead.
- Do not put water in the ear if the foreign body is of organic matter; it will cause the object to swell.

- If an insect is the foreign body, lidocaine or mineral oil can be used to immobilize the insect before removal.
- Irrigation (use room temperature sterile water or normal saline) if TM is intact.
- After removal of foreign body, otic topical antibiotics with steroid can be prescribed.

C. Neoplasm
1. Etiology
- Chronic irritation.
- Sun exposure.

2. Pathology
- Most common carcinomas of ear canal are squamous cell.

3. Clinical Features
- Can mimic a persistent otitis externa.
- Extremely high 5-year mortality rate.
- The neoplasm spreads to the cranial base lymphatics rapidly.
- May cause conductive hearing loss from buildup of debris and exudates.
- Biopsy is warranted if otitis externa does not resolve with appropriate therapy.

4. Diagnostic Studies
- Biopsy.

5. Management
- Proper and timely referral to the ENT department.
- Wide surgical resection.
- Radiation therapy.

D. Hearing Impairment (Table 1-1)
1. Etiology
CONDUCTIVE
- Foreign body, cerumen impaction, otitis media, perforation or immobilization of the TM, otosclerosis, ossicular discontinuity/fixation, or tumors.
- Usually has a history of previous ear disease.
- Onset in childhood to age 40.

SENSORINEURAL
- Common causes include natural aging (presbycusis), drugs (e.g., aspirin, aminoglycosides, gentamycin), head trauma, excessive noise exposure, acoustic neuroma.
- Onset from middle to late years.

2. Pathology
CONDUCTIVE LOSS
- Disruption of the external or middle ear, impairing sound conduction to the inner ear.
- Sound wave conduction is obstructed by canal obstruction, fluid in middle ear, or ossicular disease such as otosclerosis.

SENSORINEURAL LOSS
- Impaired nerve impulse transmission to the brain; inner ear or cochlear nerve disorder losses of both air and bone thresholds are diminished.

TABLE 1-1.   Patterns of Hearing Loss

	Conductive Loss	Sensorineural Loss
Impaired understanding of words	Minor	Often troublesome
Effect of noisy environment	May help	Increases the hearing difficulty
Usual age of onset	Childhood, young adulthood	Middle and old age
Ear canal and drum	Often a visible abnormality	Problem not visible
Weber test (in unilateral hearing loss)	Lateralizes to the impaired ear	Lateralizes to the good ear
Rinne test	BC > AC or BC = AC	AC > BC
Causes	Plugged ear canal, otitis media, immobile or perforated drum, otosclerosis, foreign body	Sustained loud noise, drugs, inner ear infections, trauma, hereditary disorder, aging

From Bickley LS, Szilagyi PG. *Bates' Pocket Guide to Physical Examination and History Taking.* 5th ed. Philadelphia, PA: Lippincott Williams & Wilkins; 2007:114, with permission.

- Seen in damage or dysfunction to cochlea/hair cells and eighth cranial nerve disease/trauma, tumors such as acoustic neuroma or CNS disease.
- Systemic causes such as diabetes mellitus.

3. **Clinical Features**

CONDUCTIVE
- Examination of auditory canal may disclose foreign body, cerumen impaction, otitis externa, or exostosis.
- Examination of TM may disclose bulging, perforation, scarring, inflammation, fluid levels, or hemotympanum.

CONDUCTIVE LOSS
- Weber test—sound lateralizes to affected ear (Figure 1-9).
- Rinne test—BC > AC or BC = AC (negative Rinne) (Figure 1-10).

SENSORINEURAL
- Upper tones are lost.
- Gradually progressive.

- May occur suddenly and needs immediate attention by an otolaryngologist.
- Usually bilateral and symmetric, but one side may start first or be worse than the other.
- More difficult to hear in noisy environment.
- Patient has difficulty hearing own voice.
- May have a history of excessive noise exposure, inner ear infections, trauma, and use of medications such as salicylates, aminoglycosides, quinine derivatives, and loop diuretics.
- Nothing can be found on physical examination of the ear.

SENSORINEURAL LOSS
- Weber test—sound lateralizes to the good ear.
- Rinne test—AC > BC (positive Rinne).

4. **Diagnostic Studies**
- **Audiogram:** Establishes pattern of hearing loss. Normal hearing: 0 to 20 dB. Severe loss by a threshold of 60 to 80 dB.
- **MRI:** Used to rule out multiple sclerosis or acoustic neuroma in certain cases.
- **CT scans:** Used in middle-ear and mastoid problems.

FIGURE 1-9. **Weber test.** (From Bickley LS, Szilagyi PG. *Bates' Guide to Physical Examination and History Taking.* 8th ed. Philadelphia, PA: Lippincott Williams & Wilkins; 2003, with permission.)

Conductive phase
Air conduction →
Bone conduction ⇢
Sensorineural phase →

FIGURE 1-10. **Rinne test.** (From Bickley LS, Szilagyi PG. *Bates' Guide to Physical Examination and History Taking.* 8th ed. Philadelphia, PA: Lippincott Williams & Wilkins; 2003, with permission.)

5. **Management**
   - Conductive hearing loss usually can be resolved with medical and/or surgical measures (cerumen or foreign-body removal, topical antibiotics for otitis externa).
   - ENT referral for conditions not responsive to treatment and for sensorineural hearing losses, especially sudden hearing loss.
   - Sensorineural hearing losses may be stabilized.
   - Routine audiograms for those exposed to high levels of noise.
   - Amplification or hearing aids.
   - Cochlear implant for those with significant sensorineural hearing loss.

E. Hematoma of the External Ear

1. **Etiology**
   - Due to trauma.
   - Hematoma develops between the cartilage and the perichondrium.

2. **Clinical Features**
   - Purplish swelling of the upper part of the ear.
   - Obscured cartilage folds.

3. **Management**
   - Refer to an ENT physician.
   - Aspiration of the area with specifically applied pressure dressing.
   - Recurrent hematomas require surgical drainage.

THE MIDDLE EAR

A. Otitis Media

1. **Etiology**
   - Common in children (90% before the age of 6), although it can occur in an adult.
   - Adults usually develop otitis media when they have had several infections as a child.
   - Higher risk for children with cleft palates, immune disorders, or Down syndrome.
   - Children feeding in less than an upright position are more predisposed to infections.
   - Upper respiratory infection (URI) predisposes, as well as day-care attendance.
   - Peaks in winter and spring.
   - Children with allergies (particularly those with large adenoids).
   - Exposed to smoking, including wood-burning stoves.
   - Familial.
   - Bacterial infection of middle ear.
   - Incidence decreases with age.
   - If unilateral in adult, ENT referral to rule out nasopharyngeal tumor.

2. **Pathology**
   - Eustachian tubes are narrow, more horizontal, and short.
   - Eustachian tubes can be obstructed secondary to large adenoids, causing poor drainage.

   - Most common causative organisms include *S. pneumoniae, H. influenzae, S. pyogenes*, and *M. catarrhalis.*
   - Acute otitis media, viral in nature (respiratory syncytial virus [RSV]), can cause 25% of the cases seen.
   - Eustachian tube malfunction causes a buildup of mucus and fluid, which becomes secondarily infected by bacteria.

3. **Clinical Features**
   - In younger patients, can be associated with conductive hearing loss, resulting in cognitive learning problems and deficiency in verbal abilities.
   - URI with runny nose and congestion may be associated.
   - Conjunctival inflammation.
   - May be asymptomatic.
   - Sometimes systemic with diarrhea and/or vomiting.
   - Difficulty hearing.
   - Otalgia.
   - Check for dental problems, tonsillitis, cervical lymphadenopathy, retropharyngeal cancer.
   - Infection may present as irritability and fever.
   - TM is often bulging and erythematous with decreased or poor light reflex.
   - Decreased visible landmarks.
   - May see cloudy, purulent fluid behind TM.
   - Possibility exists for rupture of the TM.
   - Decreased TM mobility on pneumatic insufflation.
   - Pain may precede redness.
   - Check gross hearing and whisper tests.
   - Otalgia should resolve after 24 hours.

4. **Diagnostic Studies**
   - No studies are necessary unless the child is appearing ill; refer to ENT for tympanocentesis.
   - Check for iron-deficiency anemia if the child has had multiple episodes of acute otitis media.
   - Tympanometry, if available.
   - ENTs will order a CT or MRI to check for tumors, nerve damage.

5. **Management**
   - Analgesics/antipyretics (i.e., Tylenol, codeine if necessary).
   - Auralgan every 2 hours (q2h) may be used topically for ear pain.
   - Antibiotics (amoxicillin, amoxicillin/clavulanate potassium).
   - In the case of a penicillin allergy, use trimethoprim-sulfamethoxazole (TMP-SMZ) or azithromycin.
   - Reevaluate if pain and fever persist after 3 days of treatment.
   - Decongestants (e.g., oral pseudoephedrine or oxymetazoline 0.05% topical in nose) relieve URI or Eustachian tube blockage.

- Avoid antihistamines—may cause thickened secretions.
- Myringotomy—use in patients with increased hearing loss, poor response to medical therapy, or intractable pain.

B. Serous Otitis Media

1. Etiology
- Common in children because Eustachian tube is smaller and more horizontal.
- In adults with unilateral serous otitis media, must rule out nasopharyngeal carcinoma.
- Viral.
- Mycoplasmal.
- May occur in adults after flying due to a baro-trauma, allergens, or an URI.

2. Pathology
- Serous or mucoid secretions filling middle ear and interfering with the TM movement and ossicular chain function, resulting in conductive hearing loss.
- Often due to Eustachian tube blockage or dysfunction resulting in negative pressure.
- Common in adults after having viral URI or barotrauma.

3. Clinical Features
- No acute symptoms. In children, usually discovered when the child first goes to school and hearing loss is suspected by the teacher.
- Conductive hearing loss.
- TM may be retracted, clear, or dull with bony landmarks intact.
- May have clear fluid behind TM or air bubbles.
- Decreased tympanic mobility.
- Fever and pain are not present.

4. Diagnostic Studies
- Tympanogram diagnostic, and should be done in all suspected cases.

5. Management
- Oral/topical decongestants used in Eustachian tube blockage.
- Some practitioners use short courses of oral steroids (prednisone) and/or antibiotics (amoxicillin, Augmentin, or TMP-SMZ).
- Laser expansion via endoscopy in recalcitrant cases.
- Ventilation tubes if medical treatment fails.

C. TM Rupture

1. Etiology
- Usually due to acute otitis media.

2. Clinical Features
- Discharge noted.
- Possible conductive hearing loss.

3. Diagnostics
- None.

4. Management
- Most perforations heal within 2 weeks.
- Surgical repair for those perforations that do not heal in 3 to 6 months.
- Refer to ENT for surgical repair and timing.

D. Cholesteatoma

1. Etiology
- Prolonged dysfunction of the Eustachian tube.

2. Clinical Features
- Squamous epithelium lined sac develops and then fills with desquamated keratin when obstructed.
- Chronically infected.
- Erodes bone.
- Penetrates mastoid and ossicular chain.
- Can cause facial paralysis if left untreated.
- Retraction pocket of epitympanic.
- Keratin or granulation tissue from perforated TM.

3. Diagnostic Studies
- Refer to ENT.

4. Management
- Refer to ENT.
- Surgery.

E. Mastoiditis

1. Etiology
- Inflammation of the mastoid.
- Mainly in children under 2 years of age.
- Inadequate treatment of acute otitis media.

2. Pathology
- *S. pneumoniae*.
- *S. pyogenes*.
- *S. aureus*.
- *H. influenze*.
- Occasionally gram-negative bacilli and anaerobes.

3. Clinical Features
- Preauricular pain.
- Fever.
- Erythema and tenderness of the mastoid process.
- Pinna displaced outward.
- Acute otitis media.
- Meningitis and brain abscess are complications.

4. Diagnostic Studies
- CT scan.

5. Management
- IV antibiotics.
- Myringotomy with drainage and culture.
- Mastoidectomy if treatment fails.

THE INNER EAR

A. Labyrinthitis

1. Etiology
- Mainly viral.
- Can be caused by bacteria, although unusual.
- Common in adolescents to young adults.
- Familial and/or seasonal.
- History of URI, otitis media, or sinusitis.
- Paralysis of the vestibular nerve.

2. Pathology
- Vestibular neural input disrupted to the cerebral cortex and brain stem.
- Secondary to a URI that consists of infection of the labyrinth.
- Vertigo is caused by edema and inflammation.

- Viral infection that affects the cochlea and labyrinth.

3. **Clinical Features**
   - History of URI.
   - Self-limiting.
   - May last 7 to 10 days.
   - During recovery period, sudden rapid movements of head can bring on transient vertigo.
   - Vital signs—may have orthostatic changes.
   - Nausea and vomiting.
   - Subsequent episodes can occur 12 to 18 months after the initial episode. Each episode is less severe and shorter in duration.
   - Vertigo.
   - Nystagmus (rotary away from affected ear).
   - Neurologic deficits are uncommon; CNS assessment usually is normal.
   - CNS abnormality suggests a central process.
   - Detailed history to rule out psychiatric, cardiovascular, pulmonary, CNS, or metabolic disorders.
   - Comprehensive physical examination including Head, Ears, Eyes, Nose and Throat (HEENT), neuro with mental-status examination, hearing and speech evaluation.

4. **Diagnostic Studies**
   - Audiologic testing.
   - Electronystagmography (ENG), depending on findings.
   - CT scan or MRI may be warranted on the basis of undetermined or determined neurologic findings.

5. **Management**
   - Use of methyprednisolone is possible to decrease inflammation.
   - Antihistamines, antiemetics, anticholinergics.
   - If ill, may require hospitalization.
   - Patient reassurance.

B. **Ménière Syndrome**
   1. **Etiology**
      - Malfunction of the endolymphatics.
      - Condition affecting the inner ear.
      - May be associated with trauma, syphilis, or may be idiopathic.
      - Occurs mainly in middle age.
      - Males > females.
      - Caucasians have the syndrome more frequently.
      - Inherited, history of allergies, or exposure to noise.
      - No differentiation between ears.
      - Bilateral in 20% of patients.
   2. **Pathology**
      - Imbalance in secretion and absorption of endolymphatic fluid that causes buildup of fluid in cochlea.
      - Associated hair-cell damage as a result of semicircular duct swelling.
      - Distention of endolymphatic compartment of inner ear.

3. **Clinical Features**
   - Vertigo is sudden, lasting 1 to 8 hours, and can be debilitating. Patient feels as if everything is moving.
   - Vestibular nystagmus.
   - Fullness or pressure in the ears.
   - Nausea and vomiting are possible.
   - Tinnitus.
   - Fluctuant sensorineural hearing loss.
   - HEENT, hearing acuity, speech discrimination, neurologic examination with reflexes, mental status examination, and gait should be checked. Also, the cardiovascular, pulmonary, endocrine, and psychological status of the patient should be evaluated.

4. **Diagnostic Studies**
   - ENG.
   - Audiometry.
   - EEG.
   - Rotational testing.
   - CT or MRI to rule out lesions.

5. **Management**
   - Decrease the endolymphatic hydrops.
   - Valium 5 mg IM or 10 mg PO.

   ANTICHOLINERGICS
   - Antivert 25 to 50 mg q6h.
   - Low-sodium diet (goal of therapy is to decrease endolymphatic pressure).
   - Most cases can be corrected with the diuretic and low-sodium diet.
   - Avoid caffeine, alcohol, and smoking.
   - Advise patient to get enough sleep.
   - ENT referral.
   - If medical therapy is not effective, surgical intervention may be considered.

   VESTIBULAR NEURECTOMY
   - Labyrinthectomy is the "gold standard" if hearing is already lost.
   - Resection of the eighth cranial nerve is possible, but has complications.

C. **Tinnitus**
   1. **Etiology**
      - A symptom present in ear disease.
      - Abnormal noises are heard in the head or ears.
      - Characterized as a "ringing" in the ears.
      - Important but nonspecific, and has many causes.
      - Can be caused by pathology of external ear with extension to the inner ear and CNS pathology.
      - Cause also may be psychogenic, cerebrovascular (e.g., aneurysm), or musculoskeletal (e.g., temporomandibular joint dysfunction).
   2. **Pathology**
      - Condition may originate in outer, middle, or inner ear, or within the nerve supply of the ear (CN III).
      - Also consider glomus tumors, cerebral vascular disease, carotid bruit, flow impedance disorders, arteriovenous malformation, and aneurysm if pulsatile.

3. **Clinical Features**
   - May have a history of occupational exposure to noise.
   - May have a history of use of ototoxic drugs.
   - May find cerumen impaction, foreign body, otitis media, or ruptured TM.
   - Often have accompanied sensory hearing loss.
   - Occasional high-pitched ringing is normal.
   - If severe, concentration or sleep may be affected.
4. **Diagnostic Studies**
   - ENT referral.
   - Audiogram.
   - MRI.
   - Venography.
5. **Management**
   - Treat underlying cause.
   - Change ototoxic medicines.
   - Noise protection.
   - Several drugs have been tested, but a question of efficacy exists; may try antidepressants (e.g., nortriptyline) in severe cases.
   - May need ENT referral, especially if basic measures are not successful or if tinnitus becomes debilitating.
   - Hearing aid.
   - IV lidocaine or antidepressants have been effective in treatment.

D. Vertigo
1. **Etiology**
   - Symptom of vestibular disease.
   - Sensation of motion, spinning, or tilting.
   - Perception of things spinning around the patient.
   - Can be due to peripheral or central lesions.
   - Peripheral causes usually have sudden onset.
2. **Pathology**
   - Pathology of inner ear (e.g., labyrinthitis, Ménière syndrome).
   - Pathology of eighth cranial nerve (i.e., acoustic neuroma, vasculitis, metastatic disease).
   - CNS pathology (i.e., occlusion of vertebral and posterior inferior cerebellar artery), cerebellar disease, brain stem lesions.
   - Triggers: high-sodium diet, fatigue, stress, bright lights.
   - Must rule out systemic disease—hypoglycemia, headache disorder (migraine), postural hypotension, seizure disorder, anemia, electrolyte abnormalities.
   - Can be part of a side effect of medications including tranquilizers, antibiotics, anticonvulsants, and analgesics.
3. **Clinical Features**
   - May be so severe that the patient cannot stand or walk.
   - May have associated nausea and vomiting.
   - May have nystagmus; in peripheral lesions, nystagmus is usually horizontal or rotational; in central lesions, nystagmus can be bidirectional or vertical.

- Patient may have associated tinnitus with hearing loss.
- Systemic causes may have palpitation, irregular pulse, signs consistent with congestive heart failure, and decreased cardiac volume; symptoms usually improve upon lying down.
- Need to look at gait, conduct the Romberg test, and evaluate for nystagmus.
4. **Diagnostic Studies**
   - ENG, MRI, vestibular-evoked myogenic potentials, caloric stimulation, and audiometry.
5. **Management**
   - Diagnose underlying cause.
   - In acute situations, Meclizine, Dramamine, scopolamine; these drugs may slow down long-term recovery.
   - Antidepressants—in some cases.
   - Otolaryngologic consult.

E. Acoustic Neuroma
1. **Etiology**
   - Schwannoma of the eighth cranial nerve.
   - Unilateral.
   - Hereditary syndrome possibly associated.
2. **Pathology**
   - Internal auditory canal benign lesions.
3. **Clinical Features**
   - Unilateral hearing loss.
   - Deterioration of speech discrimination.
   - Vestibular dysfunction more as disequilibrium rather than vertigo.
4. **Diagnostic Studies**
   - Enhanced MRI.
5. **Management**
   - Observation.
   - Excision or stereotactic radiotherapy.
   - Vascular endothelial growth factor blocker for those with hereditary syndrome.

F. Dysfunction of the Eustachian Tubes
1. **Etiology**
   - URI.
   - Allergies.
   - Trapped air in the middle ear results in negative pressure.
2. **Clinical Features**
   - Ear fullness.
   - Decreased hearing.
   - Retraction and decreased mobility of the TM.
   - If partial block, ears will pop and crackle.
3. **Management**
   - Systemic decongestants.
   - Intranasal decongestants.
   - Allergy patients can use intranasal corticosteroids.

G. Barotrauma
1. **Etiology**
   - Inability to equalize pressure in the ears.
   - Attributed to flying, underwater diving, or rapid change in altitude.
2. **Clinical Features**
   - Ear fullness.
3. **Management**
   - Attempt to yawn, swallow, or autoinflate.
   - Decongestant.
   - If on the ground and the above treatment fails, myringotomy or insertion of tubes.
   - Avoid diving if URI or allergies.

III. Nose

INFLAMMATORY DISEASE

A. Allergic Rhinitis
1. **Etiology**
   - Common.
   - Nasal mucosa membranes affected.
   - Affects all ages, mostly during adolescence and early adulthood.
   - Airborne particles inhaled, causing immuno-globulin E (IgE)-mediated response in the nasal mucosa.
   - Two subgroups: perennial and seasonal.
   - Most common in spring to late summer.
   - Mold spores/plant pollens.
2. **Pathology**
   - Allergen enters through the nose, is trapped by mucosa of turbinates, eliciting IgE-mediated response; mast cells release mediators and histamines.
   - Tissue edema and eosinophil infiltration results, causing itching, increased nasal secretions, sneezing.
   - Allergens: tree pollens, ragweed, grass.
   - Present in work or home environment: dust, animal dander, mold spores, mites, chemical agents occasionally.
   - Antigen exposure causes degranulation of mast cells, releasing histamine as well as various other inflammatory mediators, which set off a cascade of inflammatory responses.
   - Allergens usually are small particles (<50 μm), which enables them to be airborne easily.
   - These allergens are usually present in the environment in large amounts.
   - Ragweed is the most significant cause in the midwestern and eastern United States in late summer through early fall, whereas grass pollen is most significant in late spring through early summer.
3. **Clinical Features**
   - Clear, watery nasal discharge.
   - Sneezing—more apt to occur in early morning hours.
   - Sensation of plugged ears, postnasal drip, and nasal congestion.
   - Itching of nose, palate, and throat.
   - Nasal mucosa pale or blue in color, boggy, and edematous.
   - Conjunctival injection with tearing.
   - Alteration or loss of smell.
4. **Diagnostic Studies**
   - Allergy skin testing.
   - Radioallergosorbent testing—usually reserved for children, patients, or both, who cannot undergo skin testing (e.g., dermatographism, eczematoid dermatitis); may be used as screening examination if skin testing is not available.
   - Nasal smear examination for eosinophils.
5. **Management**
   - Intranasal corticosteroid sprays (fluticasone propionate, flunisolide, beclomethasone).
   - H_1 receptor antagonists (fexofenadine, cetirizine, loratadine).
   - H_1 receptor antagonist sprays can also be effective (azelastine, levocabastine), or adjunct therapy such as intranasal anticholinergic agents.
   - Attempt to maintain allergen-free environment (e.g., cover pillows and mattresses with plastic covers, avoid or get rid of household pets, avoid damp environments).
   - Air purifiers may help.
   - Keep humidity low (<50% prevents mold and dust mites).
   - Use air conditioners, especially in sleeping areas.
   - Antihistamines, topical nasal steroids.
   - Cromolyn sodium can be used as an adjunct.
   - Treat any concurrent sinusitis.
   - Immunotherapy for pharmacotherapy failures.

B. Nasal Polyposis
1. **Etiology**
   - Associated with allergies in 40% of patients with sinus infection.
   - Exact cause unknown, although strangulation of the swollen mucosa as it bulges through the small ostia of the ethmoid sinuses may be the cause.
   - The mucosa will swell due to infection, viruses, allergens, and environmental conditions.
   - Genetic predisposition exists.
   - If present in children, suspect cystic fibrosis.
   - Polyps can recur postsurgical excision.
2. **Pathology**
   - Composed of edematous stroma; within this stroma, numerous eosinophils, lymphocytes, neutrophils, and plasma cells are present.
   - Recurrent episodes of rhinosinusitis can cause development of polyps.
   - Frequently polyps are a primary phenomenon and cause secondary rhinosinusitis.

3. **Clinical Features**
   - Mucosal covered, pale, edematous mass.
   - May be multiple.
   - Hyposmia/anosmia.
   - Nasal mucosa may be boggy.
   - Nasal obstruction.
   - If polyp is extremely large, the patient may be a mouth breather.
   - Occasionally, polyps become so edematous they protrude from the nostril.

4. **Diagnostic Studies**
   - Nasal endoscopy.
   - CT scan.

5. **Management**
   - Topical nasal corticosteroid sprays 1 to 3 months for small polyps.
   - Oral steroid therapy—short course.
   - Treat allergies, if present.
   - Refer to otolaryngologist.
   - If patient has polyps and asthma, do not give acetylsalicylic acid (ASA) for any reason, because this can cause bronchospasm.
   - If medical management fails, surgical removal may be necessary. If the patient has recurrent polyps or is at high risk, an ethmoidectomy may be indicated.

TRAUMA

A. Epistaxis

1. **Etiology**
   - Nose bleeding from infection, trauma, allergic rhinitis, foreign body, renal failure, abnormal anatomical features, coagulation problems, alcohol abuse, inhaling street drugs, some medications (e.g., nasal corticosteroid spray, nosteroidal anti-inflammatory drugs [NSAIDs]), nasal defects, hypertension, atherosclerotic cardiovascular disease, heredity hemorrhagic telangiectasis, or tumors.
   - Use of blood thinners and anticoagulants.

2. **Pathology**

   ANTERIOR EPISTAXIS
   - Originates from the anterior aspect of the nose; Kiesselbach plexus bleeding is the most common location.

   POSTERIOR EPISTAXIS
   - Usual source is from a nasal branch of the sphenopalatine artery and associated with hypertension and atherosclerotic disease.

3. **Clinical Features**

   ANTERIOR EPISTAXIS
   - Patient may have a history of recent URI, trauma, or allergy exacerbation.
   - May have a history of recent use of inhaled irritants (i.e., cocaine, nasal sprays).
   - Bleeding from anterior nares, usually unilateral, with no sensation of blood dripping down the back of the throat.
   - Blood is bright red.

   POSTERIOR EPISTAXIS
   - An anterior site of bleeding is not visualized.
   - Patient has blood dripping down the back of the throat.
   - Patient expectorates blood.
   - Blood is dark red.

4. **Diagnostic Studies**
   - Hemoglobin and hematocrit for baseline.
   - If patient is under the age of 2 or has a family history of bleeding disorders, full workup is needed.

5. **Management**

   ANTERIOR EPISTAXIS
   - Direct pressure.
   - Use of vasoconstrictive and anesthetic agents.
   - Chemical, electrical, or thermal cautery.
   - Anterior nasal packing with petroleum jelly gauze with antibiotic prophylaxis (e.g., Augmentin).
   - Short-acting topical nasal decongestant.
   - Epistat if no mucosal tear.
   - Gelfoam or Surgicel may be used.
   - Avoid NSAIDs, ASA, and nose blowing.

   POSTERIOR EPISTAXIS
   - Posterior balloon with petrolatum gauze packed in the anterior nose.
   - Posterior nasal packing.
   - Immediate referral to otolaryngologist.
   - Check arterial blood gas.
   - Hospitalization for observation.
   - Continuous oxygen (O_2) saturation monitoring due to the possibility of respiratory failure leading to death.

B. Foreign Body of the Nose

1. **Etiology**
   - Usually a bead or seed is placed in the nose.

2. **Clinical Features**
   - Foul-smelling discharge from affected nostril.
   - Rhinorrhea.
   - Bleeding.
   - Halitosis.
   - Possible nasal obstruction.

3. **Management**
   - Older children can try to blow their nose to dislodge foreign body.
   - Removal of foreign body with the use of topical anesthesia, nasal decongestion, restraints, and good lighting.
   - If foreign body is wedged in, refer to ENT.
   - If a battery-operated foreign body is in the nose, it has to be removed within 4 hours. A battery itself is a true emergency.

IV. Sinuses

INFLAMMATORY DISEASE

A. Rhinosinusitis

1. **Etiology**
   - Inflammation or infection of the paranasal sinuses (one or both) affecting both adults and children.
   - Viral URI is the most common cause.
   - Predisposing factors: allergic sinusitis, nonallergic sinusitis, immune deficiency, anatomical anomalies.
   - Poor draining abilities result in bacterial overgrowth secondary to mucus accumulation.
   - Maxillary sinuses are the most common site of infection, 25% of which is a result of dental causes.
   - More difficult to drain maxillary sinuses, because the cilia are moving against gravity toward the upper-placed sinus ostium.

2. **Pathology**
   - The four paranasal sinuses (ethmoid, maxillary, sphenoid, frontal) drain into the nasal cavity.
   - Partial or complete obstruction due to mucosal swelling that narrows the ostia.
   - Respiratory mucosa and cilia line the sinuses enabling the mucous to be sent toward the ostia to drain.
   - The ostiomeatal complex is the most common site for obstruction.
   - Main pathogens are *S. pneumoniae* and *H. influenzae*.
   - Increase in β-lactamase producing *H. influenzae*.
   - *S. pneumoniae*, *M. catarrhalis*, and *H. influenzae* most common organisms in children.
   - Bacterial sinusitis can develop from a viral sinusitis.
   - *S. aureus* and respiratory anaerobes more frequently present in chronic sinusitis.

3. **Clinical Features**

   ACUTE
   - Headache, facial pain/pressure over sinus area, nasal congestion, cough, purulent nasal drainage or postnasal drip, pain/pressure on bending over or lying down. Halitosis and low-grade fever are possible.
   - Dental pain, ear popping, fatigue, fever (children).
   - History of recent URI or allergic rhinitis.
   - On physical examination—examination of the nose, ears, throat, lungs, and neuro is important for headache/facial pain complaints. Check dentition. Percussion for tenderness over frontal and/or maxillary sinuses. Percussion may or may not elicit pain; transillumination does not work well.

   CHRONIC
   - Persistent infection or inflammation; subtle, nonspecific signs and symptoms.
   - Purulent postnasal drip, headache, nasal congestion, sinus pressure, coughing, clearing of throat, sore throat, decrease or loss of smell, malaise.
   - Symptoms longer than 12 weeks.

4. **Diagnostic Studies**
   - Sinus X-rays—Caldwell (frontal), submentovertical (ethmoid), Waters (maxillary), and lateral (sphenoid); check for air–fluid levels, mucosal thickening, or opacification; films may be normal despite diagnosis of sinusitis.
   - CT scan of coronal plane can be used only in acute complicated sinusitis, recurrent or chronic sinusitis; cost is equal to that of four plain sinus X-rays.
   - If suspect malignancy, MRI with gadolinium.

5. **Management**
   - Fourteen days of oral antibiotics for acute sinusitis; 4 to 6 weeks for chronic disease.
   - In treatment, consider the severity, duration, and frequency of the infection; age of the patient; underlying conditions; history; and response to previous treatment.
   - Amoxicillin 250 to 500 mg PO TID; macrolides for penicillin allergic.
   - Bactrim or Septra 80 to 160 trimethoprim, 400 to 800 sulfamethoxazole PO BID.
   - Augmentin 250 to 500 PO TID for β-lactamase-inhibiting properties.
   - Fluoroquines if treatment failure.
   - Oral or nasal decongestants.
   - Mucolytics.
   - Avoid antihistamines.
   - Acetaminophen or ibuprofen can be used for headache/facial pain.
   - Topical corticosteroids for chronic (not acute).
   - IV antibiotics if frontal sinuses infected and not responding to treatment.
   - Surgery if all other treatments fail.
   - Otolaryngologic evaluation if no response to medical regimen, disease suspected outside the sinus cavity, or for chronic disease.

V. Mouth

INFLAMMATORY LESIONS

A. Herpetic Stomatitis

1. **Etiology**
   - Common viral infection of the mouth.
   - Most often occurs in children and young adults.

2. **Pathology**
   - Caused by the herpesvirus (HSV-1 or HSV-2).
   - Herpes simplex virus infects the trigeminal nerve ganglion and can remain dormant for long periods.
   - **Triggers:** Immunosuppression, trauma, fatigue, fever, cold, UV light, stress.

3. **Clinical Features**
   - Widespread gingivostomatitis.
   - Painful lesions.
   - Burning sensation.
   - Multiple vesicles that rupture to form ulcer.
   - Fever.
   - Headache.
   - Drooling.
   - Difficulty swallowing.
   - Arthralgias.
   - Pharyngitis.
   - Cervical lymphadenopathy.
   - Repeated recurrences.
4. **Diagnostic Studies**
   - None.
5. **Management**
   - Self-limited.
   - Analgesics.
   - Hydration.
   - Acyclovir can be used.
   - Viscous lidocaine if severe pain.

B. Herpes Simplex
1. **Etiology**
   - Viral infection.
2. **Pathology**
   - HSV, type 1 or type 2.
   - Occurs 2 to 20 days postexposure.
3. **Clinical Features**
   - Grouped vesicles on the lips, buccal mucosa, or both, which erupt, producing flat ulcers.
   - Most commonly seen at the vermillion border.
   - Fever.
   - Headache.
   - Malaise.
   - Repeated recurrences.
4. **Diagnostic Studies**
   - Tzanck smear of lesion confirmatory.
   - Smear shows multinucleated giant cells.
5. **Management**
   - Self-limited.
   - Can consider giving acyclovir 200 mg five times a day for 5 days, famciclovir 125 mg BID for 5 days, or valacyclovir 500 mg BID for 5 days.
   - Patient education regarding prevention of transmission.

C. Oral Candidiasis
1. **Etiology**
   - Represents an opportunistic infection in infants, leukocyte disorders, denture wearers, patients with anemia, nutritional deficiencies, use of corticosteroids or antibiotics, and immunocompromised persons (i.e., patients with AIDS, chemotherapy or radiation therapy recipients, patients with diabetes).
2. **Pathology**
   - Inflammation and edema of the underlying epithelium.

3. **Clinical Features**
   - Occurs when defenses are lowered in the host.
   - Difficult to tolerate hot and cold beverages and solid food.
   - Tongue may be depapillated, shiny, and smooth.
   - Can occur on any mucosal surface.
   - Usually painful.
   - White patches that leave a raw, inflamed area if rubbed off.
   - Mucosa may be normal or erythematous.
4. **Diagnostic Studies**
   - Potassium hydroxide prep if unsure of diagnosis.
   - Prep will disclose spores.
5. **Management**
   - Topical (clotrimazole troches) or systemic antifungal therapy (fluconazole by mouth, particularly if the esophagus is involved).
   - If the above therapy fails or patient is immunocompromised, Amphotericin B can be given intravenously.

D. Aphthous Ulcers (Figure 1-11)
1. **Etiology**
   - Common disorder of oral mucosa.
2. **Pathology**
   - Caused by nonspecific acute inflammation, possibly herpesvirus 6.
   - Trauma.
   - Systemic disorders.
   - Nutritional deficiencies particularly B and C vitamins.
   - Hormonal fluctuations.
   - Poor oral hygiene.
3. **Clinical Features**
   - Painful, round, shallow ulcers with yellow–gray fibrinoid centers and erythematous halos.
   - Present on nonkeratinized mucosa (buccal and labial mucosa).
   - Repeated recurrences.
   - May be associated with stress.

FIGURE 1-11. Aphthous stomatitis. (From Goodheart HP. *Goodheart's Photoguide of Common Skin Disorders.* 2nd ed. Philadelphia, PA: Lippincott Williams & Wilkins; 2003, with permission.)

4. **Diagnostic Studies**
   - Biopsy if no clear-cut diagnosis or if large and persistent ulcer.
5. **Management**
   - Self-limited.
   - Topical analgesics (i.e., Anbesol gel, viscous lidocaine).
   - Avoidance of spicy, hot, and citrus foods.
   - Possible use of corticosteroid gels or ointments (puts patient at risk for oral candidiasis).
   - Cimetidine can be used for maintenance if recurrent ulcers.
   - If unresponsive to treatment, laser therapy can be utilized.
   - Vitamin supplementation.
   - Biopsy if unclear diagnosis.

E. **Gingivitis**
   1. **Etiology**
      - An inflammatory periodontal disease.
   2. **Pathology**
      - Accumulation of plaque between the gingiva and teeth.
      - Misaligned teeth.
      - Trauma.
   3. **Clinical Features**
      - Bleeding gums with light contact.
      - Swollen, erythematous, and/or tender gingiva.
      - Bulbous interdental papillae.
      - Halitosis may be present.
   4. **Diagnostic Studies**
      - None.
   5. **Management**
      - Referral to dentist for dental cleaning.
      - Repair of teeth or orthodontics.
      - Treat related illnesses.
      - Brush teeth at least twice daily.
      - Floss teeth nightly.
      - Use an antibacterial mouth rinse.

F. **Necrotizing Ulcerative Gingivitis (Trench Mouth)**
   1. **Etiology**
      - Occurs in young adults under stress, in malnourished persons, or underlying systemic disease.
   2. **Pathology**
      - Caused by a wide variety of spirochetes and fusiform bacilli that normally inhabit the mouth.
   3. **Clinical Features**
      - Erythema, edema, and ulceration of the gingiva.
      - Grayish membrane forms over the inflamed and ulcerated gingival margins.
      - Halitosis, fever, cervical lymphadenopathy, malaise, fever.
   4. **Diagnostic Studies**
      - None.

5. **Management**
   - Correction of dietary inadequacies.
   - Alter or remove underlying factors.
   - Warm half-strength peroxide rinses.
   - Oral penicillin or tetracycline if needed.
   - Two percent viscous lidocaine.
   - Avoid irritants.
   - Dental curettage.
   - Dental follow-up.

DISEASES OF THE TEETH

A. **Dental Caries**
   1. **Etiology**
      - Decay of the tooth enamel causing exposure of the pulp.
   2. **Pathology**
      - Caused most commonly by *Streptococcus mutans*, *Streptococcus sobrinus*, or any other acid-producing bacteria.
      - Pulp exposure if left untreated.
      - Usually fever, swelling, and pain if abscess forms from necrotic pulp.
   3. **Clinical Features**
      - Asymptomatic in early stages.
      - Toothache.
      - Sometimes tooth is decayed.
      - First visible as a chalky white deposit in the enamel surface.
      - Teeth may become brown or black and soft.
      - Percuss on tooth to pinpoint correct tooth.
   4. **Diagnostic Studies**
      - X-rays.
   5. **Management**
      - Referral to dentist for repair or extraction.
      - I & D of abscess if present.
      - Root canal with crown if needed.
      - Oral antibiotics.
      - Saline rinses.
      - Sealants.
      - Fluoride application.
      - Instruct patient on proper oral/dental hygiene.
      - Follow up with dentist.

B. **Dental Abscess**
   1. **Etiology**
      - Decay of tooth extending beyond the enamel into the dentin and finally into the tooth pulp.
      - Trapped debris and plaque between gingiva and tooth.
   2. **Pathology**
      - Polymicrobial.
      - Most commonly caused by *Bacteroides*, *Fusobacterium*, *Peptococcus*, *Peptostreptococcus*, *Streptococcus viridans*.
   3. **Clinical Features**
      - Severe toothache.
      - Swelling.
      - Redness.

- Difficulty opening mouth and swallowing.
- Heat sensitivity.
- Fluctuant mass.
- Lymphadenopathy.
- Possible nausea, vomiting, chills, fever.
- Could have respiratory difficulty.

4. **Diagnostic Studies**
  - X-rays.
5. **Management**
  - Referral to dentist.
  - I & D if necessary, or aspiration.
  - Oral antibiotics.
  - May require root canal therapy.
  - NSAIDs.

C. Parotitis

1. **Etiology**
  - Risk factors generally unknown.
  - Guanethidine or iodides can cause swelling.
  - Chronic cases are due to autoimmune processes.
  - Dehydration.
2. **Pathology**
  - Depends on the cause.
3. **Clinical Features**
  - Pain caused by chewing.
  - Progressive swelling and pain of the gland.
  - Fever.
  - Viral: present bilaterally, malaise, fever, anorexia.
  - Tender to palpation, erythema and swelling noted at gland on visual exam.
  - Purulent saliva.
4. **Diagnostic Studies**
  - Saliva culture.
  - Check rheumatoid factor, anti-SS-B, and anti-SS-A.
  - Sialography.
  - Ultrasound.
  - If suspected malignancy, CT scan and MRI with gadolinium enhancement.
5. **Management**
  - Treat underlying condition.
  - Interventional sialoendoscopy.
  - Incisional biopsy.
  - Surgery.
  - Dental care.

D. Sialadenitis

1. **Etiology**
  - Inflammation of the submandibular or parotid gland.
2. **Pathology**
  - *S. aureus.*
3. **Clinical Features**
  - Swelling of the gland.
  - Duct opening tenderness and erythema.
  - Swelling and pain when eating.
  - Usually occurs when patient in dehydrated state or has chronic illness.
  - Purulent drainage.

4. **Diagnostic Studies**
  - CT or ultrasound if no response to treatment.
5. **Management**
  - Hydration.
  - Gland massage.
  - IV antibiotics. Less severe, oral antibiotics.
  - Warm compresses.

PREMALIGNANT AND MALIGNANT LESIONS

A. Leukoplakia/Erythroplakia of Mouth and Tongue (Figure 1-12)

1. **Etiology**
  - Chronic irritation of tissue (e.g., from trauma, alcohol, tobacco).
  - Erythroplakia more likely to be cancer than leukoplakia.
2. **Pathology**
  - Increased thickness of the keratin layer, neovascularization.
  - If epithelial dysplasia is present, the lesion is considered precancerous.
3. **Clinical Features**
  - Leukoplakia is a flat or raised white lesion on the oral mucosa or tongue and cannot be removed by rubbing the surface.
  - Erythroplakia is a reddish, velvety lesion on the oral mucosa or tongue and presents with erythema.
  - Most cases of erythroplakia are precancerous or cancerous.
  - Thorough examination of the mouth.
  - Check for lymph node enlargement.
  - Fiber-optic examination.
4. **Diagnostic Studies**
  - Biopsy or exfoliative cytologic examination.
5. **Management**
  - Otolaryngologic referral.
  - Some clinical trials support the use of β-carotene, retinoids, and vitamin E.

FIGURE 1-12. Oral hairy leukoplakia. (From Goodheart HP. *Goodheart's Photoguide of Common Skin Disorders.* 2nd ed. Philadelphia, PA: Lippincott Williams & Wilkins; 2003, with permission.)

- Fine-needle aspiration biopsy of enlarged lymph nodes.
- If biopsy is positive for oral squamous cell carcinoma, surgery/radiation therapy.

B. Neoplasms of the Tongue
1. **Etiology**
   - Most common carcinoma of the tongue is squamous cell carcinoma; more common in men than women, a family history of aerodigestive cancers, older age.
   - Most common on lateral tongue.
2. **Pathology**
   - Caused by carcinogenic agents such as tobacco, alcohol, environmental exposures, geographic location, and betel nuts.
3. **Clinical Features**
   - Begins as a painful, indurated plaque on the tongue that ulcerates.
   - Presents as a nonhealing ulcer or exophytic lesion.
   - Patient may also have associated lymphadenopathy.
   - May have referred ear pain.
   - Hemoptysis.
   - Dysphagia.
   - Odynophagia.
   - Feeling of a mass in the throat.
   - Mass in the neck region.
   - In advanced disease, the tongue may be fixed.
4. **Diagnostic Studies**
   - Biopsy.
   - CT with contrast.
   - Chest X-ray.
   - Liver function tests.
   - Bone scan if indicated.
   - Positron emission tomography scan if unclear diagnosis, primary site of cancer not located, or for pretreatment assessment.
5. **Management**
   - Surgery, radiation therapy alone or with brachytherapy, and chemotherapy.
   - Consult oncologist.
   - Follow-up imaging if nonsurgical treatment.

VI. Throat
INFLAMMATORY DISEASES
A. Laryngitis
1. **Etiology**
   - Laryngeal mucous membrane infection.
2. **Pathology**
   - Usually viral.
   - Can be caused by adenovirus or influenza.
   - **Other viruses:** RSV, Coxsackie virus, rhinovirus.
   - **Bacterial causes:** *H. influenzae, M. catarrhalis.*
   - Caused by URI, trauma to the throat, vocal abuse, toxic exposure, gastrointestinal or pulmonary

complications, smoking, laryngopharyngeal reflux, and, occasionally, allergy.
3. **Clinical Features**
   - Hoarseness, cough, sore throat.
   - Possible pain and difficulty swallowing.
   - Fever if infective causes.
   - Possible vesicles on the soft palate.
   - Lymphadenopathy.
   - May be associated with URI if acute.
   - If lasts >2 weeks, needs otolaryngologic evaluation.
4. **Diagnostic Studies**
   - Laryngoscopy if suspected masses, infection, structural abnormality, vocal cord dysfunction.
5. **Management**
   - Voice rest.
   - Do not clear throat.
   - Smoking and alcohol cessation.
   - Humidifier.
   - Hydration.
   - Treat underlying cause.
   - Surgery may be indicated in chronic cases.

B. Bacterial Pharyngitis/Tonsillitis
1. **Etiology**
   - Inflammation of the oropharynx.
2. **Pathology**
   - Eighty percent are viral: adenovirus, herpesvirus, rhinovirus, coronavirus.
   - Bacterial: group A β-hemolytic streptococci (GABHS), mycoplasma, Group G and C *Streptococcus, Neisseria gonorrhoeae, Chlamydia.*
   - Usually occurs in the winter/spring.
   - Spread by droplets.
3. **Clinical Features**
   - GABHS: Tender cervical lymphadenopathy, fever over 38° C, no cough, pharyngotonsillar exudate.
   - Headache.
   - Acute onset of sore throat with difficulty swallowing.
   - Fever >101° F.
   - Malaise, anorexia.
   - Arthralgias, myalgias.
   - Nausea/vomiting, abdominal pain in children.
   - Patient appears ill.
   - Tachycardic.
   - Tender, enlarged lymph nodes.
   - Erythema with or without exudate.
   - Petechiae of soft palate and strawberry tongue with strep. Scarlatiniform rash may be present.
4. **Diagnostic Studies**
   - Rapid strep-antigen testing.
   - Throat culture.
   - CBC with differential.
5. **Management**
   - Oral antibiotics (PenVK or cefuroxime axetil; erythromycin as an alternative to penicillin or for suspected mycoplasma or chlamydial bacteria).

- Amoxicillin or Azithromycin if compliance concern.
- Steroids may be necessary, although rarely used.
- Decadron 10 mg IM for rapid resolution of symptoms.
- Hydration, rest, ibuprofen for pain and decrease fever.
- Patient not infectious after 24 hours of antibiotic therapy.
- Otolaryngologic referral if history of recurrent symptomatic infections.

C. Viral Pharyngitis/Tonsillitis
1. Etiology
- Inflammation of the pharynx or tonsils.
2. Pathology
- Respiratory viruses are the most common cause of sore throat.
- Adenovirus, herpesvirus, rhinovirus, and coronavirus.
3. Clinical Features
- Acute onset of sore throat.
- May be accompanied by conjunctivitis, rash, cough, sputum production, rhinitis, and systemic symptoms.
- Pharyngeal erythema, exudates, tonsillar enlargement, and cervical adenopathy may be present.
- Look for ulcers in the mouth.
4. Diagnostic Studies
- Check liver/spleen size.
- CBC count for atypical lymphocyte.
- Monospot.
5. Management
- Hydration, gargles, and appropriate analgesics.
- Lozenges also may be helpful.

D. Epiglottitis
1. Etiology
- Acute inflammation of the supraglottic larynx, including epiglottitis that can progress rapidly to upper airway obstruction.
- Occurs in children 2 to 7 years old, but may also occur in adults.
- More common in patients with diabetes.
- In pediatric patients, symptoms can progress in 12 to 24 hours after onset.
2. Pathology
- Usually caused by *H. influenzae* type b (this organism is rare in adults).
3. Clinical Features
- Acute onset of high fever, sore throat, odynophagia, irritability, hoarseness, and restlessness.
- Rapid development of a sore throat with subjective complaints of odynophagia that outweigh the physical findings.
- Moderate-to-severe respiratory distress.
- Drooling, inspiratory stridor.
- Patient prefers sitting, leaning forward with elbows on knees.

4. Diagnostic Studies
- Lateral X-ray of the upper airway shows epiglottic swelling.
- Laryngoscopy in adults.
5. Management
- Immediate otolaryngologic/pediatric evaluation.
- Secure airway.
- Do not instrument patient.
- Preferred approach is nasotracheal intubation in operating room by otolaryngologist with a pediatric anesthesiologist present. Oral intubation for adults as indicated.
- Hospitalize in ICU.
- Oxygen saturation with pulse oximetry.
- IV antibiotics (ceftizoxime, cefuroxime) with possible steroids (dexamethasone).

INFECTION

A. Peritonsillar Abscess
1. Etiology
- Infection from the tonsil to the peritonsillar fascial planes.
2. Pathology
- Complications of mononucleosis, tonsillitis, and peritonsillar cellulitis.
- Polymicrobial.
- Usually *Streptococcus* or *Staphylococcus*.
- Anaerobic bacteria: *Bacteroides*.
3. Clinical Features
- Symptoms usually begin while patient is on the antibiotic.
- Young adults <30 years.
- Increased incidence in winter months.
- Follows a 2- to 3-day history of a sore throat.
- Inflammation, cellulitis, pocket of pus in the supratonsillar space.
- Can produce trismus.
- Fever, odynophagia, headache, malaise.
- Referred pain to the ear.
- Sore throat is more on one side.
- Drooling.
- Mild tachycardia.
- Deviated uvula with peritonsillar swelling, erythema of posterior pharynx.
- Exudate may or may not be present.
- Ipsilateral lymph node enlargement of the anterior chain.
4. Diagnostic Studies
- CT is used for diagnosis between a peritonsillar abscess and peritonsillar cellulitis.
5. Management
- Pediatrics: IV hydration and antibiotics.
- Surgery if no relief.
- Most cases can be handled outpatient.
- Admit patient if severe pain, dyspnea, trismus, drooling.
- Consult otolaryngologist.
- I & D or aspiration of the abscess.

- Consider immediate tonsillectomy.
- Broad spectrum cephalosporin.
- Before abscess formation, Clindamycin with oral amoxicillin may clear a peritonsillar cellulitis and prevent abscess formation.

SELECTED REFERENCES

Andreoli CM, Gardiner MF. Traumatic hyphema: clinical features and management. UpToDate. 2010. http://www.uptodate.com. Accessed May 5, 2011.

Andreoli TE, Benjamin IJ, Griggs RC, et al, eds. *Andreoli and Carpenter's Cecil Essentials of Medicine*. 8th ed. Philadelphia, PA: Saunders/Elsevier; 2010.

Bickley LS, Szilagyi PG, eds. *Bates' Guide to Physical Examination and History Taking*. 10th ed. Philadelphia, PA: Wolters Kluwer/LippincottWilliams & Wilkins; 2009.

Braverman RS. Eye. In: Hay WW, Levin MJ, Sondheimer JM, et al, eds. In: *Current Diagnosis and Treatment of Pediatrics*. 20th ed. New York, NY: McGraw-Hill; 2011:401–441.

Greenberg RD, Castleberry J. Eye emergencies. In: Stone CD, Humphries RL, eds. *Current Diagnosis and Treatment Emergency Medicine*. 6th ed. New York, NY: McGraw Hill; 2008:487–512.

Jacobs DS. Pterygium. UpToDate. 2010. http://www.uptodate.com. Accessed May 5, 2011.

Kaplan JL, Beers MH, Berkwits M, et al, eds. *Merck Manual of Diagnosis*. 18th ed. Whitehouse Station, NJ: Merck Research Laboratories; 2006.

Lustig LR, Schindler JS. Ear, nose & throat disorders. In: McPhee SJ, Papdakis MA, eds. *Current Medical Diagnosis and Treatment*. 50th ed. New York, NY: McGraw Hill-Medical; 2011:198–238.

Riordan-Eva P. Disorders of the eyes and lids. In: McPhee SJ, Papdakis MA, eds. *Current Medical Diagnosis and Treatment*. 50th ed. New York, NY: McGraw Hill-Medical; 2011:166–197.

Stallard TC. Emergency disorders of the ear, nose, sinuses, oropharynx, & mouth. In: Stone CD, Humphries RL, eds. *Current Diagnosis and Treatment Emergency Medicine*. 6th ed. New York, NY: McGraw Hill; 2008:513–539.

Templer JW, Liess BD. Parotitis. Emedicine. 2009. http://emedicine.medscape.com/article/882461-overview. Accessed May 4, 2011.

Washington University School of Medicine Department of Medicine, Cooper DH, Krainik AJ, Lubner SJ, et al. *The Washington Manual of Medical Thearpeutics*. 32nd ed. Philadelphia, PA: Lippincott Williams & Wilkins; 2007.

Wright KW. Strabismus. In: McInerny TK, ed. *Textbook of Pediatrics*. Elk Grove Village, IL: American Academy of Pediatrics; 2009. http://online.statref.com/document.aspx?fxid=357&docid=837. Accessed May 9, 2011.

Yoon PJ, Kelley PE, Friedman NR. Ear, nose, & throat. In: Hay WW, Levin MJ, Sondheimer JM, et al, eds. *Current Diagnosis and Treatment of Pediatrics*. 20th ed. New York, NY: McGraw-Hill; 2011:452–486.

Pulmonary Disorders

Diane Abercrombie • Torry Grantham Cobb • Todd Phillip Smith

I. Pulmonary Thromboembolism

A. Etiology

- Thrombi originating in the venous circulation or the right side of the heart.
- Most commonly affecting but not limited to the femoral and popliteal vessels of the lower extremities.
- Estimated US incidence of venous thromboembolism is 1,000,000 cases annually with 10% (400,000 to 650,000) developing pulmonary thromboembolism (PTE) and 10% (50,000) of those succumbing.
- Mortality much greater when diagnosis is not established.

B. Pathophysiology

- Nearly all pulmonary emboli originate in the peripheral venous circulation, particularly the pelvis and lower extremities.
- Emboli transported to the pulmonary circulation lodge in vessels relative to their size.
- Emboli predominantly consist of intravascular thrombotic material. Less common embolic sources include fat, foreign bodies, tumor, air, amniotic fluid, and bone marrow.
- "Massive pulmonary emboli" refer to those large enough to lodge near the central pulmonary arterial circulation.
- Pulmonary infarction more typically results from multiple smaller emboli, but is common due to the collateral flow maintained by pulmonary circulation redundancy.
- Hemodynamically, PTE may result in increased pulmonary vascular resistance, pulmonary hypertension, and right ventricular failure. Local bronchoconstriction and physiologic dead space also may occur.

C. Clinical Features

- Peripheral venous thrombus findings are notoriously nonspecific.
- Dorsiflexion of the foot with resulting calf pain (Homan sign) is a classic finding of lower extremity thromboembolism, but is non-specific.
- Many conditions mimic venous thrombosis, which may also be asymptomatic, and only 50% of patients with PTE have clinical findings of venous thrombosis of the lower extremities.
- PTE typically presents abruptly with tachypnea, pleuritic chest pain, apprehension, and dyspnea. Less common symptoms include hemoptysis, diaphoresis, cough, and syncope.

- Massive PTE may present as right ventricular failure and systemic hypotension. However, the presentation can be subtle complicating the diagnostic picture.
- The classic triad (Virchow's) of venous stasis, hypercoagulable state, and venous endothelial injury predisposes to venous thrombus development and PTE (Table 2-1).
- History is of critical importance. Physical examination may be normal or reveal a variety of findings or exhibit signs of pulmonary hypertension like right ventricular heaves or increased pulmonary component of S2.
- Clinical risk factors include cancer, oral contraceptives, smoking, prolonged immobility, surgery (specifically, the postoperative state), myocardial infarction, congestive heart failure (CHF), obesity, and orthopedic injury of pelvis, hips, or lower extremities (Table 2-1).
- Genetic predisposition to hypercoagulability is now recognized in the form of antithrombotic protein deficiencies (rare) including antithrombin III, protein C, and protein S, or abnormal variants of clotting factors.
- Individuals heterozygous for factor V Leiden have at least three to five times increased risk of developing venous thrombosis and homozygous patients have even higher risk.
- Because factor V Leiden is so common among known thrombophilic factors, it accounts for 20% of patients with new venous thrombosis incident.

TABLE 2-1.	Risk Factors for Thromboembolism
Immobilization	
Lower extremity/pelvic trauma or surgery	
Malignancy	
Pregnancy and postpartum state	
Oral contraceptives and estrogens	
Obesity	
CHF	
Nephrotic syndrome	
Hematologic disorders (polycythemia vera, paroxysmal nocturnal hemoglobinuria, Waldenstrom macroglobulinemia)	
Coagulation abnormalities (lupus anticoagulant, anticardiolipin antibodies, protein C or S deficiency, antithrombin III deficiency, factor V Leiden)	

From Hume HD, ed. *Kelley's Essentials of Internal Medicine.* 2nd ed. Philadelphia, PA: Lippincott Williams & Wilkins; 2001:718, with permission.

- Patients with elevated levels of plasma homocysteine are also at increased risk. However, in as many as half of the cases no predmoninat risk factor is identified.

D. Diagnostic Studies

- Ninety percent of patients with proven PTE have a partial pressure of oxygen in arterial blood (PaO_2) <80 mm Hg.
- Respiratory alkalosis with hypocapnia is common. In severe cases profound acidemia, hypercapnia, and hypoxemia may be present.
- Electrocardiographic (ECG) findings include tachycardia, atrial arrhythmias, and nonspecific ST-T wave changes, but are transient and nonspecific.
- Chest X-ray (CXR) abnormalities frequently nonspecfic due to underlying disease state with no pathognomonic findings related to PTE.
- Up to 30% of patients with PTE may have small effusion, which is typically exudative and often hemorrhagic.
- Ventilation/perfusion (V/Q) scan may be useful, but low probability result does not rule out PTE.
- The D-Dimer test is useful if negative, but nonspecific if positive.
- Use of contrast computed tomography (CT) angiography is becoming more commonplace and is the standard in some facilities.
- Venous thrombosis studies of the lower extremities, including both noninvasive (Doppler, plethysmography, duplex scan, etc.) and invasive (^{125}I fibrinogen scan, venography).
- Pulmonary angiography may be diagnostic is the gold standard and should be used when other modalities are inconclusive.

E. Management

- Measures to minimize the risk of venous thrombosis or the propagation of existing thrombus.
- Anticoagulation is preventative rather than definitive.
- Standard therapy consists of intravenous (IV) heparin followed by 3 to 6 months of warfarin therapy.
- Low molecular weight heparin may be used in place of standard heparin therapy and may also be used prophylactically.
- Thrombolysis is still controversial in clinical practice.
- Surgical or percutaneous (filter) interruption of the inferior vena cava when anticoagulation is contraindicated or for repeated events despite anticoagulation.
- Surgical embolectomy is rarely employed.
- Key feature of management is prophylaxis.

II. Bronchogenic Carcinoma (Lung Cancer)

A. Etiology

- Rare in nonsmokers. Other implicated factors include air pollution, ionizing radiation, asbestosis, exposure to heavy metals, and industrial carcinogens.
- Cigarette smoking is the most important etiologic factor in the United States (85% of all cases—87% of male cases and 85% of female cases).

- Risk is proportional to pack year history with ex-smokers maintaining increased risk through-out life.
- Study of genetic predisposition is ongoing, focusing on smokers who do not develop lung cancer.
- Genetic mutations affecting proteins like k-ras, c-erb, and p53 which function as proto-oncogenes are also being investigated.

B. Pathology

- More than 20 benign or malignant primary lung neoplasms have been identified. Major cell types are small cell lung cancer (SCLC), representing <20% of reported cases and nonsmall cell lung cancers (NSCLCs) including squamous cell carcinoma (30% to 35%), adenocarcinoma (30% to 35%), and large cell carcinoma (3-5%), small cell carcinoma (10-15%), and bronchiolalveolar cell carcinoma (2%)
- Squamous cell carcinoma is amenable to early detection (in sputum) because of its tendency to originate in central bronchi. Due to slow growth rate have lower risk of matastasis, but is still possible to metastasizes to adjacent structures and regional lymph nodes in the hilum or mediastinum.
- Small cell also occurs centrally with widespread metastasis, usually before initial diagnosis.
- Adenocarcinoma has recently equaled or surpassed squamous cell as the most frequent cell type and usually presents in the periphery.
- Adenocarcinoma tends to be glandular and mucus-producing and is frequently associated with pleural effusions.
- Large cell tends to originate peripherally and is not amenable to early sputum detection.

C. Clinical Features

- History of cigarette smoking.
- Nonspecific symptoms such as cough, weight loss, dyspnea, chest pain, increased sputum production and hemoptysis, frequently related to other comorbidities.
- A change in the above symptoms may suggest bronchogenic carcinoma.
- Specific symptoms usually occur late.
- Asymptomatic presentation may be in the form of a solitary pulmonary nodule found incidentally on chest radiograph.
- Physical findings absent or nonspecific.
- Local metastasis may result in symptoms associated with mediastinal structures such as phrenic nerve, superior vena cava, recurrent laryngeal nerve.
- Common distant metastatic sites include bone, brain, adrenal glands, kidney and liver.
- Cervical and supraclavicular lymphadenopathy occurs frequently.
- Presence of paraneoplastic syndromes grouped as endocrine, systemic, neurologic, cutaneous, hematologic, and renal.
- Clubbing is commonly associated with bronchogenic carcinoma.

- Asymptomatic radiologic finding is a common presentation.

D. Diagnostic Studies

- CXR, CT, complete blood count (CBC), liver function, electrolytes, calcium.
- Cytology of sputum.
- Analysis of pleural fluid.
- CT scan useful.
- Necessary histologic examination of tissue retrieved by bronchoscopy, lymph node biopsy, metastatic tumor biopsy, open biopsy, needle aspirates, etc.
- Increasing interest in positron emission tomography (PET) scanning is becoming more common place in the evaluation process. Offers good negative predictive value, but less sensitive for small lesions and high false positive rate in certain benign lesions that metabolize FDG.
- Routine screening, even of smoking population, not currently recommended.

E. Management

- Staging by tissue-type diagnosis. NSCLC staged through TNM (tumor, node, metastasis) classification. SCLC staged through limited (one hemithorax) or extensive disease.
- NSCLC treatment options include surgical resection and/or combined modality therapy or palliative therapy to minimize airway obstruction.

- Chemotherapy is controversial in NSCLC. Adjuvant therapies have been suggested in patients with high risk for surgical failure. Five-year survival rate for all NSCLC is about 15%. SCLC therapy focuses on chemotherapy.
- Five-year survival for SCLC is about 7% with limited-stage disease and 1% for extensive-stage disease. Surgery for bronchogenic carcinoma of all types is most successful in very localized tumors—5-year survival of such patients approaches 50%. The cornerstone of long-term treatment is to prevent smoking.

III. Mediastinal Diseases

A. Etiology

- Mediastinal masses are commonly of metastatic origin. Of those originating in the mediastinum, about 75% are benign.
- The most common tumor originating in the mediastinum is thymoma, although lymphatic tumors, teratomatous tumors, and intrathoracic goiters may also appear in the mediastinum. Vascular tumors may also originate in the mediastinum.
- Hernias through the diaphragm may also present as mediastinal masses (Table 2-2).

B. Pathology

- Mediastinum is divided into three compartments—anterior, middle, and posterior.

TABLE 2-2. Clinical Features of Mediastinal Masses

	Incidence	Peak Age (y)	Common Clinical Findings	Diagnostic Studies
Anterior				
Thymoma	Most common anterior mediastinal mass	40–60	Myasthenia gravis in 35%	CT, needle aspiration, surgical biopsy
Lymphoma	Common	20–30	Cough, pain, fever, weight loss	CT, needle aspiration, surgical biopsy
Thyroid	Uncommon	Any age	Asymptomatic, airway obstruction, hyperthyroidism, and hypothyroidism	Physical examination: enlarged thyroid, deviated trachea, ^{131}I scan
Teratoma	Uncommon	<35	Asymptomatic	CT, surgical biopsy
Middle				
Hiatal hernia	Very common	>40	Asymptomatic	Esophagram
Metastatic cancer	Very common	>35	Asymptomatic or symptoms of primary tumor	Needle aspiration, surgical biopsy
Sarcoidosis	Common	<35	Asymptomatic or systemic symptoms	Tissue biopsy—skin, lung (transbronchial)
Aortic aneurysm	Common	>50	Asymptomatic or chest pain with dissection	CT or angiogram
Pericardial cyst	Most common mediastinal cyst	Any age	Asymptomatic	CT, surgical resection
Bronchogenic cyst	Rare	<35	Asymptomatic, rare compression, or infection	CT, surgical resection
Posterior				
Neurogenic tumors	20% of all primary mediastinal tumors	Any age	Asymptomatic or rare neurologic symptoms	CT, myelogram, surgical resection

From Hume HD, ed. *Kelley's Essentials of Internal Medicine.* 2nd ed. Philadelphia, PA: Lippincott Williams & Wilkins; 2001:713, with permission.

- Differential of anterior tumors includes thymoma, teratoma, thyroid lesions, parathyroid lesions, lymphoma, germ cell tumor including teratoma, and other miscellaneous mesenchymal tumors.
- Middle mediastinal masses include lymphadenopathy (benign or malignant), pulmonary artery enlargement, great vessel aneurysm, developmental cysts, dilated azygous/hemiazygous vein, some diaphragmatic hernias, and foramen of Morgagni hernias.
- Posterior compartment tumors are primarily neurogenic or diaphragmatic hernias. Most mediastinal masses occupy the anterior or middle compartments.

C. Clinical Features
- Most patients are asymptomatic with incidental findings on CXR.
- Symptoms may be related to the site of original involvement rather than mediastinal condition.
- About 50% of patients with thymoma present initially with myasthenia gravis.
- Physical findings are usually nonspecific.
- There may be a mass effect causing superior vena caval compression with resultant facial and upper extremity edema and prominent venous pattern.

D. Diagnostic Studies
- CXR.
- CT scan helpful in delineating anatomy.
- Angiography and/or venography in suspected vascular conditions.
- Barium swallow if esophageal involvement.
- Magnetic resonance imaging (MRI) to visualize planes other than axial, and to better delineate hilar structures.
- Tissue diagnosis necessary in neoplastic conditions.

E. Management
- Varied depending on underlying cause of mass.

IV. Pleural Conditions
A. Anatomy and Physiology
- Collection of fluid with-in the virtual space created by visceral and parietal pleura.
- Pleura consists of two components—visceral (covering the lungs) and parietal (covering the inner surface of the chest wall, diaphragm, and mediastinum).
- Pulmonary circulation supplies blood to the visceral pleura, which has no sensory nerves.
- Systemic circulation supplies parietal pleura, which also contains sensory nerves.
- The two layers create a virtual space, which is normally lubricated by 5 to 10 mL of pleural fluid.
- Pleural fluid is produced in the parietal pleura and resorbed through the lymphatic drainage of the visceral pleura at a rate of 15 to 20 mL per day.

V. Pleural Effusion
A. Etiology
- Transudative (low protein) effusions predominantly result from CHF—also cirrhosis and nephrotic syndrome—conditions that do not directly affect the pleural tissue.
- Exudative (high protein) effusions arise due to changes in vascular permeability that results in fluid accumulation, typically result from inflammatory or malignant processes such as tuberculosis (TB), pneumonia, carcinoma, infarction, trauma with possible hemothorax, and the interruption of lymphatic channels and/or the thoracic duct resulting in direct accumulation of lymph (chylothorax) in pleural space and rheumatic disorders.
- Less common etiologies include asbestosis, Meigs syndrome, uremia. Empyema is a special case in which frank pus is located within the pleural space (Table 2-3).

B. Pathophysiology
- Pleural fluid is normally drained through the lymphatic channels of the parietal pleura.
- Noninflammatory effusions can occur in any condition that causes ascites, obstruction to venous or lymphatic drainage, or CHF.
- Inflammatory effusions typically result from conditions that cause inflammation of the pleura or adjacent structures.
- Worsened by obstruction of lymphatic drainage.
- Unless iatrogenically introduced, air in the pleural space indicates bronchopleural fistula.
- Empyema is an occasional complication of bacterial pneumonia or lung abscess.

C. Clinical Features
- Depending on the amount of fluid, underlying cause, and ability to compensate, symptoms and physical findings may be absent. Symptoms, when present, may include dyspnea, cough, and pleuritic pain. Dyspnea is related to volume of fluid accumulation.
- Physical examination may reveal decreased breath sounds, decreased diaphragmatic excursion on the affected side(s), decreased tactile fremitus, dullness to percussion, and "E to A" change (egophony).
- Empyema should be suspected in the presence of persistent or recurrent fever after treatment of bacterial pneumonia.

D. Diagnostic Studies
- CXR with blunting of costophrenic angle (gutter). Up to 300 mL of fluid may be undetectable in posterior/anterior (PA) CXR. Lateral decubitus radiograph is more sensitive to smaller fluid amounts. Thoracentesis is both diagnostic and potentially therapeutic in terms of volume reduction.
- Fluid should be evaluated for total protein, lactase dehydrogenase (LDH), white blood cell (WBC) with differential, glucose, and/or pH.
- Also include acid-fast, Gram's stain, aerobic and anaerobic cultures, and cytology.
- Other diagnostic studies include pleural biopsy for undiagnosed exudative effusions.
- Larger specimens may be obtained through thoracoscopy or open pleural biopsy.

TABLE 2-3. Differential Diagnoses of Pleural Effusions

Transudative pleural effusions
CHF
Cirrhosis
Nephrotic syndrome
Myxedema
Pulmonary emboli
Urinothorax
Atelectasis
Constrictive pericarditis
Exudative pleural effusions
Neoplastic diseases
Infectious diseases
Bacterial infections
Tuberculosis
Fungal infections
Viral infections
Parasitic infections
Pulmonary emboli
GI disease
Esophageal perforation
Pancreatic disease
Intra-abdominal abscesses
Diaphragmatic hernia
Collagen vascular disease
Rheumatoid pleuritis
Systemic lupus erythematosus
Drug-induced lupus
Wegener granulomatosis
Churg–Strauss syndrome
Postcardiac injury (Dressler) syndrome
Asbestos exposure
Meigs syndrome
Drug-induced pleural disease
Nitrofurantoin
Dantrolene
Methysergide
Bromocriptine
Procarbazine
Amiodarone
Radiation therapy
Hemothorax
Chylothorax
Uremic pleuritis
Lymphangiomyomatosis

From Light RW. *Pleural Diseases*. Philadelphia, PA: Lea & Febiger; 1990, with permission.
From Hume HD, ed. *Kelley's Essentials of Internal Medicine*. 2nd ed. Philadelphia, PA: Lippincott Williams & Wilkins; 2001:711 , with permission.

- Chest CT better at defining pleural space than plain CXR and beneficial in determining anatomical extent of pleural and lung lesions.

E. Management
- Establish cause of effusion and treat appropriately. Thoracentesis for therapeutic reasons should be considered when large effusions result in pulmonary dysfunction. Limit fluid removal to 1,000 to 1,500 mL at a time due to the possibility of pulmonary edema in reexpanded lung.
- Empyema or persistent effusion of other origin may require chest tube to water seal drainage.

VI. Pneumothorax

A. Etiology
- Air is not normally present in the pleural space, but can be introduced by a break in either pleural membrane, resulting in a pneumothorax.
- Entry through parietal pleura caused by trauma or iatrogenic means.
- Entry through visceral pleura caused by rupture of bleb, cyst, bulla, etc., or by necrosis of adjacent lung tissue. Termed *primary spontaneous pneumothorax* when etiology not readily apparent—more common in tall, thin, young adult male smokers.
- Regardless of etiology result is positive pleural pressure that compresses lung tissue.

B. Clinical Features
- Acute onset of dyspnea and chest pain, although may be asymptomatic, especially if small pneumothorax.
- If large enough, diminished breath sounds, diminished tactile fremitus, and increased resonance on percussion tachycardia, pleural friction rub, and tracheal shift to contralateral side.
- Patient with tension pneumothorax presents in acute distress.

C. Diagnostic Studies
- CXR confirms presence of pneumothorax.

D. Management
- Small pneumothorax may resolve spontaneously. Larger pneumothorax may require evacuation of air by catheter or large-bore drainage tube to sealed water drainage. Hemodynamic compromise in a tension pneumothorax can be relieved with immediate decompression by placing a needle or catheter in the pleural space.

VII. Pulmonary Function and Diagnosis (Figure 2-1)

A. Pulmonary Function Testing

PATHOLOGY
- A group of tests designed to measure the lungs capacity to take in and release air, as well as the volume and rate of air on inspiration and expiration.
- Objective method to evaluate functional change in a patient with known or suspected lung disease.
- In addition, pulmonary function testing (PFT) allows for the determination of whether the patient has lung disease significant enough to result in respiratory impairment and dysfunction.
- PFT **provides three main categories of information:**
  - Lung volumes.
  - Measurement of the size of the assorted compartments within the lung.

FIGURE 2-1. Flow-volume curve (FVC) and spirometry tracing (volume-time curve) from a normal subject, with both curves from the same expiratory effort. FVC, forced vital capacity; FEV1, forced expiratory volume in the first second of expiration; PEFR, peak expiratory flow rate; FEF$_{25\%}$, forced expiratory flow rate at 25% VC. For this and other flows, the subscript indicates that the flow is measured at the volume expired, usually expressed as a percentage of the vital capacity. (Reprinted with permission from Hume HD (Ed), KELLEY'S TEXTBOOK OF INTERNAL MEDICINE, 4th ed. Philadelphia, PA: Lippincott Williams & Wilkins, 2000, p 2580.)

- Flow rates, measurement of maximal flow within the airways and diffusing capacity, measurement of gas transfer between alveoli and pulmonary capillary blood.
- PFT varies based on a patient's age, gender, height, weight, and ethnicity.
- During the testing, maximal respiratory effort is required since suboptimal respiratory effort may result in difficulty with test interpretation.
- **Indications:**
  - Although indications for PFT are varied, it is indicated in the basic evaluation of lung function pattern.
  - Serial PFT allows for quantification of improvement/deterioration in functional lung status, evaluation for initiation and response to therapeutic interventions, disability evaluations, longitudinal surveillance in the occupational setting, and determination of possible significant preoperative and postoperative respiratory problems.
- **Contraindications:**
  - There are certain medical conditions where PFT may be contraindicated: acute severe—asthma, respiratory distress, angina aggravated by testing, pneumothorax, ongoing hemoptysis, and active pulmonary tuberculosis.

B. Patterns of Impairment

- Spirometry, documentation of exhaled volume versus time during a forced exhalation (with or without response to an inhaled bronchodilator for possible reversible airflow), allows for the basic assessment of obstructive and restrictive pulmonary dysfunction.
- In a restrictive pattern (i.e., neuromuscular and chest wall diseases), there is a reduction in lung volumes—total lymphatic count (TLC), respiratory volume (RV), vital capacity (VC), functional residual capacity (FRC)—and normal expiratory airflow—maximum midexpiratory flow rate (MMFR), forced expiratory volume in 1 second (FEV_1) to forced vital capacity (FVC) ratio. With severe disease MMFR is decreased.
- An obstructive pattern (i.e., asthma, chronic bronchitis, and emphysema) results in a decrease in rates of expiratory airflow (decrease FEV_1/FVC and MMFR) with high RV, increased RV/TLC ratio depicting air trapping (Figure 2-2).
- A mixed obstructive/restrictive pattern results in difficulty in test interpretation and would show decreased FEV_1 and FVC, decreased FEV_1/FVC ratio, and decreased TLC.
- **Interpretation:**
  - Normal standards (predicted value) have been established.
  - As aforementioned, normality is based on patient demographic variables and may vary between laboratories.
  - Normal values are defined between 95% and 80% of predicted value.
  - FEV_1/FVC, however, confers a normal test if value is >80% of predicted value.

VIII. Chronic Obstructive Pulmonary Disease

- Chronic disorders that disturb airflow either within the airways or within the lung parenchyma.
- Obstruction is generally progressive, may coincide with airway hyper-reactivity, and may be partially reversible.
- Generally refers to chronic bronchitis or emphysema; however, patients often exhibit features of both.
- Does not commonly include bronchial asthma.
- Estimated that at least 16 million persons in the United States suffer from chronic obstructive pulmonary disease (COPD); with another 16 million Americans undiagnosed.

	Normal	Obstruction-hyperinflated	Restriction
VC (liters)	6.0	4.0	4.0
TLC (liters)	8.0	10.0	5.0
FRC (liters)	4.0	7.0	3.0
RV(liters)	2.0	6.0	1.0

FIGURE 2-2. Absolute lung volumes in a normal person, a patient with hyperinflation secondary to obstructive airway disease, and a patient with restrictive lung disease. *VC*, vital capacity, the volume expired from a maximal inspiration (*TLC*, total lung capacity) to full expiration (*RV*, residual volume); *FRC*, functional residual capacity, volume at end of a normal tidal breath; *IC*, inspiratory capacity; *TV*, tidal volume; *ERV*, expiratory reserve volume. In obstruction, FRC and RV are both increased at the expense of the VC; thus, TLC is only minimally increased. In restriction, the FRC, RV, and VC are all decreased proportionally, resulting in a decrease in the TLC, which defines restriction. (From Hume HD (Ed). KELLEY'S ESSENTIALS OF INTERNAL MEDICINE. 2nd ed. Philadelphia, PA: Lippincott Williams & Wilkins, 2001, p 632.)

- Fourth most common cause of death and continues to rise in prevalence and mortality.
- Elderly men are at greatest risk for mortality from the disease.
- Fifteen percent of patients with COPD exhibit progressively disabling symptoms as early as their fifth and sixth decades.
  - Up to 15% of patients with established COPD have not been direct consumers of tobacco.
- Due to the presence of cigarette smoking, the World Health Organization (WHO) predicts that COPD will be the third most common cause of death by the year 2020—12.5 million from chronic bronchitis and 1.65 million from emphysema. Thus, nearly all smokers exhibit an accelerated decline in lung function that is dose and duration dependent (Figure 2-3).

A. Etiology and Pathogenesis
- **Risk factors for the development of COPD:**
  - Cigarette smoking (80% risk) most important risk factor; however, only 15% of smokers develop severe disease.
- The remaining 20% of patients with COPD frequently are exposed to a combination of environmental tobacco smoke (exposure of nonsmokers to cigarette smoke), occupational dusts and chemicals, indoor air pollution from biomass fuel used for cooking, and heating in poorly ventilated buildings.
- Genetics (<1% risk); deficiency of the protein α_1-antitrypsin (AAT) may lead to premature emphysema, chronic bronchitis, and occasionally bronchiectasis; severity of lung disease varies.
- Air or environmental pollution—role unclear, low significance, primarily important due to its potential for causing exacerbations of preexisting COPD, pollutants secondary to occupational exposure (i.e., miners).
- Infection (i.e., viral upper respiratory infection) does not initiate disease, but may lead to a transient worsening of symptoms and pulmonary functioning in those with preexisting COPD. In those patients with acute viral infection, bacterial infections may lead to superinfection. Emerging data suggest that upper respiratory infection during childhood may be a risk factor for later development of COPD because of its impact on lung growth and function,

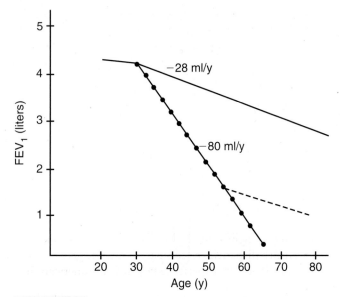

FIGURE 2-3. Loss of forced expiratory volume in 1 second (FEV1) of a 6-foot-tall man in a lifetime (*solid line*). FEV1 is on the vertical axis and age by decade is on the horizontal axis. The dotted line projects the accelerated rate of loss of FEV_1 in patients with emphysema. The broken line shows the mean effect of smoking cessation. (From Hume HD (Ed). KELLEY'S ESSENTIALS OF INTERNAL MEDICINE. 2nd ed. Philadelphia, PA: Lippincott Williams & Wilkins, 2001, p 673.)

possibly accounting for nonuniformity of development of COPD in smokers.

- Hyperresponsive airways, Dutch hypothesis (1960): asthma, atopy, nonspecific airway hyperresponsiveness, and serum deficiency of protein AAT may underlie the development of chronic airflow obstruction.
- **Presentation Types:**
  - Type A (pink puffer): Emphysema predominates with arterial PO_2 preserved; thus patient is pink, thin, cachectic appearing. Usually not cyanotic and typically works hard to get air (puffing). Major complaint is often severe shortness of breath. Presentation typically after age 50. Cough is rare, with scant clear, mucoid sputum. No peripheral edema, no adventitious lung sounds.
  - Type B (blue bloater): Bronchitis predominates with significant hypoxemia resulting in cyanosis, obesity, and peripheral edema secondary to right ventricular failure. Major complaint is chronic, productive cough with mucopurulent sputum and frequent exacerbations of disease due to chronic chest infections. Often presents by 30s and 40s. Chest noisy with wheezing and rhonchi common.
  - Most patients do not fall into one category, but rather, exhibit symptoms of both.

B. Clinical Features

CHRONIC BRONCHITIS

- Enlargement of mucus-secreting glands and increased number of goblet cells; quantity of airway mucus is increased.

- Cough and sputum production 3 months of the year for 2 consecutive years.
- Rhonchi, sputum production.
- Wheezing.
- Dyspnea.
- Prolonged expiration.
- Obesity.
- Cyanosis and cor pulmonale, consisting of leg edema, elevated jugular venous pressure, right ventricular heave, and tricuspid insufficiency.

EMPHYSEMA

- Dyspnea on exertion.
- Minimally productive cough.
- Pursed-lip breathing.
- Thin appearance.
- Depressed diaphragm.
- Hyperresonant to percussion.
- Prolonged expiration.
- Diminished breath sounds.
- Wheezing.
- Cor pulmonale.

C. Diagnostic Studies and Approach

CHRONIC BRONCHITIS

- CXR in chronic bronchitis may reveal increased anteroposterior (AP) diameter, thickened bronchial markings, enlarged right side of heart.
- PFT may reveal reduced FEV_1 and/or FVC; maybe some reversibility after bronchodilator therapy, normal to elevated TLC/RV; normal diffusing capacity.
- Arterial blood gases (ABGs): Hypoxemia and hypercapnia. However, chronic bronchitis is a clinical diagnosis; thus patient history is crucial.

EMPHYSEMA

- CXR in emphysema may reveal low, flat diaphragm; increased retrosternal airspace; "pruning" of vascular markings; long, narrow heart shadow; bullae (radiolucent, >1 cm, arcuate hairline shadows).
- PFT: Fixed reduction in FEV_1 and/or FVC, increased TLC and/or RV, reduced diffusing capacity.
- ABGs: Normocapnia, mild to moderate hypoxemia. AAT serum level may be low. Although high-resolution CT is more sensitive as an imaging method for detecting emphysema, it is not routinely performed in the diagnostic evaluation.
- Lung biopsy is not performed to make the diagnosis. True pathologic confirmation is typically obtained through postmortem examination.
- PFT and ABG analyses remain the most useful physiologic adjuncts in evaluating patients with COPD.

D. Management

- To date, the only treatment strategies shown to reduce mortality is smoking cessation and supplemental oxygen to ensure oxygen saturation >90% as measured by pulse oximetry. Pharmacologic therapy should be approached via stepwish approach.
- Numerous modalities of treatment available.

- Treatment varies from patient to patient.
- New long-acting β-agonist Brovana (Sepracor) for the long-term maintenance treatment of bronchoconstriction due to COPD.
- Consider referring the patient to a pulmonologist if the COPD onset occurs before the age of 40, there are frequent exacerbations (two or more a year) despite optimal treatment, there is severe or rapidly progressive COPD, symptoms are disproportionate to the severity of airflow obstruction, or there is a need for long-term oxygen therapy.

CHRONIC BRONCHITIS

- Smoking cessation, exercise (20 minutes, 3x weekly), healthy lifestyle, immunization (pneumococcal and influenza vaccines).
- **Pharmacologic intervention:**
  - May include β_2-agonist (e.g., albuterol), anticholinergic aerosols (ipratropium or tiotropium [Spiriva]); many physicians consider these drugs now as first-line agents in the treatment of COPD.
  - Long-acting sympathomimetics (salmeterol or formoterol) may be considered in those with more severe disesae.
  - Short-course corticosteroids (inhaled, oral, or parenteral), although use is controversial and most useful in bronchitis with some reversibility.
  - Antibiotics for acute exacerbations or to treat acute bronchitis and/or prevent acute exacerbations of chronic bronchitis. However, there is little data to support use of prophylactic antibiotics.
  - Supplemental oxygen if PO_2 >55 mm Hg at rest, exercise, nocturnally, or if cor pulmonale is present.
  - Diuretics if cor pulmonale present.
  - Pulmonary rehabilitation focusing on patient education and exercise training.
  - Chest physiotherapy, postural drainage in those patients with excessive amounts of retained secretions who cannot clear by coughing or other methods. To date, outcome data has not supported the use of expectorant and mucolytic therapies.
  - New long-acting β-agonist Brovana for the long-term maintenance treatment of bronchoconstriction due to COPD.

EMPHYSEMA

- As above, theophylline, AAT replacement if deficient.
- Corticosteroids minimally effective.
- Lung volume reduction surgery (severe disease only).
- Lung transplantation (end-stage COPD).
- Mechanical ventilation to support gas exchange and maintain acceptable ABG values.
- Bullectomy, an older pulmonary procedure, may prove useful in those patients with severe bullous emphysema.

IX. Asthma

- According to The National Asthma Education and Prevention Program (NAEPP) guidelines, asthma is a chronic inflammatory disease characterized by airway narrowing and obstruction, hyper responsiveness of airways and airway inflammation. Airflow obstruction is reversible spontaneously or with pharmacotherapy.
- Can occur at any age, but probably the most common chronic disease in children and young adults. Fifty to eighty percent of children with asthma develop symptoms prior to age 5 years. , Affectings 3 to 5 percent of population.
- Results in over 470,000 hospitalizations per year, with an estimated 5,000 deaths in the United States. There is a health disparity noted among African Americans and asthma.
  - Hospitalization rates have been highest among black and children, and death rates for asthma are consistently highest among blacks aged 15 to 24 years.
- Health disparities as compared with the general population are experienced by African Americans in childhood asthma.

A. Etiology

- The strongest identifiable predisposing factor for the development of asthma is atopy; however, obesity is increasingly recognized as a risk factor.
- Potential risk factors for the development of asthma may be classified as inherited or acquired.
- Inherited or allergic asthma characterized by symptoms that occur with exposure to an allergen to which patients have been previously sensitized.
- Patients exhibit markers for allergic disease (positive skin testing, elevated serum immunoglobulin, IgE, levels), a strong positive family history of allergic conditions (e.g., allergic rhinitis and eczema), and exacerbations based on allergen exposure.
- Acquired or environmental asthma is generally seen in patients who have no history of allergies. There may be no family history of asthma.
- Acquired asthma may be precipitated by exposure to a variety of environmental stimuli such as house dust mites, domestic animals, and cockroaches. These irritants are commonly found indoors, centralized in bedding and carpets, and present throughout the year.
- Maternal cigarette smoking has been implicated as a predisposing factor for the development of childhood asthma.
- Sinusitis, upper respiratory tract infections, or psychological stress are known to precipitate airway inflammation.
- Exercise-induced bronchoconstriction and inhalation of cold air during winter months may result in asthma exacerbations and/or worsening of symptoms in some patients, as well as aspiration and gastroesophageal reflux.
- Some patients may experience asthma symptoms after ingestion of certain medications like aspirin, nonsteroidal anti-inflammatory drugs, or tartrazine dyes.
- There are also reports of women experiencing catamenial asthma at predictable times during menses.
- Occupational asthma is triggered by various agents in the workplace; may occur weeks to years after initial exposure and sensitization.

B. Pathology

- Asthma results from a combination of process that results in airway obstruction, hyperinflation, and airway limitation.
- Chronic airway obstruction characterized by infiltration of the airway wall, mucosa, and lumen by activated eosinophils, mast cells, macrophages, and T lymphocytes.
- Bronchial smooth muscle contraction results from mediators released by inflammatory, local neural and epithelial cells.
- Epithelial damage manifested by denudation and desquamation of the epithelium, leading to mucous plug.
- This airway inflammation underlies disease chronicity and contributes to airway hyperresponsiveness and airflow limitation.
- Airway remolding characterized by:
  - Subepithelial fibrosis.
  - Smooth muscle hypertrophy and hyperplasia.
  - Goblet cell and submucosal gland hypertrophy and hyperplasia resulting in mucus hypersection.
  - Possible airway wall thickening due to acute edema and cellular infiltration during asthma exacerbations.

C. Clinical Features

- Classified according to frequency of symptoms, FEV1/FVC, nighttime awakenings and interference with normal activity.
- Key symptoms include wheezing, cough, dyspnea, and chest tightness. However, these symptoms are highly variable. Symptoms are typically worse at night, may occur spontaneously, or may be precipitated or exacerbated by many different triggers.
- Patients experiencing an asthmatic attack may exhibit tachypnea, prolonged expiratory and/or inspiratory phases of respiration or silent chest, and use of accessory muscles of respiration.
- Symptoms may occur singularly or in combination, and patients may not exhibit a classic presentation with several or all of these complaints.
- Chest may be hyperresonant on percussion.
- Fatigue and pulsus paradoxus (inspiratory decline in systolic blood pressure of at least 10 mm Hg) are late signs and may signal the need for critical types of intervention, including intubation and ventilatory support.
- Wheezing is more pronounced during expiration rather than inspiration. Status asthmaticus (tachycardia, tachypnea, accessory muscle use, pulsus paradoxus, wheezing or silent chest, altered mental status, paradoxic abdominal and diaphragmatic movement on inspiration) may result from a severe acute asthmatic attack refractory to treatment with bronchodilators. Cardiac asthma is defined as wheezing triggered by decompensated congestive heart failure.
- **Classification of asthma severity for ≥12 years of age and recommended treatment:**
  - *Mild intermittent asthma*
    - Characterized by mild asthma symptoms two or fewer times a week; nocturnal awakening fewer than two times a month; ≤2 days per week use of short-acting β_2-agonist (SABA) for symptom control (not prevention of exercise-induced bronchospasm [EIB]); no interference with normal activity; initial peak expiratory flow (PEF) ≥70%, normal or personal best; normal FEV$_1$ between exacerbations; FEV$_1$ of >80% predicted and FEV$_1$/FVC normal.
    - Recommend treatment: Step 1: usually cared for at home, Step 2: prompt relief with a inhaled SABA on an as-needed basis.
  - *Mild persistent asthma*
    - This is characterized by asthma symptoms more than 2 days per week, but not daily; three to four times per month of nighttime awakening; PEF 40% to 60% predicted or personal best; FEV$_1$ > 80% of personal best, >2 days per week use of SABA for symptom control (not for EIB), but not daily and not more than one time on any day; minor interference with normal activity; FEV$_1$/FVC normal.
    - Recommended treatment: In addition to the SABA, a long-term controller medication is required. A low dose of inhaled is recommended long-term controller medication for this degree of severity. Alternative treatment (listed alphabetically): cromolyn, leukotriene modifier, nedocromil, OR sustained release theophylline to serum concentration of 5–15 g/mL.
  - *Moderate persistent asthma*
    - This is characterized by daily asthma symptoms; nighttime awakenings >1 time per week, but nightly; >1 day per week use of SABA for symptom control (not for EIB daily, but not nightly; impairment; some limited interference with normal activity; FEV$_1$ >60%, but <80% predicted; FEV$_1$/FVC reduced 5%; PEF of <60% to <80% of personal best.
    - Recommended treatment: The use of a low to a medium dose of inhaled corticosteroid together with a long-acting bronchodilator is the preferred therapy. Alternative treatments include increasing to a medium dose of inhaled corticosteroid or adding a leukotriene antagonist or theophylline to low to medium dose of inhaled corticosteroid.
  - *Severe persistent asthma*
    - This is characterized by asthma symptoms throughout the day; nighttime awakenings often seven times per week; several times per day use of SABA for symptom control (not for EIB) daily; extremely limited interference with normal daily activity; FEV$_1$<60%; FEV$_1$/FVC reduced >5%; PEF of <60 of personal best.
    - Recommended treatment: A high dose of inhaled corticosteroid and a long-acting bronchodilator are the preferred therapies. These patients may require long-term oral corticosteroids, although repeated attempts should be made to reduce the dose while they are receiving high-dose inhaled corticosteroids.

D. Diagnostic Studies

- Laboratory studies in asthma may provide both diagnostic and prognostic data. Spirometry (FEV1, FVC, FEV1/FVC) is recommended at initial assessment, when symptoms and peak flow measurements have stabilized, both before and after bronchodilator challenge.

PULMONARY FUNCTION TESTING

- The evaluation of asthma should include spirometry (FEV_1, FVC, FEV_1/FVC) before and after administration of short-acting bronchodilator.
- Airflow obstruction is indicated by reduced FEV_1/FVC.
- Significant reversibility of airflow obstruction is defined by an increase of ≥12% and 200 mL in FEV_1 or ≥15% and 200 mL in FVC after inhaling a short-acting bronchodilator.
- A positive bronchodilator response strongly confirms the diagnosis. Bronchial provocation testing with inhaled histamine or methacholine is useful when asthma is suspected but spirometry is nondiagnostic.
  - Bronchial provocation test is not recommended if the FEV_1 is <65% of predicted.
  - A positive methacholine test is defined as a ≥20% fall in the FEV_1 at an exposure to a concentration of 8 mg per mL or less.
  - Exercise challenged testing may be useful in patients with symptoms of exercise-induced bronchospasms.

PEAK EXPIRATORY FLOW

- A 20% change in the PEF values from morning to afternoon or from day to day suggests inadequately controlled asthma.
- PEF values <200L per minute indicated severe airflow obstruction.
- IgE determination: May indicate allergic/inherited asthma, complete blood count, and sputum cytology showing eosinophilia.
- Sweat test in chronic childhood asthma, immunoglobulins to assess for immunodeficiency as indicated, and IgE (allergic aspergillosis) as indicated.
- Skin testing to assess sensitivity to environmental allergens.
- Evaluation for paranasal sinus or gastroesophageal reflux should be considered in asthma patients with pertinent symptoms and in those with severe or refractory symptoms.
- **The following may be helpful in acute situations:**
  - ABG analysis looking for hypoxemia, normal or increased $PaCO_2$, and acidosis.
  - Chest/sinus radiography: not particularly useful. Typically reveals normal findings. Chest imaging is indicated when pneumonia or complication of asthma is suspected.
  - Pulse oximetry to monitor oxygen saturation.

E. Management

- The 2007 NAEPP guidelines classify the treatment of asthma in broad categories based upon age. The goals of the asthma therapy are as follows: to minimize chronic symptoms that interfere with normal activity (including exercise) guidelines to prevent exacerbations; no missed days at work school for both the parent and the child; minimal or no chronic symptoms day or night; peak flow measurements >80% of patients personal best; minimal or no adverse effects from medications; and minimal use of short-acting inhaled β_2-agonist (<1 time per day, <1 canister per month) to reduce or prevent underlying airway inflammation and the series of chemical mediators that contribute to bronchospasm. Thus, treatment is geared toward the level of control based upon the most severe impairment or risk category. The new stepwise approach to the diagnosis and management of asthma was developed in an effort to assist with clinical decision-making to meet individual patient needs and improve patient perceived control of asthma, to reduce or eliminate emergency department visits and hospitalizations.
- The stepwise approach to the diagnosis and management of asthma was developed in an effort to assist with clinical decision making to meet individual patient needs. The trend has been to use glucocorticoid preparations sooner and more frequently. Inhaled preparations are considered first-line and preferred in all patients identified with persistent disease.
- The small risk of delayed growth in children with chronic inhaled corticosteroid use is well balanced by the effectiveness of these medications.

LONG-TERM CONTROL MEDICATIONS

- Anti-inflammatory agents: inhaled corticosteroids are preferred first-line agents for all patients with persistent asthma; systemic corticosteroids (oral or parenteral) most effective in achieving prompt control of asthma during exacerbations or when initiating long-term asthma therapy in patients with severe symptoms.
- Long-acting bronchodilators; mediator inhibitors, such as cromolyn sodium and nedocromil, are long-term medications that prevent asthma symptoms and improve airway function in patients with mild persistent asthma or exercise-induced symptoms; β-adrenergic agonists, such as salmeterol and formoterol, provide bronchodilation for up to 12 hours after a single dose; phosphodiesterase inhibitors, such as theophylline, provides mild bronchodilation in asthmatic patients.
- Leukotriene modifiers; zileuton is a 5-lipoxygenase inhibitor that decreases leukotriene production, and zafirlukast and montelukast are cysteinyl leukotriene receptor antagonists.
- Desensitization immunotherapy for specific allergens can be considered in asthma patients who have exacerbations of asthma symptoms when exposed to allergens to which they are sensitive.
- Vaccination, specifically Pneumovax, annual influenza vaccinations, including seasonal and epidemic influenza A (H1N1). Immunotherapy for specific allergens should be considered in selected asthma patients.

QUICK-RELIEF MEDICATIONS

- β Adrenergic agonists; short-acting inhaled β_2-agonists, including albuterol, levalbuterol, bitolterol, pirbuterol, and terbutaline, are effective bronchodilators during exacerbations.
- Anticholinergic agents (e.g., ipratropium bromide) reverse vagally mediated bronchospasm but not allergen-or exercise-induced bronchospasm, and decrease mucus gland hypersection seen in asthma.
- Phosphodiesterase inhibitors (e.g., methylxanthines) are not recommended for therapy of asthma exacerbations. Theophylline provides mild bronchodilation in asthmatics. Sustained-release theophylline may be useful in adjunct therapy. It is essential that serum concentrations of theophylline be monitored.
- Corticosteroids (e.g., methylprednisolone, prednisolone, and prednisone) effective for primary treatment for patients with moderate to severe asthma exacerbations and for patients with exacerbations who do not respond promptly and completely to inhaled β_2-agonist therapy.
- Diet for patients with food allergies, maintain normal exercise and activity except for those patients with exercise-induced asthma, patient education and use of a written action plan regarding the nature of asthma, goals of therapy, warning signs of impending attack, correct use of medication, and peak flow meters are highly recommended, especially for those patients exhibiting moderate or severe persistent asthma, as well as patients with a history of severe exacerbations.
- Communication with family, school, and work where appropriate.
- Antibiotics are not recommended for the treatment of acute asthma exacerbations except in cases where the patient has comorbid conditions (i.e., pneumonia and bacterial sinusitis).

X. Pulmonary Arterial Hypertension

- Refers to elevation of intravascular pressure within the pulmonary circulation.
- May be acute or chronic.
- Prevalence is estimated at 15 cases per one million adults. The development of this disorder is based upon right heart catheterization measurements. Defined as mean pulmonary artery pressure >25 mmHg at rest (normal 8-20 mmHg), or >30 mmHg with exercise.
- Classification Change: World Health Organization Functional class (2008 Dana Point classification) is one way of describing the severity of Pulmonary Arterial Hypertension (PAH) and reflects the impact the condition has on a patient's life in terms of physical activity and symptoms. There are five classes of PAH based on the underlying pathophysiology associated with the disesae: Pulmonary arterial hypertension (PAH), pulmonary hypertension with left heart disease which is more common than PAH, pulmonary hypertension associated with lung disease and/or hypoxemia, pulmonary hypertension from chronic thrombotic and/or embolic disease, and pulmonary hypertension whose origin is either multifactorial or unclear. The WHO also describes four classes of PAH based on patient's ability to function. Class I is the least severe, classified as diseases that localize to small pulmonary muscular arterioles. Class IV is the most complicated. Typically occurs in patients with hematologic disorders, Sarcoidosis, glycogen storage disorders, and other miscellaneous causes. Patients with Class I Pulmonary Arterial Hypertension (PAH) are not limited in terms of physical activity. Patients with class IV PAH are unable to perform any physical activity without symptoms and may experience symptoms during rest.
- Central physiologic abnormality of pulmonary hypertension is increased right ventricular afterload due to elevated pulmonary vascular resistance. The development of right ventricular hypertrophy, and intimal proliferation are the consequences of pulmonary hypertension, as the pulmonary pressure rises to a level inappropriate for a given cardiac output, despite the etiology. As a consequence, patients may develop atheromatous changes and in situ thrombosis which leads to further narrowing of the arterial bed. Thus, left untreated, pulmonary hypertension has a poor prognosis, (15% annual mortality rate), and considered a life-threatening condition.
- Idiopathic (formerly Primary) idiopathic pulmonary hypertension, or plexogenic pulmonary arteriography, is a rare disorder, occurring mainly in young and middle-aged women. Characterized by histopathologic plexiform lesion found in muscular pulmonary arteries. There may be some genetic history. Typically no identifiable cardiopulmonary or connective tissue disorder. Risk factors include hepatic cirrhosis, portal hypertension, HIV infection, and use of anorectic drugs. Clinical presentation consist of progressive shortness of breath with lethal outcome.
- Secondary pulmonary hypertension is caused by varied mechanisms such as emphysema and pulmonary fibrosis and obstruction of the pulmonary vascular bed as seen with chronic pulmonary thromboembolic disease.
- Pulmonary veno-occlusive disease (fibrotic occlusion of pulmonary veins and venules, secondary hypertensive changes in pulmonary arterioles and muscular pulmonary arteries) is a rare cause of postcapillary pulmonary hypertension also seen in children and young adults.
- The etiology is unknown, but is associated with conditions such as viral infection, bone marrow transplantation, chemotherapy, and malignancy (Table 2-4).
- Patients exhibit progressive fibrotic occlusion of pulmonary veins and venules, coupled with secondary hypertensive changes in the pulmonary arterioles and muscular pulmonary arteries.

A. Etiology

- Causes of PAH pulmonary arterial hypertension can be placed into five broad categories: 1) reduction in cross-sectional area of the pulmonary arterial bed,

TABLE 2-4.	Classification of Pulmonary Hypertension

Postcapillary
Left heart failure
Aortic or mitral valve disease
Pulmonary venous disease
Left atrial myxoma
Precapillary
Chronic respiratory disease
Congenital heart disease
Pulmonary vasculitis
Primary pulmonary hypertension
Occlusive pulmonary vascular disease

From Hume HD (Ed). KELLEY'S ESSENTIALS OF INTERNAL MEDICINE 2nd ed. Philadelphia, PA: Lippincott Williams & Wilkins, 2001, p 136.

e.g., emphysema, interstitial lung disease, sickle cell disease, collagen-vascular disease, acidosis, lung resection hypoxemia from any cause; 2) increased pulmonary venous pressure, e.g., constrictive pericarditis, LVF or reduced compliance, Mitral stenosis, Pulmonary veno-occlusive disease, mediastinal diseases compressing pulmonary veins; 3) increased pulmonary blood flow, e.g., congenital L-R intracardiac shunts; 4) Increased blood viscosity, e.g., polycythemia; 5) Miscellaneous, e.g., HIV, PAH in conjunction with hepatic cirrhosis, portal hypertension.

B. Pathology
- Abnormalities most frequently observed in the small muscular arteries and arterioles include intimal hyperplasia and medial hypertrophy, ensuing destruction of the lumen leading to pulmonary vascular resistance and a decrease in the number of small vessels (arteries and arterioles).
- Severe pulmonary hypertension leads to further changes in the larger (elastic) pulmonary arteries: thickening of the artery wall, notably the media layer; in situ thrombosis in the pulmonary vasculature; and hypertrophy of right ventricular wall, with or without dilation.

C. Clinical Features
- **Symptoms:** Dyspnea, dull, retrosternal chest pain usually triggered by exertion, exertional fatigue, syncope. Symptoms of right-sided heart failure (e.g., syn lower extremity swelling, ascites and hoarseness due to impingement of recurrent laryngeal nerve by enlargpulmonary artery).
- **Physical examination findings:** Narrowing and splitting of S_2, accentuation of the pulmonary component of S_2, cardiac lift/heave in left lower sternal border (LLSB), right-sided presystolic gallop (S_4), mid-diastolic gallop (S_3), systolic ejection click, jugular venous distension (JVD), peripheral edema, occasional pulmonic or tricuspid insufficiency murmurs.

D. Diagnostic Studies
- CXR and high-resolution CT scans: Increased pulmonary artery vasculature, enlarged cardiac silhouette with bulging of the anterior cardiac border, redistribution of blood flow from lower to upper lung zones, interstitial or alveolar edema, dilation of the right and left main and lobar pulmonary arteries.
- Perfusion lung scan: Reveals focal perfusion defects (e.g., recurrent pulmonary emboli).
- PFT: To detect underlying airflow obstruction or restricted lung volumes, and a decreased diffusing capacity.
- ABG analysis: To determine hypoxemia or acidosis.
- Echocardiography and electrocardiography: Demonstration of right ventricular hypertrophy and estimation of pulmonary arterial pressure.
- Doppler ultrasonography: A reliable noninvasive means of estimating pulmonary artery systolic pressure.
- Cardiac catheterization: To definitively determine the degree of pulmonary hypertension.
- Laboratory analysis should be conducted to assess for secondary pulmonary hypertension—for example, LFTs, HIV, and collagen-vascular serology.

E. Management
- Management of pulmonary hypertension is dependent on the associated specific disorder leading to symptomatology and the severity of disease.
- Focus is placed on correction of cardiac disease and/or decreasing pulmonary venous and capillary pressures.

TREATMENT MODALITIES
- For idiopathic PAH without underlying cause, pharmacotherapy is used. The goal is dilation of pulmonary arteries, thereby, reducing pulmonary arterial pressures, as well as reducing pulmonary arterial hypertrophy. Three main categories of drugs are used: 1)prostaglandins, e.g., epoprostenol (Flolan), treprostinil (Remodulin), and iloprost (Ventavis); short-acting, IV or inhalation, must be given frequently or on continuous basis; Long-term effect suggest a reversal of vascular remodeling and proliferative changes in the pulmonary arterial system in addition to its vasodilator effect 2) Phosphodiesterase type 5 inhibitor, e.g., sildenafil (Revatio, Viagra. Less effective than prostaglandins but have a more favorable dosing regimen of one to three times daily, po; 3) endothelium antagonist, e.g. bosentan (Tracleer and Ambrisentan (Letairis). Given po, one to two times daily. In rare cases, calcium channel blockers may be of benefit.
- For PAH with underlying etiology, the goal is treatment of the primary problem, e.g., treatment of left-sided heart failure, causes of hypoxia like COPD, chronic lung disease, treatment of scleroderma by rheumatologist. Long-term anticoagulation therapy is warranted if patient has some type of clotting disorder

such as chronic thromboembolic pulmonary hypertension. Surgical removal of blood clots may be warranted.

- Continuous intravenous infusion of prostacyclin (PGI_2) or epoprostenol. There has been therapeutic success with prostacyclin; Treatment of polycythemia via repeated phlebotomy, diuretics, salt restriction, supplemental oxygen for cor pulmonale. For end-stage disease, combined heart-lung transplantation or lung transplantation alone (considered unrealistic for most patients), thromboendarterectomy, supplemental O_2 for correction of alveolar hypoxia and hypoxemia.
- Patients are also generally placed on long-term anti-coagulation therapy with warfarin.

XI. Sleep Apnea Syndrome

Repetitive episodes of airflow cessation (apnea) during sleep.

- The syndrome includes three types of sleep apnea: primary central sleep apnea (lack of respiratory drive), obstructive sleep apnea (transient obstruction) and mixed (a combination of both).
- Obstruction occurs at the level of the pharynx.
- Apnea often terminates with short gasps or snorting.
- Typically a chronic condition that results in excessive daytime sleepiness.

A. Etiology

Primary central sleep apnea characterized by the absence of respiratory effort is rare and not well understood.

- Obstructive sleep apnea due to narrowing or obstruction of the upper airway may be the result of:
  - Obesity or excessive soft tissue in the soft palate.
  - Alcohol or sedative ingestion prior to sleep.
- Neuromuscular disorders that cause a loss of normal pharyngeal muscle tone resulting in the passive collapse of the pharynx.
- Craniofacial abnormalities such as micrognathia.
- Macroglossia, adenotonsillar hypertrophy, or enlarged uvula.
- Nasal obstruction, upper respirator infections, smoking or hypothyroidism may precipitate or worsen obstructive sleep apnea.

B. Epidemiology

- Prevalence of primary central sleep apnea is less than 1%.
- Prevalence of obstructive sleep apnea is 4% in men and 2% in women.
- Prevalence of obstructive sleep apnea is higher in obese and hypertensive patients.

C. Clinical Features

- Disturbed sleep pattern.
- Loud snoring.
- Snorting.
- Agitation during sleep.
- Violent movements during sleep with the sleep partner complaining of being hit or injured because of these random, violent movements.
- Severe headache upon awakening.
- Excessive daytime sleepiness (may fall asleep during daily activities).
- Sore or dry throat.
- Cognitive impairment.
- Personality disorder.
- Morning headaches.
- Decreased libido.
- Depression.

D. Associated Conditions

- Cardiac arrhythmias.
- Conduction disturbances.
- Pulmonary hypertension.
- Unexplained cor pulmonale.
- Systemic hypertension.

E. Diagnostic Studies

Polysomnography (PSG), a nighttime sleep study, is the diagnostic test of choice.

- Apneic episodes must last a minimum of 10 seconds and occur 10–15 times an hour to be considered clinically significant.
- The apnea/hypoapnea index (AHI), total number of apneas and hypopneas divided by the total sleep time, is used to categorize sleep apnea in to mild: AHI = 5–15; moderate: AHI = 15–30; severe: AHI >30.
- Multiple sleep latency test (MSLT) is a diagnostic tool to measure daytime somnolence.
- ABG analysis may reveal daytime hypercapnia.
- CXR and electrocardiography may reveal signs of pulmonary hypertension or cor pulmonale. Serum thyroid-stimulating hormone to detect unsuspected hypothyroidism.
- Erythrocytosis is common; thus, a hemoglobin level should be obtained.
- Other diagnostic studies performed in selected patients include fiber-optic examination of upper airway to rule out obstructing tumors and cephalometric radiography to define the anatomy of the upper airway if surgical treatment is considered.

F. Management

Treatment is aimed at treating the underlying condition and may include weight loss and avoidance of alcohol, sedatives and smoking.

- The most effective treatment for obstructive sleep apnea is nasal continuous positive airway pressure (nasal C-PAP).
- Bilevel positive airway pressure (BIPAP) is effective for treating central sleep apnea.
- Oral and dental appliances such as Snore Guard have been used for obstructive sleep apnea when patients are unable to tolerate CPAP.
- Various surgical procedures: Uvulopalatopharyngoplasty (UPPP), tracheostomy, and craniofacial surgery may be recommended to patients with obstructive sleep apnea who fail CPAP.
- Pharmacologic therapy has not proven beneficial for sleep apnea.

XII. Pneumonia and Infections of the Lung

A. Etiology

- Pneumonia is an inflammation of the lung parenchyma characterized by consolidation of the affected area and filling of the alveolar air spaces with exudate, inflammatory cells, and fibrin.
- Pneumonias are grouped into two categories: community-acquired pneumonias and healthcare-related pneumonias (hospital-acquired and ventilator associated).
- Age, environmental exposure(s), underlying disease processes, and seasonal factors may affect etiology and pathology of pneumonia.
- Infection by bacteria or viruses is the most common cause; however, trauma to the chest wall, inhalation of chemicals, or infection by other infectious agents such as rickettsiae, fungi, parasites, and yeasts can occur (Table 2-5).
- In addition to the above causes, events surrounding September 11, 2001 have brought to light organisms uncommonly seen in clinical practice.
- Age, environmental exposure(s), underlying disease processes, and seasonal factors may affect etiology and pathology of pneumonia.

TABLE 2-5.	**Organisms that Cause Pneumonia**
Common	**Uncommon**
Outpatient Pneumonia	
Streptococcus pneumoniae	*Legionella* species
Mycoplasma pneumoniae	*Staphylococcus aureus*
Respiratory viruses	*Mycobacterium tuberculosis*
Chlamydia pneumoniae	Fungi
Haemophilus influenzae	*Klebsiella pneumoniae*
Community-Acquired Pneumonia Requiring Hospitalization	
S. pneumoniae	*M. pneumoniae*
H. influenzae	*Moraxella catarrhalis*
Polymicrobial	*M. tuberculosis*
Anaerobic bacteria	Fungi
Aerobic Gram-negative bacilli	
Legionella species	
S. aureus	
C. pneumoniae	
Respiratory viruses	
Severe Community-Acquired Pneumonia Requiring Hospitalization	
S. pneumoniae	*H. influenzae*
Legionella species	*M. tuberculosis*
Aerobic Gram-negative bacilli	Fungi
M. pneumoniae	
Respiratory viruses	

From Fauci AS, Harrison TR, eds. *Harrison's Principles of Internal Medicine.* 17th ed. New York, NY: McGraw-Hill; 2008, with permission.

B. Pathophysiology

- Factors that may affect the lung's defenses include age; chronic lung diseases such as cystic fibrosis, asthma, and chronic obstructive pulmonary disease (COPD); immunocompromised states such as chemotherapeutic medications and HIV/AIDS; cigarette smoking; allergens; anesthesia; and alcohol abuse.
- Two main routes of infection of the lungs are aspiration of oropharyngeal flora and inhalation of airborne pathogens.
- Two other less-common routes of infection include systemic bacteremia (blood borne) and direct extension from a focus of infection adjacent to the lung.
- Previously, pneumonias were classified by the anatomic structure invaded but the current classification system categorizes them by etiologic agent.: bacterial, mycoplasma, pneumosystic, viral etc.
- Necrotizing pneumonia or lung abscesses, or both, occur when necrotic lung tissue is released into small, adjacent airways, creating multiple abscesses (<2 cm in diameter), or into larger airways or bronchopulmonary segments, creating larger abscesses (>2 cm in diameter).

C. Clinical Features

- Depending on the pathogen, route of exposure, age of the patient, and environment, presentation of a patient with pneumonia may be classified as typical or atypical.
- A typical (obvious or classical) presentation might include sudden onset of fever, single shaking chill, productive cough (usually with purulent sputum), and pleuritic chest pain.
- Signs of consolidation may include egophony, dullness to palpation, and increased fremitus.
- Auscultatory findings may include bronchial breath sounds and crackles over the affected areas.
- An atypical (obscure or unusual) presentation may be characterized by a gradual onset of nonspecific symptoms (headache, myalgia, fatigue, nausea, vomiting, diarrhea, loss of appetite), and a dry cough.
- Physical findings tend to be minimal (crackles or scattered rhonchi) without overt signs of consolidation.

SIGNS AND SYMPTOMS OF PULMONARY DISEASE CAUSED BY BIOTERRORISM (TABLE 2-6)

- Pulmonary anthrax (etiologic agent, *Bacillus anthracis*)—Patients are first seen with flu-like illness. Symptoms can include malaise, low-grade fever, myalgia, nonproductive cough, and chest discomfort. Several days after the initial presentation, patients become acutely ill and can have high fever, severe respiratory distress, shock, and coma.
- Pneumonic plague (etiologic agent, *Yersinia pestis*)—Patients become acutely ill after a 2- to 3-day incubation period. High fever, rigors, tachycardia, headache, myalgias, dyspnea, cough, malaise, and/or cyanosis are common features.

TABLE 2-6.	Historic Clues to Unusual Pneumonias	
Type of Pneumonia	**Exposure History**	**Occupational or Risk Population**
Anthrax	Cattle, horses, swine, wools, hides	Butchers, tanners, wool carders, agricultural workers
Brucellosis	Cattle, swine, goats, raw milk products	Abattoir workers, recent Mexican immigrants, veterinarians, agricultural workers
Coccidioidomycosis	Travel to San Joaquin Valley, southern California, southwest Texas, New Mexico, Arizona	Agricultural workers, construction workers
Cryptococcosis	Pigeon droppings, HIV	AIDS
Histoplasmosis	Chicken or bat droppings, travel to Ohio or Mississippi River valley	Agricultural workers, construction workers
Legionnaires disease	Contaminated air coolers or hospital water supply	Office workers, maintenance workers, hospitalized patients
Melioidosis	Travel to southeast Asia, Australia, South and Central America, Guam	Military personnel
Plague	Ground squirrels, prairie dogs, rabbits, rats in endemic areas (western United States)	Hunters, campers, agricultural workers
Psittacosis	Budgerigars, cockatoos, parrots, parakeets, pigeons, turkeys	Bird fanciers, agricultural workers
Q fever	Cattle, sheep, or goat milk, placentas, or feces	Agricultural workers
Sporotrichosis	Rose thorns	Gardeners, florists
Tularemia	Tissue of rabbits or squirrels, bite of infected ticks or flies	Hunters, campers

From Fauci AS, Harrison TR, eds. *Harrison's Principles of Internal Medicine*. 17th ed. New York, NY: McGraw-Hill; 2008, with permission.

- Pulmonary tularemia (etiologic agent, *Francisella tularensis*)—Patients clinically complain of fever, chills, drenching sweats, severe weakness, cough, and/or headache.
- Bioterrorism has become a reality after spores of *B. anthracis* sent through the mail caused skin lesions or lung infections, or both, in some citizens of the United States.
- Other organisms the Pentagon recognizes as agents of bioterrorism that can infect the skin or lung, or both, include *Y. pestis* (etiologic agent of the plague) and *F. tularensis* (etiologic agent of tularemia).
- Pneumonias are classified by infecting or causative agents, each of which will have differing etiology, clinical manifestation, clinical course, and treatment regimen.

PATHOPHYSIOLOGY

- Pneumonia typically occurs when host defense mechanisms are incapable of contending with a pathogenic challenge by bacteria, fungus, rickettsia, etc.
- Defense mechanisms include the mucociliary lining of lung, phagocytic cells (alveolar macrophages, neutrophils), lung surfactant, specific antibodies (immunoglobulin G[IgG]), chemoattractive/tactic agents (C5a, interleukin-8).

COMPLICATIONS OF PNEUMONIA

- The inflammatory process of pneumonia can have the potential to extend from the parenchyma to the pleural surface. If this occurs, an empyema, or collection of pus in the pleural space, develops.
- CXR shows a pleural effusion, and empyema is diagnosed when a thoracentesis demonstrates pleural fluid containing significant amounts of leukocytes, bacterial organisms, or both.
- Staphylococci also have been implicated along with other aerobic organisms in cases of empyema.
- Treatment includes antibiotics and placement of a chest tube into the pleural space for drainage.
- Another complication of pneumonia is the formation of a lung abscess, or a localized collection of pus, which typically causes tissue destruction and complicates pneumonia.
- CXR will generally reveal the lung abscess.
- Treatment consists of prolonged antibiotic treatment. Surgical intervention is rarely needed because the abscess usually drains through the tracheobronchial tree.

D. Diagnostic Studies

- CXRs are used most often to confirm the presence and extent of involvement of the inflammatory process.
- CXRs may not be diagnostic if patients are unable to mount an inflammatory response (e.g., patients with HIV/AIDS, agranulocytosis) or if CXR is taken at an early phase of an infiltrative process (pneumocystis pneumonia in a patient with HIV/AIDS).

- The American Thoracic Society consensus panel recommends sputum gram stain and culture for suspected resistant organisms.
- Techniques (such as transtracheal aspiration, transthoracic lung puncture, and bronchoscopically obtained specimens) through use of protected brush or bronchoalveolar lavage can yield noncontaminated results for viral, aerobic, anaerobic, and mycobacterium cultures, as well as Gram, acid-fast, Gomori, and fluorescent antibody staining.
- Open lung biopsy is reserved for suspicious (cancerous) focal lesions that cannot be reached through bronchoscopy, or when a definitive diagnosis is not forthcoming after other techniques have been used, or both.
- Two blood cultures from different venipuncture sites should be obtained when evaluating patients with pneumonia.
- Culture of pleural fluid should be obtained if empyema is suspected.
- Antibody titer (IgG, IgM, *Legionella*) can be helpful for diagnosing *Mycoplasma pneumoniae*, *Chlamydia pneumoniae*, and *Legionella pneumophila*.
- A urine antigen test highly specific and sensitive for *L. pneumophila* can also be obtained, as appropriate.
- Viral studies are available to detect influenza A and B as well as severe acute respiratory syndrome (SARS) coronavirus.

E. Management
- In general, pharmacologic treatment of patients with pneumonia begins empirically.
- Patient history, medication allergies, mechanism, as well as environmental site of exposure, age, and underlying disease states guide the clinical decision making process.
- Common empiric oral antibiotics used to treat community-acquired pneumonia can include macrolide antibiotics such as azithromycin or clarithromycin, amoxicillin + clavulanate, second- or third-generation cephalosporins, fluoroquinolones, co-trimoxazole, and erythromycin in combination with either a cephalosporin or amoxicillin + clavulanate.
- Antibiotics used to empirically treat hospital-acquired pneumonia are usually given IV and can include choices from the following classes: penicillins, cephalosporins, and aminoglycosides.
- Other drugs used for this type of pneumonia are metronidazole, chloramphenicol, fluoroquinolones, clotrimazole, clindamycin, and vancomycin.
- Rickettsial infections are commonly treated with doxycycline, and fungal infections are treated with either fluconazole or amphotericin B.
- Influenza A or B can be treated with oseltamivir or zanamivir within the first 48 hours, but these drugs are only effective in reducing symptoms and duration of illness. No treatment has proven efficacious for respiratory syncytial virus in adults, parainfluenza

virus, adenovirus, metapneumovirus, SARS coronavirus, or hantavirus. Treatment is supportive care (oxygen and ventilator support).

CURRENT TREATMENT RECOMMENDATIONS FOR PATHOGENS USED IN BIOTERRORISM
- *B. anthracis*—ciprofloxacin or doxycycline.
- *Y. pestis*—streptomycin or doxycycline.
- *F. tularensis*—streptomycin.

XIII. Diffuse Parenchymal Lung Disease (Also Called Interstitial Lung Disease)

A. Etiology
Diffuse parenchymal lung disease, also known as interstitial lung disease, is a clinical term for a heterogenous group of lower respiratory tract disorders that affect the alveolar interstitium: capillaries, alveolar spaces, connective tissue, larger blood vessels, lymphatics, and airways.

- Incidence has been estimated as high as 80.9 per 100,000 men and 67.2 per 100,000 women in the U.S.
- Causes of ILD are diverse and range from idiopathic to genetic. Drugs, environmental factors, alveolar-filling disorders, rheumatologic disorders, and vasculitides are included as possible causes.
- Classifying the diseases into clinical categories can aid in the clinical decision-making process and narrow of the differential diagnosis (Table 2-7).

B. Pathophysiology
- Although causes of ILD are numerous (approximately 150 separate diseases are characterized by some interstitial diffuse parenchymal lung tissue damage), the reason so many diseases are couched under that title is the common pathophysiologic, radiographic, and clinical features of the affected patients.
- The basis for these common findings is extensive disruption of alveolar tissue, loss of functional alveoli, and replacement of functional tissue by scar tissue.
- Immunopathologic response of lung tissue to irritants causes an initial inflammation that heals by scar tissue formation. If the irritant/disease is persistent, a chronic phase of the disorder causing disruption of pulmonary function and gas exchange.
- Larger airways, such as the bronchioles, can be involved in the inflammatory process, leading to bronchiolitis obliterans and an organizing pneumonia. This occurrence also is thought to be a part of interstitial diffuse parenchymal lung disease.

C. Clinical Features
ASSESSMENT
- The most common presenting complaint is development of progressive dyspnea. Initially, the shortness of breath is felt only with exertion and worsens as the inflammatory process progresses.

TABLE 2-7. Etiologic Classification of ILD

Idiopathic Interstitial Pneumonias	Associated with Collagen Vascular Disease
Idiopathic pulmonary fibrosis	Progressive systemic sclerosis
Desquamative interstitial pneumonia	Ankylosing spondylitis
Acute interstitial pneumonia (Hamman–Rich syndrome)	Rheumatologic and autoimmune diseases
Respiratory bronchiolitis associated ILD	Systemic lupus erythematosus
Cryptogenic organizing pneumonia (Idiopathic bronchiolitis obliterans with organizing pneumonia)	Rheumatoid arthritis
	Progressive systemic sclerosis
Occupational and environmental exposures	Sjögren syndrome
Alveolar Filling Disorders	Polymyositis and dermatomyositis
Goodpasture syndrome	Mixed connective tissue disease
Pulmonary alveolar proteinosis	**Associated with Pulmonary Vasculitis**
Pulmonary hemosiderosis	Wegener granulomatosis
Pulmonary hemorrhage	Churg–Strauss syndrome
Chronic eosinophilic pneumonia	**Hypersensitivity Pneumonitis**
Inherited Forms	Occupational and environment ILD
Familial idiopathic pulmonary fibrosis	Drug-induced/ iatrogenic ILD
Tuberous sclerosis	**Other Forms**
Neurofibromatosis	Sarcoidosis
Gaucher disease	Langerhans cell histiocytosis
Niemann–Pick disease	
Hermansky–Pudlak syndrome	

From Goldman L, Ausiello D, eds. *Cecil Medicine.* 23rd ed. Philadelphia, PA: Saunders Elsevier; 2008:641, with permission.

- Nonproductive, dry cough and fatigue are common complaints of patients with ILD.
- If pneumonia is present (as with bronchiolitis obliterans), cough will be a major complaint.
- In patients with ILD diffuse parenchymal lung disease from a rheumatic source, a common complaint may be pleuritic chest pain.
- Any symptom that worsens or is out of the ordinary must be taken seriously.
- If pleuritic chest pain and sudden worsening of shortness of breath should occur, spontaneous pneumothorax in association with lymphangioleiomyomatosis, neurofibromatosis, tuberous sclerosis, or Langerhans cell histiocytosis could be suspected.
- Hemoptysis should alert the clinician to malignancy, diffuse alveolar hemorrhage syndromes, pulmonary embolus, and superimposed infection.

HISTORY
- Obtaining a thorough history with specific attention to duration and progression of illness is of utmost importance in discovering the cause.
- Obtaining and reviewing prior patient records will help toward this end. Evaluation should include a detailed, lifelong occupational and environmental history; known exposures to inhaled agents (including hobbies); specific questions related to medications that induce ILD; smoking history; and family history.

PHYSICAL FINDINGS
- Physical examination can disclose findings ranging from a normal pulmonary examination to bilateral crackles, wheezing, rhonchi, or coarse rales. Clubbing (pulmonary osteoarthropathy) of the nails (both fingers and toes) may be present, but physical examination findings rarely aid in establishing the diagnosis.

D. Diagnostic Studies

CXR
- Usually has an important role in establishing the diagnosis of interstitial diffuse parenchymal lung disease.
- As with patient history, evaluation of previous CXRs to ascertain disease progression in a given patient is most important.
- Infiltrates in lower-lung zones provide a clue to the presence of an ILD process; they will have a "ground-glass" appearance in the early stage of the disease, and a nodular, linear, and/or honeycombed appearance in the later stages.

HIGH-RESOLUTION COMPUTED TOMOGRAPHY
- High-resolution CT scan can distinguish reversible lung disease from irreversibly damaged areas and thus establish a diagnosis and provide staging of the disease.

MORE INVASIVE PROCEDURES
- Fiber-optic bronchoscopy and open-lung biopsy are reserved for disease processes that remain undiagnosed (malignancy, sarcoidosis, infection, etc.) despite other less-invasive procedures.

LABORATORY AND OTHER STUDIES
- Laboratory studies rarely point to a specific diagnosis and more often suggest a diagnosis.
- Erythrocyte sedimentation rate is usually elevated in ILD diffuse parenchymal lung disease.
- Tests for cryo-Igs and serologic tests for collagen vascular disease, rheumatoid factor, antinuclear antibodies, and complement levels offer clues to the presence of underlying disease processes.
- ECG may show right ventricular and atrial strain.
- ABG measurements can show mild hypoxemia, although arterial blood pH is usually normal unless the patient is exercising, in which case it will fall.

- In most cases, pulmonary function test (PFT) can provide useful information when trying to document physiologic changes associated with ILD diffuse parenchymal lung disease and responses (or lack thereof) to treatment.
- PFT should be used with caution, especially in current or former smokers who might have ILD and emphysema.

E. Management

GOALS OF TREATMENT

- Remove/discontinue exposure of pulmonary irritants such as smoke, dust, and medication.
- Prevent destruction of lung tissue by inhibiting the inflammatory reaction within the lung.
- Relieve symptoms of these disease processes.
- Every effort should be made to ascertain the underlying disease process and treat accordingly; otherwise, corticosteroids are the mainstay of treatment for ILD diffuse parenchymal lung disease.
- In patients who cannot tolerate corticosteroids, or whose symptoms progress despite steroid treatment, cyclophosphamide, or azathioprine can be tried.
- Supplemental oxygen can be administered in patients whose oxygen tension is <55 mm Hg at rest or with exercise.
- Pneumococcal and influenza vaccines should be administered prophylactically.
- When therapeutic measures fail, lung transplantation has been authorized as a treatment in patients with end-stage ILD diffuse parenchymal lung disease.
- Selection guidelines and relative contraindications for transplantation are fairly stringent.
- Two-year survival rates are currently between 60% and 80%, with failures usually occurring from infections that complicate immunosuppressive therapy or from tissue rejection.

XIV. Respiratory Failure

A. Etiology

- Respiratory failure can be divided into acute or chronic stages, depending on evolution of the process; each stage has specific physiologic, pathogenic, and therapeutic characteristics.
- Respiratory failure can be further categorized into (a) type I—hypoxemic respiratory failure (a failure of gas exchange) and (b) type II—hypercapnic with or without hypoxemic respirature failure (a failure of ventilation).
- It is important to note that respiratory failure can be the result of extrapulmonary processes such as sepsis, shock, or trauma.
- Increased dead space—refers to conditions that cause areas of the lung to be ventilated but not perfused, or when the decrease in perfusion exceeds decreases in ventilation, as in COPD, asthma, cystic fibrosis, or interstitial lung fibrosis.
- Decreased minute ventilation—refers to processes or diseases that affect the patient's normal ventilation/metabolism of gases, specifically CO_2, and may be the result of chest wall abnormalities, neurologic abnormalities, metabolic abnormalities, drug overdose, or airway obstruction.
- Patients usually have more than one disease or process that precipitates respiratory failure.
- Age at onset and overall patient health are two important prognostic factors for recovery from respiratory failure.
- The most common cause of death in patients with respiratory failure is multisystem organ failure.

B. Clinical Features

- Depending on the pathogenesis of respiratory failure (hypoxia vs. hypercapnia), patients can have specific symptomatology. The severity of symptoms (a patient's ventilatory response) depends on the degree of the patient's physiologic ability to sense and respond to hypoxia or hypercapnia (Table 2-8).
- Typical initial presentations of both types can include complaints of sudden breathlessness, palpitations, dizziness, and mild confusion.
- Physical examination may disclose diffuse crackles, signs of consolidation, decreased breath sounds, weakness, hypotension, tachycardia, wheezing, altered mental status, and lower-extremity edema.

TABLE 2-8. Pulmonary and Extrapulmonary Causes of ALI and ARDS

Direct or primary pulmonary causes

Aspiration of gastric contents
Diffuse pneumonia
Pulmonary contusion
Inhalation injury
Chest trauma
Near-drowning

Extrapulmonary causes

Sepsis
Bacteremia without sepsis
Severe sepsis/systemic inflammatory response syndrome
Major trauma
Hypertransfusion
Postcardiopulmonary bypass
Shock and hypotension
Drug overdose
Severe burns
Pancreatitis

From Goldman L, Ausiello D, eds. *Cecil Medicine.* 23rd ed. Philadelphia, PA: Saunders Elsevier; 2008:778, with permission.

C. Diagnostic Studies

HYPOXIA

- CXR may show small "white" lungs, patchy, diffuse infiltrates, signs of consolidation, and/or lobar atelectasis.

HYPERCAPNIA

- CXR may show hyperinflation, large "black" lungs, bullae, and increased vascular markings (COPD); in addition, hypoinflation and small "black" lungs with neuromuscular disease or drug toxicity may be present.

D. Pathophysiology

HYPOXIC RESPIRATORY FAILURE

- Any acute or chronic condition that produces PaO_2 <60 mm Hg or arterial oxygen saturation (SaO_2) <90% is considered hypoxic respiratory failure.
- Acute lung injury (ALI) and acute respiratory distress syndrome (ARDS) both fall into this category. The most common risk factor for developing ARDS is sepsis. Other risk factors for developing ARDS include: systemic inflammatory response syndrome, shock, truma, aspiration, near-drowning, pancreatitis, DIC and burns
- Can occur as a result of:
  - *Shunting*—refers to anatomic- or physiologic-acquired defect that causes venous blood to mix with arterial blood after bypassing functional pulmonary architecture.
  - *Ventilation/perfusion mismatch*— refers to diseases that decrease or inhibit normal ventilation-to-perfusion ratios such as COPD, interstitial inflammation, and vascular inflammation.
  - *Low inspired oxygen tension*—refers to a combination of conditions that can lead to hypoxia (e.g., low oxygen levels such as those seen at high altitudes or inhalation of toxic gases in combination with cardiopulmonary disease processes).
  - *Hypoventilation*—refers to processes that might elevate the $PaCO_2$, thus displacing the alveolar oxygen.
  - *Diffusion impairment*—refers primarily to patients who have ILD that decreases the diffusion of gases in the alveoli.
  - *Low mixed venous oxygenation*—refers to factors that cause a decrease in mixed venous oxygen tension, which in turn affects the PaO_2, especially in the presence of intrapulmonary shunting or ventilation/perfusion mismatch.

HYPERCAPNIC-(HYPOXIC) RESPIRATORY FAILURE

- Any disease or process that causes acute CO_2 retention in which the $PaCO_2$ tension is 45 to 50 mm Hg and respiratory acidosis (pH <7.35) is present is considered hypercapnic (hypoxic) respiratory failure.
- Increased $PaCO_2$ is the result of increased CO_2 production, decreased tidal ventilation or increased dead space ventilation. Hypermetabolic states such

exercise, fever, sepsis, trauma, burns, excessive carbohydrate intake and hyperthryoidsim can increase CO_2 production.

E. Diagnostic Studies

- ECG findings can range from sinus tachycardia, acute myocardial infarction, and left ventricular hypertrophy to normal ECG, right ventricular hypertrophy, and low voltage.
- Blood studies also are cause dependent and range from nonspecific findings to elevated hemoglobin, respiratory acidosis, mixed metabolic and respiratory acidosis, and hypokalemia.

F. Management

- Treatment is etiology dependent. A thorough patient history is essential and should include events leading up to and after the onset of respiratory problems, past and present pulmonary diseases/conditions. The physical examination and laboratory/radiographic findings are necessary to pinpoint a diagnosis.
- Treatment is then based on the condition identified and type of failure (hypoxia vs. hypercapnia).
- Hypoxic respiratory failure treatment includes treating the predisposing condition and administering supportive therapy, including maintaining an open airway (possible intubation), administering O_2, and ventilatory support (placing patients on a mechanical ventilator).

Hypoxic respiratory failure treatment includes treating the predisposing condition and administering supportive therapy, including maintaining an open airway (possible intubation), administering O_2, and ventilatory support (placing patients on a mechanical ventilator).

- No increase in survival rates have been demonstrated in randomized, controlled clinical trials with the use of early administration of high-dose corticosteroids, prostagladin E_1, NSAIDs, antiendotoxin and anticytokine thereapy, inhaled nitric oxide, surfactant therapy, antioxidant therapy, positional changes or partial liquid ventilation.
- The main goal of therapy is to maintain adequate PaO_2 levels while remaining aware of therapeutic complications such as O_2 toxicity, volume overload, gastrointestinal (GI) bleeding, malnutrition, sepsis, thromboembolism, and mechanical ventilator-associated problems.
- Weaning patients from mechanically-assisted ventilation devices should be accomplished as soon as possible after they are stabilized.
- Treatment of hypercapnic respiratory failure is similar to hypoxic respiratory failure with some slight variation in ventilatory support. The main goal continues to be maintenance of adequate PaO_2 and decreasing the elevated levels of $PaCO_2$.
- In patients who have high baseline $PaCO_2$ (such as patients with COPD), normalization of $PaCO_2$

should not be the primary goal; rather, adequate PaO_2 levels should be maintained. Patients with COPD can be difficult to wean from ventilatory devices.

- Complications such as infection, thromboembolism, GI bleeding, agitation, and volume overload become accentuated due to the prolonged time on mechanical ventilatory support.
- Antibiotics, heparin, H_2-blockers, antianxiolytics, and maintenance of electrolyte balance are strategies to use as the situation warrants.

SELECTED READINGS

American Thoracic Society: Medical Section of the American Lung Association. Standards for the diagnosis and care of patients with chronic obstructive pulmonary disease. *Am J Respir Crit Care Med.* 1995;152:S77–S120.

Ball WC Jr. Pleural effusions. In: Stobo JD, Hellmann DB, Ladenson PW, Petty BG, Traill TA, eds. *The Principles and Practice of Medicine.* 23rd ed. Stamford, CT: Appleton & Lange; 1996:184–188.

Beers MH, ed. *Merck Manual.* 18th ed. Whitehouse Station, NJ: Merck Research Laboratories; 2006.

Bell WR. Venous thrombosis and pulmonary embolism. In: Stobo JD, Hellmann DB, Ladenson PW, Petty BG, Traill TA, eds. *The Principles and Practice of Medicine.* 23rd ed. Stamford, CT: Appleton & Lange; 1996:171–176.

Celli BR. Diseases of the diaphragm, chest wall, pleura, and mediastinum. In: Bennett JC, Plum F, eds. *Cecil Textbook of Medicine.* 20th ed. Philadelphia, PA: WB Saunders; 1996:442–448.

Disease syndromes. In: Isada CM, Kasten BL Jr, Goldman MP, Gray LD, Aberg JA, eds. *Infectious Disease Handbook.* 2nd ed. Ohio, OH: Lexi-Comp; 1996:42–44.

Drazen JM, Weinberger SE, McFadden ER, Disorders of the respiratory system. In: Fauci AS, Braunwald E, Isselbacher KJ, Wilson JD, Martin JB, Kasper DL, Hauser SL, Longo DL, eds. *Harrison's Principles of Internal Medicine.* 14th ed. New York, NY: McGraw-Hill; 1998:1407–1491.

Domino FJ, ed. *The 5-Minute Clinical Consult.* 19th ed. Philadelphia, PA: Lippincott, Williams & Wilkins; 2011.

Expert Panel Report 2. *Clinical Practice Guidelines. Guidelines for the Diagnosis and Management of Asthma.* National Institutes of Health. National Heart, Lung and Blood Institute; 1997 Oct. Report No.: NIH 97–4051.

Fauci AS, Harrison TR, eds. *Harrison's Principles of Internal Medicine.* 17th ed. New York, NY: McGraw-Hill; 2008.

Goldman L, Ausiello D, eds. *Cecil Medicine.* 23rd ed. Philadelphia, PA: Saunders Elsevier; 2008:641.

Jankowich MA, Aliotta JM. Neoplastic disorders of the lung. In: Andreoli TE, Benjamin IJ, Griggs RC, Wing EJ, eds. *Cecil Essentials of Medicine.* 8th ed. Philadelphia, PA: Saunders Elsevier; 2010:266–270.

Johanson WG Jr. Overview of pneumonia. In: Bennett JC, Plum F, eds. *Cecil Textbook of Medicine.* 20th ed. Philadelphia, PA: WB Saunders; 1996:411–413.

Kollef MH. Critical care. In: Carey CF, Lee HH, Woeltje KF, eds. *The Washington Manual of Medical Therapeutics.* 29th ed. Philadelphia, PA: Lippincott-Raven; 1998:170–188.

McCool FD. Disorders of the pleura, mediastinum, and chest wall. In: Andreoli TE, Benjamin IJ, Griggs RC, Wing EJ, eds. *Cecil Essentials of Medicine.* 8th ed. Philadelphia, PA: Saunders Elsevier; 2010:266–270.

Miller YE. Pulmonary neoplasms. In: Bennett JC, Plum F, eds. *Cecil Textbook of Medicine.* 20th ed. Philadelphia, PA: WB Saunders; 1996:436–441.

Rounds S. Pulmonary vascular disease. In: Andreoli TE, Benjamin IJ, Griggs RC, Wing EJ, eds. *Cecil Essentials of Medicine.* 8th ed. Philadelphia, PA: Saunders Elsevier; 2010:241–243.

Runge MS, Greganti MA, eds. *Netter's Internal Medicine.* 2nd ed. Philadelphia, PA: Saunders Elsevier; 2009.

Schapira RM, Varkey B, Kutty K. Bronchogenic carcinoma. In: Kutty K, Schapira RM, Ruiswyk JV, eds. *Kochar's Concise Textbook of Medicine.* 4th ed. Philadelphia, PA: Lippincott Williams & Wilkins; 2003:953–955.

Schuller D. Pulmonary disease. In: Carey CF, Lee HH, Woeltje KF, eds. *The Washington Manual of Medical Therapeutics.* 29th ed. Philadelphia, PA: Lippincott-Raven; 1998:190–211.

Senior RM. Pulmonary embolism. In: Bennett JC, Plum F, eds. *Cecil Textbook of Medicine.* 20th ed. Philadelphia, PA: WB Saunders; 1996:422–429.

Stauffer JL. Lung. In: Tierney LM Jr, Mcphee SJ, Papadakis MA, eds. *Current Medical Diagnosis and Treatment.* 36th ed. Stamford, CT: Appleton & Lange; 1997:236–319.

Summer WR. Respiratory failure. In: Bennett JC, Plum F, eds. *Cecil Textbook of Medicine.* 20th ed. Philadelphia, PA: WB Saunders; 1996:452–459.

Terry PB. Nodules and masses in the lung and mediastinum. In: Stobo JD, Hellmann DB, Ladenson PW, Petty BG, Traill TA, eds. *The Principles and Practice of Medicine.* 23rd ed. Stamford, CT: Appleton & Lange; 1996:177–183.

Toews GB. Interstitial lung disease. In: Bennett JC, Plum F, eds. *Cecil Textbook of Medicine.* 20th ed. Philadelphia, PA: WB Saunders; 1996:390–399.

Turino GM. Approach to the patient with respiratory disease. In: Bennett JC, Plum F, eds. *Cecil Textbook of Medicine.* 20th ed. Philadelphia, PA: WB Saunders; 1996:368–370.

Varkey B, Schapira RM, Kutty K. Pleural effusion. In: Kutty K, Schapira RM, Ruiswyk JV, eds. *Kochar's Concise Textbook of Medicine.* 4th ed. Philadelphia, PA: Lippincott Williams & Wilkins; 2003:957–961.

Weinberger SE. *Principles of Pulmonary Medicine.* 3rd ed. Philadelphia, PA: WB Saunders; 1998.

Weinberger SE. *Principles of Pulmonary Medicine.* 4th ed. Philadelphia, PA: WB Saunders; 2004.

Heart and Blood Vessel Disorders

Matt Dane Baker

I. Heart Failure

A. Etiology

HIGH-OUTPUT HEART FAILURE (HF) (LESS COMMON THAN LOW-OUTPUT HF)

- Anemia.
- Hyperthyroidism.
- Arteriovenous (A-V) fistula with shunting.
- Beriberi (thiamine deficiency).
- Paget disease.

LOW-OUTPUT HF

- Chronic hypertension—common etiology.
- Ischemic heart disease—common etiology.
- Cardiomyopathies.
- Valvular heart disease (VHD).
- Dysrhythmias.

RIGHT-SIDED HF

- Pulmonary disease (chronic obstructive pulmonary disease with cor pulmonale).
- Pulmonary hypertension.
- Right ventricular infarction.
- Mitral stenosis (MS).
- Simultaneous with left-sided HF—common etiology.

LEFT-SIDED HF

- Myocardial infarction (MI) with left ventricular (LV) infarction—common etiology.
- Systemic hypertension—common etiology.
- Cardiomyopathy.
- Endocarditis.
- Aortic valve disease and mitral regurgitation (MR).

SYSTOLIC HF (HF with Decreased or Impaired Ejection Fraction [EF])

- Dilated cardiomyopathies.
- MI—common etiology.
- Chronic hypertension—common etiology.

DIASTOLIC HF (HF with Normal or Preserved EF)

- Restrictive, infiltrative cardiomyopathies (amyloidosis, sarcoidosis).
- Pericardial effusion.
- Hypertrophic cardiomyopathy.
- Myocardial ischemia and infarction—common etiology.
- Hypertension—common etiology.

B. Pathology

- HF refers to an abnormal state characterized by failure of the heart to pump enough blood to meet the metabolic demands of the body tissues.
- Congestive heart failure (CHF) is the state of circulatory congestion secondary to HF, which can be divided into high- or low-output failure, left- or right-sided failure, systolic or diastolic failure. Often, substantial crossover exists between these pathophysiologic categories because left- and right-sided failure, and systolic and diastolic dysfunction, often occur simultaneously.
- High-output failure results from excessive demand for cardiac output or abnormally high tissue demands. Myocardial function itself may be normal but inadequate to meet increased demands. This is uncommon.
- Low-output failure occurs secondary to disorders of the heart that result in diminished cardiac output.
- Right-sided failure involves impairment of the right side of the heart and, thus, leads to systemic venous congestion seen in the liver and periphery.
- Left-sided failure results from insults to the left atrium and ventricle and, consequently, results in pulmonary congestion.
- Simultaneous left- and right-sided failure is often referred to as biventricular failure.
- Systolic failure involves a decrease in cardiac contractility and EF, whereas diastolic dysfunction results from poor ventricular compliance and relaxation, and impaired ventricular filling. Diastolic failure is now referred to as HF with normal or preserved EF.
- Diminished cardiac output can be caused by conditions that alter preload, afterload, and contractility; most therapies are designed to correct these physiologic derangements or address the compensation mechanisms.
- Compensation mechanisms in HF include adrenergic autonomic stimulation; activation of the rennin–angiotensin–aldosterone system; ventricular hypertrophy, then remodeling; secretion of antidiuretic hormone; and secretion of atrial or brain natriuretic peptides (BNPs).

- Obesity is now known to be an independent risk factor for HF, as is obstructive sleep apnea.

C. Precipitating Factors
- Myocardial ischemia or infarction.
- Dysrhythmia, especially atrial fibrillation due to loss of atrial kick (contraction).
- Infection.
- Shock/trauma.
- Thyroid disease (hyper or hypo).
- Pulmonary embolism.
- Dietary indiscretion (excess salt intake).
- Medication nonadherence.
- Drugs—β-blockers, nonsteroidal anti-inflammatory drugs (NSAIDs), calcium channel blockers, thiazolidinediones.

D. Demographics
- Five million persons have HF in the United States, with 550,000 new cases diagnosed each year.
- Most common admitting diagnoses in hospitalized elderly individuals.

E. Clinical Features

HISTORY
- Fatigue.
- Anorexia.
- Dyspnea, initially dyspnea on exertion.
- Orthopnea.
- Paroxysmal nocturnal dyspnea (PND).
- Coughing (pink, frothy sputum), wheezing.
- Minimal right upper quadrant abdomen discomfort.
- Ankle edema.
- Nocturia.
- **Symptoms classified using New York Heart Association (NYHA) scale:**
  - Class I: Cardiac disease but no limitations. Asymptomatic on ordinary activities.
  - Class II: Slight limitation. Comfortable at rest, but experience symptoms with ordinary activities.
  - Class III: Marked limitation. Comfortable at rest, but symptomatic with less than ordinary activities.
  - Class IV: Inability to perform any physical activity without symptoms. Symptoms at rest.
- HF is also classified using the American Heart Association/American College of Cardiology (AHA/ACC) staging system. This system acknowledges HF as a progressive disorder that should be addressed from a preventative perspective with intervention before structural damage or symptoms appear.
  - Stage A: At high risk for HF but without structural heart disease or symptoms of HF.
  - Stage B: Structural heart disease but without signs or symptoms of HF.
  - Stage C: Structural disease with prior or current symptoms of HF.
  - Stage D: Refractory HF requiring specialized interventions.

PHYSICAL FINDINGS
- Early or mild HF may have no signs.
- Tachypnea.
- Jugular venous distention (JVD).
- Hepatojugular reflux.
- Pulmonary rales or crackles (bibasilar).
- Wheezing ("cardiac asthma").
- Pleural effusion with diminished breath sounds and dullness to percussion (bilateral or right).
- Lateral displacement of apical impulse.
- Third heart sound (S_3 gallop).
- Cardiac murmurs as etiology or MR murmur from dilated ventricle.
- Paradoxical splitting of second heart sound (S_2).
- Hepatomegaly.
- Ascites.
- Cyanosis.
- Peripheral edema (ankle, pedal, pretibial, sacral if bedfast patient, anasarca).
- Hypotension, cool extremities, and mental status changes (in severe CHF).
- Cheyne–Stokes respiration (in severe failure).

F. Diagnostic Studies
- Chest X-ray (CXR): Cardiomegaly, pleural effusions (right or bilateral), Kerley B lines, increased pulmonary vascular markings and cephalization of pulmonary vascular markings (increase in upper lobes), interstitial edema, butterfly or bat-wing pattern of pulmonary edema (Figure 3-1).
- Echocardiography (two-dimensional [2-D] and cardiac Doppler)—This is the most useful test in diagnosis. Can see wall/chamber hypertrophy or dilatation, ventricular wall akinetic or dyskinetic areas, reduced estimated LVEF (<50%) in systolic failure, valvular lesions.
- BNP or N-terminal pro-BNP—elevated. Used in emergency department and inpatient settings.
- Multigated acquisition (MUGA) scan (nuclear ventriculography)—reduced LVEF. Used if echocardiogram (Echo) results are not optimal.
- Cardiac catheterization with ventriculography—reduced LVEF. Used if concurrent coronary artery disease (CAD) is suspected.
- Electrocardiogram (ECG)—sinus tachycardia, LV hypertrophy (LVH), evidence of MI (not specific for HF).
- Arterial blood gas studies—respiratory alkalosis. Used in emergency department and inpatient settings.
- Blood urea nitrogen (BUN)—mild azotemia.
- Creatinine—mildly increased.
- Electrolyte—dilutional hyponatremia.
- Complete blood cell (CBC)—anemia.
- Aspartase aminotransferases (AST; alanine aminotransferase)—sometimes increased.
- Urine analysis (UA)—proteinuria.
- Albumin and thyroid-stimulating hormone (TSH)—to look for underlying etiology.

FIGURE 3-1. Chest PA (A) and lateral (B) radiographs. CHF with pulmonary edema. (From Erkomen WE. Diagnostic radiology chest. In: Erkomen WE, ed. *Radiology 101: The Basics and Fundamentals for Imaging.* Philadelphia, PA: Lippincott-Raven; 1998:122, with permission.)

G. Management (Based on AHA/ACC System)

STAGE A: PREVENTION IN HIGH-RISK PATIENTS

- Treat hypertension—thiazide diuretics, angiotensin-converting enzyme (ACE) inhibitors, or angiotensin receptor blockers (ARBs) are good choices—lipid disorders, diabetes, obstructive sleep apnea, and metabolic disorder.
- **Lifestyle changes:**
  - Salt (sodium) restriction.
  - Smoking cessation.
  - Exercise—avoid deconditioning or overexercise.
  - Weight reduction, if appropriate.
  - Alcohol avoidance.

STAGE B: PREVENTION OF PROGRESSION IN PATIENTS WITH STRUCTURAL DAMAGE BUT NO SYMPTOMS

- **All measures in Stage A plus:**
  - ACE inhibitor or ARB.
  - Consider β-blocker in CAD patients with angina or past MI.

STAGE C: SYMPTOMATIC HF

- Lifestyle changes (see above).
- Daily weight monitoring.
- Assessment for precipitating, treatable causes.
- Antiembolism stockings.
- ACE inhibitors (ACE-I)—the mainstay of therapy because these have been proved to reduce mortality.
- Diuretics, especially loop diuretics (furosemide) initially; can add metolazone. These are for symptomatic control.
- Angiotensin II (AII) receptor antagonists (e.g., valsartan, candesartan); consider if patient develops cough on ACE inhibitors. Have been shown to decrease mortality.
- β-Blockers—carvedilol, extended release metoprolol succinate, bisoprolol (use when stable, start with low dose, increase slowly). Have been shown to decrease mortality.
- All Stage C patients should be on an ACE-I or ARB, and a β-blocker if tolerated.
- **Can then add:**
  - Combination hydralazine and isosorbide dinitrate. Shown to be effective in African American patients.
  - Spironolactone–aldosterone antagonist or eplerenone (Inspra; G.D. Searle, Peapack, NJ), a selective aldosterone receptor antagonist. Has been shown to decrease mortality.
  - Digoxin—in systolic failure, especially in patients with atrial fibrillation. Keep digoxin level between 0.5 and 0.8 ng per mL.
  - Implantable cardioverter-defibrillators (ICDs) in patients with NYHA Class II or III and LVEF <35%.
  - Biventricular pacemaker in patients with cardiac dyssynchrony and QRS duration >0.12 milliseconds; LVEF ≤35%; and NYHA Class III or IV.
  - Nesiritide (Natrecor; Scios, Sunnyvale, CA)—recombinant BNP. Used only in inpatient or emergency department setting.
  - Nitroglycerin (NTG) intravenously (IV). Used only in inpatient or emergency department setting.
  - Anticoagulants—useful in atrial fibrillation.
- In severe HF hospitalized patients—nitroprusside, IV morphine, amrinone, milrinone, dopamine, dobutamine, left ventricular assist devices (LVADs).
- **NOTE:** Calcium channel blocker may be helpful in HF with normal EF.

STAGE D: REFRACTORY HF

- Younger patients and patients of all ages with few comorbidities should be referred for LVADs, and transplant.

- Older patients with significant comorbidities and poor prognosis should be considered for hospice care and ICD deactivation.

H. Monitoring
- Weights.
- Electrolytes (especially potassium because of diuretic-induced hypokalemia).
- BUN, creatinine.
- CXR.

II. Hypertension

A. Etiology

PRIMARY OR ESSENTIAL
- Idiopathic; has genetic component and environmental precipitating factors such as salt intake, obesity, stress, sedentary lifestyle, and alcohol intake. This is by far the most common etiology for hypertension. Sympathetic hyperactivity, the Renin-Angiotensin-Aldosterone system, and defects in natriuresis play a role.

SECONDARY
- Glomerulonephritis.
- Pyelonephritis.
- Polycystic kidney disease.
- Renal artery stenosis or renovascular hypertension.
- Coarctation of the aorta.
- Hyperaldosteronism.
- Cushing disease.
- Hyperthyroidism.
- Pheochromocytoma.
- Acromegaly.
- Hyperparathyroidism.
- Preeclampsia.
- Obstructive sleep apnea.
- Drugs—cocaine, oral contraceptives, NSAIDs, decongestants, corticosteroids, sympathomimetics.

B. Pathology
- Hypertension—defined as a state of sustained elevated systemic arterial blood pressure.
- Essential or primary hypertension—idiopathic disorder without established etiology.
- Secondary hypertension—less common and caused by disorders in other organ systems (see II. A.).
- Malignant hypertension—currently called hypertensive crisis; presents with severe elevation of blood pressure (BP) (diastolic >140 mm Hg), funduscopic changes (hemorrhages, exudates, papilledema), often with manifestations of hypertensive encephalopathy such as confusion and stupor. Hypertensive emergency is defined by BP >220/125.
- Systolic hypertension is a greater risk for cardiovascular disease than diastolic in those over the age of 50.

C. Complications and End-Organ Damage from Hypertension
- Retinopathy.
- CAD.
- HF.
- Peripheral vascular disease (peripheral arterial disease [PAD]).
- Nephropathy, chronic renal disease, end-stage renal disease.
- Cerebrovascular disease—transient ischemic attack (TIA), cerebrovascular accident (CVA), vascular dementia.
- Aortic dissection.

D. Demographics
- About 15% of US Caucasian population and 20% of African American population.
- Increased frequency with aging.

E. Clinical Features
- Silent or mostly asymptomatic disease. History, physical examination, laboratory evaluation designed to establish diagnosis, rule out secondary etiologies, identify end-organ damage, uncover concurrent atherosclerosis risk factors.

HISTORY
- Occipital headache with high BP.

PHYSICAL FINDINGS
- BP—two or more readings on two or more office visits (systolic ≥140 mm Hg, diastolic ≥90 mm Hg).
- Eye—funduscopic-narrowed arteries, A-V nicking, copper or silver wiring of arterioles, hemorrhages, exudates, papilledema.
- Increased S_2.
- Also should do neck, lung, heart, abdomen, peripheral pulses, extremity, neurologic examinations to identify end-organ damage.

F. Diagnostic Studies (Table 3-1)
- None needed for diagnosis—ambulatory BP monitoring may be useful.
- CBC count or hemoglobin/hematocrit.
- UA (assess for proteinuria).
- Electrolytes (sodium, potassium).
- Creatinine.
- Lipids: cholesterol—total, high-density lipoprotein (HDL-C), low-density lipoprotein (LDL-C), triglycerides.
- Twelve-lead ECG (assess for LVH).
- BUN.
- Fasting blood glucose.
- Calcium.
  - CXR and Echo looking for cardiomegaly and ventricular hypertrophy may be helpful.

G. Management
- Salt restriction—2.4 g sodium (Na) or 6 g sodium chloride per day. Dietary Approaches to Stop Hypertension (DASH) diet with increased fruits and vegetables and decreased salt.

TABLE 3-1. Classification of BP for Adults of Age 18 and Older[a]

Category	Systolic (mm Hg)		Diastolic (mm Hg)
Normal	<120	—	<80
Prehypertension	120–139	or	80–89
Hypertension[b]	—	—	—
Stage I	140–159	or	90–99
Stage II	≥160	or	≥100

From *The Seventh Report of The Joint National Committee on Prevention, Detection, Evaluation, and Treatment of High Blood Pressure*. National Institutes of Health, National Heart, Lung, and Blood Institutes: NIH Publications 03–5233; 2003:3, with permission.

[a]Not taking antihypertensive drugs and not acutely ill. When systolic and diastolic BPs fall into different categories, the higher category should be selected to classify the individual's BP status. Optimal BP with respect to cardiovascular risk is ≤115/75 mm Hg. However, unusually low readings should be evaluated for clinical significance.

[b]Based on the average of two or more readings taken at each of two or more visits after an initial screening.

- Weight reduction.
- Decreased alcohol (<1 ounce per day).
- Tobacco cessation.
- Adequate potassium, magnesium, calcium intake.
- Aerobic exercise program.
- Stress reduction—biofeedback, relaxation exercises.

PHARMACOLOGIC
- Goal: <140/90 or <130/80 for those with diabetes mellitus (DM) or chronic kidney disease.
- Most will need at least two agents for optimal control.
- Diuretics—thiazides such as hydrochlorothiazide (HCTZ), potassium sparing, loop. Low-dose thiazides (e.g., HCTZ 12.5 to 25 mg) are excellent starting agents.
- ACE inhibitors (e.g., captopril, enalapril, lisinopril). Useful in patients with concurrent DM, HF, or old MI.
- AII receptor antagonists (e.g., losartan, valsartan, candesartan).
- β-Blockers (e.g., metoprolol, propranolol). Useful in patients with old MI or with concurrent tachycardia.
- α-Blockers (e.g., prazosin, terazosin, doxazosin). Useful in male patients with concurrent benign prostatic hyperplasia.
- Mixed α- and β-blockers (e.g., labetalol).
- Calcium channel blockers (e.g., amlodipine). Verapamil and diltiazem useful in patients with concurrent supraventricular tachycardia (SVT).
- Vasodilators (e.g., hydralazine).
- Centrally and peripheral-acting adrenergic inhibitors (e.g., clonidine, methyldopa, reserpine).
- Selective aldosterone receptor antagonists (e.g., eplerenone).
- Renin inhibitors (e.g., aliskiren).

H. Monitoring
- BP—home, office, and ambulatory monitors.
- Potassium level if on diuretics.
- Periodic UA, creatinine.

III. Angina Pectoris

A. Etiology
- Atherosclerotic stenosis of coronary arteries—most common.
- Coronary artery spasm.
- Congenital coronary artery anomalies.
- Aortic stenosis (AS), regurgitation.
- Hypertrophic cardiomyopathy.
- Myocardial muscle bridge.
- Pulmonary hypertension.
- Severe systemic hypertension.
- Collagen vascular disease.
- Syndrome X (possible microvascular disease).

B. Pathology
- Symptom complex of chest discomfort or equivalent secondary to myocardial ischemia because of mismatch of supply and demand.
- Classic stable angina—substernal pressure or heaviness sensation precipitated by exertion or anxiety; relieved in a predictable pattern by rest.
- Unstable angina—chest discomfort at rest, or new and severe (within 2 months and brought on by minimal exertion), or has changed in pattern with increased frequency, duration, and intensity.
- Crescendo angina—angina occurring with increasing frequency.
- Variant angina (Prinzmetal)—rest or nocturnal chest pain with ST segment elevation on ECG; thought to be caused by coronary artery spasm.
- Postprandial angina—angina occurring after meals.
- Anginal equivalent—dyspnea on exertion caused by myocardial ischemia.
- Syndrome X—typical exertional or stress-induced angina in the absence of coronary artery stenosis on angiography.
- Silent ischemia—evidence of myocardial ischemia on stress ECG, thallium, or echocardiography without

chest discomfort; thought to be more common in patients with diabetes.

C. Risk Factors for Atherosclerosis

- Advancing age.
- Male gender (female begins to equal male after menopause).
- Smoking tobacco.
- Hypertension.
- Genetic (family history: CHD in male first-degree relative <55 years; CHD in female first-degree relative <65 years).
- Increased total cholesterol and LDL-C, decreased HDL-C, increased apolipoprotein (a) (Lp(a)), increased small, dense LDL particles, increased triglycerides.
- DM.
- Obesity.
- Sedentary lifestyle.
- Increased homocysteine.
- Increase C-reactive protein (inflammation).
- Low-glutathione peroxidase (antioxidant enzyme).
- Proteinuria.

D. Clinical Features

HISTORY

- Precordial pressure or heaviness radiating to back, neck, shoulders, arms, lower jaw, or teeth brought on by exertion, eating large meal, cold air exposure, or emotional stress, and relieved by rest or NTG; usually lasts minutes.
- May present as dyspnea on exertion.
- Levine sign—patient describes pain using clenched fist over his or her anterior chest (sternum).
- May be accompanied by dyspnea, dizziness, palpitations, and infrequently syncope.

PHYSICAL FINDINGS

- May be normal.
- Fourth heart sound (S_4) and sometimes S_3.
- Paradoxical splitting of S_2 during angina episode.
- May have signs of atherosclerosis (e.g., xanthelasma, decreased peripheral pulses).
- May have signs of hypertension as risk factor (e.g., increased BP, retinopathy).
- Murmur of AS or aortic regurgitation (AR) as etiology, or MR from papillary muscle dysfunction.
- Signs of HF as complication.

E. Diagnostic Studies

- ECG—can frequently be normal or may show ST segment depression or T-wave inversion during attack; Q waves seen in patients with previous MI.
- Cholesterol may be elevated with elevated LDL-C, increased Lp(a), decreased HDL-C, increased triglycerides.
- C-reactive protein—increased.
- Homocysteine—increased.

- Ambulatory ECG may show transient ST segment depression with exertion.
- Stress testing is usually done as the second step after the resting ECG and can include the following:
  - Stress or exercise ECG—may disclose temporary ST segment depression.
  - Myocardial perfusion scintigraphy after exercise (or pharmacologic stress testing with IV dipyridamole or adenosine) with thallium-201, technetium-99m, tetrofosmin, or sestamibi using planar or single-photon emission computed tomography imaging—may show reversible perfusion defects.
  - Stress echocardiography using exercise or pharmacologic agents (dipyridamole, dobutamine, adenosine)—may show stress-induced global or regional wall motion abnormalities.
  - Stress gated blood-pool scintigraphy (technetium-99m) using exercise or pharmacologic agents—may show stress-induced global or regional wall motion abnormalities.
- Positron emission tomography.
- Cardiac magnetic resonance imaging (MRI).
- Ultrafast electron-beam computed tomography scan for coronary artery calcification.
- Cardiac arteriography—cardiac catheterization with angiography is a definitive study to diagnose, quantify, and anatomically define CAD ("gold standard").

F. Management

- Smoking cessation.
- Weight reduction, low-fat/low-cholesterol diet.
- Cardiac rehabilitation or supervised exercise program to improve exercise capacity.
- Treat hypertension, diabetes, and hypercholesterolemia (goal—LDL <100 mg per dL, ideal would be <70 mg per dL).

PHARMACOLOGIC

- Aspirin—81 to 325 mg per day, or clopidogrel.
- Sublingual (SL) NTG spray or tablets—as needed or before exertion.
- Long-acting oral nitrates (e.g., isosorbide dinitrate and isosorbide 5-mononitrate) with 8- to 12-hour nitrate-free period to avoid tolerance.
- Long-acting transdermal nitrates by way of paste or patches with 8- to 12-hour nitrate-free period to avoid tolerance.
- IV NTG in unstable angina.
- IV heparin in unstable angina.
- β-Adrenergic blockers.
- Calcium channel blockers (i.e., diltiazem or verapamil). Avoid short-acting nifedipine as this may increase the risk of cardiac event.
- Ranolazine (Ranexa)—can cause QT prolongation.
- Folic acid to decrease homocysteine. This has not been proved to yield absolute benefit.
- Statin to decrease LDL and C-reactive protein.

INVASIVE REVASCULARIZATION PROCEDURES
(PERCUTANEOUS CORONARY INTERVENTIONS [PCI])
- Percutaneous transluminal coronary angioplasty (PTCA).
- Directional coronary atherectomy.
- Coronary laser angioplasty.
- Coronary stenting, including drug-eluting stents (used with PTCA).

SURGICAL PROCEDURES
- Coronary artery bypass grafting surgery.

OTHERS
- Mechanical extracorporeal counterpulsation—limited data.

IV. Acute Myocardial Infarction (AMI)

A. Etiology/Pathology
- Most AMI events occur in patients with preexisting atherosclerotic coronary artery stenosis when endothelial plaque becomes unstable by rupturing or fissuring, which stimulates adhesion of platelets and deposition of fibrin. Platelets release vasoconstrictors such as thromboxane A2. These factors lead to occlusion of coronary vessels and subsequent myocardial ischemia and necrosis. A small percentage (2% or less) of AMIs are secondary to pure vasospasm, congenital anomalies, vasculitis, or embolism.

B. Demographics
- Age—usually over age 40.
- Gender—age 40 to 70: men > women; age >70: men = women.

C. Complications
- HF.
- Cardiogenic shock.
- Papillary muscle dysfunction or rupture with MR.
- Ventricular aneurysm.
- Ventricular rupture, ventricular septal defect (VSD).
- Dysrhythmias, heart blocks.
- Pericarditis.
- Dressler syndrome—post-MI pericarditis, fever, pulmonary infiltrates.
- Mural thrombus.

D. Clinical Features

HISTORY
- Severe squeezing retrosternal pain or tightness lasting >30 minutes. Radiation of pain to neck, jaw, and left arm is common. Radiation to right arm or back occurs less frequently. Unrelieved by NTG or rest.
- Dyspnea.
- Anxiety.
- Generalized weakness.
- Lightheadedness.
- Nausea, vomiting.
- Diaphoresis.

- Syncope—occasional.
- Silent AMIs are rare but do occur; elderly patients and patients with diabetes can have atypical presentations.

PHYSICAL FINDINGS
- May be normal.
- Clammy skin.
- Increased or decreased BP.
- JVD with HF.
- S_4.
- S_3 with CHF.
- Apical systolic murmur of MR with papillary muscle dysfunction.
- Dysrhythmias.
- Wheezing or rales.

E. Diagnostic Studies
- ECG in Q wave MI: inverted T waves, elevated ST segments (concave downward), Q waves usually within 12 to 36 hours, dysrhythmias common. ECG in non-Q-wave MI: ST segment elevation or depression. ECG in non-ST segment elevation MI: ST segment depression. All MIs can have dysrhythmias, AV blocks, and bundle-branch blocks.
- Elevated cardiac enzymes: creatine kinase-MB (CK-MB) isoenzymes rise within 4 to 8 hours, peak at 12 to 20 hours, and return to normal in 2 to 3 days. Lactase dehydrogenase isoenzymes rise within 14 to 24 hours, total LDH peak at 2 to 3 days, and return to normal in 8 to 14 days. AST rises within 12 hours, peaks at 36 hours, and returns to normal in 3 to 4 days.
- Troponin T and I rise within 4 hours, and return to normal in 7 days for I, and 10 to 14 days for T; can also be elevated in unstable angina.
- Most MIs are diagnosed with ECG, CK-MB, and troponin.
- Leukocytosis—nonspecific.
- Plasma myeloperoxidase (inflammation marker)—can detect early AMI before necrosis, but not widely.
- Elevated erythrocyte sedimentation rate (ESR)—nonspecific.
- Elevated myoglobin—nonspecific.
- Tecnetium-99m infarct imaging and thallium perfusion imaging.
- Echo to evaluate valve and LV function.
- MRI with gadolinium.

F. Management
- Oxygen.
- Nitrates—SL and IV.
- Morphine sulfate.
- Aspirin—162 to 325 mg.
- Clopidogrel (Plavix) or Prasugrel (Effient) for Segment Elevation Myocardial Infarction (STEMI).
- β-Adrenergic blocking agents (metoprolol or carvedilol) PO if no HF.

- ACE inhibitors (captopril, enalapril, lisinopril).
- Thrombolytic therapy—if patient has pain ≤12 hours (some studies have shown benefit up to 24 hours), ST segment elevation, and no contraindications (e.g., recent bleed). *Drugs*: Tissue plasminogen activator, streptokinase, reteplase, tenecteplase, anistreplase, or anisoylated plasminogen-streptokinase activator complex with heparin.
- Glycoprotein IIb/IIIa antagonists or inhibitors: abciximab (ReoPro; Eli Lilly, Indianapolis, IN), tirofiban (Aggrastat; Merck, West Point, PA), eptifibatide (Integrillin; Millenium, San Francisco, CA and Schering, Kenilworth NJ)—used for unstable angina, and AMI sometimes with thrombolytics or PTCA.
- Heparin: unfractionated or low-molecular-weight heparin (LMWH)—enoxaparin and others. Usually used in conjunction with thrombolytics or PTCA.
- Emergency or primary PCI if center equipped properly.
- Cardiac monitoring.

POST-AMI CARE
- Submaximal stress test within 1 to 3 weeks.
- Holter monitoring.
- Echocardiography and MUGA to determine LVEF.
- Cardiac rehabilitation.
- Address high lipids with statin (LDL <100 mg per dL, ideal <70), glucose, or BP.
- Stop smoking.
- Continue aspirin, clopidogrel, or both, and β-blocker or ACE inhibitor as prophylaxis against recurrent AMI.
- Folic acid if homocysteine level is high. Benefit not fully established.

V. Pericarditis

A. Etiology
- Idiopathic.
- Viral—coxsackie virus, echovirus, HIV, adenovirus, Epstein-Barr virus, mumps virus.
- Bacterial—*Staphylococcus*, *Pneumococcus*, *Mycoplasma*, tuberculosis.
- Fungal.
- Lyme disease.
- Parasites.
- Collagen vascular diseases—rheumatoid arthritis (RA), systemic lupus erythematosus (SLE), scleroderma.
- AMI.
- Cardiac surgery.
- Uremia.
- Neoplasm (lung, lymphoma, mesothelioma).
- Trauma.
- Radiation.
- Myxedema.
- Sarcoidosis.
- Pancreatitis.
- Inflammatory bowel disease.
- Aortic dissection.

- Drugs—procainamide, hydralazine, minoxidil, bleomycin, phenytoin, mesalamine.

B. Pathology
- Inflammation of pericardial sac. Can cause effusion. When effusion is large enough to decrease cardiac output, it is called cardiac tamponade and is a medical emergency. Constrictive pericarditis—caused by chronic pericardial inflammation leading to fibrosis, scarring, and calcification.

C. Demographics
- Men > women.

D. Clinical Features

HISTORY
- Sharp retrosternal chest pain with radiation to back and shoulder, intensifies with inspiration and lying supine, relieved by sitting up and leaning forward.
- Odynophagia.
- Anorexia.
- Anxiety.
- Myalgia.

PHYSICAL FINDINGS
- Fever.
- Splinted breathing.
- Pericardial friction rub (three components—systolic, early diastolic, late diastolic).
- Dysrhythmias—SVT.
- Tachypnea.

PERICARDIAL TAMPONADE
- Dyspnea.
- Tachycardia.
- Cyanosis.
- JVD.
- Hypotension.
- Pulsus paradoxus.
- Muffled heart tones.

CONSTRICTIVE PERICARDITIS
- Can be asymptomatic early in course.
- Dyspnea.
- Fatigue.
- JVD.
- Peripheral edema.
- Hepatomegaly, ascites.

E. Diagnostic Studies
- ECG—acute phase with concave-up ST elevation in precordial leads, especially with absence of reciprocal ST depression seen in AMI. Intermediate phase ST segment returns to baseline and T waves invert. In late phase, ECG can return to normal. In constrictive pericarditis and cardiac tamponade, ECG may disclose low QRS voltage. In cardiac tamponade, electrical alternans may be seen.
- Echo to detect pericardial effusion.
- Leukocytosis.
- Elevated ESR.

- CXR may show large effusion, but not nearly as sensitive or specific as Echo.
- May see mildly elevated cardiac enzymes, especially CK-MB.
- Viral titers, antinuclear antibody, rheumatoid factor, purified protein derivative, antistreptolysin O (ASO) titers, BUN, creatinine, and blood cultures may be helpful in elucidating the cause.
- Cardiac catheterization should be considered in constrictive pericarditis.

F. Management

UNCOMPLICATED ACUTE PERICARDITIS
- Acetylsalicylic acid (ASA), NSAIDs, or prednisone.
- Analgesia (e.g., codeine).
- Rest.
- Observation for signs/symptoms of evolving tamponade.
- Treat underlying etiology.

CHRONIC CONSTRICTIVE PERICARDITIS
- Cardiothoracic surgery referral for possible stripping.

CARDIAC TAMPONADE
- Immediate pericardiocentesis.
- Cardiothoracic surgery referral for pericardial window drainage, if recurrent.

VI. Valvular Heart Disease

A. Pathology
- Cardiac valves maintain unidirectional forward flow of blood through the heart. VHD presents with cardiac and pulmonary symptoms, or with heart murmur. It causes cardiac murmurs, although all murmurs do not reflect VHD. All VHDs cause derangement of blood flow in the heart. This derangement causes turbulent flow across valves, which often leads to fibrosis and calcifications of valves that can eventually cause hemodynamic compromise. When confronted with the possibility of VHD, five questions must be asked.
  - *What valve is affected?* Disorders of aortic and mitral valve are more common, although pulmonic and tricuspid lesions do occur.
  - *What is the hemodynamic derangement?* VHD usually presents as either stenosis or regurgitation. In stenosis, the valve fails to open completely, and subsequent outflow obstruction can occur, often causing backflow circulatory congestion. In regurgitation or insufficiency, the valve fails to remain completely closed when it should, thus allowing for backward reflux of blood.
  - *How severe is the hemodynamic compromise?* Lesions in VHD can vary from minimal to severely life threatening.
  - *What is the etiology of the lesion?*
  - *How has the VHD lesion affected the patient's circulation, especially in regard to ventricular function and pulmonary circulation?*

B. Aortic Stenosis
- Valvular narrowing with resistance to LV outflow.

1. Etiology
- Congenital unicuspid, bicuspid, or tricuspid valve with commissural fusion.
- Rheumatic fever—was the most common cause 50 years ago; now congenital and degenerative are more common. Usually involves both aortic and mitral valves but AS can occur alone.
- Degenerative calcific disease in elderly patients, which may be an autoimmune reaction.

2. Clinical Features

HISTORY
- Angina pectoris (occurs in 50% to 70% of patients with severe AS).
- Syncope and presyncope (with severe AS).
- Dyspnea on exertion.
- PND.
- Orthopnea.
- Fatigue.
- Palpitations.
- Sudden death.

PHYSICAL FINDINGS
- Narrowed pulse pressure.
- Hypertension in elderly patients with AS.
- Delayed and diminished carotid upstroke (pulsus parvus et tardus).
- Systolic thrill felt over base or carotids.
- LV heave or lift.
- Crescendo-decrescendo systolic murmur best heard at second intercostal space (ICS), right sternal border with radiation into carotids, down left parasternal border to the apex.
- Early systolic ejection click.
- Paradoxical splitting of S_2 may occur (suggests severe disease).
- Delayed, decreased intensity, or absent aortic second sound (A_2).
- S_4 gallop.
- Early diastolic murmur of AR.
- Can have irregular–irregular cardiac rhythm if atrial fibrillation is present.

3. Diagnostic Studies
- Echo/Doppler—decreased valve excursion (<1.0 cm^2 significant stenosis, <0.8 cm^2 indicates severe AS compromising CO), calcification of valve, LVH, decreased LVEF, increased valve gradient.
- ECG—LVH, dysrhythmias, conduction defects.
- CXR—normal or cardiomegaly.
- Cardiac catheterization.

4. Management
- Cardiothoracic surgery referral for valve replacement in patients with symptomatic disease.
- Balloon valvuloplasty may be considered for pediatric congenital disease and for elderly patients who may not tolerate valve replacement surgery.

C. Aortic Regurgitation

- Incompetent valve causing retrograde flow from aorta into left ventricle that may lead to HF. There are both acute and chronic forms of AR.

1. **Etiology**
   - Congenital bicuspid valve.
   - Bacterial endocarditis (acute AR).
   - Rheumatic fever.
   - Syphilis.
   - Dissecting aortic aneurysm.
   - Marfan syndrome.
   - Ankylosing spondylitis.
   - Giant cell arteritis.
   - Osteogenesis imperfecta.
   - SLE.
   - RA.
   - Reiter syndrome.
   - Aneurysm of sinus of Valsalva.
   - Severe systemic hypertension.

2. **Clinical Features**

   HISTORY
   - May be asymptomatic in mild and moderate disease.
   - Dyspnea on exertion.
   - Orthopnea.
   - PND.
   - Palpitations.
   - Fatigue.

   PHYSICAL FINDINGS
   - Widened pulse pressure with increased systolic BP and reduced diastolic BP.
   - Korotkoff sounds persisting until zero.
   - Abrupt rise of upstroke, quick collapse of peripheral pulses (water-hammer or Corrigan pulse).
   - Bisferious pulse with double pulsation.
   - Pistol shot sounds over femoral artery (Traube sign).
   - Thrill felt at carotids, base of heart.
   - Single S_2 (A_2 absent).
   - S_3 may be heard.
   - Early decrescendo high-frequency blowing diastolic murmur best heard at left sternal border/third and fourth ICS; accentuated by having patient sit up, lean forward, and hold breath after deep expiration, or by squatting, or isometric exercise such as handgrip. Some can be heard at right parasternal border. In severe disease, murmur may be holodiastolic or an Austin Flint murmur (rumbling mid- and late-diastolic heard at apex) may be identified.
   - Midsystolic murmur may be heard at base due to augmented stroke volume and rates of ejection.

3. **Diagnostic Studies**
   - Echo/2-D and Doppler—regurgitation, aortic leaflet thickening, calcification of valve.
   - ECG—left axis deviation (LAD) and/or LVH.
   - CXR—normal or cardiomegaly.
   - Cardiac catheterization.

4. **Management**
   - Endocarditis treatment if required in acute AR.
   - Cardiothoracic surgery referral for valve replacement in patients with symptomatic disease.

D. Mitral Stenosis

- Valvular narrowing with resistance to LV filling causing left atrial enlargement, dysthymias (atrial fibrillation), HF with pulmonary edema, and eventually right-sided symptoms.

1. **Etiology**
   - Rheumatic fever most common; most commonly develops in third or fourth decades.

2. **Clinical Features**

   HISTORY
   - Fatigue.
   - Dyspnea on exertion.
   - Orthopnea.
   - PND.
   - Palpitations.
   - Cough.
   - Hoarseness due to compression on left recurrent laryngeal nerve by dilated left atrium.
   - Hemoptysis due to rupture of bronchial vein.
   - Chest pain.
   - Edema.

   PHYSICAL FINDINGS
   - Early- to mid-diastolic low-pitch rumble murmur best heard at apex in left lateral decubitus position; presystolic murmurs also may be present.
   - Apical diastolic thrill can sometimes be felt in patients with loud murmurs in left lateral decubitus position.
   - Right ventricular lift in pulmonary hypertension.
   - Accentuated S_1 early in disease.
   - Single or closely split and accentuated S_2 can occur later in disease.
   - Opening snap after S_2.
   - Malar flush over cheeks.
   - Clubbing.
   - Rales.
   - Peripheral edema.
   - JVD.
   - Irregular–irregular rhythm of atrial fibrillation.
   - Graham Steell murmur (high-pitched decrescendo diastolic murmur at left sternal border) of pulmonic regurgitation (PR) can be heard in patients with severe pulmonary hypertension.

3. **Diagnostic Studies**
   - Echo/2-D and Doppler—thickening and calcification of valve, reduced leaflet excursion and doming, decreased mitral orifice (severe if valve area is <1.0 cm^2), enlarged left atrium, increased valve gradient.

- ECG—left atrial enlargement, atrial fibrillation, right axis deviation (RAD) may be seen.
- CXR—left atrial enlargement, cephalization of pulmonary markings, Kerley B lines, pulmonary edema with CHF.
- Cardiac catheterization.

4. **Management**
   - Patient should avoid unnecessary stress or exertion.
   - Treat atrial fibrillation, usually with digoxin.
   - Treat CHF as needed.
   - Balloon valvuloplasty and commissurotomy may be considered in younger symptomatic patients.
   - Cardiothoracic surgery referral for valve replacement in patients with severe disease.

E. Mitral Regurgitation
- Disorders of leaflets, chordae tendineae, papillary muscles, anulus, and LV myocardium can cause failure of complete valve closure with reflux into left atrium during systole. Acute pulmonary edema occurs less frequently with MR than with MS.

1. **Etiology**
   - Mitral valve prolapse (MVP).
   - Rheumatic fever.
   - Ruptured chordae tendineae from endocarditis, MVP, rheumatic disease, trauma.
   - Infective endocarditis (IE).
   - Papillary muscle dysfunction or rupture from ischemic heart disease and AMI.
   - Calcified mitral anulus.
   - Congenital heart disease (CHD).
   - Marfan syndrome.
   - Dilated cardiomyopathy.

2. **Clinical Features**

   HISTORY
   - May be asymptomatic in mild and sometimes moderate disease.
   - Fatigue.
   - Dyspnea on exertion.
   - Orthopnea.
   - PND.
   - Palpitations.
   - Symptoms of MVP (see VI. F. 2.).

   PHYSICAL FINDINGS
   - High-frequency blowing holosystolic murmur best identified at apex with radiation to axilla in chronic MR; can be accentuated by squatting; can be decrescendo in acute MR; can have late-systolic murmur with click in MVP.
   - Soft S_1.
   - S_3.
   - Irregular–irregular rhythm of atrial fibrillation.
   - JVD in long-standing disease.
   - Pulmonary rales can occur.
   - Peripheral edema in severe disease.

3. **Diagnostic Studies**
   - Echo/2-D and Doppler—MR.
   - ECG—left atrial enlargement, atrial fibrillation.
   - CXR—left atrial and ventricular enlargement and increased pulmonary markings can be seen.
   - Cardiac catheterization.

4. **Management**
   - Treat atrial fibrillation usually with digoxin.
   - Cardiothoracic surgery referral for valve replacement in patients with progressive disease.

F. MVP Syndrome
- Bulging or billowing of mitral valve leaflets into left atrium during systole with or without MR. Many patients have benign course but some have significant MR, dysrhythmias, and rare cases of sudden death have been reported. Women > men under age 20, and women = men over age 20.

1. **Etiology**
   - Primary—genetic, autosomal dominant with variable expression.
   - Primary—Marfan syndrome and other connective tissue diseases.
   - Secondary to CAD, rheumatic heart disease, or cardiomyopathies.

2. **Clinical Features**

   HISTORY
   - May be totally asymptomatic.
   - Can have left precordial atypical chest pain.
   - Palpitations.
   - Dyspnea.
   - Panic attacks/anxiety.
   - Fatigue.
   - Dizziness, presyncope, rarely syncope.
   - Rare transient cerebral ischemic episodes.

   PHYSICAL FINDINGS
   - Low BP and orthostasis.
   - Midsystolic click.
   - Late-systolic murmur best heard at apex, increases in intensity with standing and handgrip.
   - Thoracic skeletal abnormalities such as scoliosis, pectus excavatum, and straight thoracic spine.
   - Dysrhythmias such as SVT sometimes noted.

3. **Diagnostic Studies**
   - Echo/2-D and Doppler—MVP and determine whether MR is present.
   - ECG—usually normal; can show ST segment depression or T wave inversion in inferior leads III and aVF.
   - Cardiac catheterization may be needed in patients with significant MR.

4. **Management**
   - Most patients require only education.
   - β-Blockers helpful if palpitations are problematic.
   - Cardiothoracic surgery referral for valve replacement in patients with severe MR.

G. Pulmonic Stenosis
- Narrowing of pulmonic valve leading to right ventricular outflow obstruction and right-sided HF.
1. Etiology
- Almost always congenital and disease of the young.
- Severe disease may present as HF in neonatal period. Disease may also progress with time and become symptomatic in late childhood and adolescence.
- Rubella embryopathy.
2. Clinical Features

HISTORY
- Fatigue.
- Dyspnea on exertion.
- Dizziness.
- Occasional syncope.
- Chest pain.
- Edema.

PHYSICAL FINDINGS
- Harsh midsystolic crescendo-decrescendo murmur loudest at left upper sternal border with radiation to neck, increased with inspiration. The longer the murmur, the more severe the stenosis.
- Right ventricular heave felt at epigastrium.
- Thrill with louder murmurs (IV/VI or greater).
- Pulmonic ejection sound.
- Wide split S_2 with soft delayed pulmonic second sound (P_2).
- S_4 can be heard.
- JVD may be present.
- Hepatomegaly and ascites with right-sided HF.
- Peripheral edema later in course.
3. Diagnostic Studies
- Echo/2-D and Doppler—PS, thickened valve.
- ECG—RAD and right ventricular hypertrophy (RVH) may be seen.
- CXR—right ventricular enlargement can be seen.
- Cardiac catheterization.
4. Management
- Balloon valvuloplasty is the preferred treatment.
- Cardiothoracic surgery referral for valve replacement in patients with progressive disease.

H. Pulmonic Regurgitation
- Incomplete valve closure with retrograde flow into right ventricle during systole.
1. Etiology
- Pulmonary hypertension from left VHD.
- Pulmonary hypertension from pulmonary disease.
- Congenital.
- Idiopathic pulmonary artery dilatation.
- Complication of corrective surgery for tetralogy of Fallot.
- Infectious endocarditis.

2. Clinical Features
- Most cases well tolerated with few, if any, symptoms. Can see decreased exercise tolerance in patients with severe disease.
- Graham Steell murmur (high-pitched decrescendo early-diastolic murmur at second left ICS and mid-left sternal border) in patients with PR secondary to severe pulmonary hypertension.
- PR secondary to congenital etiology may be lower-pitched, late-diastolic best heard at third and fourth left ICS.
- Loud P_2 with pulmonary hypertension.
- Right ventricular heave.
3. Diagnostic Studies
- Echo/2-D and Doppler—PR.
- Cardiac catheterization.
4. Management
- Many patients do not require specific treatment for PR, but pulmonary hypertension should be treated.
- Cardiothoracic surgery referral in patients with severe progressive disease.

I. Tricuspid Stenosis (TS)
- Narrowing of valvular orifice obstructing flow from right atrium to right ventricle.
1. Etiology
- Rheumatic fever most common; mostly seen in conjunction with mitral and aortic lesions.
- Congenital.
- Right atrial myxoma.
- Carcinoid syndrome.
- Endomyocardial fibroelastosis.
- Bacterial endocarditis.
2. Clinical Features

HISTORY
- Fatigue.
- Pulsation or fluttering sensation in neck.

PHYSICAL FINDINGS
- Low-pitched mid-diastolic or presystolic rumbling murmur best heard at fourth and fifth ICS left sternal border or below xiphoid process. Intensified by inspiration (Carvallo sign). Also can be higher pitched and can be identified at apex.
- Sometimes opening snap can be heard.
- Diastolic thrill can sometimes be palpated.
- Split S_1 with loud tricuspid first sound (T_1).
- Single S_2.
- S_3 can be heard over the jugular veins.
- Prominent presystolic venous wave and JVD.
- Hepatomegaly and hepatic pulsations.
- Ascites. Peripheral edema.
3. Diagnostic Studies
- Echo/2-D and Doppler—TS.
- ECG—right atrial hypertrophy.
- CXR—right atrial enlargement.
- Cardiac catheterization.

4. Management
- Sodium restriction.
- Diuretics.
- Valvotomy.
- Cardiothoracic surgery referral in patients with severe progressive disease.

J. Tricuspid Regurgitation (TR)
- Inadequate closure of valve with retrograde flow from right ventricle into right atrium.

1. Etiology
- Dilatation of annulus secondary to right ventricular dilation (functional).
- Rheumatic fever.
- Congenital.
- Myxoma.
- Carcinoid syndrome.
- Bacterial endocarditis especially in IV drug abuse.
- Tricuspid valve prolapse.

2. Clinical Features

HISTORY
- Dyspnea.
- Pulsation sensation in neck.
- Abdominal pain and bloating.
- Peripheral edema.

PHYSICAL FINDINGS
- Parasternal lift.
- High-pitched blowing holosystolic or pansystolic murmur best heard at left sternal border fourth ICS. Intensified by inspiration and squatting. Decreases with standing and Valsalva.
- Right ventricular S_3.
- Irregular–irregular rhythm of atrial fibrillation.
- JVD and pulsatile neck veins.
- Palpable liver pulsations.
- Ascites.
- Peripheral edema.

3. Diagnostic Studies
- Echo/2-D and Doppler—TR, right atrial enlargement.
- ECG—right atrial hypertrophy.
- CXR—right atrial and ventricular enlargement.
- Cardiac catheterization.

4. Management
- Treat underlying condition.
- Annuloplasty.
- Cardiothoracic surgery referral for valve replacement in patients with severe disease.

VII. Aortic Aneurysm

A. Etiology
- Atherosclerosis—most common etiology.
- Marfan syndrome, especially with thoracic aneurysms.
- Aortitis—mycotic, salmonella, and other infections.

B. Pathology
- Aneurysm—localized area of dilatation or increased diameter of vessel. Most aortic aneurysms are located in abdominal aorta just below the level of renal arteries. Aneurysms can also be located in ascending aorta, aortic arch, and descending aorta. Complications of aortic aneurysms include rupture (chance higher if >5.5 cm), thromboembolism, and distal ischemia.

C. Clinical Features

HISTORY
- Most cases are asymptomatic until large or rupturing.
- Abdominal fullness or pulsation sensation.
- Back pain.

PHYSICAL FINDINGS
- Pulsatile mass in epigastric area if abdominal with aortic width >3 cm.

D. Diagnostic Studies
- Ultrasound (U/S).
- Computed tomography (CT) scan.
- Aortography used before surgical intervention.
- CXR may disclose calcifications.

E. Management
- If abdominal aortic aneurysm is <4 cm and asymptomatic, can watch and follow with serial U/Ss.
- If >4 cm, surgical referral warranted; consider elective surgery if >5.5 cm.

VIII. Aortic Dissection

A. Etiology
- Hypertension.
- Marfan syndrome.
- Cystic medial necrosis.
- Iatrogenic complication of catheterization.

B. Pathology
- Aortic dissection—caused by tear in intima with formation of false channel in media by hematoma. Mostly occur in ascending aorta several centimeters from aortic valve or descending aorta just distal to origin of left subclavian. Ascending aortic dissections have high mortality rate without treatment as opposed to dissections of descending aorta that have a much better prognosis.
- **DeBakey has classified these into three types:**
  - Type I: involves aortic root, aortic arch, and descending aorta.
  - Type II: involves only ascending aorta.
  - Type III: involves only distal aorta beyond the origin of left subclavian artery.

C. Demographics
- Most common between the sixth and eighth decade; men > women.

D. Clinical Features

HISTORY

- Sudden onset of tearing, severe anterior chest pain with radiation to interscapular region.
- Back pain.
- CHF symptoms—dyspnea.
- Syncope.
- Abdominal pain.
- CVA symptoms.

PHYSICAL FINDINGS

- Increased BP or hypotension.
- Wide pulse pressure.
- Aortic insufficiency murmur in dissections of ascending aorta.
- Diminished or asymmetric peripheral pulses.
- Left pleural effusion sometimes seen with decreased breath sounds and dullness at left base.
- Focal neurologic deficits may be seen.

E. Diagnostic Studies

- CXR—widening of superior mediastinum, displacement of trachea, left pleural effusion, enlargement of aortic knob.
- Transesophageal echocardiography (TEE).
- CT scan with contrast.
- Aortic angiogram ("gold standard").
- MRI.

F. Management

- Immediate surgical referral for all ascending aortic dissections (types I and II).
- Medical therapy can be used in uncomplicated descending dissections (type III) including IV propranolol or nitroprusside.

IX. Rheumatic Fever and Heart Disease

A. Etiology

- Group A—β-hemolytic streptococcal pharyngitis.

B. Pathology

- An inflammatory immunologic response to streptococcal infection affecting the heart (endocardium and valves, myocardium, pericardium), skin, joints, and central nervous system (CNS); recurrences are common.

C. Demographics

- Children of ages 5 to 15.
- Incidence in United States dropping.

D. Clinical Features

- Symptoms of rheumatic fever commonly occur 1 to 3 weeks after pharyngitis episode.
- Symptoms of VHD from childhood infection can be delayed until third or fourth decade.

MODIFIED JONES CRITERIA FOR DIAGNOSIS OF INITIAL ATTACK

- With documented preceding group A streptococcal infection (throat culture, throat rapid antigen detection test, elevated or rising strep antibody titers), two major manifestations or one major and two minor manifestations.

MAJOR MANIFESTATIONS

- Carditis (pericarditis, myocarditis, VHD that can affect any valve, but mitral and aortic lesions are most common).
- Polyarthritis (medium to large joints; knees, ankles, wrists). Migratory and disappear within 3 to 4 weeks.
- Chorea (late finding).
- Erythema marginatum.
- Subcutaneous nodules (painless over bony prominences).

MINOR MANIFESTATIONS

- Arthralgia (this cannot be used as minor criterion a part of the Modified Jones Criteria if polyarthritis is used as a major criterion).
- Fever (101° to 104° F).
- Prolonged PR interval.
- Elevated acute phase reactants.

OTHER MANIFESTATIONS OUTSIDE OF JONES CRITERIA

- Abdominal pain.
- Facial tics or grimace.
- Epistaxis.

E. Diagnostic Studies

- Acute phase reactants (e.g., ESR, C-reactive protein) elevated.
- Antistreptolysin O (ASO), antideoxyribonuclease B (DNase), rapid strep antigen test, or throat culture bacteriologic or serologic evidence group A strep infection.
- ECG—prolonged PR interval.
- Echo—pericardial effusion or valvular lesions (cannot use as a sole diagnostic method).
- CBC—anemia.

F. Management

- Penicillin to treat streptococcal infection.
- Prednisone for carditis with cardiomegaly.
- Aspirin if no cardiomegaly.
- Haloperidol to treat chorea.

X. Infective Endocarditis

A. Etiology

ACUTE BACTERIAL ENDOCARDITIS (ABE)

- *Staphylococcus aureus*—most common.
- Group A, B, C, and G streptococci.
- *Haemophilus influenzae.*
- *Streptococcus pneumoniae.*
- *Neisseria gonorrhea.*
- *Enterococcus.*

SUBACUTE BACTERIAL ENDOCARDITIS (SBE)

- *Streptococcus viridans* and *S. bovis*—most common.
- *Streptococcus fecalis* and *S. faecium* (i.e., enterococci).
- *S. aureus.*

- HACEK organisms (*Haemophilus, Actinobacillus, Cardiobacterium, Eikenella, Kingella*).

ENDOCARDITIS WITH IV DRUG ABUSE
- *S. aureus*—frequently methicillin-resistant *S. aureus*.
- *Pseudomonas aeruginosa* and *P. cepacia*.
- *Enterococcus*.
- *Candida* fungal species.

PROSTHETIC VALVE ENDOCARDITIS
- *S. aureus*.
- *Staphylococcus epidermidis*.
- *Candida* and *Aspergillus* fungal species.
- *S. viridans*.
- *Enterococcus*.

B. Pathology
- Infection with inflammation affecting valvular endocardium and occasionally mural endocardium. May lead to vegetations, valve destruction, systemic embolization.
- Can be classified into ABE, SBE, endocarditis with IV drug abuse, and early (within 60 days of implantation) or late (60 days or longer after implantation) prosthetic valve endocarditis. ABE is caused by virulent organisms and has an aggressive course. SBE usually occurs in patients with preexisting VHD and has a slower, more indolent course. Endocarditis in IV drug abusers has predilection for tricuspid valve.

C. Risk Factors
- Prosthetic cardiac valves.
- Congenital cardiac anomalies.
- Previous IE.
- Rheumatic heart disease.
- Any VHD, including MVP when with MR.
- Hypertrophic cardiomyopathy.
- Indwelling intravascular devices.
- Dental or surgical procedures that cause transient bacteremia.
- IV drug abuse.

D. Clinical Features
- Classic triad—fever, heart murmur, positive blood culture; however, all of these do not have to be present.

HISTORY
- Fever.
- Anorexia and weight loss.
- Night sweats.
- Fatigue.
- Arthralgias, myalgias.
- Cephalgia.
- Delirium.
- Muscle weakness, paralysis.
- Cold painful extremity with embolism.
- Gross hematuria.

PHYSICAL FINDINGS
- Murmurs—mostly mitral and aortic involvement, but tricuspid lesions seen in IV drug abuse.

- Fever (ABE—102° to 105° F; SBE—99° to 100° F).
- Conjunctival hemorrhage.
- Petechiae (particularly oropharynx, lower extremity).
- Splinter hemorrhages (on nail beds).
- Osler nodes (subcutaneous nodules of fingers).
- Janeway lesions (small nonpainful hemorrhagic patches on palms, soles of feet).
- Roth spots (oval white areas surrounded by hemorrhage) on funduscopy.
- Pericardial friction rub.
- JVD, rales, gallops with HF.
- Cold, pale extremity with absent pulse in septic emboli.
- Focal neurologic signs in septic emboli.

E. Diagnostic Studies
- Positive blood cultures (multiple 2 to 3; 2 by Duke criteria) for typical organisms.
- Echo disclosing vegetations; TEE may be especially sensitive.
- Leukocytosis.
- Elevated ESR or C-reactive protein.
- Microscopic hematuria on UA.
- Anemia (normocytic) in SBE on CBC.
- Positive rheumatoid factor in SBE.
- Circulating immune complexes, decreased C3 and C4.
- CXR—infiltrates, pleural effusion.

F. Management
- IV antibiotics for 4 to 6 weeks; penicillin G for penicillin-susceptible *S. viridans*, and others as indicated by culture and sensitivity results.
- Surgical consultation for valve replacement should be considered in complicated cases (e.g., with HF, emboli, dehiscence of prosthetic valve, or resistance to antibiotics).
- Prophylaxis—In 2007 the AHA, in conjunction with the professional organizations representing dentistry (ADA), infectious disease (IDSA), and pediatrics (AAP), published updated recommendations for the prevention of IE. The new guidelines recommend that antibiotic prophylaxis be administered only to patients undergoing dental procedures who are at the highest risk of adverse outcomes from IE (see X.G. below). They no longer recommend prophylaxis for lower-risk patients (such as those with most types of VHD including MVP), or for patients undergoing genitourinary or gastrointestinal (GI) procedures. Patients at highest risk should receive antibiotic prophylaxis—amoxicillin 2 g PO 30 to 60 minutes prior to the procedure (cephalexin, clindamycin, azithromycin, or clarithromycin may be used for penicillin-allergic patients.)

G. Cardiac Conditions Requiring IE Prophylaxis
- (Adapted from Wilson W, Taubert KA, Gewitz M, et al. Prevention of infective endocarditis. *Circulation*. 2007;155, May 8).

- Prosthetic cardiac valves.
- Previous IE.
- Cardiac transplantation recipients who develop VHD.
- **Congenital Heart Disease:**
  - Unrepaired cyanotic CHD, including palliative shunts and conduits.
  - Completely repaired CHD defects with prosthetic material or device during the first 6 months after the procedure.
  - Repaired CHD with residual defects at the site or adjacent to the site of the patch or device.

XI. Chronic Occlusive Arterial Disease/PAD

A. Etiology
- Atherosclerosis (arteriosclerosis obliterans)—most common etiology.
- Thromboangiitis obliterans (Buerger disease)—occurs in young (<50 years) male smokers.
- Trauma.
- Arteritis.
- Extrinsic compression.

B. Pathology
- Obstruction or narrowing of lumen of peripheral arteries, most commonly in lower extremity, causing interruption of blood flow. These patients are at high risk for CAD.

C. Risk Factors
- Advancing age.
- Smoking tobacco.
- DM.
- Hypertension.
- Hyperlipidemia.
- Obesity.

D. Demographics
- Increases with age.
- Men > women.

E. Clinical Features
HISTORY
- Intermittent claudication—reproducible exercise-induced pain, commonly in calf with femoral obstruction, relieved with rest.
- Foot ulcers.
- Rest pain in severe disease.
- Erectile dysfunction.

PHYSICAL FINDINGS
- Diminished or absent peripheral pulses.
- Absent hair on toes, feet.
- Atrophic skin changes.
- Lower-extremity rubor on dependency, pallor on elevation.
- Decreased temperature of affected limb.
- Ischemic ulcers on toes, heels, or foot.
- Gangrene in severe disease.

F. Diagnostic Studies
- Doppler U/S.
- Arteriography.
- Magnetic resonance angiography.

G. Management
- Smoking cessation.
- Low-fat/low-cholesterol/low-calorie diet.
- Optimal diabetes, hypertension control.
- Foot care.
- Graduated exercise program.
- Aspirin—162 to 325 mg per day.
- Cilostazol (Pletal; Otsuka America, Rockville, MD). Now the mainstay of drug therapy.
- Pentoxifylline (Trental; Aventis, Bridgewater, NJ). Not widely used but may help.
- Clopidogrel (Plavix; Sanofi-Synthelabo, New York, NY and Bristol-Myers Squibb, New York, NY).
- Propionyl-L-carnitine may be helpful.
- Surgical and invasive measures (e.g., angioplasty, bypass grafting, arthrectomy, stents) for rest pain, intolerable or disabling claudication, or changes that may lead to gangrene (e.g., nonhealing ulcers) especially in patients with diabetes.

XII. Acute Arterial Occlusion
ARTERIAL DISEASE
A. Etiology
- **Embolism:**
  - VHD.
  - Atrial fibrillation.
  - IE.
  - AMI.
  - Cardiomyopathy.
  - Myxoma.
  - Myocardial aneurysm.
  - Proximal atherosclerotic plaques.
  - Proximal arterial aneurysms.
  - Thrombosis.

B. Pathology
- Acute arterial occlusions may be caused by all the same etiologies as chronic disease (see XI.), but may also be caused by embolic events from thrombi in heart disease or aneurysms, arterial spasm, myeloproliferative disorders (polycythemia vera), or hypercoagulability states (neoplastic disease).

C. Clinical Features
FIVE P'S
- Pain.
- Pallor.
- Paresthesia.
- Pulselessness.
- Paralysis.

OTHER MANIFESTATIONS
- Livedo reticularis (with arteriolar occlusions).
- Cyanosis.

D. Diagnostic Studies
- Arteriography.

E. Management
- Embolism—heparin.
- Thrombosis—thrombocytotics (e.g., alteplase).
- Surgical referral—embolectomy.
- Treat underlying cause.

XIII. Varicose Veins

A. Etiology
- Hereditary faulty or incompetent venous valves and weak vein walls. Incompetence at saphenofemoral junction common.
- Congenitally absent venous valves.
- Deep vein thrombophlebitis (DVT).
- Increased with dependency, obesity, right-sided HF, pregnancy.

B. Pathology
- Dilated, torturous superficial veins mostly in lower extremities; medial fibrosis and valve atrophy in veins are noted.

C. Clinical Features

HISTORY
- Often asymptomatic other than cosmetic concerns.
- Lower-extremity muscle cramps, aching.

PHYSICAL FINDINGS
- Dilated, torturous superficial veins in lower extremities.
- Edema of affected limb.
- Varicose, stasis ulcers.
- Trendelenburg test.

D. Diagnostic Studies
- None helpful.

E. Management
- Elevate legs.
- Elastic compression stockings.
- Avoid girdles.
- Surgical treatment with ligation, stripping, stab evulsion phlebectomy, or sclerotherapy.
- Encourage ambulation.

XIV. Chronic Venous Insufficiency

A. Etiology
- Hereditary faulty or incompetent venous valves, weak vein walls.
- DVT.

B. Pathology
- Dysfunction or incompetence of venous valves both in superficial and deep venous systems.

C. Clinical Features

HISTORY
- Lower-extremity aching.

PHYSICAL FINDINGS
- Edema of lower extremities.
- Stasis skin changes including hyperpigmentation (often brownish), dermatitis, ulceration.
- Stasis ulcers.
- Trendelenburg test.

D. Diagnostic Studies
- Venous Doppler studies of lower extremities.

E. Management
- Elevate legs.
- Elastic compression stockings.
- Avoid girdles.
- Treat ulcers with dressings, skin grafting, or hyperbaric oxygen when large and nonhealing.
- Encourage ambulation.

XV. Superficial Thrombophlebitis

A. Etiology
- Septic—*Staphylococcus aureus*, *Klebsiella*, *Candida*, cytomegalovirus in HIV.
- Malignancy.
- Oral contraceptives.
- Pregnancy.
- Hypercoagulability states.
- Behçet disease.
- Buerger disease.

B. Pathology
- Inflammation of superficial veins with thrombosis.

C. Risk Factors
- Immobilization.
- Obesity.
- Advanced age.
- IV catheter in place for >2 days.
- Burns.
- Steroids.
- AIDS.
- Varicose veins.
- Postoperative.
- Pregnancy.

D. Clinical Features
- Fever.
- Local pain.
- Edema, erythema, warmth, tenderness along course of vein.
- Tender palpable cord.

E. Diagnostic Studies
- In septic etiology—leukocytosis, culture blood, and IV site.
- Duplex Doppler U/S.

F. Management
- Extremity elevation.
- Apply heat.
- In aseptic—NSAIDs, also consider heparin, warfarin.

• In septic—IV synthetic penicillin, aminoglycoside; consider excision of vein.

XVI. Deep Vein Thrombosis and Thrombophlebitis/Venous Thromboembolic Disease

A. Etiology
• Venous stasis.
• Coagulopathies.
• Genetic.

B. Pathology
• Thrombosis in deep veins of lower extremities or pelvis causing inflammation. Major complication—pulmonary embolism.

C. Risk Factors
• Virchow triad (stasis, vascular injury, hypercoagulable state).
• Immobility, prolonged bed rest.
• Pregnancy.
• Oral contraceptives.
• Surgery, especially hip surgery.
• Long bone fractures of legs.
• Increased age.
• Varicose veins.
• Cancer.
• Central venous pressure lines.
• Antiphospholipid antibodies.
• Protein C deficiency.
• Protein S deficiency.
• Factor V Leiden mutation and activated protein C resistance.
• Antithrombin III deficiency.
• Connective tissue disorders.
• Polycythemia vera.

D. Clinical Features
• Lower-extremity pain.
• Lower-extremity edema.
• Calf tenderness.
• Erythema, warmth in some cases.
• Positive Homans sign (pain on dorsiflexion of foot).

E. Diagnostic Studies
• Venogram ("gold standard").
• Noninvasive venous studies—duplex Doppler U/S and B-mode U/S or impedance plethysmography.

F. Management
• Heparin (unfractionated or LMWH: e.g., enoxaparin) followed by outpatient warfarin for 3 to 6 months. Consider lifetime warfarin if protein C or S or antithrombin III deficient or for factor V Leiden mutation. Direct thrombin inhibitors may replace warfarin in the future as primary treatment for DVT.
• Monitor for pulmonary embolus.

XVII. Hyperlipidemia and Dyslipoproteinemia

A. Etiology

PRIMARY
• Dietary.
• Genetic.
• Obesity.
• Sporadic.

SECONDARY
• DM.
• Uremia.
• Metabolic syndrome.
• Nephrotic syndrome.
• Hypothyroidism.
• Pregnancy.
• Acromegaly.
• Cushing disease.
• Drugs: β-blockers (nonintrinsic sympathomimetic activity, ISA), diuretics, corticosteroids, oral contraceptives, progestins, alcohol for triglyceride.

B. Pathology
• Plasma lipids (triglyceride, cholesterol ester)—transported in blood by lipoproteins, classified by their density; chylomicrons are largest and least dense and carry mostly triglycerides, very low-density lipoprotein (VLDL) carry mostly triglycerides, LDL transports cholesterol as its major function, and HDL transports cholesterol from peripheral tissues to the liver.
• Lipoproteins—composed of lipids and protein (called apoproteins). Lipoprotein (a) or Lp(a) is an LDL-like particle. Increased total cholesterol, LDL, Lp(a), small dense LDL particles, and decreased levels of HDL have been associated with atherosclerosis and CAD.
• High triglyceride levels have been associated with increased risk of CAD in women and patients with DM. High triglyceride levels (>1,000) can cause pancreatitis.

C. Types
• The six types of dyslipoproteinemia are shown in Table 3-2.

TABLE 3-2.   Types of Hyperlipidemia

Type	Lipid Elevation	CAD Risk
I	Triglyceride (chylomicrons)	Normal
IIA	Cholesterol (LDL)	Very high
IIB	Cholesterol and triglyceride (LDL and VLDL)	Very high
III	Cholesterol and triglyceride (β-VLDL and LDL)	Very high
IV	Triglycerides (VLDL)	Varied
V	Triglycerides (VLDL and chylomicrons)	Moderate

β-VLDL, beta-very low density lipoproteins.

D. Clinical Features

- Usually asymptomatic until atherosclerosis develops (CAD, TIA/CVA, PAD).
- Xanthelasma, xanthomas.
- Corneal arcus before age 50.

E. Diagnostic Studies

- Fasting lipid studies (Table 3-3). Some also now test for Lp(a) and LDL particle size.
- Triglycerides.
- TSH if hypothyroidism suspected.
- Fasting glucose if DM suspected.
- BUN, creatinine, UA if nephrotic syndrome suspected.

F. Management

- Weight-loss diet.
- Low-fat/low-cholesterol diet—AHA or National Cholesterol Education Program (NCEP) Step I diet <30% total calories from fat with 8% to 10% saturated fat. Cholesterol intake should be ≤300 mg per day. Dietary changes should be initiated in all patients with elevated lipid levels.
- Aerobic exercise program.
- **Therapeutic recommendations from the NCEP–Adult Treatment Panel III based on LDL level (ATP IV will be out in 2012):**
  - Patients with CHD or CHD risk equivalent (i.e., DM): Goal—<100 mg per dL (optional <70), lifestyle modification for 3 to 6 months—100 to 129 mg per dL, or drugs—especially if ≥130 mg per dL.
  - Patients with ≥2 CHD risk factors with Framingham 10-year coronary heart disease risk of ≤20%: Goal—<130 mg per dL, lifestyle modification for 3 to 6 months—130 to 159 mg per dL, drugs—≥130 mg per dL if 10-year risk 10% to 20% or >160 mg per dL if 10-year risk <10%.
  - Patients with 0 to 1 CHD risk factors: Goal—<160 mg per dL, lifestyle modification for 3 to 6 months—160 to 189 mg per dL, drugs—≥190 mg per dL.

MEDICATIONS

- Hydroxymethylglutaryl coenzyme A reductase inhibitors or statin drugs are excellent for reduction of LDL-C. They can also cause modest reduction in triglycerides and small increase in HDL-C. Hepatic toxicity and myositis are major side effects, and liver enzymes should be monitored.
- Fibric acid derivatives (e.g., gemfibrozil) are used primarily to lower triglycerides and increase HDL-C and are effective in this regard. They only show small reductions in LDL-C and should not be used primarily to treat elevated LDL-C. Major side effects of these agents are GI. Liver function abnormalities may occasionally be noted.
- Nicotinic acid (niacin) is effective at lowering triglycerides and elevating HDL-C. It also can lower LDL-C moderately. This medication is inexpensive but use is limited due to side effects such as severe flushing. Flushing can be limited if started at low doses (50 mg TID), increasing slowly and gradually, and by giving aspirin simultaneously. GI side effects and hyperuricemia are also reported with this agent.
- Bile acid sequestrants or resins (e.g., cholestyramine, colestipol) can lower LDL-C effectively. These agents are not widely used since the introduction of statin drugs because this class is unpalatable and causes significant annoying GI side effects (e.g., bloating, constipation).
- Probucol—related to antioxidants; can lower LDL-C modestly, but may also lower HDL-C; not widely used currently.
- Ezetimibe (Zetia; Merck, Schering-Plough, North Wales, PA)—inhibits intestinal cholesterol absorption.

TABLE 3-3.	Fasting Lipid Studies
NCEP ATP III Lipid Result Classification LDL	
Optimal	<100
Near or above optimal	100–129
Borderline high	130–159
High	160–189
Very high	≥190
Total cholesterol	
Desirable	<200
Borderline high	200–239
High	<240
HDL	
Low	<40
High	>60

XVIII. Cardiomyopathy

A. Pathology

- Primary cardiomyopathies—disorders of myocardium that negatively affect its pumping capability and can lead to HF.
- They can be classified into three types—dilated cardiomyopathy, hypertrophic cardiomyopathy, and restrictive cardiomyopathy.
- Myocardial dysfunction caused by ischemic heart disease (CAD), hypertensive disease, or VHD are classified as secondary cardiomyopathies.

B. Dilated Cardiomyopathy

- Damage to myocardium causing dilated left ventricle, decreased EF, systolic HF. HF, emboli, dysrhythmia, and sudden death are major complications.

1. **Etiology**
   - Idiopathic (to 50% of cases).
   - Infective myocarditis—commonly caused by enterovirus, specifically coxsackie virus group B; also can be caused by Lyme disease and HIV.
   - Drugs—cocaine, Adriamycin.
   - Alcohol.
   - Autoimmune—SLE, scleroderma.
   - Peripartum.
   - Hemochromatosis.
   - Thyroid dysfunction (hypo or hyper).

2. **Clinical Features**

   HISTORY
   - Flulike symptoms a few weeks before cardiac failure symptoms in viral myocarditis.
   - Dyspnea on exertion and rest in severe disease.
   - Orthopnea.
   - PND.
   - Fatigue.
   - Syncope.
   - Palpitations.

   PHYSICAL FINDINGS
   - Tachycardia.
   - Tachypnea.
   - Pulsus alternans.
   - Cyanosis.
   - Cool extremities.
   - JVD, hepatojugular reflux.
   - Bibasilar rales.
   - S_3 gallop.
   - S_4 gallop.
   - Hepatomegaly.
   - Ascites.
   - Peripheral edema.
   - Systolic murmur of functional MR.

3. **Diagnostic Studies**
   - Echo, cardiac Doppler—chamber size dilation, reduced LVEF.
   - ECG—nonspecific ST-T wave abnormalities, LVH, left bundle branch block (LBBB).
   - CXR—cardiomegaly, pulmonary congestion, pleural effusions.
   - Nuclear ventriculography (MUGA scan)—reduced LVEF.
   - Catheterization.
   - Myocardial biopsy.

4. **Management**
   - Rest.
   - Sodium restriction.
   - Diuretics.
   - ACE inhibitors or ARBs.
   - Nitrates.
   - Hydralazine.
   - Digoxin.
   - Consider warfarin.
   - Dopamine in hospital.
   - Treat arrhythmias carefully.
   - Surgery referral—transplant.

C. Hypertrophic Cardiomyopathy

- Massive hypertrophy of left ventricle, often more pronounced at septum, leads to delayed cardiac relaxation, impaired ventricular filling, diastolic dysfunction, small LV cavity, and often LV outflow obstruction. Hypertrophy may be asymmetric or concentric. Usually presents in young adulthood.

1. **Etiology**

   PRIMARY
   - Genetic (autosomal dominant) familial hypertrophic cardiomyopathy (previously called idiopathic hypertrophic subaortic stenosis).

   SECONDARY
   - Hypertension.
   - AS.

2. **Clinical Features**

   HISTORY
   - Dyspnea on exertion.
   - Angina pectoris.
   - Presyncope and syncope on exertion.
   - Fatigue.
   - Palpitations.
   - PND.
   - Sudden death.

   PHYSICAL FINDINGS
   - Bisferious carotid pulsation.
   - Prominent A wave of jugular vein.
   - S_4 gallop.
   - Harsh crescendo-decrescendo systolic murmur best heard at left sternal border, apex; increases with Valsalva and standing; decreases with squatting.
   - May have concurrent MR.

3. **Diagnostic Studies**
   - Echo—often diagnostic.
   - ECG—LVH, nonspecific ST-T abnormalities, deep septal Q waves in inferior leads, or tall narrow R waves in V1 and V2.
   - Twenty-four-hour Holter monitor to assess for ventricular tachycardia (VT) if syncope or palpitations present.
   - Cardiac catheterization.

4. **Management**
   - Avoid overly vigorous exercise.
   - β-Blockers.
   - Verapamil, a calcium channel blocker.
   - Surgical referral for myectomy in refractory cases.
   - Digoxin—contraindicated except for atrial fibrillation with uncontrolled rate.
   - Nitrates and diuretics should usually be avoided.

D. Restrictive Cardiomyopathy
- Decreased elasticity and compliance of ventricles usually from infiltrative process, causing high filling pressures and diastolic dysfunction, and failure.
- Less common than hypertrophic or dilated type.

1. **Etiology**
   - Amyloidosis.
   - Sarcoidosis.
   - Hemochromatosis.
   - Scleroderma.
   - Friedreich ataxia.

2. **Clinical Features**

   HISTORY
   - Dyspnea on exertion.
   - Fatigue.
   - PND.
   - Orthopnea.
   - Edema.

   PHYSICAL FINDINGS
   - JVD.
   - S_3 gallop.
   - S_4 gallop—occasional.
   - Pulmonary rales.
   - Pedal, ankle edema.

3. **Diagnostic Studies**
   - Echo—often diagnostic.
   - Cardiac biopsy—occasionally necessary.

4. **Management**
   - Diuretics (loop).
   - Vasodilators (ACE inhibitors, nitrates).
   - Digoxin may be of benefit.
   - Referral or transplant if refractory.

XIX. Congenital Heart Disease
- There are a variety of congenital structural abnormalities of the heart. Many are diagnosed in infancy, but some do not become symptomatic until adulthood. Etiology of most is unknown. Some are caused by known genetic factors, intrauterine rubella syndrome, and medications (e.g., lithium with Ebstein anomaly).

A. Atrial Septal Defect (ASD)
1. **Pathology**
   - Except for MVP and bicuspid aortic valve, ASD is the most common type of CHD.
   - Defect in atrial septum causing opening between left and right atria.
   - Shunting—typically left to right.
   - Symptoms may not appear until adulthood.
   - Ostium secundum—most common type of ASD.

2. **Clinical Features**
   - Usually minimal in childhood, but can exhibit failure to thrive.
   - Adults may have dyspnea on exertion and fatigue.
   - Right ventricular lift.
   - Fixed widely split S_2.
   - Early systolic flow murmur can be heard at left second to third ICS. Later, a low-pitched diastolic murmur at upper left sternal border can sometimes be identified.
   - Clubbing.
   - Cyanosis.

3. **Diagnostic Studies**
   - Echocardiography.
   - ECG—RAD, RVH, rSR' pattern.
   - Cardiac catheterization.

4. **Management**
   - Surgical repair.

B. Ventricular Septal Defect
1. **Pathology**
   - Defect in ventricular septum causing opening between left and right ventricles.
   - Mostly congenital in origin, but may be acquired as a complication of AMI.
   - Shunting—typically left to right.
   - Can lead to pulmonary hypertension.
   - Symptoms may not appear until adulthood.

2. **Clinical Features**
   - Failure to thrive in infancy.
   - Dyspnea.
   - JVD.
   - Left lower sternal thrill.
   - S_3.
   - High-pitched holosystolic murmur at left sternal border.
   - Diastolic murmur of PR.
   - Clubbing.
   - Cyanosis.

3. **Diagnostic Studies**
   - Echocardiography.
   - ECG—LVH, RVH, atrial enlargement.
   - CXR—may have enlarged heart.
   - Cardiac catheterization.

4. **Management**
   - Endocarditis prophylaxis.
   - Surgical repair in significant impairments.

C. Coarctation of the Aorta
1. **Pathology**
   - An area of narrowing of aorta usually located distal to left subclavian artery.

2. **Clinical Features**
   - Failure to thrive in infancy.
   - Bilateral claudication.
   - Headache.
   - Hypertension.
   - Delayed femoral pulse compared with brachial pulse.
   - Decreased leg BP.
   - Murmurs (AS, AR).
   - S_4.

3. **Diagnostic Studies**
   - Echocardiography (transthoracic, TEE).
   - ECG—LVH.
   - CXR—rib notching.
   - Cardiac catheterization, angiogram.
4. **Management**
   - Balloon angioplasty.
   - Surgical correction.

D. Patent Ductus Arteriosus
1. **Pathology**
   - Failure of ductus arteriosus (shunt from pulmonary artery to aorta) to close as it usually does in the first or second day of life.
   - Common in infants and children, but relatively rare in adults.
   - Can occur as a result of maternal rubella.
2. **Clinical Features**
   - Failure to thrive in infancy.
   - Recurrent respiratory infections.
   - Fatigue.
   - Dyspnea on exertion.
   - Angina and syncope can occur in adults.
   - With left-to-right shunt—continuous machine murmur or systolic murmur, thrill can occur.
   - With right-to-left shunt—cyanosis, clubbing, diastolic Graham Steell murmur.
3. **Diagnostic Studies**
   - Echocardiography/cardiac Doppler.
   - ECG—LVH, left atrial hypertrophy.
   - Cardiac catheterization, angiogram.
4. **Management**
   - Catheter plug procedure.
   - Surgical correction.

E. Tetralogy of Fallot
1. **Pathology**
   - Most common cyanotic CHD in older children and adults.
   - Can have five characteristics including large VSD, right ventricular infundibular stenosis and obstruction, pulmonic stenosis (PS), RVH, overriding aorta.
   - Right-to-left shunting typical.
2. **Clinical Features**
   - Cyanosis, retarded growth in childhood.

   ADULTS WITHOUT CORRECTION
   - Clubbing.
   - Fatigue.
   - Dyspnea on exertion.
   - Edema and syncope can be late findings.
   - Thrill at left sternal border.
   - Single S_2.
   - Systolic ejection murmur.
3. **Diagnostic Studies**
   - CBC—polycythemia.
   - Echocardiography/cardiac Doppler.
   - ECG—RVH, RAD.

- CXR—in children, a small boot-shaped heart may be seen.
- Cardiac catheterization, angiogram.
4. **Management**
   - Good dental hygiene.
   - Endocarditis prophylaxis.
   - Surgical repair.

XX. Giant Cell Arteritis (Also Called Cranial Arteritis and Temporal Arteritis)

A. Etiology
- Idiopathic, may be autoimmune.

B. Pathology
- Systemic granulomatous inflammation of medium and large arteries, mostly affecting cranial arteries.
- Blindness—significant complication if untreated.
- Usually occurs in people older than 60 years and associated with polymyalgia rheumatica.

C. Clinical Features
HISTORY
- Headache—usually unilateral temporal.
- Jaw claudication with mastication.
- Visual disturbances (scotoma, diplopia, amaurosis fugax, blindness).
- Sore throat.
- Fever.
- Arthralgias, myalgias.
- TIA/CVA symptoms.

PHYSICAL FINDINGS
- Swollen, tender temporal artery.
- Scalp tenderness.
- Focal neurologic signs with TIA/CVA.

D. Diagnostic Studies
- Elevated ESR—sometimes >100.
- Temporal artery biopsy—diagnostic.
- May have to biopsy contralateral side if initially negative.

E. Management
- Prednisone—high dose (60 mg) for approximately 6 weeks, then taper over months to years, guided by symptoms and ESR.

XXI. Conduction Disorders

A. Etiology
- Drugs (digoxin, β-blockers, and some calcium channel blockers such as diltiazem and verapamil).
- Ischemia, AMI.
- CHD.
- Thyroid disorders.

B. Pathology
- Interruptions in cardiac conduction pathways that can occur between atria and ventricles

(atrioventricular [AV] blocks), or at ventricular bundle branches (bundle branch blocks [BBB]).

- These conditions are often related to fibrosis of conduction tissue.

C. Clinical Features

- Many, such as first-degree AV block, second-degree AV block (type I), right bundle branch block (RBBB), and LBBB, may be asymptomatic.
- Some second-degree type II AV blocks and third-degree AV blocks with significant bradycardia can cause lightheadedness, angina, and syncope.

D. Diagnostic Studies

- Most diagnosed on 12-lead ECG.

E. Management

- First-degree AV blocks frequently require no treatment.
- Underlying causes should be determined and treated.

- Offending drugs should be discontinued, when possible.
- Second-degree type II AV block and third-degree AV block require temporary pacemaker; if persistent, require permanent pacemaker.

F. Types

AV BLOCKS

- **First-degree AV block**—Impulse from SA node delayed conducting to ventricles at AV node. PR interval on ECG >0.20 seconds. Every P wave followed by normal ventricular impulse (QRS) complex (Figure 3-2).
- **Second-degree AV block type I (Mobitz type I or Wenckebach)**—Characterized by progressively lengthening PR intervals until complete block occurs and QRS complex dropped, and cycle repeats itself. QRS complexes are normal (Figure 3-3).
- **Second-degree AV block type II (Mobitz type II)**—This rhythm involves intermittent complete block with dropped QRS complex without lengthening

FIGURE 3-2. **First-degree AV block ECG.** (From Huff J. AV junctional arrhythmias and AV blocks. In: Huff J, ed. *ECG Workout, Exercises in Arrhythmia Interpretation.* 3rd ed. Philadelphia, PA: Lippincott-Raven; 1997:58, with permission.)

FIGURE 3-3. **Second-degree AV block, Type I or Wenckebach.** (From Huff J. AV junctional arrhythmias and AV blocks. In: Huff J, ed. *ECG Workout, Exercises in Arrhythmia Interpretation.* 3rd ed. Philadelphia, PA: Lippincott-Raven; 1997:59, with permission.)

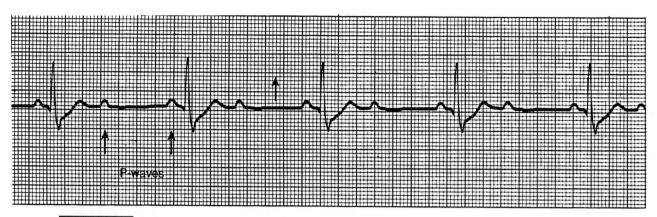

FIGURE 3-4. Second-degree AV block type II ECG. (From Huff J. AV junctional arrhythmias and AV blocks. In: Huff J, ed. *ECG Workout, Exercises in Arrhythmia Interpretation.* 3rd ed. Philadelphia, PA: Lippincott-Raven; 1997:59, with permission.)

PR interval. PR intervals are uniform, but atrial rate faster than ventricular rate. This often has a regular pattern with one QRS for every two or three atrial impulses (P wave), as in a 2:1 or 3:1 block. This type of AV block can progress to complete or third-degree AV block (Figure 3-4).

- **Third-degree AV block**—Complete AV block or complete disassociation between atria and ventricles with no atrial impulses reaching ventricles. Independent atrial and ventricular rates are present. Ventricle must pace itself independently through an ectopic pacemaker in nodal areas or ventricles. If ectopic pacemaker is ventricular, QRS complexes are wide (Figure 3-5).

BUNDLE BRANCH BLOCKS AND PREEXCITATION

- **RBBB**—Interruption of cardiac impulse at right bundle branch causing left ventricle to be depolarized slightly before right ventricle, which causes widened QRS (>0.12 seconds) with the RSR′ configuration seen in right precordial leads (V$_1$ and V$_2$) on ECG

(Figure 3-6). Biphasic QRS with broad S wave is also seen in lead I.

- **LBBB**—Interruption of cardiac impulse at left bundle branch causing right ventricle to be depolarized slightly before left ventricle, which causes widened QRS (>0.12 seconds) with RSR′ configuration seen in left precordial leads (V$_5$ and V$_6$) on ECG. BBB almost always related to pathologic condition. LBBB may interfere with interpretation of ischemia and AMI on ECG.

- **Left anterior hemiblock or left anterior fascicular block**—Interruption of conduction at anterior division or fascicle of left bundle branch, which has the following characteristics on ECG:
  - LAD (lead I positive, lead aVF negative).
  - Lead II dominantly negative.
  - Slightly widened QRS (0.10 to 0.12).
  - Small Q waves can be seen in leads I and aVL.
  - Small R waves seen in leads II, III, and aVF.

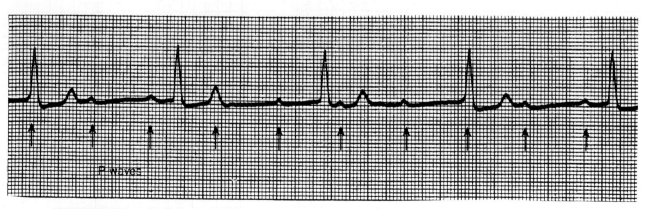

FIGURE 3-5. Third-degree AV block ECG. (From Huff J. AV junctional arrhythmias and AV blocks. In: Huff J, ed. *ECG Workout, Exercises in Arrhythmia Interpretation.* 3rd ed. Philadelphia, PA: Lippincott-Raven; 1997:59, with permission.)

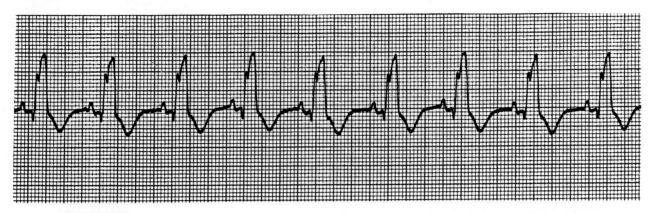

FIGURE 3-6. **Bundle branch block ECG.** (From Huff J. AV junctional arrhythmias and AV blocks. In: Huff J, ed. *ECG Workout, Exercises in Arrhythmia Interpretation*. 3rd ed. Philadelphia, PA: Lippincott-Raven; 1997:60, with permission.)

- **Wolff–Parkinson–White (WPW)**—Condition characterized by accessory conduction pathway or bypass tract that may bypass normal conduction delay to ventricles occurring at AV node, which can lead to preexcitation and paroxysmal tachycardias. ECG features of WPW are as follows:

- δ Wave, slurred upstroke of QRS (Figure 3-7).
- Widened QRS of >0.10 seconds (Figure 3-7).
- Shortened PR interval of <0.12 seconds.
- Symptomatic WPW with tachycardia can be treated with catheter ablation of accessory pathways

FIGURE 3-7. **WPW ECG.** (From Zipes DP. Cardiac arrhythmias. In: Kelley WN, ed. *Textbook of Internal Medicine*. 3rd ed. Philadelphia, PA: Lippincott-Raven; 1997:60, with permission.)

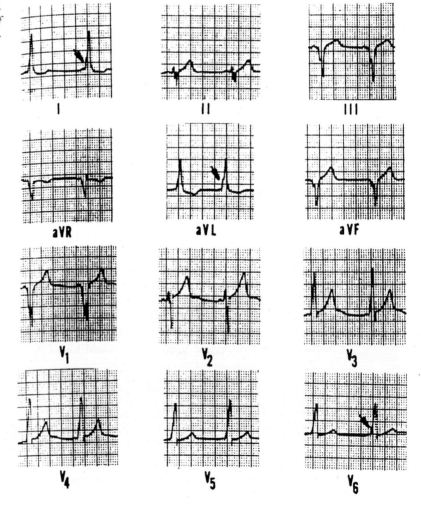

XXII. Cardiac Dysrhythmias

A. Etiology

- Ischemia and AMI.
- Drugs.
- Electrolyte imbalances (especially potassium).
- Thyroid disease.
- CHDs.
- Inflammatory conditions (myocarditis, endocarditis).
- Cardiomyopathies.
- VHD.

B. Pathology

- Cardiac dysrhythmias—abnormalities of cardiac rhythm and can include ectopic beats, slow heart rates (bradycardias), rapid heart rates (tachycardias), and disorganized or erratic rhythms (fibrillation).
- These disturbances can arise from abnormalities of impulse formation, abnormalities of impulse conduction, triggered activity, or reentry phenomenon.

C. Clinical Features

- Many dysrhythmias (e.g., sinus arrhythmia, sinus brady-cardia, mild sinus tachycardia) can be asymptomatic.
- Many dysrhythmias (e.g., tachycardias, atrial fibrillation, ectopic beats) present with palpitations.
- Severe bradycardias (with rate <40 per minute) and tachycardias may cause decreased cerebral perfusion with mental status changes, dizziness, and syncope.
- Severe bradycardias and tachycardias may lead to decreased cardiac output and CHF symptoms and signs; atrial fibrillation may also cause CHF due to loss of atrial contraction or "kick."
- Severe bradycardias and tachycardias can cause diminished coronary perfusion in patients with CAD and may precipitate angina pectoris.
- Lethal dysrhythmias (e.g., ventricular fibrillation) cause sudden death.
- Cardiac auscultation is the major step in diagnosing.

D. Diagnostic Studies

- ECG—12-lead ECG and rhythm strips are the main studies used to diagnose dysrhythmias.

- Twenty-four-hour ambulatory Holter monitoring; event recorders may be needed to disclose intermittent dysrhythmias.
- Signal-averaged ECGs are used to uncover late potentials seen in patients susceptible to VT.
- Autonomic tilt-table testing can be performed for syncope of unknown etiology.
- Electrophysiologic studies use electrode catheters in the heart to stimulate and map dysrhythmias; these can also be used to test the effectiveness of certain medications and ablate accessory pathways.
- Other studies (e.g., serum electrolytes, thyroid function tests, echocardiography, stress testing, cardiac catheterization) may be needed to delineate the etiology of dysrhythmia.

E. Types

- **Sinus tachycardia**—Sinus rhythm originating from SA node with resting heart rate of >100 per minute, but almost always <160 per minute (can rarely go as high as 200 per minute).
  - Normal for infants and young children, and often caused by noncardiac conditions in adults such as drugs (cocaine, sympathomimetics, decongestants, bronchodilators, nicotine, caffeine), anxiety, anemia, fever, hypovolemia, hypoxemia, exercise, and thyrotoxicosis.
  - Management—usually aimed at delineating and treating cause.
- **Sinus bradycardia**—Sinus rhythm originating from SA node with a rate of <60 per minute, which can be caused by vagal stimulation, hypothyroidism, medications (β-blockers), high levels of aerobic fitness, and inferior AMI.
  - Management—usually no treatment required unless CNS symptoms develop secondary to cerebral hypoperfusion; in those cases, IV atropine and pacing can be used.
- **Paroxysmal supraventricular tachycardia (PSVT)**—characterized by abrupt onset of increased heart rate of 200 to 250 per minute from atrial or junctional foci; common presentation of WPW and reentry phenomenon (Figure 3-8).

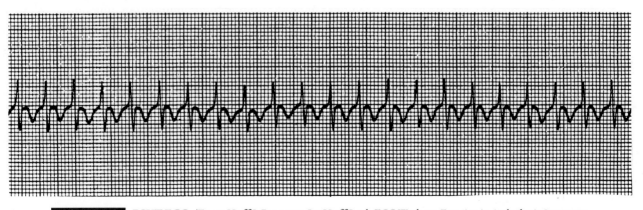

FIGURE 3-8. **PSVT ECG.** (From Huff J. Post-test. In: Huff J, ed. *ECG Workout, Exercises in Arrhythmia Interpretation.* 3rd ed. Philadelphia, PA: Lippincott-Raven; 1997:62, with permission.)

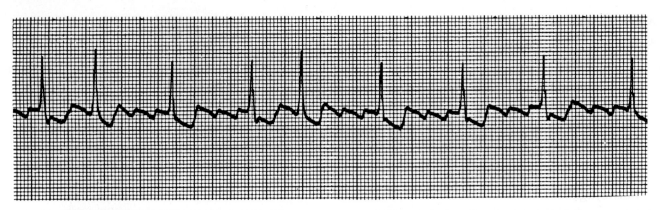

FIGURE 3-9. Atrial flutter ECG. (From Huff J. Post-test. In: Huff J, ed. *ECG Workout, Exercises in Arrhythmia Interpretation.* 3rd ed. Philadelphia, PA: Lippincott-Raven; 1997:62, with permission.)

MANAGEMENT

- Carotid sinus massage.
- Vagal stimulation.
- Synchronized direct current (DC) electrical cardioversion for hemodynamically unstable patients.
- Adenosine IV.
- Calcium channel blockers (i.e., verapamil or diltiazem).
- β-Blockers (e.g., propranolol, metoprolol, esmolol).
- Amiodarone.
- Digoxin IV (unless caused by digoxin toxicity).
- Overdrive pacing.
- Radiofrequency ablation can be used in preexcitation syndromes with an accessory pathway such as WPW.
- **Atrial flutter**—Tachycardia with atrial rate of 250 to 350 per minute and some atrioventricular block causing ventricular rate usually half or one-third of atrial rate (2:1, 3:1 AV block). P waves occur in rapid succession and form characteristic "sawtooth" pattern or "flutter waves." These flutter waves may not be apparent until rate is slowed by carotid sinus massage. Atrial flutter can be caused by HF and pulmonary disease and sometimes seen alternating with atrial fibrillation ("fib-flutter") (Figure 3-9).

MANAGEMENT

- Rate control: β-blockers, calcium channel blockers, or digoxin.
- Cardioversion: use with anticoagulation if >48 hours. Synchronized DC cardioversion. Can use with ilbutilide.
- Chronic: amiodarone, dofetilide, or EPS with ablation.
- **Atrial fibrillation**—Dysrhythmia caused by rapid erratic atrial impulse firing from multiple foci. Ventricular response irregular–irregular and may have slow, normal, or fast rate. Distinct P waves usually not discernible; can be caused by chronic hypertension, HF, WPW, pericarditis, S/P cardiac surgery, heavy alcohol use, sick sinus syndrome, rheumatic heart disease, pulmonary disease, thyrotoxicosis, VHD/mitral valve disease, hypokalemia, CAD/AMI, or pulmonary embolus (Figure 3-10). Can also be seen in normal heart (Lone A. Fib).

MANAGEMENT

- Search for cause Thyroid function tests (TFTs), Echo, cardiac enzymes, electrolytes).
- Control rate: digoxin, β-blockers, verapamil, or diltiazem can be given to control ventricular response rate.

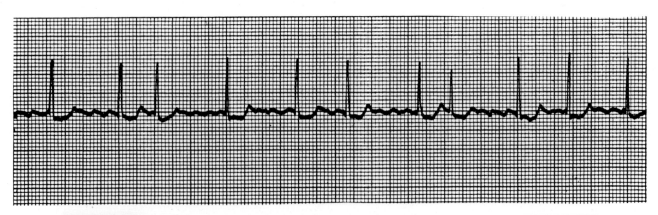

FIGURE 3-10. Atrial fibrillation ECG. (From Huff J. Post-test. In: Huff J, ed. *ECG Workout, Exercises in Arrhythmia Interpretation.* 3rd ed. Philadelphia, PA: Lippincott-Raven; 1997:63, with permission.)

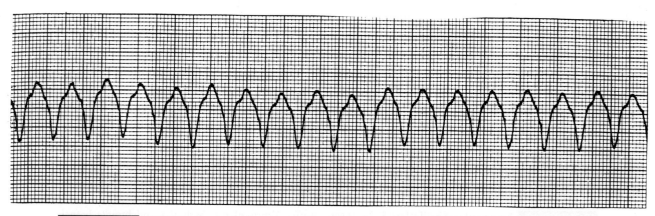

FIGURE 3-11. **VT ECG.** (From Huff J. Ventricular arrhythmias and bundle branch blocks. In: Huff J, ed. *ECG Workout, Exercises in Arrhythmia Interpretation*. 3rd ed. Philadelphia, PA: Lippincott-Raven; 1997:63, with permission.)

- Cardioversion can be attempted using drugs such as amiodarone. If unstable, synchronized electrical cardioversion should be done with or without ibutilide; followed by anticoagulation. If stable and in A. Fib >48 hours, a TEE should be performed prior to cardioversion to look for an atrial thrombus. If present, the patient should be treated with anticoagulant for 4 weeks prior to cardioversion followed by 4 weeks after.
- Anticoagulation with warfarin to the international normalized ratio of 2:3 will reduce the risk of embolic stroke. Dabigatran (Pradaxa) can also be used and may have lower risk of bleeding. Rivaroxaban (Xarelto) can also be used in nonvalvular A. Fib. For Lone A. Fib in young (<65 years old) patients with no history of heart disease, hypertension, or diabetes ASA can be used.
- Dronedarone (Maltaq), amiodarone, propafenone, flecainide, and dofetilide have been used to maintain patients in Normal Sinus Rhythm (NSR).
  - Recent studies show rate control with anticoagulation may be as efficacious as cardioversion.

- Radiofrequency ablation also has been successful in refractory cases.
- **VT**—Characterized by a rapid rate (150 to 250 per minute) originating from ectopic ventricular focus. Can be caused by CAD, AMI, or antiarrhythmic drugs. Antiarrhythmic drugs (e.g., quinidine, procainamide, disopyramide, flecainide, encainide, amiodarone, Stadol) can cause polymorphic form of VT (called torsades de pointes) usually by prolonging the QT interval. VT can cause hemodynamic instability and even pulseless state. Even when the patient appears hemodynamically stable, VT is an emergent condition because it can progress to ventricular fibrillation and death. Important to differentiate VT from SVT with aberrancy, although sometimes difficult without slowing the rate (Figures 3-11 and 3-12).

MANAGEMENT
- Unstable and pulseless VT should be defibrillated.
- Synchronized DC cardioversion for stable VT.
- Lidocaine IV can also be used in stable VT.
- Magnesium can be given to treat torsades de pointes.
- Overdrive pacing also can be used in VT.

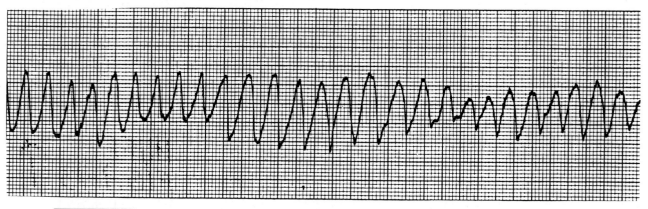

FIGURE 3-12. **Torsades de pointes ECG.** (From Huff J. Ventricular arrhythmias and bundle branch blocks. In: Huff J, ed. *ECG Workout, Exercises in Arrhythmia Interpretation*. 3rd ed. Philadelphia, PA: Lippincott-Raven; 1997:63, with permission.)

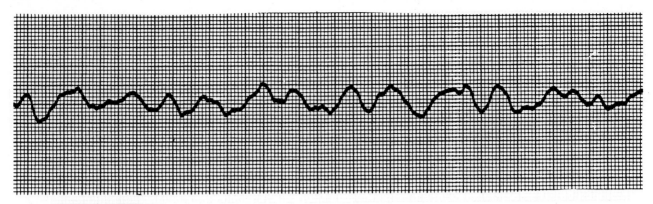

FIGURE 3-13. **Ventricular fibrillation ECG.** (From Huff J. Ventricular arrhythmias and bundle branch blocks. In: Huff J, ed. *ECG Workout, Exercises in Arrhythmia Interpretation.* 3rd ed. Philadelphia, PA: Lippincott-Raven; 1997:64, with permission.)

- **Ventricular fibrillation**—Totally disorganized rapid ventricular firing from multiple ectopic foci causing no effective cardiac output, pulseless state, and death (Figure 3-13).

  MANAGEMENT
  - Immediate cardiopulmonary resuscitation.
  - Defibrillation.
  - Automatic implantable cardioverter defibrillators can be surgically installed in patients at high risk for ventricular fibrillation.

- **Premature atrial contractions (PAC, APC, APB)**—Caused by impulse originating in ectopic focus in atrium outside of SA node that occurs earlier than expected in cardiac cycle. P wave has different morphology than normal sinus beats, but QRS usually appears normal. These can be idiopathic or related to caffeine, tobacco, or myocardial ischemia (Figure 3-14).

  MANAGEMENT
  - PACs usually require no treatment other than correcting potential underlying etiologies.
  - Persons with no underlying heart disease can have PACs.

- Patients should be instructed to avoid tobacco, alcohol, and caffeine products.

- **Premature ventricular contractions (PVC, VPC, VPB)**—Caused by ectopic focus in ventricle with impulse that occurs earlier than expected in cardiac cycle. QRS complex appears wide; they can occur in pairs (couplets), can occur after every other normal beat (bigeminy), can originate from one ectopic focus with a similar morphology (unifocal), or can originate from multiple foci with different morphology (multifocal). They can be idiopathic and occur in people without disease, or can be caused by myocardial ischemia, cardiomyopathy, or structural abnormalities (Figure 3-15).

  MANAGEMENT
  - In patients with no underlying heart disease, PVCs are usually not treated. The Cardiac Arrhythmia Suppression Trial study disclosed higher mortality in patients with ventricular ectopy treated with class IC antiarrhythmic drugs in comparison with placebo groups.
  - Patients with ventricular ectopy and LV dysfunction with an EF <30% may also benefit from antiarrhythmic medication.

FIGURE 3-14. **Premature atrial contraction ECG.** (From Huff J. Atrial arrhythmias. In: Huff J, ed. *ECG Workout, Exercises in Arrhythmia Interpretation.* 3rd ed. Philadelphia, PA: Lippincott-Raven; 1997:64, with permission.)

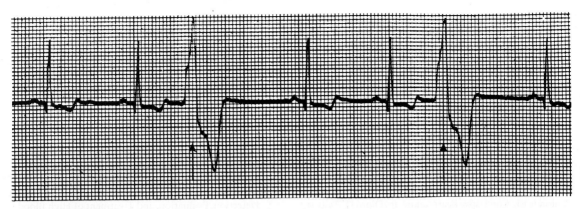

FIGURE 3-15. **Premature ventricular contraction ECG.** (From Huff J. Ventricular arrhythmias and bundle branch blocks. In: Huff J, ed. *ECG Workout, Exercises in Arrhythmia Interpretation*. 3rd ed. Philadelphia, PA: Lippincott-Raven; 1997:65, with permission.)

- Patients should be instructed to avoid caffeine, tobacco, and alcohol.
- β-Blockers can be used in low-risk patients with symptoms.
- **Premature junctional contractions (PJC)**—Ectopic premature beats originating from AV node or AV junction; characterized by retrograde conducted P waves that may be inverted, buried in the QRS, or appear after the QRS and narrow QRS complex.
- **Escape beats and rhythms**—At times when SA node fails to function properly or AV conduction is interrupted, as seen with pauses, severe bradycardia, and higher level AV blocks (second-degree type II or third degree), an ectopic pacemaker takes over. If pacemaker is at the AV junction, the patient exhibits PJCs or develops junctional escape or idiojunctional rhythm with rate usually about 60 per minute, retrograde P wave, and narrow QRS. They also have accelerated junctional rhythm with a rate of 70 to 130 per minute that can occur after cardiothoracic surgery, with digoxin toxicity, or with myocarditis. If pacemaker is in the ventricles, PVCs, ventricular escape rhythm, or idioventricular rhythm is seen with wide QRS complex and at a rate of about 30 to 40 per minute. Accelerated ventricular rhythms can also occur.

MANAGEMENT
- Treat underlying cause.
- Symptomatic bradycardias can be treated temporarily with IV atropine.
- Second-degree type II or third-degree AV blocks require pacemaker insertion.
- **Sick sinus syndrome**—Includes various disorders affecting SA node and conduction system. Occurs commonly in elderly persons and can cause sinus arrest or intermittent episodes of bradycardia alternating with tachycardia ("brady–tachy syndrome"). Pacemaker insertion is sometimes required.

SELECTED REFERENCES

Abbott JA, Cheitlin MD. Cardiac arrhythmias. In: Saunders CE, Ho MT, eds. *Current Emergency Diagnosis and Treatment*. 6th ed. Stamford, CT: Appleton & Lange; 2008:578–607.

American Heart Association. *Acls Provider Manual*. Dallas, TX: American Heart Association; 2001:123–144.

Bashore TM, Granger CB, Hranitzky P, et al. Heart disease. In: McPhee S, Papadakis M, Rabow MW, eds. *2011 Current Medical Diagnosis and Treatment*. New York, NY: McGraw-Hill; 2011:317–415.

Bates B. The cardiovascular system. In: Bates B, ed. *A Guide to Physical Examination and History Taking*. 6th ed. Philadelphia, PA: Lippincott-Raven; 1995:259–312.

Blankenberg A, Rupprecht HJ, Bickel C, et al. Glutathione peroxidase 1 activity and cardiovascular events in patients with coronary artery disease. *New Engl J Med*. 2003;349:1605–1613.

Branch WT, Alexander RW, Schlant RC, et al. *Cardiology in Primary Care*. New York, NY: McGraw-Hill; 2000.

Braunwald E, Goldman L. *Primary Cardiology*. 2nd ed. Philadelphia, PA: WB Saunders; 2003.

Brennan ML, Penn MS, Van Lente F, et al. Prognostic value of myeloperoxidase in patients with chest pain. *N Engl J Med*. 2003;349:1595–1604.

Caruso AC. Arrhythmias. In: Noble J, Greene HL, Levinson W, Modest GA, Young MJ, eds. *Textbook of Primary Care Medicine*. 2nd ed. St. Louis, MO: Mosby; 1996:199–210.

Dambro MR. Aortic dissection. In: Dambro MR, ed. *Griffith's 5 Minute Clinical Consult*. Baltimore, MD: Williams & Wilkins; 1998:66–67.

Dambro MR. Aortic valvular stenosis. In: Dambro MR, ed. *Griffith's 5 Minute Clinical Consult*. Baltimore, MD: Williams & Wilkins; 1998:68–69.

DeGowin EL, DeGowin RL. The thorax and cardiovascular system. In: De-Gowin EL, DeGowin RL, eds. *Bedside Examination*. 4th ed. New York, NY: Macmillan; 1981:229–471.

Diprio JT, Talbert RL, Yee GC, et al. *Pharmacotherapy: A Pathophysiologic Approach*. 5th ed. New York, NY: McGraw-Hill; 2002:chaps 15 and 17.

Dubin D. Infarction. In: Dubin D, ed. *Rapid Interpretation of EKG'S*. 3rd ed. Tampa, FL: Cover Publishing; 1981:204–245.

Executive Summary of the Third Report of the National Cholesterol Education Program Expert Panel on Detection, Evaluation, and Treatment of High Blood Cholesterol in Adults (Adult Treatment Panel III). National Institutes of Health, National Heart, Lung, and Blood Institutes. *JAMA*. 2001;285:2486–2509.

Geraets DR. The heart and myocardial infarction. In: Traub SL, ed. *Basic Skills in Interpreting Laboratory Data*. 2nd ed. Bethesda, MD: American Society of Health-System Pharmacists; 1996:187–212.

Gotto AM. Hyperlipidemia. In: Rakel RE, ed. *Conn's Current Therapy*. Philadelphia, PA: WB Saunders; 1998:567–574.

Huff J. Atrial arrhythmias. In: Huff J, ed. *ECG Workout, Exercises in Arrhythmia Interpretation*. 3rd ed. Philadelphia, PA: Lippincott-Raven; 1997:89–132.

Huff J. AV junctional arrhythmias and AV blocks. In: Huff J, ed. *ECG Workout, Exercises in Arrhythmia Interpretation*. 3rd ed. Philadelphia, PA: Lippincott-Raven; 1997:133–180.

Huff J. Post-test. In: Huff J, ed. *ECG Workout, Exercises in Arrhythmia Interpretation*. 3rd ed. Philadelphia, PA: Lippincott-Raven; 1997:247–284.

Huff J. Ventricular arrhythmias and bundle branch blocks. In: Huff J, ed. *ECG Workout, Exercises in Arrhythmia Interpretation*. 3rd ed. Philadelphia, PA: Lippincott-Raven; 1997:181–226.

Johnson JA, Lalonde RL. Congestive heart failure. In: Dipro JT, Talbert RL, Yee GC, Matzke GR, Wells BG, Posey LM, eds. *Pharmacotherapy: A Pathophysiologic Approach*. 3rd ed. Stamford, CT: Appleton & Lange; 1997:219–256.

Lowering plasma homocysteine. *Med Lett Drugs Ther*. 2003;45(1168):85–86.

Margolis S. Disorders of plasma lipids and lipoproteins. In: Stobo JD, Traill TA, Hellman DB, Ladenson PW, Petty BG, eds. *The Principles and Practice of Medicine*. 23rd ed. Stamford, CT: Appleton & Lange; 1996:338–347.

Michael TAD. Systolic and diastolic murmurs. In: Tap M, ed. *Auscultation of the Heart, A Cardiophonetic Approach*. New York, NY: McGraw-Hill; 1998:161–218.

Miles NM, Williams ES, Zipes DP. Acquired valvular heart disease. In: Andreoli TE, Bennett JC, Carpenter CCJ, Plum F, eds. *Cecil Essentials of Medicine*. 4th ed. Philadelphia, PA: WB Saunders; 1997:45–52.

Miles NM, Williams ES, Zipes DP. Congestive heart failure. In: Andreoli TE, Bennett JC, Carpenter CCJ, Plum F, eds. *Cecil Essentials of Medicine*. 4th ed. Philadelphia, PA: WB Saunders; 1997:40–44.

Pagana KD, Pagana TJ. *Manual of Diagnostic and Laboratory Tests*. 2nd ed. St. Louis, MO: Mosby; 2002:123.

Pederson D. Infectious endocarditis. In: Labus JB, ed. *The Physician Assistant Medical Handbook*. Philadelphia, PA: WB Saunders; 1995:378–388.

Rahimtoola SH. Valvular heart disease. In: Stein JH, ed. *Internal Medicine*. 5th ed. St. Louis, MO: Mosby; 1998:239–262.

Schwartz B, O'Brien KL. Streptococcal infections. In: Kelly WN, ed. *Textbook of Internal Medicine*. 3rd ed. Philadelphia, PA: Lippincott-Raven; 1997:1614–1622.

Segal BL. Clinical recognition of rheumatic heart disease. In: Chizner MA, ed. *Classic Teachings in Clinical Cardiology; A Tribute to W. Proctor Harvey*. Cedar Grove, NJ: Laennec Publishing; 1996:991–1016.

Seventh Report of the Joint National Committee on Prevention, Detection, Evaluation, and Treatment of High Blood Pressure. National Institutes of Health, National Heart, Lung, and Blood Institutes. *JAMA*. 2003;289:2560–2572.

Spittell PC, Spittell JA. Diseases of the peripheral arteries and veins. In: Stein JH, ed. *Internal Medicine*. 5th ed. St. Louis, MO: Mosby; 1998:305–312.

Stanley VR. Fascicular blocks. In: Stanley VR, ed. *12-Lead ECG Interpretation for Emergency Personal; A Systematic Analytical Approach*. Fayetteville, WV: Independently Published ISBN 0-9635759-3-7; 1995:71–75.

Tierney LM, McPhee SJ, Papadakis MA. *Lange Current Medical Diagnosis and Treatment*. New York, NY: McGraw-Hill; 2004:chap 10.

Zipes DP. Cardiac arrhythmias. In: Kelly WN, ed. *Textbook of Internal Medicine*. 3rd ed. Philadelphia, PA: Lippincott-Raven; 1997:410–435.

Zipes DP. Management of cardiac arrhythmias: pharmacological, electrical, and surgical technique. In: Braunwald E, ed. *Heart Disease, A Textbook of Cardiovascular Medicine*. Philadelphia, PA: WB Saunders; 1992:628–666.

Gastrointestinal Disorders

Rosalie G. Coppola • Julie J. Kinzel

I. Disorders of the Esophagus

A. Gastroesophageal Reflux Disease

1. **Etiology**
   - Etiology multifactorial.
   - Multiple defects contribute to the development of gastroesophageal reflux disease (GERD).

2. **Pathology**
   - Major pathogenesis appears to be transient or sustained inappropriate relaxation of the lower esophageal sphincter (LES), not associated with swallowing.
   - Acid-rich stomach contents reflux into esophagus, resulting in esophageal tissue damage.
   - Contributing factors—abnormal esophageal epithelial resistance, abnormal gastric emptying, characteristics of the gastric reflux.
   - Other factors influencing LES tone include foods, increased intra-abdominal pressure, and medications.
   - Foods decreasing LES tone include fatty foods, chocolate, ethanol, peppermint, and onions.
   - Factors increasing intra-abdominal pressure include pregnancy, obesity, bending, lifting, straining, coughing, vomiting, and tight-fitting clothes.
   - Common drugs or medications known to decrease LES tone include caffeine, nicotine, calcium channel blockers, nitrates, theophylline, and some sedatives.
   - When associated with a hiatal hernia, delayed esophageal clearance can lead to significant esophageal tissue damage and Barrett esophagus.

3. **Clinical Features**
   - Heartburn and/or regurgitation—hallmark symptom.
   - Pain—often described as burning, substernal, radiating upward, usually worse 30 to 60 minutes after meals, and when lying supine, and typically relieved with sitting up and antacids.
   - Ten percent of patients present with atypical "anginal" type chest pain.
   - Sour taste in mouth, sore throat, laryngitis, hoarseness, cough, and wheezing may be presenting symptoms.
   - Dysphagia and regurgitation may indicate concurrent motility dysfunction or development of complications (e.g., esophageal stricture or Barrett metaplasia).
   - Esophagitis may result in peptic stricture, esophageal obstruction, esophageal perforation, or Barrett metaplasia.
   - Severity of symptoms does not correlate well with degree of esophageal mucosal damage.
   - Physical examination findings are nonspecific in uncomplicated cases.

4. **Diagnostic Studies**
   - Indicated in patients with atypical symptoms such as dysphagia, regurgitation, vomiting, or patients unresponsive to empiric therapy.
   - Upper endoscopy with biopsy documents type and extent of esophageal tissue damage.
   - Barium esophagography—is of limited value and may fail to identify reflux disease or esophageal mucosal damage. May be useful in patients with severe dysphagia to evaluate for peptic stricture before endoscopy.
   - Ambulatory esophageal pH monitoring—optimal study to document pathologic reflux and indicated in patients with normal endoscopy results and symptoms nonresponsive to proton pump inhibitors, when considering antireflux surgery in patients with normal endoscopy, and with atypical symptoms such as noncardiac chest pain and cough nonresponsive to antireflux therapy.
   - Esophageal manometry—useful in documenting evidence of motility disorders and LES pressures, and recommended when surgical intervention is planned.

5. **Management**
   - Mild, intermittent symptoms may be treated with trial of antacids, along with lifestyle modifications.
   - Lifestyle modifications should include weight loss, low-fat diet, and smaller serving portions.
   - Avoidance of foods (citrus fruits, tomatoes, and soft drinks) or medications known to decrease LES tone or cause direct mucosal irritation.
   - Avoidance of cigarette smoking and limited alcohol intake.
   - Elevation of head of bed, refraining from lying down after meals, not eating at least 3 hours before bedtime, avoiding tight-fitting clothes.

- Pharmacologic therapy indicated in moderate-to-severe disease and when attempts at lifestyle modification fail.
- Histamine-2 (H_2) receptor antagonists decrease gastric acid secretion; in higher doses, facilitate esophagitis healing.
- Promotility agents enhance esophageal clearance, increase LES pressure, and are more effective in patients with nocturnal symptoms and predominantly dyspeptic symptoms (e.g., abdominal bloating, nausea, early satiety).
- Proton pump inhibitors are the drugs of choice in severe cases, documented esophagitis, or failure with H_2 receptor antagonists, and are frequently used as a first-line choice because of ease of dosing, availability, and efficacy.
- Surgical fundoplication indicated when medical therapy fails.

B. Functional or Nonulcer Dyspepsia
1. Etiology
- Prevalence ranges from 25% to 40%.
- Estimated to be 27% in children.
2. Risk Factors
- Smoking.
- Use of aspirin or high-dose acetaminophen.
  - History often includes
  - Postprandial fullness.
  - Early satiety.
  - Epigastric pain or burning.
  - No documented structural disease or damage.
3. Treatment
- Evaluate for predominant symptom.
- Trial of proton pump inhibitor or H_2 blocker.
- Avoid exacerbating foods such as caffeine, alcohol.
- Counseling, psychological interventions.

C. Infectious Esophagitis
1. Etiology
- Common in immunosuppressed patients (e.g., in patients with AIDS, solid organ transplants, leukemia, lymphoma).
- Candidal infections often associated with uncontrolled diabetes, systemic antibiotic, corticosteroid, and radiation therapies.
- Eosinophilic esophagitis is a rare idiopathic disorder seen in children and adults. Results in esophageal infiltrates of eosinophils associated with food allergies, asthma, and other atopic diseases.
2. Pathology
- Common opportunistic pathogens include *Candida albicans*, herpes simplex, and cytomegalovirus (CMV).
- Herpes simplex may be seen in immune-competent patients.
3. Clinical Features
- Odynophagia, dysphagia, and retrosternal chest pain.

- Oral thrush may be seen in 75% of patients with candidal esophagitis and in 25% to 50% of patients with viral esophagitis.
- Physical examination may disclose signs of underlying immune deficiency (e.g., fever, generalized lymphadenopathy, skin lesion, or rashes).
4. Diagnostic Studies
- Endoscopy with biopsy yields high diagnostic accuracy.
- Endoscopic findings suggestive of candidal esophagitis include linear or diffuse yellow–white plaques.
- Endoscopic findings suggestive of CMV include single and multiple large superficial ulcers.
- Upper gastrointestinal (GI) symptoms with mucosal biopsy show >15 intraepithelial eosinophils per high-power field.
- Endoscopic findings consistent with herpes simplex include multiple small deep ulcers.
5. Management
- Dependent on the pathogen isolated, severity of illness, and immune status of the patient.
- Candidal esophagitis in immune-competent patients may be treated with topical antifungal agents; in immunosuppressed patients, oral or intravenous (IV) antifungal agents are required.
- Initial treatment of choice for CMV esophagitis is IV ganciclovir; when side effects are intolerable or response is poor, IV foscarnet is indicated.
- Eosinophil esophagitis treatment—topical steroids swallowed ± esophageal dilatation.

D. Pill-induced Esophagitis
1. Etiology
- Commonly implicated drugs include nonsteroidal anti-inflammatory drugs (NSAIDs), iron, antibiotics, vitamin C, potassium chloride, quinidine, zalcitabine, zidovudine, and alendronate.
2. Pathology
- Inflammation of esophageal mucosa presumed secondary to direct prolonged contact with various medications.
- Risk factors include swallowing pills without water or while lying supine, hospitalized or bedridden patients, and concurrent intestinal motility disorders.
3. Clinical Features
- Sudden retrosternal chest pain, odynophagia, and dysphagia typically occurring several hours after taking a pill.
- Elderly more often present with dysphagia and minimal pain.
- Complications include esophagitis with stricture, hemorrhage, and perforation.
- Physical examination findings are nonspecific in uncomplicated cases.
4. Diagnostic Studies
- Endoscopy typically discloses one or more discrete ulcers.

5. **Management**
   - Remove offending agent.
   - Drink at least 4 oz of water with medications.
   - Remain upright at least 30 minutes after ingestion of medication.

E. Esophageal Achalasia

1. **Etiology**
   - Progressive motor disorder of unknown etiology.
2. **Pathology**
   - Thought to result from degeneration of the myenteric plexus and enteric nervous system, along with defective LES innervation.
   - LES remains tonically contracted, failing to relax during swallowing.
   - Often associated with loss of normal peristalsis in distal two-thirds of esophageal smooth muscle.
3. **Clinical Features**
   - Symptoms typically seen between the ages of 25 and 60 years.
   - Gradual progressive dysphagia for solids and liquids.
   - Regurgitation of undigested food.
   - Nocturnal regurgitation results in cough and possible aspiration pneumonia.
   - Substernal discomfort and fullness after eating.
   - Anorexia and weight loss.
   - Complications include esophageal dilation, ulceration, infection, and rupture.
   - Physical examination findings are typically nonspecific in uncomplicated cases.
4. **Diagnostic Studies**
   - Esophageal manometry confirmatory. Findings on manometry include absence of peristalsis, low amplitude waves associated with swallowing, and incomplete relaxation of the LES on swallowing.
   - Barium esophagography may disclose esophageal dilation "sigmoid esophagus," absent peristalsis, and classic "birds beak" narrowing of distal esophagus.
   - Endoscopy should be performed to evaluate presence of esophageal inflammation, carcinoma, or other possible causes of obstruction.
   - Chest X-ray may disclose enlarged dilated esophagus.
5. **Management**
   - Endoscopic-guided injections of botulinum toxin into the LES result in relaxation of LES and symptomatic relief in two-thirds of patients for 6 to 12 months.
   - Fluoroscopic-guided pneumatic dilation of gastroesophageal junction results in symptomatic relief in over two-thirds of patients.
   - Surgical myotomy is indicated when conservative methods have failed.

F. Diffuse Esophageal Spasm

1. **Etiology**
   - Uncommon motility disorder seen equally in all ages and sexes.
2. **Pathology**
   - Motor disorder of the esophageal smooth muscle characterized by high-amplitude, nonperistaltic spontaneous esophageal contractions.
3. **Clinical Features**
   - Nonprogressive, mild intermittent dysphagia to solids and liquids.
   - Dysphagia may be provoked by stress, extremes in temperature of liquids, or large food boluses.
   - Intermittent chest pain described as dull, stabbing, or crushing that may radiate to neck, back, or arms and may be provoked by certain foods, hot or cold beverages, often unrelated to meals.
   - Chest pain may last minutes to hours and may awaken patient from sleep.
   - Pain may be confused with angina, although typically not exertional.
4. **Diagnostic Studies**
   - Barium esophagography discloses uncoordinated simultaneous contractions below the aortic arch, taking on characteristic "corkscrew" or "rosary bead" appearance.
   - Esophageal manometry may show characteristic prolonged large amplitude intermittent simultaneous esophageal contractions.
5. **Management**
   - Goal of therapy—reassurance and reduction of symptoms.
   - Sublingual nitroglycerin, longer-acting nitrates, and calcium channel blockers are effective in eliminating symptoms in some patients.
   - Dilation with Maloney bougies reported to relieve symptoms, and a long surgical myotomy may be required in debilitated patient with intractable symptoms.

G. Scleroderma Esophagitis

1. **Etiology**
   - Commonly associated with progressive systemic sclerosis or calcinosis, Raynaud phenomenon, esophageal dysmotility, sclerodactyly, and telangiectasia (CREST) syndrome.
   - May be the presenting patient complaint leading to diagnosis of scleroderma.
2. **Pathology**
   - Atrophy and fibrosis of the esophageal smooth muscle lead to low-amplitude peristaltic waves and eventual aperistalsis.
   - Marked decrease in LES pressures results in free gastroesophageal reflux and severe esophagitis.
   - Some studies suggest neural defect rather than primary myogenic disorder.
3. **Clinical Features**
   - Major symptoms include heartburn and dysphagia.
   - Complications include severe erosive esophagitis, peptic stricture, and Barrett metaplasia.

4. **Diagnostic Studies**
   - Barium esophagography discloses loss of peristalsis in distal esophagus and patulous LES.
   - Esophageal manometry discloses low LES pressures and decreased or absent peristalsis in distal two-thirds of esophagus.
   - Upper endoscopy with biopsy confirms degree of esophagitis, presence of Barrett metaplasia, or peptic stricture.
5. **Management**
   - Antireflux therapy including H_2 receptor antagonists, proton pump inhibitors, and promotility agents to prevent reflux complications.
   - Dilation may be required in presence of peptic stricture.

H. Esophageal Webs and Rings

1. **Etiology**
   - Webs are thin, weblike constrictions typically located in the proximal esophagus.
   - Webs associated with iron deficiency common in middle-aged women constitute Plummer–Vinson syndrome.
   - Schatzki ring—lower weblike constriction located at the squamocolumnar mucosal junction.
2. **Pathology**
   - Exact pathogenesis is unclear; lesions are typically congenital or inflammatory in nature.
   - Some evidence suggests GERD may be predisposing factor for the development of Schatzki ring.
3. **Clinical Features**
   - Usually asymptomatic unless marked esophageal narrowing occurs.
   - Intermittent dysphagia to solid foods may occur as large boluses of food lodge.
   - Obstructing food may spontaneously clear with ingestion of liquids or regurgitation.
   - Occasionally, impacted food may require endoscopic extraction.
4. **Diagnostic Studies**
   - Barium esophagography may disclose esophageal stricture.
   - Upper endoscopy may differentiate other causes of obstruction.
5. **Management**
   - Reassurance.
   - Instruct patients to chew food well.
   - Webs associated with iron deficiency anemia resolve well with treatment of anemia.
   - Mechanical disruption of the web or ring with bougienage dilation.

I. Zenker Diverticulum

1. **Etiology**
   - Esophageal diverticula.
2. **Pathology**
   - Weakness in posterior pharyngeal wall at pharyngoesophageal junction, possibly due to loss of elasticity of the upper esophageal sphincter.

3. **Clinical Features**
   - Symptoms result when undigested food particles lodge in the diverticula.
   - Gradual onset dysphagia.
   - Spontaneous regurgitation of undigested food particles.
   - Halitosis.
   - Nocturnal choking.
   - Neck mass on physical examination may be noted.
   - Complications include obstruction, aspiration pneumonia, bronchiectasis, and lung abscess.
4. **Diagnostic Studies**
   - Barium esophagography—diagnostic procedure of choice to visualize diverticula.
   - Upper endoscopy—should be used cautiously due to risk of perforation.
5. **Management**
   - Cricopharyngeal myotomy with or without diverticulectomy or surgical excision may be required.

J. Esophageal Varices

1. **Etiology**
   - Dilated submucosal veins.
2. **Pathology**
   - Venous collateral circulation secondary to portal hypertension seen in approximately 50% of patients with cirrhosis.
   - One-third of patients with varices develop upper GI bleeding.
   - Bleeding commonly occurs in varices located in gastroesophageal junction.
   - Factors believed to be related to bleeding include size of the varix, presence of red weal markings on endoscopy, current alcohol abuse, and severity of liver disease.
3. **Clinical Features**
   - Typically present with painless, massive upper GI bleeding.
   - Bright red or "coffee ground" hematemesis.
   - Melena: massive bleeds may present with hematochezia.
   - Postural hypotension, tachycardia, and shock.
4. **Diagnostic Studies**
   - Upper endoscopy localizes bleeding.
   - Complete blood cell (CBC) count, platelet count, prothrombin time (PT), partial thromboplastin time (PTT), electrolytes, liver function tests (LFTs), and albumin.
   - Evaluate for coagulopathies, liver function, and hemodynamic state.
5. **Management**
   - Emergency stabilization of patients.
   - Treat underlying coagulopathy, if present.
   - Endoscopic evaluation with therapeutic banding or sclerotherapy of varix.
   - When hemorrhage is too vigorous or endoscopy is unavailable, balloon tube tamponade may be used.

- Pharmacologic management includes use of vaso-constrictive drugs (e.g., vasopressin, somatostatin).
- Antibiotic prophylaxis (norfloxacin 400 mg BID or ciprofloxacin IV).
- When endoscopic or pharmacologic therapy fails, portal decompressive procedures may be necessary.

K. Mallory–Weiss Syndrome

1. **Etiology**
   - Superficial mucosal tear at the gastroesophageal junction.
2. **Pathology**
   - Presumed to occur secondary to sudden elevation of intra-abdominal pressure, as seen in vomiting or retching.
3. **Clinical Features**
   - Acute upper GI bleeding with hematemesis and occasionally melena.
   - Accounts for 5% to 10% of acute upper GI bleeding.
   - History of preceding vomiting, retching, or alcohol abuse may be obtained.
4. **Diagnostic Studies**
   - Upper endoscopy confirms the tear.
5. **Management**
   - Emergency stabilization, if necessary.
   - Bleeding typically resolves spontaneously.

II. Disorders of the Stomach and Intestines

A. Peptic Ulcer Disease

1. **Etiology**
   - Common disorders include gastric and duodenal ulcers.
   - Approximately 10% of adults develop peptic ulcer disease (PUD) in their lifetime.
   - Ulcers are slightly more common in men than in women, in the ratio of 1.3:1.
   - Duodenal ulcers are five times more common than gastric ulcers and typically seen in younger patients.
   - Gastric ulcers are more common in the elderly and have a high association with gastric cancer.
   - PUD is the most common cause of acute upper GI bleeding.
2. **Pathology**
   - Ulcers are typically 5 mm in diameter and extend through the muscularis mucosae.
   - Peptic ulcers result from disruption of gastric or duodenal mucosa secondary to an overproduction of acid or defects in the protective mucous barrier of the stomach.
   - Three major causes have been implicated in the development of PUD: *Helicobacter pylori*, NSAIDs, and hypersecretory peptic states.

- *H. pylori*—noninvasive spiral gram-negative bacillus, residing in the mucous gel coating the epithelial cells of the stomach, seen in approximately one in six patients with PUD. Exact pathogenesis of ulcer formation remains unclear, but may reflect disruption of the protective mucous barrier.
- NSAIDs inhibit prostaglandin synthesis. Prostaglandins are known to increase mucosal blood flow, increase bicarbonate and mucus secretion, and stimulate mucosal repair. Aspirin is the most ulcerogenic NSAID.
- Zollinger–Ellison (ZE) syndrome—benign gastrin-secreting tumor usually located in the pancreas that results in uninhibited secretion of gastrin and constant acid production.

3. **Clinical Features**
   - Hallmark symptom—epigastric pain (dyspepsia).
   - Dyspepsia—often characterized as gnawing, dull, "hunger-like" discomfort localized to the epigastrium.
   - Pain typically fluctuates in intensity throughout the day and night (rhythmicity) and may last for weeks with long intervals of pain-free periods (periodicity).
   - Pain relieved with food or antacids, recurring 2 to 4 hours after meals, with strong nocturnal component, suggestive of duodenal ulcers.
   - Pain aggravated by food and associated with weight loss, suggestive of gastric ulcers.
   - Many patients deny provocative or palliative relationship with food or antacids.
   - Associated symptoms include nausea, anorexia, and abdominal bloating.
   - Vomiting, weight loss, early satiety, hematemesis, melena, hematochezia; change in intensity, quality, radiation, rhythmicity, or periodicity; may indicate complicated PUD.
   - Complications include bleeding, perforation, penetration, and obstruction.
   - Physical examination findings may disclose epigastric tenderness.
   - Rigid, board-like abdomen and rebound tenderness—suggestive of perforation; pallor, weakness, dyspnea, orthostatic changes—suggestive of bleeding; abdominal distention with positive "succussion" splash—suggestive of gastric outlet obstruction; change in quality and radiation of pain to the back may indicate penetration.

4. **Diagnostic Studies**
   - Upper endoscopy provides optimal visualization and opportunity for biopsy, and is a procedure of choice.
   - Barium esophagography limited due to poor visualization of ulcers hidden in duodenal folds and inability to differentiate between benign or malignant ulcers. When used to screen uncomplicated

dyspepsia, follow-up endoscopy should be performed.
- Tests to diagnose *H. pylori* include endoscopic gastric mucosal biopsy for rapid urease testing and histology, noninvasive urease breath test, and serology.
- Laboratory studies—usually normal in uncomplicated PUD.

5. **Management**
- Pharmacotherapy directed at reduction of acid secretion, preserving mucosa defenses, and eradication of *H. pylori* infection.
- Proton pump inhibitors inactivate acid-secreting enzymes.
- Proton pump inhibitors are currently the treatment of choice for PUD, given their high safety and efficacy profile.
- H_2-receptor antagonists bind to H_2 receptors on gastric parietal cells and inhibit cyclic adenosine monophosphate and acid secretion.
- Sucralfate, bismuth, antacids, and prostaglandin analogs enhance mucosal barrier defenses and promote ulcer healing.
- Combination antibiotic regimes with bismuth or proton pump inhibitors are most effective in eradication of *H. pylori* and decrease the incidence of antibiotic resistance associated with monotherapy.
- Regular, well-balanced diets.
- Discontinuation of smoking increases the rate of healing.

B. **Erosive and Hemorrhagic Gastritis**
1. **Etiology**
- Commonly associated with stress seen in critically ill, hospitalized patients; patients taking medications such as aspirin and NSAIDs, and heavy alcohol consumption.
- Also associated with portal hypertension and, less commonly, radiation, ingestion of caustic agents, drugs such as potassium chloride, iron supplements.

2. **Pathology**
- Characterized by superficial inflammation and erosions of gastric mucosa without penetration into the submucosa and muscularis.
- Multiple factors implicated in the development of gastritis include hypersecretion of acid, diminished mucus secretion, epithelial growth, tissue mediators, decreased intramucosal pH, and intramucosal energy deficits.

3. **Clinical Features**
- Usually asymptomatic.
- When symptomatic, hematemesis and melena are often the presenting symptoms, indicating upper GI bleeding.
- Bleeding—usually minimal and results in <5% of upper GI bleeding.

- Associated symptoms may include anorexia, nausea, vomiting, and dyspepsia.

4. **Diagnostic Studies**
- Upper endoscopy discloses classic mucosal erythema, subepithelial hemorrhages, and erosions.

5. **Management**
- Pharmacologic prophylaxis for patients at high risk for stress-related gastritis including trauma, burns, sepsis, coagulopathy, respiratory failure, central nervous system injury, liver, and renal failure.
- Prophylactic agents such as IV proton pump inhibitors, sucralfate, or H_2-receptor antagonists given routinely to high-risk patients have been shown to reduce incidence of significant bleeding by 50%.
- Discontinuation of NSAIDs, aspirin, and alcohol.
- Reduction of portal hypertension.

C. **Malabsorption**
1. **Etiology**
- Comprises multiple disease entities.
- May result from pancreatic enzyme deficiency, pancreatic enzyme inactivation, primary mucosal disease, celiac disease, extensive intestinal resections, defective bile formation, disruptive enterohepatic circulation, ingestion of nutrient-binding agents, bacterial overgrowth, and lymphatic obstruction.

2. **Pathogenesis**
- Impaired intraluminal digestion prevents adequate digestion of dietary fats, proteins, and carbohydrates as seen in pancreatic insufficiency and liver and biliary tract disorders.
- Disruption of the intestinal mucosal function due to inadequate absorptive surface area as seen in short-bowel syndrome; primary mucosal absorptive defects as in Crohn disease, tropical sprue, and celiac disease; isolated brush border enzyme deficiency as seen in lactase deficiency, prevents fats, proteins, amino acids, and specific nutrients from being absorbed.

3. **Clinical Features**
- Symptoms vary depending on etiology, pathogenesis, severity, location, and length of intestines involved. Celiac disease may be more common than previously thought. Peak incidence in adults aged between 40 and 50 years, more common in women than in men.
- Diarrhea may reflect increased secretion and decreased absorption of water and electrolytes; malabsorption of fatty acids and bile salts.
- Steatorrhea reflects malabsorption of fats.
- Weight loss, malnutrition, and weakness reflect malabsorption of fats, proteins, and carbohydrates.
- Anemia may reflect defects in absorption of iron, vitamin B_{12}, or folic acid.

- Paresthesia, tetany, and bone pain may denote malabsorption of calcium, vitamin D, and magnesium.
- Muscle cramps and weakness may reflect excess potassium loss.
- Bleeding tendency may reflect malabsorption of vitamin K–dependent coagulation factors.
- Edema and muscle wasting reflect hypoalbuminemia secondary to malabsorption of protein.
- Classical presentation of celiac disease is malabsorption and failure of infants to thrive after cereal is added to their diet. In adults, more nonspecific symptoms such as fatigue, iron deficiency anemia, change in bowel habits, infertility, and bone weakness may be presenting signs or symptoms.

4. **Diagnostic Studies**
- Routine studies for suspected malabsorption—CBC, serum iron, vitamin B_{12} and folate levels, serum calcium, alkaline phosphatase (ALK-P), albumin, β-carotene, and PT. For celiac disease, findings include positive serology of tissue transglutaminase or antiendomysial antibody tests with distal duodenal biopsy for confirmation.
- Specific studies—Sudan stain for fecal fat (falsely negative in 25%); excretion of 10 g per day of fat by way of quantitative 72-hour stool collection is a more sensitive means of detecting fat malabsorption.
- Several serologic studies to detect antibodies are useful in screening for sprue, although mucosal biopsies of distal duodenum or proximal jejunum remain the standard for the diagnosis of celiac sprue.
- Hydrogen breath test—readily available for the diagnosis of lactase deficiency.
- Normal D-xylose test—suggests pancreatic insufficiency, reduced bile salts, and lymphatic obstruction.
- Elevated serum amylase and lipase—indicate pancreatic insufficiency; response to pancreatic enzyme supplementation by an N-benzoyl-L-tyrosyl-p-aminobenzoic acid test or secretin stimulation test is confirmatory.
- Plain films or computed tomography (CT) scan of abdomen may disclose calcification of the pancreas.
- Endoscopic retrograde cholangiopancreatography may show dilated ducts, intraductal stones, strictures, or pseudocyst.

5. **Management**
- Treatment—dependent on etiology of the malabsorption.
- Dietary restriction of gluten—essential in the treatment of celiac disease; restriction of lactose-containing products dramatically decreases symptoms associated with lactase deficiency.

- Malabsorption secondary to short-bowel syndrome may require supplementation with enteral supplements, total parenteral nutrition (TPN), parenteral vitamins, and lactose restriction.
- Antidiarrheal may reduce episodes of diarrhea.
- Malabsorption secondary to chronic pancreatic disease requires supplementation with pancreatic enzymes and concurrent bicarbonate administration; H_2-receptor antagonists or protein pump inhibitors reduce steatorrhea by decreasing acid and uninhibiting the activity of lipase.

D. **Irritable Bowel Syndrome**
1. **Etiology**
- Chronic functional intestinal disorder characterized by abdominal pain, altered bowel habits not related to a detectable organic pathology.
- Symptoms typically begin in late teens or early 20s.
- More common in women than in men.

2. **Pathology**
- Multiple pathophysiologic mechanisms have been identified—dysmotility, heightened visceral nociception, and psychosocial disorders.

3. **Clinical Features**
- Symptoms should be present 3 to 6 months before diagnosis is considered.
- Abdominal pain may be characterized as intermittent, crampy, sharp, burning, often localized to one quadrant—usually the lower left quadrant, typically nonradiating, often aggravated by stress and worse 1 to 2 hours after meals, not interfering with sleep, often relieved by defecation.
- Constipation, diarrhea, or more often alternating constipation and diarrhea.
- Characteristic stool patterns—first morning stool is usually normal followed by frequent episodes of increasingly loose stool; formed pencil-sized hard pellet stools reflect rectosigmoid spasms.
- Explosive defecation is seen in 20% of patients with irritable bowel syndrome (IBS).
- Mucus may cover stools or pass separately.
- Abdominal bloating and flatulence.
- Physical examination may disclose mild lower abdominal tenderness.
- Presence of hematochezia, weight loss, fever, and nocturnal diarrhea—inconsistent with IBS—warranting further investigation.

4. **Diagnostic Studies**
- CBC, serologic test, serum albumin, erythrocyte sedimentation rate (ESR), and stool for occult blood are normal in patients with IBS.
- When diarrhea predominates thyroid functions, stool for ova and parasites, 24-hour stool collection is warranted.
- Patients younger than 40 years—consider flexible sigmoidoscopy; those older than 50 years not evaluated previously—consider barium enema or colonoscopy.

5. **Management**
- Patient reassurance, education on the functional and chronic nature of the disease process is essential.
- Daily record of specific food intake, concurrent psychosocial stressors, along with symptoms, may be helpful for some patients.
- Foods found to provoke symptoms should be avoided. Common flatulogenic foods—brown beans, cabbage, Brussels sprouts, raisins, coffee, red wine, and beer.
- Trial of high-fiber diet.
- Pharmacotherapy targeted at specific symptoms reserved for refractory cases.
- Antispasmodic agents—dicyclomine given 30 to 60 minutes before meals may relieve postprandial bloating, loperamide for diarrhea, lubiprostone 8 μg BID for females older than 18 years, an intestinal chloride channel activator, or polyethylene glycol 3350 may benefit constipation refractory to fiber supplementation. Probiotics may reduce IBS symptoms.
- Psychotropic agents—amitriptyline may be helpful in patients with intractable pain.
- Behavioral modification, biofeedback, and hypnotherapy benefit some patients.

E. **Antibiotic-Associated Colitis**
1. **Etiology**
- Diarrhea related to antibiotic use. Common culprits—ampicillin, clindamycin, tetracycline, and cephalosporins.
2. **Pathogenesis**
- Diarrhea is often mild, dose related, and rarely occurring up to 3 weeks after discontinuation of antibiotic and is more often resolving after discontinuation of antibiotic.
- Significant diarrhea almost always caused by intestinal proliferation of *Clostridium difficile* and elaboration of its toxin.
3. **Clinical Features**
- Mild-to-moderate watery diarrhea.
- Crampy, lower abdominal pain.
- Profuse, watery, bloody diarrhea and fever may be seen in more severe cases.
- Complications—dehydration, electrolyte imbalance, toxic megacolon, perforation, and death.
4. **Diagnostic Studies**
- Demonstration of cytotoxin B in stool—definitive but takes 24 hours.
- Rapid enzyme-linked immunosorbent assays for both enterotoxin A and cytotoxin B are faster, but less sensitive.
- Cultures are expensive and timely, and do not differentiate from toxigenic strains.
- Fecal leukocytes may be seen in 50% of patients.
- Flexible sigmoidoscopy may disclose nonspecific inflammation; yellow adherent colonic plaques (pseudomembranes) may be noted in severe disease. Pseudomembranes localized in the proximal colon may be missed by sigmoidoscopy.
5. **Management**
- Discontinue antibiotics, if possible.
- Drug of choice for severe cases—metronidazole.
- Vancomycin is equally effective, more expensive, and associated with the development of antibiotic-resistant organisms.
- Multiple relapses consider tapering and pulsed antibiotic therapy.
- Twenty percent of patients may relapse within 1 to 2 weeks after discontinuation of therapy. Relapses respond well to second course of metronidazole or vancomycin.

F. **Crohn Disease**
1. **Etiology**
- Idiopathic chronic inflammatory bowel disease (IBD) of unknown etiology.
- More common in Caucasians than African Americans and Asians.
- Men and women are affected equally.
- Peak incidence between the ages of 15 and 35.
- Evidence suggests some familial basis along with environmental component.
2. **Pathogenesis**
- Transmural inflammatory process involving any area of the GI tract from the mouth to the anus, most commonly affecting the terminal ileum.
- Characterized by exacerbations and periods of remission.
- Chronic inflammation results in ulceration, stricture, fistula, and abscess formation.
3. **Clinical Features**
- Symptoms and signs are dependent on the site and severity of inflammation.
- Low-grade fever, malaise, weight loss, and generalized fatigability.
- Abdominal pain may be steady, localized to the right lower quadrant.
- Usually nonbloody diarrhea.
- Associated perianal fissures, fistulas, and abscesses.
- Extraintestinal infestations—oral aphthous ulcers, erythema nodosum, pyoderma gangrenosum, episcleritis, iritis, uveitis, nondeforming arthritis, pericholangitis, and sclerosing cholangitis.
- Extensive ileal disease results in malabsorption of bile salts, increasing incidence of gallstones, steatorrhea, deficiency in fat-soluble vitamins, and increased colonic oxalate absorption increasing the incidence of nephrolithiasis.
- Anemia of chronic disease, iron deficiency, and vitamin B_{12} or, rarely, folate deficiency.
- Increase in colon cancer has been noted in the presence of colonic disease.
- Physical findings may show right lower quadrant tenderness with palpable mass. Other findings

vary depending on severity of involvement and degree of inflammation.

4. **Diagnostic Studies**
   - Laboratory findings correlate poorly with patient's clinical status.
   - CBC may disclose anemia, leukocytosis; serum albumin may show hypoalbuminemia secondary to intestinal protein loss or malabsorption; ESR or C-reactive protein may be elevated during active inflammation.
   - Stool for occult blood, white blood cells (WBCs), culture, ova and parasites, and *C. difficile* toxin.
   - Upper GI series with small bowel follow-through may show ulcerations, strictures, or fistulas.
   - Colonoscopy to evaluate colonic disease. Colonoscopy allows for mucosal biopsies and may disclose ulcers, alternating with area of normal mucosa, giving the mucosa a cobblestone appearance and rectal sparing.
   - CT scanning may distinguish thickened, matted bowel loops, intra-abdominal abscess.
   - Presence of granulomas on biopsy—highly suggestive of Crohn disease.

5. **Management**
   - Well-balanced diet, high-fiber supplementation is helpful in patients with mainly colonic involvement, patients with obstructive symptoms do best with low-roughage diet, and a trial lactose-free diet is helpful because lactose deficiency is common.
   - Four-week course of enteral therapy may induce remissions; TPN may be required in the presence of severe malnutrition or preoperatively to improve nutritional status.
   - Pharmacotherapy includes antispasmodics and antidiarrheals for symptomatic relief; 5-acetylsalicylic acid (5-ASA) agents—sulfasalazine may improve active disease in patients with primarily colonic involvement, but is of limited value in patients with small intestinal disease; corticosteroids are effective in suppressing both small- and large-bowel inflammation, serious side effects often limit their use; mercaptopurine (6-MP) indicated in patients with unresponsive disease, chronic steroid use, or symptomatic fistulas. Patients on 6-MP require weekly CBCs to evaluate for neutropenia. Tumor necrosis factor inhibitors adalimumab, certolizumab, and infliximab IV infusion promote rapid symptom improvement in patients unresponsive to other therapies and those with fistula disease.
   - Indications for surgery—intractability, abscess, stricture, and severe bleeding.

G. Ulcerative Colitis
1. **Etiology**
   - Idiopathic chronic IBD of unknown etiology.
   - Occurs in all age groups with peaks in both the third and the seventh decades.
   - More common and may be more severe in non-smokers and former smokers.

2. **Pathogenesis**
   - Inflammation of mucosal surface of the colon and rectum resulting in erosions, friability, and bleeding.
   - Lesions typically involve the rectum and extend proximally in a continuous process.
   - Characterized by exacerbations and periods of remission.
   - Approximately 50% of patients have disease localized to the rectosigmoid colon; approximately 10% to 15% of patients have extensive pancolitis.

3. **Clinical Features**
   - Although the clinical picture is highly variable, certain clinical features appear to correlate with the extent of disease.
   - Disease may be classified as mild, moderate, and severe (Table 4-1).
   - Bloody diarrhea is hallmark.
   - Mucus and pus in stools.
   - Crampy abdominal pain.
   - Fecal urgency, constipation, and tenesmus with predominately rectal involvement.
   - Fever, weight loss, anemia, hypovolemia, and hypoalbuminemia in severe disease.
   - Extracolonic manifestations—erythema nodosum, pyoderma gangrenosum, episcleritis, thromboembolism, and oligoarticular nondeforming arthritis.
   - Complications—fulminant colitis, toxic megacolon; risk of colon cancer after 10 years increases from 0.5% to 1% per year.

4. **Diagnostic Studies**
   - Test of choice in evaluation of acute disease is sigmoidoscopy. Endoscopic findings—mucosal edema, friability, mucopus, and erosions.
   - Colonoscopy should not be performed during acute severe illness because of the risk of bowel perforation. When symptoms improve, colonoscopy is useful to evaluate disease extent and cancer surveillance.
   - Plain film radiographs identify colonic dilation in acute severe disease.
   - Barium enemas are contraindicated in evaluation of acute disease and may precipitate toxic megacolon.
   - Low hemoglobin and hematocrit reflect anemia; elevated ESRs indicate inflammation; decreased albumin in the presence of protein loss indicates enteropathy.

5. **Management**
   - Regular diet, avoidance of caffeine and flatulogenic foods. Fiber supplementation decreases diarrhea and rectal symptoms. Antidiarrheals contraindicated during acute disease, but may be helpful in patients with mild chronic symptoms.

TABLE 4-1.   Spectrum of Clinical Severity of Ulcerative Colitis

Feature	Mild	Moderate	Severe or Fulminant
Bowel movements per day	≤5	>5	Hourly
Rectal bleeding	Intermittent	Usual	Continuous and severe
Weight loss	Minimal	<10 lb	10–20 lb
"Toxic" appearance	No	No	Yes
Fever	No	Perhaps	Yes
Tachycardia	No	Frequently	Yes
Abdominal tenderness	No	Frequently	Yes
Bowel sounds	Normal	Normal or increased	Reduced or silent
Anemia	No	Hematocrit >30	Hematocrit <25–30
Leukocytosis	No	Yes	Yes
Left shift	No	Yes	Yes
Albumin	Normal	Normal	Reduced
Bacteremia	No	Seldom	Frequently

From Yamada T, Hasler W. Inflammatory bowel disease. In: Kelly WN, ed. *Inflammatory Bowel Disease*. Philadelphia, PA: JB Lippincott Company; 1994:128, with permission.

- Goals of pharmacotherapy—symptomatic relief, suppression of inflammation, termination of acute exacerbation, and prevention of relapse.
- Acute disease—topical mesalamine rectal suppositories or enemas are the recommended treatment of choice for distal colitis. Topical corticosteroids are less effective. Systemic corticosteroids or immunosuppressive agents are recommended when topical therapy fails.
- Acute disease extending above the sigmoid colon—oral sulfasalazine and oral mesalamine are recommended.
- Failure to respond after a 2- to 3-week course of oral agent—consider an adjunctive 2-week trial of topical corticosteroid foam or enemas. Continued failure requires systemic corticosteroids. Cyclosporine, 4 mg/kg/day intravenously, improves 60-75% of patients with severe colitis who do not improve with 7-10 days of intravenous corticosteroids. Infliximab used as an outpatient when unresponsive to oral prednisone, oral 5-ASA and rectal medications should be considered before colectomy.
- Maintenance therapy with sulfasalazine, mesalamine, and olsalazine generally decreases relapse rate from 75% to 25%.
- Surgical therapy recommended in severe disease unresponsive to systemic corticosteroids.

H. Diverticular Disease

1. Etiology

- Herniations of colonic mucosa through the muscularis, typically at a site of least resistance, usually where the nutrient artery penetrates the muscularis. Diverticula vary in sizes and numbers and are most often located in sigmoid colon with approximately one-third present in proximal colon.
- Incidence increases with age. More than one-third of patients older than 60 years have diverticular disease.

2. Pathogenesis

- High prevalence in Western countries and low incidence in underdeveloped countries and vegetarians suggest a strong dietary influence in the pathogenic development.
- Diverticular disease believed to be secondary to long-term diet deficient in fiber.
- It is believed that decreased fecal bulk, narrowed, contracted bowel, and high intraluminal pressures to move along smaller hard fecal mass over time result in thickening, hypertrophy, and fibrosis of the colonic musculature and herniation of the colonic mucosa.
- Inherited weakness in colonic wall; intestinal dysmotility also may have a role in the development of diverticulosis.
- Hardened fecaliths within the diverticula may erode through the nutrient vessel, resulting in hemorrhage.
- Fecaliths, invasion of colonic bacteria may result in inflammation of the diverticular sac with subsequent microperforation, pericolic abscess, or generalized peritonitis.

3. Clinical Features

- Uncomplicated diverticulosis is most often asymptomatic. Nonspecific chronic constipation, alterations in bowel habits, and abdominal pain may be noted.
- Bleeding diverticulosis typically presents with an acute onset of painless, large-volume hematochezia.
- Bleeding complicates diverticulosis in 3% to 5% of the cases and is the most common cause of acute lower-GI bleeding.

- Diverticulitis presents as aching left lower quadrant abdominal pain, tenderness, and palpable mass; fever, nausea, vomiting, constipation, or loose stools. Hematochezia—rare; occult blood loss—common.

4. **Diagnostic Studies**
   - Plain films may be used to evaluate for free abdominal air.
   - CT scan of the abdomen and pelvis can be diagnostic as well as document the presence of an abscess and inflammation.
   - Colonoscopy and sigmoidoscopy (although contraindicated during acute diverticulitis) may be helpful in confirming presumptive diagnosis and excluding others.
   - Diverticular hemorrhage may be evaluated by colonoscopy after bleeding subsides. Continued active bleeding may be evaluated with 99mTc-labeled red blood scan, mesenteric angiography, and scintigraphy.

5. **Management**
   - Uncomplicated diverticulosis should be treated with high-fiber diet or fiber supplements.
   - Patients with mild diverticulitis may be treated as outpatients with low-residue diet, metronidazole, in addition to ciprofloxacin or trimethoprim–sulfamethoxazole.
   - Patients unresponsive to outpatient therapy require hospitalization, nothing by mouth, IV antibiotics.
   - Failure to respond within 72 hours necessitates surgical consultation.
   - Massive diverticular bleeding with hypovolemia requires emergent hospitalization, evaluation, and resuscitation.
   - Bleeding ceases spontaneously in 90% of patients.
   - Therapeutic options for unresponsive bleeding—surgery or intra-arterial vasopressin.

I. Vascular Ectasis (Angiodysplasia and Arteriovenous Malformations)

1. **Etiology**
   - Etiology unknown.
   - Associated with congenital disorders.
   - Hereditary hemorrhagic telangiectasis and scleroderma.
   - May result in acute or chronic upper- or lower GI bleeding.
   - Located throughout the GI tract, most commonly in the cecum and ascending colon.
   - One-fourth of patients older than 60 years have lower GI bleeding secondary to angiodysplasia.
   - Responsible for 5% to 10% cases of lower GI bleeding.

2. **Pathology**
   - Degenerative lesion consisting of distorted, dilated vessels lined with vascular endothelium.

3. **Clinical Features**
   - Hematochezia, typically massive, resolving spontaneously, often recurring.
   - Occult blood in chronic bleeds.
   - Iron-deficiency anemia.
   - Hematemesis and melena may be seen with upper GI tract involvement.

4. **Diagnostic Studies**
   - Panendoscopy and small bowel capsule endoscopy are the diagnostic studies to identify lesions in the colon, stomach, and duodenum.
   - Occasionally, laparotomy and intraoperative endoscopy of the small bowel are required to control bleeding.

5. **Management**
   - Chronic bleed—iron supplements, intermittent transfusions; hormonal therapy with estrogen and progesterone is currently under investigation.
   - Minor active bleeding lesions may be treated by way of endoscopic cauterization or laser therapy.
   - Severe active bleeding may require angiography with vasopressin to control bleeding.
   - Uncontrolled or recurrent bleeding may require right hemicolectomy.

III. Anorectal Disorders

A. Hemorrhoids

1. **Etiology**
   - Hemorrhoids are seen in 50% of persons older than 50 years and are uncommon in persons younger than 25 to 30 years.
   - Five percent of persons over age 50 have symptoms.
   - Hemorrhoids may become symptomatic secondary to increased systemic venous pressures as seen with pregnancy, prolonged sitting, straining, constipation, obesity, and increased portal pressure associated with congestive heart failure (CHF) and cirrhosis.

2. **Pathology**
   - Hemorrhoidal venous plexuses, along with arterial plexuses, smooth muscle, and connective tissue, comprise anal cushions that allow variable stool sizes to pass without damaging the rectal mucosa. Hemorrhoidal disease is believed to arise when the internal or external hemorrhoidal plexus enlarges, resulting in venous swelling and displacement of vascular anal cushions.
   - Enlargement and redundancy of anal cushions over time may result in protrusion or bleeding.

3. **Clinical Features**
   - Internal hemorrhoids—most often present with intermittent rectal bleeding described as painless bright red, seen on toilet paper, coating stool, or dispersed in toilet water following defecation.

- If occult bleeding occurs, massive bleeding is rare.
- Vague anal discomfort may be associated.
- Discomfort increases with progressive enlargement or prolapse through the anus.
- Prolapse can become chronic leading to soiling, mucoid anal discharge, pruritus ani, infection, thrombosis, and strangulation.
- Presence of rectal pain associated with internal hemorrhoids suggests complication and requires surgical consult.
- External hemorrhoids—covered by pain-sensitive skin most commonly manifest as perianal pain aggravated by defecation.
  - A tender anal mass may be palpated.
  - Thrombosis may be precipitated by coughing and heavy lifting, and result in a perianal hematoma.

4. **Diagnostic Studies**
   - Typically made on inspection, digital examination, and direct visualization by way of anoscope or proctoscope.
   - Proctosigmoidoscopy or colonoscopy should be performed in all patients with hematochezia, especially in the presence of anemia, to rule out disease proximal to the sigmoid colon.
   - Colonoscopy is preferred in patients older than 40 years with anemia.
   - External hemorrhoids appear as soft, painless mass outside the anal verge or when thrombosed firm, tender, bluish mass.
   - Internal hemorrhoids are typically not visible, but may protrude through the anus with straining.
   - Prolapsed hemorrhoids appear as purple nodules covered by mucosa.
   - Uncomplicated internal hemorrhoids on digital rectal examination are neither palpable nor tender.

5. **Management**
   - Often, hemorrhoidal symptoms, even associated with thrombosis, abate spontaneously within days to weeks.
   - Symptoms often recur.
   - Conservative therapy—high-fiber diet, increased fluid intake, warm sitz baths, and topical rectal hydrocortisone preparations for relief of pruritus and discomfort.
   - Analgesic rectal preparation or systemic analgesics are useful when pain is problematic.
   - Surgical referral—failure to respond to conservative treatment, debilitating pain, evidence of infection, strangulation, or ulceration.

B. **Anorectal Abscess and Fistulas**
   1. **Etiology**
      - Anorectal abscesses are more common in men.
      - Often result from a bacterial infection of anal glands and ducts.
      - Typical organisms isolated—*Staphylococcus aureus, Escherichia coli, Bacteroides, Proteus*, and *Streptococcus species*.
      - Most abscesses are located in the posterior rectal wall.
      - Most anorectal fistulas result from abscesses of the anal glands.
      - Some are not pyogenic in nature and are due to IBD, tuberculosis, diverticular, or neoplastic disease and trauma.
   2. **Pathology**
      - Abscesses are speculated to result when discharge from anal glands is inhibited due to anal muscle tone causing stasis, dilation, and eventual infection.
   3. **Clinical Features**
      - Anorectal abscess—sudden onset of throbbing perianal pain aggravated by sitting, coughing, defecating, and walking.
      - Draining abscess produces mucopurulent discharge and scant blood.
      - Fever, malaise, and chills may be present.
      - Complication—systemic and necrotizing infection.
      - Uncomplicated fistulas most commonly present with intermittent painful perianal swelling, followed by relief with onset of purulent discharge.
      - Tenesmus and painful defecation may occur with high intramuscular fistulas.
   4. **Diagnostic Studies**
      - Diagnosis is frequently made by inspection and digital rectal examination.
      - Anoscopy also allows for better visualization.
   5. **Management**
      - Surgical referral for incision and drainage.

IV. Disorders of the Liver and Pancreas

A. **Viral Hepatitis**
   1. **Etiology**
      - Hepatitis A virus (HAV), a ribonucleic acid (RNA) virus primarily transmitted by way of the oral-fecal route, typically by contamination of food or water.
        - Risk factors include poor sanitation; closed communities sharing toilet and eating facilities—schools, daycare facilities, or military bases; ingestion of raw, contaminated shellfish.
        - Children younger than 6 years in a household have been reported to be the most common source of infection in adults without other identifiable risk factors. Most likely because 70% of children with hepatitis A are asymptomatic.
        - Incubation period is 2 to 6 weeks—average 30 days.
        - Mortality rate is 0.1%, fulminant course uncommon, and carrier state and chronic disease absent.

- Hepatitis B virus (HBV) is a double-stranded DNA virus with eight different genotypes.
  - Transmitted by way of inoculation of infected blood or body fluids—transfusions, unprotected sexual intercourse, needle sharing, and in children, close personal contact in endemic areas through open cuts or sores.
  - High-risk populations include healthcare workers, men who have sex with men, and IV drug abusers.
  - Incubation period—6 weeks to 6 months.
  - Mortality rate—up to 60%; fulminant disease—less than 1%; chronic disease and cirrhosis occur in 3% to 5% of patients with hepatitis B.
  - Chronic hepatitis B has become more prevalent in the United States largely because of immigration from more endemic countries. Chronic HBV is defined as persons with a positive Hepatitis B surface antigen (HBsAg) for >6 months. They are at increased risk for developing cirrhosis and hepatocellular cancer.
- Hepatitis C virus (HCV) is a single-stranded RNA virus, transmitted by infected blood and body fluids with six major genotypes identified.
  - Approximately 50% of cases are related to IV drug use, 4% attributed to blood transfusions, 6% by sexual or household exposure, and 4% by way of occupational exposure to contaminated blood; in the remaining cases, the source is unclear.
  - Additional risk factors identified include intranasal cocaine use, hemodialysis and body piercing. Maternal-perinatal transmission is low.
  - Incubation period—6 to 7 weeks.
  - Mortality rate—1%, with chronic disease seen in approximately 50% of patients.
- Hepatitis D (delta agent) is defective RNA virus requiring assistance with hepatitis B, specifically the presence of HBsAg, to illicit infection.
- Hepatitis E virus is an RNA virus typically transmitted by the fecal-oral route, responsible for epidemic outbreaks in developing countries.
  - Incubation period—35 to 40 days; mortality rate—approximately 0.5%, with a mortality rate of 20% seen in pregnant women.
  - No carrier state exists.

2. **Pathogenesis**
   - The exact pathogenesis remains unclear and may be more a result of immunologic host response than direct cytopathic effect of the virus.
   - Histologic findings include focal liver necrosis, mononuclear infiltration, hyperplasia of Kupffer cells, and cholestasis.

3. **Clinical Features**
   - Variable ranging from asymptomatic disease, chronic progressive symptoms, fulminant disease, and death.
   - Prodromal phase (2 to 14 days) characterized by malaise, fatigue, migratory arthralgias, anorexia, coryza, low-grade fever, skin rash, right upper quadrant pain, pruritus, nausea, and abdominal fullness; loss of taste for cigarette smoking; amber-colored urine; acholic stools appear 1 to 4 days before the onset of jaundice. Hepatitis A is the only viral hepatitis causing spiking fevers.
   - Icteric stage often absent; peaks approximately during the second week, but may persist 6 to 8 weeks. Onset of jaundice typically signals clinical improvement.
   - Convalescent stage with improvement of appetite, resolution of jaundice, and abdominal pain.
   - Physical findings include hepatomegaly seen in 50% of patients; splenomegaly in 15%; posterior cervical and epitrochlear lymphadenopathy.
   - Sequelae—acute fulminant disease characterized by encephalopathy, coagulopathy, jaundice, edema, ascites, electrolyte abnormalities, asterixis, spasticity, hyperreflexia, fetor hepaticus. Chronic hepatitis characterized by a prolonged course (>3 to 6 months) of persistent elevated serum aminotransferase levels, with hepatic inflammation, necrosis, fibrosis, and eventual cirrhosis.
   - Hepatitis B and C viruses carry a high risk of hepatocellular cancer.

4. **Diagnostic Studies**
   - WBC count usually low or normal, with occasional predominance of large atypical lymphocytes.
   - Mild proteinuria and bilirubinuria.
   - Elevated aspartate aminotransferase (AST) and alanine aminotransferase (ALT).
   - Elevated bilirubin (Bil) and ALK-P.
   - Prolonged PT time, hypoalbuminemia, and elevated blood ammonia levels in severe or end-stage disease.
   - Serologic markers for hepatitis A–fecal HAV rarely present beyond the first week of illness. Immunoglobulin M (IgM) antibodies to HAV (anti-HAV) indicate acute hepatitis; immunoglobulin G (IgG) antibodies peak after 1 month and may persist for years; presence of IgG anti-HAV alone indicates previous exposure, noninfectivity, and future immunity.
   - Several serologic markers are associated with hepatitis B.
   - HBsAg indicates infection with HBV and denotes infectivity.
   - Antibody to HBsAg (anti-HBs) appears after the antigen is cleared and with successful immunization, signaling recovery from acute disease.
   - Serologic gap between the time HBsAg clears and antibody to the surface antigen (anti-HBs) becomes detectable is referred to as the window period.
   - IgM antibody to the HBV core (anti-HBc) may be the only marker detectable during the window period, indicating acute infection or relapse in chronic disease.

- IgG antibody to the HBV core also appears during acute infection, but persists indefinitely. IgG antibody in the presence of HBsAg indicates chronic infection and in the absence of HBsAg indicates recovery.
- Hepatitis B envelop antigen (HBeAg) appears shortly after HBsAg is detected, indicating viral replication and infectivity.
  - Persistence beyond 3 months suggests chronic disease.
  - Clearance of HBeAg followed by antibody to the HBV envelop (anti-HBe) denotes decreased replication and decreased infectivity.
- HBV DNA closely corresponds with the presence of HBeAg in serum, but is a more precise marker of infectivity and viral replication.
- Common serologic patterns and interpretation are listed in Table 4-2.
- Hepatitis D virus (HDV) may be diagnosed by detection of hepatitis D antigen, HDV antibody (anti-HDV), or HDV RNA in serum.
- HCV may be diagnosed by enzyme immunoassay detecting antibodies to HCV. Supplemental recombinant immunoblot assay is more sensitive and specific to confirm the diagnosis, or polymerase chain reaction to detect HCV RNA.
- Liver biopsy in patients with chronic disease evaluates the extent of hepatocellular damage. HCV FibroSURE test is a six biochemical marker blood test that correlates well with liver biopsy Metavir fibrosis scoring and necroinflammation and could be substituted for liver biopsy to minimize risks associated with biopsy.

5. **Management**
   - Treatment during the acute phase is primarily supportive—hydration, rest, restricted physical activity, high-calorie diet, avoidance of hepatotoxic drugs, and evaluation for complications. Treatment of acute hepatitis B is generally not required. Treatment of acute hepatitis C may benefit from interferon α or peginterferon, which may decrease the risk of chronic hepatitis. It may be more beneficial to use in cases where serum HCV RNA levels fail to clear after 3 to 4 months since 20% of patients with acute hepatitis C will clear the virus spontaneously.
   - Patients may return to work when jaundice resolves or when no longer too fatigued to sustain activity.
   - Follow-up LFTs and seromarkers until return to normal.
   - Treatment of fulminant hepatitis requires intensive care with maintenance of fluid balance, support of circulation and respiration, correct control bleeding and hypoglycemia, restriction of protein intake, and liver transplantation.
   - Chronic hepatitis C—use of a slow-release, long-acting interferon (peginterferon) injected weekly and nucleoside analog ribavirin pills taken daily in divided doses. Recent FDA-approved treatment includes the use of protease inhibitors either boceprevir or teleprevir capsules along with peginterferon and ribavirin.
   - Chronic hepatitis B—standard therapy remains interferon α or peginterferon. Peginterferon has replaced interferon α because of its longer half-life, requiring weekly injections. Other well-tolerated treatments include entecavir and tenofovir preferred as first-line drugs and lamivudine and telbivudine when short courses of treatment may be required because of their higher rate of resistance with long-term use.

TABLE 4-2.	Serologic Screening Tests for the Diagnosis of Acute Viral Hepatitis			
Anti-HAV IgM	**HBsAg**	**Anti-HBc IgM**	**Anti-HCV**	**Interpretation**
Positive	Negative	Negative	Negative	Acute hepatitis A
Positive	Positive	Negative	Negative	Acute hepatitis A in a chronic HBsAg carrier
Negative	Positive	Positive	Negative	Acute hepatitis B
Negative	Negative	Positive	Negative	Recent hepatitis B; "serologic window" between disappearance of HBsAg and appearance of anti-HBs
Negative	Negative	Negative	Positive or negative	Acute hepatitis C[a]
Negative	Positive	Negative	Negative or positive	Chronic HBsAg carrier[b] with a superimposed hepatitis (hepatitis C, delta[c], alcohol, or drug related); possible reactivation of HBV infection

[a]Positive test may be delayed for 2 to 4 weeks; current assays may not detect all cases.
[b]Minority of HBsAg carriers with active disease exhibit low-titer IgM anti-HBc.
[c]Reflex testing with antibody to delta virus is appropriate.
From Perillo RP, Regenstein FG. Viral and immune hepatitis. In: Kelly WN, ed. *Essentials of Internal Medicine.* Philadelphia, PA: JB Lippincott Company; 1994:822–833, with permission.

- General preventative guidelines—universal precaution when handling all blood and body fluids; strict attention to hand washing when in contact with contaminated linens, clothing, and eating utensils; careful screening of all donated blood; routine hepatitis screening for all pregnant women; careful disposal of all contaminated needles; and safe sexual practices.
- Immune globulin should be administered to all household personnel and close contacts of patients with hepatitis A. Vaccines are recommended for all patients living or traveling to endemic areas.
- Hepatitis B immunoglobulin (HBIG) may provide protection if given within 7 days of exposure.
  - Newborns of HBV-infected mothers should receive HBIG and HBV vaccine at delivery.
  - Subsequent HBV vaccine should be started.
  - Currently, universal vaccinations of all infants and children are recommended.

B. Cirrhosis

1. Etiology
- In the United States, alcohol abuse remains the leading cause of cirrhosis; other causes—viral hepatitis, chronic biliary obstruction, metabolic disorders, and chronic CHF.

2. Pathogenesis
- Irreversible liver destruction characterized by hepatocellular injury, fibrosis, and nodular regeneration.

3. Clinical Features
- Onset of symptoms is typically gradual, rarely abrupt.
- Weight loss, weakness, and fatigue are common.
- Abdominal discomfort.
- Anorexia, nausea, and vomiting are noted in advanced disease.
- Menstrual disorders, impotence, testicular atrophy, gynecomastia, loss of pubic and axillary hair, spider angiomas, and palmar erythema.
- Hepatomegaly, splenomegaly, jaundice, and bleeding esophageal varices result from portal hypertension.
- Late manifestations—coagulopathy, ascites, dilated superficial abdominal veins, peripheral edema, and pleural effusions.
- Hepatic encephalopathy characterized by alterations in consciousness, disruption in the sleep–awake cycle, asterixis, tremor, hyperreflexia, eventual coma, and death.

4. Diagnostic Studies
- WBC count may be low, normal, or elevated. Anemia, typically megaloblastic reflecting folate deficiency. Thrombocytopenia secondary from alcoholic bone marrow suppression, splenic sequestration, or sepsis. Elevated PT and PTT reflect inability of liver to produce clotting factors. Elevated Bil, AST, ALT, and ALK-P. Decreased serum albumin and increased γ-globulin.

- Ultrasound (U/S) discloses hepatomegaly, splenomegaly, liver nodularity, or atrophy.
- Upper endoscopy or barium swallow identifies esophageal varices.
- CT scan may delineate nodules consistent with hepatocellular carcinoma.
- Paracentesis in the presence of ascites.
- Liver biopsy identifies characteristic histologic features.

5. Management
- Vaccinate against hepatitis A.
- Screen for esophageal varices.
- Abstinence from alcohol is the most important aspect of therapy.
- Low in protein diet—1 to 1.5 g per kg.
- Sodium restriction, fluid restriction, and diuretics for ascites and edema.
- Avoidance of drugs metabolized in the liver.
- Multivitamins, folic acid, and iron supplements for anemia.
- Evaluate and treat complications.
- Evaluation for liver transplantation.

C. Acute and Chronic Pancreatitis

1. Etiology
- Causes of acute pancreatitis include alcohol ingestion, gallstones, trauma, metabolic diseases such as renal failure, infectious agents, cystic fibrosis, certain drugs, vasculitis, penetrating peptic ulcer, congenital anomaly, and conditions that result in obstruction of the ampulla of Vater such as Crohn disease.
- In the United States, the most common cause of chronic pancreatitis is alcoholism. Other causes include cystic fibrosis, severe malnutrition, pancreatic and duodenal cancer, hyperparathyroidism, ZE syndrome, trauma, hematochromatosis, postsurgery, enzyme deficiencies; frequently idiopathic.

2. Pathology
- Exact pathogenesis of acute pancreatitis is unclear.
- Thought to result from direct injury to the pancreatic acinar cells, possibly from reflux of bile into the pancreas.
- Activated pancreatic enzymes from damaged acinar cells leak into surrounding tissue, resulting in inflammation.
- Exact pathogenesis of chronic pancreatitis is unclear.
- Chronic inflammation results in progressive fibrosis and destruction of the pancreas.

3. Clinical Features
- Acute pancreatitis—sudden onset of epigastric pain, radiating to the back or sides; described as severe, constant, boring, aggravated by walking and lying supine, and relieved by leaning forward.
  - Associated symptoms include nausea and vomiting.

- Physical examination shows epigastric tenderness, abdominal distention, low-grade fever, decreased or absent bowel sounds with associated paralytic ileus, ascites, and mild jaundice.
- Inflamed pancreas is occasionally palpable.
- Tachycardia, pallor, hypotension, and shock may be noted.
- In severe necrotizing pancreatitis with hemoperitoneum, a bluish discoloration of the skin around the umbilicus (Cullen sign) and an ecchymotic discoloration of the flanks (Turner sign) from tissue catabolism of hemoglobin may be noted.
- Ten percent to 20% of patients have pulmonary findings including basilar rales and pleural effusion.
- Complications—acute renal failure, pancreatic infection or abscess, acute respiratory distress syndrome, pseudocysts, chronic pancreatitis (10% of patients), and diabetes mellitus (DM) rarely after single acute attack.
- Chronic pancreatitis—may present similar to acute pancreatitis.
  - Typically, with persistent epigastric pain referred to the upper left lumbar region associated with anorexia, nausea, vomiting, bowel changes, and weight loss; lasting hours to weeks.
  - Malabsorption symptoms or signs such as weight loss and steatorrhea also are common.
  - Physical findings are minimal, including low-grade fever and abdominal tenderness.
  - Complications—DM, pancreatic abscess, pseudocyst, common bile duct stricture, steatorrhea, malnutrition, PUD, and narcotic addiction.

4. **Diagnostic Studies**

   ACUTE AND CHRONIC PANCREATITIS
   - Elevated serum amylase and lipase greater than three times the upper limit of normal. Lipase is the most accurate enzyme for acute pancreatitis.
   - Leukocytosis (10,000 to 30,000 per μL) in acute pancreatitis.
   - Hyperglycemia, hypocalcemia, hyperbilirubinemia, hypertriglyceridemia, proteinuria, glycosuria, abnormal coagulation studies, elevated blood urea nitrogen, and serum ALK-P.
   - Pancreatic insufficiency suggested by excess fecal fat in stool and confirmed by response to pancreatic enzyme supplements or direct or indirect stimulation of pancreatic enzymes.
   - Plain films of the abdomen may show nonspecific findings including gallstones, "sentinel loop;" although normal in >50% of patients with pancreatitis.

- Upper GI series may identify thickened duodenal folds, displaced stomach suggestive of pancreatic mass.
- U/S may identify pancreatic edema, calcification, pseudocysts, and masses, and it permits visualization for biopsy.
- CT scan is excellent for detailed visualization of the pancreas and surrounding tissue. Dynamic bolus CT scan can identify areas of pancreatic necrosis. CT-guided biopsy of necrotic area may disclose infection or malignancy.

5. **Management**

   ACUTE PANCREATITIS
   - Often responds well to bed rest, restricted solid or liquid oral feeding, nasogastric suctioning for patients with ileus or severe pain, narcotics such as meperidine for pain control.
   - Diet may be advanced to clear liquids when pain or ileus resolves.
   - Surgical consult for all patients.
   - Severe acute disease may require large amounts of IV fluids, infusions of serum albumin, or fresh frozen plasma.
   - Monitor and treat complications.
   - Antibiotics for documented infection.

   CHRONIC PANCREATITIS
   - Management is directed at controlling pain and malabsorption.
   - Nonnarcotic drugs for pain relief, avoidance of alcohol and meals rich in fat, and pancreatic enzyme replacement.
   - Endoscopic U/S is the most sensitive study to detect structural changes in chronic pancreatitis.
   - Treat associated diabetes.
   - Surgery consult for possible surgical or endoscopic treatment of persistent draining.

SELECTED REFERENCES

Ayoub WS. *Treatment of Chronic Hepatitis B and Hepatitis C.* Wayne, PA: Turner White Communications Inc; 2007. Gastroenterology Board Review Manual. Vol. 13, Part 1.

Cheskin LJ. Constipation and diarrhea. In: Barker LR, Burton JR, Zieve PD, eds. *Principles of Ambulatory Medicine.* 4th ed. Baltimore, MD: Williams & Wilkins; 1995:476–491.

Cheskin LJ. Diverticular disease of the colon. In: Barker LR, Burton JR, Zieve PD, eds. *Principles of Ambulatory Medicine.* 4th ed. Baltimore, MD: Williams & Wilkins; 1995:499–502.

Cheskin LJ. Gastrointestinal bleeding. In: Barker LR, Burton JR, Zieve PD, eds. *Principles of Ambulatory Medicine.* 4th ed. Baltimore, MD: Williams & Wilkins; 1995:469–476.

Dienstag JL, Isselbacher KJ. Acute hepatitis. In: Isselbacher KJ, Braunwald E, Wilson JD, et al, eds. *Harrison's Principles of Internal Medicine.* 13th ed. New York, NY: McGraw-Hill Inc; 1994:1458–1477.

Dienstag JL, Isselbacher KJ. Chronic hepatitis. In: Isselbacher KJ, Braunwald E, Wilson JD, et al, eds. *Harrison's Principles of Internal Medicine.* 13th ed. New York, NY: McGraw-Hill Inc; 1994:1478–1483. http://dynaweb.ebscohost.com/

Friedman LS. Liver, biliary, & pancreas. In: Tierny LM, McPhee SJ, Papadakis MA, eds. *Current Medical Diagnosis and Treatment*. 46th ed. New York, NY: Lange Medical Books, McGraw-Hill; 2007.

Glickman RM. Inflammatory bowel disease. In: Isselbacher KJ, Braunwald E, Wilson JD, et al, eds. *Harrison's Principles of Internal Medicine*. 13th ed. New York, NY: McGraw-Hill Inc; 1994:1403–1416.

Goyal RK. Diseases of the esophagus. In: Isselbacher KJ, Braunwald E, Wilson JD, et al, eds. *Harrison's Principles of Internal Medicine*. 13th ed. New York, NY: McGraw-Hill Inc; 1994:1355–1363.

Greenberger NJ, Isselbacher KJ. Disorders of absorption. In: Isselbacher KJ, Braunwald E, Wilson JD, et al, eds. *Harrison's Principles of Internal Medicine*. 13th ed. New York, NY: McGraw-Hill Inc; 1994:1386–1403.

Greenberger NJ, Toskes PP, Isselbacher KJ. Acute and chronic pancreatitis. In: Isselbacher KJ, Braunwald E, Wilson JD, et al, eds. *Harrison's Principles of Internal Medicine*. 13th ed. New York, NY: McGraw-Hill Inc; 1994:1520–1532.

Huether SE. Structure and function of the digestive tract. In: McCance KL, Huether SE, Brashers VL, et al, eds. *Pathophysiology: The Biologic Basis for Disease in Adults and Children*. 6th ed. Canada: Mobs Inc; 2010.

Katz PO. Disorders of the esophagus. In: Barker LR, Burton JR, Zieve PD, eds. *Principles of Ambulatory Medicine*. 4th ed. Baltimore, MD: Williams & Wilkins; 1995:435–446.

Katz PO. Peptic ulcer disease. In: Barker LR, Burton JR, Zieve PD, eds. *Principles of Ambulatory Medicine*. 4th ed. Baltimore, MD: Williams & Wilkins; 1995:456–468.

Kimmey MB, Silverstein FE. Gastrointestinal endoscopy. In: Isselbacher KJ, Braunwald E, Wilson JD, et al, eds. *Harrison's Principles of Internal Medicine*. 13th ed. New York, NY: McGraw-Hill Inc; 1994:1350–1355.

LaMont JT, Isselbacher KJ. Diseases of the small and large intestine. In: Isselbacher KJ, Braunwald E, Wilson JD, et al, eds. *Harrison's Principles of Internal Medicine*. 13th ed. New York, NY: McGraw-Hill Inc; 1994:1417–1424.

Lingappa VR. Gastrointestinal disease. In: McPhee SJ, Lingappa VR, Ganong WF, et al, eds. *Pathophysiology of Disease: An Introduction to Clinical Medicine*. 1st ed. Stamford, CT: Appleton & Lange; 1995:215–244.

Lingappa VR. Liver disease. In: McPhee SJ, Lingappa VR, Ganong WF, et al, eds. *Pathophysiology of Disease: An Introduction to Clinical Medicine*. 1st ed. Stamford, CT: Appleton & Lange; 1995:245–277.

Lok ASF, McMahon BJ. AASLD practice guidelines chronic hepatitis B: update 2009. *Hepatology*. 2009;50:661–662, 1–38.

Loyd RA, McClellan DA. Update on the evaluation and management of functional dyspepsia. *Am Fam Physician*. 2011;83(5):547–552.

McGuigan JE. Peptic ulcer and gastritis. In: Isselbacher KJ, Braunwald E, Wilson JD, et al, eds. *Harrison's Principles of Internal Medicine*. 13th ed. New York, NY: McGraw-Hill Inc; 1994:1363–1382.

McQuaid KR. Alimentary tract. In: Tierny LM, McPhee SJ, Papadakis MA, eds. *Current Medical Diagnosis and Treatment*. 46th ed. New York, NY: Lange Medical Books, McGraw-Hill; 2007.

McQuaid KR. Gastrointestinal disorders. In: Tierny LM, McPhee SJ, Papadakis MA, eds. *Current Medical Diagnosis and Treatment*. 50th ed. New York, NY: Lange Medical Books, McGraw-Hill; 2011.

Mezey E. Diseases of the liver. In: Barker LR, Burton JR, Zieve PD, eds. *Principles of Ambulatory Medicine*. 4th ed. Baltimore, MD: Williams & Wilkins; 1995:507–517.

Perillo RP, Regenstein FG. Viral and immune hepatitis. In: Kelly WN, ed. *Essentials of Internal Medicine*. Philadelphia, PA: JB Lippincott Company; 1994:822–833.

Podolsky DK, Isselbacher KJ. Alcohol-related liver disease and cirrhosis. In: Isselbacher KJ, Braunwald E, Wilson JD, et al, eds. *Harrison's Principles of Internal Medicine*. 13th ed. New York, NY: McGraw-Hill Inc; 1994:1483–1495.

Schuster MM. Abdominal pain. In: Barker LR, Burton JR, Zieve PD, eds. *Principles of Ambulatory Medicine*. 4th ed. Baltimore, MD: Williams & Wilkins; 1995:447–456.

Schuster MM. Irritable bowel syndrome. In: Barker LR, Burton JR, Zieve PD, eds. *Principles of Ambulatory Medicine*. 4th ed. Baltimore, MD: Williams & Wilkins; 1995:492–499.

Smith GW. Benign conditions of the anus and rectum. In: Barker LR, Burton JR, Zieve PD, eds. *Principles of Ambulatory Medicine*. 4th ed. Baltimore, MD: Williams & Wilkins; 1995:1347–1361.

Tierny LM, McPhee SJ, Papadakis MA, eds. *Current Medical Diagnosis and Treatment*. 42nd ed. New York, NY: Lange Medical Books, McGraw-Hill; 2003.

Toskes PP, Greenberger NJ. Approach to the patient with pancreatic disease. In: Isselbacher KJ, Braunwald E, Wilson JD, et al, eds. *Harrison's Principles of Internal Medicine*. 13th ed. New York, NY: McGraw-Hill Inc; 1994:1516–1520.

Tran TT. Audio-digest gastroenterology. In: *Diseases of the Liver Vaccines for the Prevention and Treatment of Liver Disease*. 17(2), February 2003.

Yamada T, Hasler W. Inflammatory bowel disease. In: Kelly WN, ed. *Inflammatory Bowel Disease*. Philadelphia, PA: JB Lippincott Company; 1994:124–128.

Behavioral Disorders

M. Rebecca Buckley • Anthony S. Zaza

This chapter is not an exhaustive review of the extensive array of behavioral and mental health disorders that may present across all populations and various demographics of individuals. Rather, the selection of clinical disorders was based on those which the physician assistant may most likely encounter during the course of his or her practice. The summaries of the disorders are meant as quick synopses of the disorder in question, differential diagnoses, common symptomatology, and potential treatment considerations. As with all areas of medical and psychiatric practice, providers are advised to consult with their colleagues and specialty-specific professionals for additional guidance when the possibility of several different diagnostic and subsequent treatment pathways exists.

Be advised that the most recent data and available information have been gleaned from the clinical literature on these disorders. However, changes and updates in prevalence rates and other statistical considerations are continuous and ongoing. Such recent changes are ongoing, therefore recent changes may not be reflected in this chapter at this time. In addition, we expect that the *Diagnostic and Statistical Manual of Mental Disorders* (Fifth Edition) (*DSM-V*) will be published in 2013 and will certainly include changes in the classification of mental disorders.

I. Childhood Disorders

A. Autism

1. Definition

- Autism is one of a complex set of pervasive developmental disorders (PDDs) which cause significant functional difficulties in a child's (and if not arrested and treated, potentially an adult's) social interactions and communication. It manifests itself differently across a "spectrum" of other developmental disorders that include Asperger syndrome and atypical (nonspecific) PDDs. Autism most typically presents during the early childhood developmental years, but may also evidence in later childhood.

2. Etiology

- Although not completely certain, a combination of biologic factors including prenatal viral exposure, immune system abnormality, and/or genetic factors are involved.
- The current prevalence of the autism spectrum disorders (ASDs) as estimated by sources such as

the Centers for Disease Control and the National Institute of Mental Health (NIMH) is 1 in 110 below the age of 8. The latter represents a potential increase of up to 57% since previous findings in 2002 (i.e., 1 in 115). Other estimates have suggested somewhere around 5 and 20 of 10,000 children may demonstrate symptoms of autism or other PDD, with an average of approximately 14 of 10,000. The latest information suggests that boys tend to exhibit the disorder in the ratio of 4:1 compared with girls. It remains unclear whether discrepancies in reported statistics are a result of sampling methodology or whether the incidence of such disorders is increasing.

3. Clinical Features

- Clinical features of the disorder are typically evidenced between the ages of 12 and 24 months, generally with onset observed before 36 months.

PRIMARY SIGNS

- **Social interactions**—Infant or toddler: exhibits physical signs of significant emotional discomfort, if not detachment (i.e., may not cuddle or respond to affection and touching; may not make eye contact).
- **Communication difficulties**—Typically demonstrates language difficulties (i.e., appears to be unable to communicate or has ability to communicate, but fails to communicate with others across a variety of settings, such as home, school, and social environments).
- **Repetitive behaviors**—May engage in repetitive, self-stimulating behavior (i.e., repetitive face scratching, head rubbing, and other behavioral tics/movements).
- May exhibit impulsivity.

OTHER SIGNS AND SYMPTOMS

- *Persistent failure* to develop sufficient and appropriate mutual social relationships in many, if not most, interactions and social situations.
- Failure to show preference for parents over other adults.
- Failure to develop friendships with other children.
- May exhibit an exquisite, if not unusual, sensitivity (even possibly extreme responses) to various visual, auditory, and olfactory stimuli, and either an

avoidance or a preoccupation with such (e.g., child overreacts when fire alarm or school bell rings).

- May also express exquisite tactile sensitivity to certain food.
- May form unusual attachments to ordinary objects (e.g., paper or rubber bands).
- Possible spinning and repetitive body movements (e.g., arm flapping).
- Extreme cases may include evidence of potential self-injurious or even self-destructive behavior.
- May experience eating and toileting problems.
- In addition to sensory difficulties (i.e., sensitivity to stimuli), may also exhibit mild signs of possible mental retardation, as well as episodic seizure activity.

4. Diagnostic Studies

- Multidisciplinary team evaluation as possible (psychiatrist, psychologist, neurologist, speech pathologist, pediatrician, etc.). Evaluations to include structured psychiatric interview, and as possible psychological/neuropsychological testing, neurologic and speech evaluations.
- Extensive family and social history.
- Physical examination.

5. Management/Treatments

- Referral to child psychiatrist, psychologist, or neuropsychologist to establish accurate autism diagnosis and degree of severity, and to determine appropriate interventions, including intensive multidisciplinary learning support (LS) services. Behavior therapy and school-based interventions/options.
- **Pharmacotherapy**—plays a minor role at this stage and used only for specific symptoms (e.g., atypical antipsychotics for aggression and stimulants for comorbid attention-deficit/hyperactivity disorder [ADHD]).
- Resources and supports for family.

B. Conduct Disorders

1. Definition

- Conduct disorders include a group of behavioral and emotional problems in children and adolescents characterized by repetitive, disruptive, and persistent age-inappropriate patterns of behavior that violate the rights of others and/or grossly violate societal rules and boundaries.
- Children and adolescents with these disorders exhibit great difficulty perceiving, acknowledging, and abiding by socially acceptable rules of behavior and interaction.
- A minority of patients with this disorder may eventually develop an antisocial personality (ASP) disorder or develop substance abuse and/or other addictive disorders in adulthood if left untreated.
- Includes at least three of the following characteristics: Aggression toward people and/or animals; destruction of property/violation of property

rights of others; a pattern of deceitfulness; chronic and consistent violation of rules (imposed by adults such as parents or other formal agents).

- Such patterns of behavior cause significant impairment in social, academic, and occupational arenas of functioning and development.
- A minority of patients with this disorder may eventually develop an ASP disorder or develop substance abuse and/or other addictive disorders in adulthood, if left untreated.

2. Etiology

- Number of causal factors implicated, but no known single cause.
- ADHD, oppositional defiant disorder (ODD), or both often precede or coincide with the development of conduct disorder.

POTENTIAL CAUSAL INTERACTIVE FACTORS

- Temperament.
- Parenting style focused on problem behavior, ignoring good behavior, and indirectly reinforcing problem behavior.
- May include association with a delinquent peer group.
- Parental modeling of impulsivity and rule-breaking behavior.
- Genetic predisposition.
- May suggest and/or evidence low IQ or brain damage (especially in violent children/adolescents).
- Parental/marital conflict may exist in the home.
- Placement in institutional settings as infant or toddler (e.g., nonparental and nonfamilial custodial care) may coincide with such diagnoses.
- Poverty.
- It is estimated that 3% to 7% of boys have a higher prevalence rate of this disorder compared to girls.
- Conduct problems are usually referred to child and adolescent mental health professionals.

3. Clinical Features

- Persistent repetitive pattern of inappropriate behaviors that have the violation of the basic rights of others and/or age-appropriate rules of society as an essential feature.
- **Demonstrates at least three of the following:**
  - Stealing.
  - Persistent lying.
  - Property destruction of varying degrees (including vandalism).
  - Running away from home.
  - Violating curfew set by parents and caregivers.
  - Deliberate fire setting.
  - Repeated truancy (beginning before age 13).
  - Cruelty to animals.
  - "Bullying" behaviors (i.e., physical and verbal aggressive behavior with other children or adults).
  - Apparent lack of appropriate feelings of guilt or remorse, empathy for others, or feeling of

responsibility for own behavior, and/or feelings of "justified" aggressive behavior.

4. Diagnostic Determinations and Differentiation
- Reports from parent, child, and/or other social/community agents (e.g., teachers and coaches).
- **Rule out of common concurrent diagnosis, especially:**
  - ADHD.
  - Anxiety and mood disorders (depression, mania, and psychosis).
  - Substance abuse.
  - Developmental disorders (especially developmental reading and expressive language disorder).
  - Mental retardation.
  - Complex partial seizures (especially children with violent conduct disorders).

5. Management/Treatment
- Multimodal treatment approach that uses all available family and community resources provides best results.
- Individual psychotherapy.
- Behavior modification.
- Parental counseling.
- Environmental intervention, including special education programs and hospitalization, for severely aggressive presentations.
- Residential treatment as indicated.
- Legal assistance/intervention as necessary to enforce cooperation with treatment.
- **Psychopharmacologic intervention for aggressive behavior as follows:**
  - Central nervous system (CNS) stimulants (methylphenidate).
  - Antidepressants (including tricyclic antidepressants [TCA], such as desipramine).
  - Antihypertensives (clonidine).
  - Mood stabilizers.
  - Antipsychotics (Table 5-1).

C. Oppositional Defiant Disorder
1. Definition
- Milder form of chronic behavior problems than seen in conduct disorder.
- Children with ODD are at risk for developing a conduct disorder.
- Behavior problems are usually present as worse at home, but may extend to school and peers.

2. Etiology
- Although unknown with certainty, hypothesized factors may include inherited predisposition, modeling of parental oppositional and defiant behavior, and parental inability to reward good behavior or set firm, fair, and consistent limits.

- The literature suggests that base prevalence rates for ODD range from 1% to 16%, although a number of surveys estimate such to be 6% to 10% in nonclinical samples (i.e., gleaned from parental reports). More stringent sampling (which includes more strict impairment criteria) suggests that the rates are lower. Before puberty, the condition is more common in boys (i.e., 2:1 to 3:1 of boys over girls). After puberty, it tends to be almost exclusively identified in boys.
- The disorder usually manifests by age 8. ODD and other conduct problems are the most prominent reasons for referrals to outpatient and inpatient mental health clinics and treatment settings for children, accounting for at least 50% of all clinical referrals.

3. Clinical Features
- Chronic pattern of stubborn, negativistic, provocative, hostile, and defiant behavior. No typical violation of others' rights.
- Often irritable, resentful, and quick to take offense.
- Loss of temper.
- Frequent arguments with adults.
- Difficulty and outright refusal to follow directives.
- Tendency to blame others for his or her own inappropriate actions.
- Exhibiting a tendency toward vindictiveness when he or she perceives "injury" to sense of self.
- Symptoms tend to be more prominent as familiarity of the patient with others increases.

4. Diagnostic Studies
- Structured psychiatric interview.
- Critical parent and teacher reports. (**NOTE:** Behavior may not seem abnormal or evidence itself during a diagnostic interview.)
- Psychological testing to rule out low IQ or learning disabilities.

5. Management
- **Psychotherapy**—behavioral therapy, individual therapy, family counseling, and behavior modification.

D. Attention-Deficit/Hyperactivity Disorder
1. Definition
- A pattern of disordered behavior characterized by persistent hyperactivity, inattention, and/or distractibility.
- Symptoms typically are evidenced before age 7 and present for at least 6 months.
- To meet criteria for ADHD, these symptoms must occur *in more than one setting* (e.g., school and home for children, and work and home for adults).
- Behavior patterns and physical activity may appear "excessive" for what is considered age appropriate, the demands of the situation, and intelligence.

TABLE 5-1. Pharmacotherapeutics

Generic (Brand Name)	Maximum Daily Dose (mg)
Typical Antipsychotic Agents	
Chlorpromazine (Thorazine)	1,000
Thioridazine (Mellaril)	800[a]
Perphenazine (Trilafon)	64
Fluphenazine (Prolixin)	40 (10 mg/day IM)
Trifluoperazine (Stelazine)	40
Thiothixene (Navane)	60
Haloperidol (Haldol)	100
Molindone (Moban)	225
Atypical Antipsychotic Agents	
Clozapine (Clozaril)	900[a]
Olanzapine (Zyprexa)	20[a]
Quetiapine (IR , XR)	800[a]
Risperidone (Risperdal)	16[a]
Ziprasidone (Geodon)	80 mg BID[a]
Aripiprazole (Ability)	30[a]
Paliperidone (Invega)	12[a]
Mood Stabilizers	
Lithium	1,800[a]
Valproic acid (Depakote, Depakene)	60 mg/kg/day[a]
Carbamazepine (Tegretol)	1,600[a]
Lamotrigine (Lamictal)	200[a]
Sedatives and Hypnotics	
Chloral hydrate (Noctec)	200 (rarely used)
Flurazepam (Dalmane)	30 (rarely used)
Zolpidem (Ambien)	10
Temazepam (Restoril)	30
Estazolam (Prosom)	2
Eszopiclone (Lunesta)	2
Ramelteon (Rozerem)	8
Antianxiety Agents and Benzodiazepines	
Alprazolam (Xanax)	4
Chlordiazepoxide (Librium)	100–300 for alcohol withdrawal
Clonazepam (Klonopin)	20
Clorazepate (Tranxene)	90
Diazepam (Valium)	40
Lorazepam (Ativan)	10
Oxazepam (Serax)	120
Hydroxyzine HCl (Atarax/Vistaril)	600
Buspirone (BuSpar)	60
Diphenhydramine (Benadryl)	400
TCA/Other	
Amitriptyline (Elavil)	300[a]
Clomipramine (Anafranil)	250[a]
Doxepin (Sinequan)	300[a]
Imipramine (Tofranil)	300[a]
Amoxapine (Asendin)	400[a]
Desipramine (Norpramin)	300[a]
Nortriptyline (Pamelor)	150[a]
Maprotiline (Ludiomil)	225[a]
Trazodone (Desyrel)	600[a]
Mirtazapine (Remeron)	45[a]
SSRIs	
Fluoxetine (Prozac)	80[a]
Sertraline (Zoloft)	200[a]
Paroxetine (Paxil)	40[a]
Citalopram (Celexa)	60[a]
Escitalopram (Lexapro)	20[a]
Selective Norepinephrine Reuptake Inhibitors	
Bupropion (Wellbutrin, SR and XL, Zyban)	450
Venlafaxine (Effexor, XR)	225
Duloxetine (Cymbalta)	120
Desvenlafaxine (Pristiq)	50
Antiparkinsonian Drugs	
Trihexyphenidyl (Artane)	15
Diphenhydramine (Benadryl)	400 (also used in adjunct with neuroleptics for EPSs)
Benztropine (Cogentin)	6 (also used in adjunct with neuroleptics for EPSs)
Carbidopa/levodopa (Sinemet)	200/2000
Amantadine (Symmetrel)	400
Alzheimer Drugs	
Memantine (Namenda)	20
Donepezil (Aricept)	10
Stimulants and Nonstimulants	
Methylphenidate HCl (Ritalin)	60[a]
Methylphenidate transdermal (Daytrana)	30[a]
Methylphenidate (Concerta)	72[a]
Lisdexamfetamine (Vyvanse)	70[a]
Dextroamphetamine sulfate (Dexedrine)	60[a]
Amphetamine (Adderall)	60[a]
Atomoxetine (Strattera)	100[a]
Drugs used in Chemical Dependency	
Acamprosate (Campral)	1998
Naltrexone (ReVia)	50

[a]Black Box Warnings.
Note: This list is not meant to be inclusive of all psychiatric medications. Doses will need to be adjusted for elderly persons, children (where indicated), and hepatic and renal function.

2. Etiology

- No clear etiology. Prevalence of approximately 3% to 7% incidence in school-aged children (*DSM-IV-TR*). However, some studies have estimated higher rates in community samples. Parental surveys suggest that 9.5% or 5.4 million children 4 to 17 years of age have ever been diagnosed with ADHD, as of 2007, suggesting an increase in parent-reported ADHD of 22% between 2003 and 2007.

- Boys (13.2%) were more likely than girls (5.6%) to have ever been diagnosed with ADHD.

3. **Clinical Features**
   - Must have *six or more* symptoms of *hyperactivity* or *inattention* for a reliable diagnosis. (**NOTE:** It is likely that the following difficulties present to children and individuals eventually diagnosed with attention-deficit disorder or ADHD, precisely because they have failed to pay attention to instructions, details, etc. initially, and consequently cannot recall or track such information or items when later called upon to do so.)

   INATTENTION
   - Difficulty following instructions.
   - Short attention span at work and play.
   - Does not appear to be listening.
   - May appear to be "daydreaming."
   - Loses things.
   - Makes careless mistakes.
   - Difficulty organizing.
   - Forgetful.
   - Avoids engaging in "effortful" mental activities, particularly when "not interested" (again, this may suggest an avoidance tactic when called upon to demonstrate something that he or she does not know what to do, given a lack of attention to instructions and directions initially).
   - Attention to an agent or an item is easily distracted by a competing stimulus (e.g., a child listening to a teacher may easily lose focus and quickly turn attention to a sound or visual image outside a nearby window).

   HYPERACTIVITY/IMPULSIVITY
   - Fidgety or restless.
   - Difficulty staying seated.
   - Difficulty waiting in lines or awaiting his or her turn.
   - Impulsive or intrusive speech.
   - Difficulty playing quietly.
   - Running about or climbing excessively in situations in which these activities are inappropriate.
   - Symptoms must be present often, but not necessarily all of the time or in every situation.
   - May display significant variability in symptom presentation across various environments and situations.
   - May display potentially dangerous, impulsive behavior episodically.
   - It is important to rule out age-appropriate behavior as well as other psychiatric disorders.

4. **Diagnostic Studies**
   - Structured psychiatric interview. Consider neuro-psychological assessment.

- Diagnosis based on specific criteria and ruling out of other causes of behavior.
- Cognitive testing is very useful in confirming inattention and impulsivity.

5. **Management**
   - Behavioral interventions at home and school, as well as the addition of pharmacologic treatment, have proved most beneficial in the treatment and management of ADHD.
   - School programs and LS systems designed to address this disorder.
   - Behavioral therapy.
   - Pharmacotherapy may include the following agents: Ensure there are no medical contraindications, such as cardiac arrhythmias or cardiac congenital defects. No active addiction issues. The latest studies seem to show that there is more risk of drug use in patients who are not treated for their ADHD than those who are treated.
   - Methylphenidate, short acting and/or long acting.
   - Dextroamphetamine sulfate.
   - Atomoxetine (Strattera). Second-line agents: antidepressants and α agonists.

E. **Mental Retardation**
   1. **Definition**
      - Mental retardation is characterized by significantly subaverage general intellectual functioning (IQ below 70), with significant limitations in adaptive functioning and associated difficulties in a variety of skill domains, most typically involving communication, self-care, social/interpersonal skills, self-direction, academic skill acquisition, occupational, leisure, and safety concerns.
      - Accompanied by significant limitations in adaptive functioning.
      - Must manifest itself before age 18.

   2. **Etiology**
      - Etiology derives from genetic chromosomal and inherited conditions.
      - Prenatal exposure to infections and toxins may be implicated fetal alcohol syndrome (FAS)/fetal alcohol effect (FAE), as would be perinatal trauma (i.e., prematurity).
      - Severity of the mental retardation is related to the timing and duration of the trauma or its exposure to the CNS.
      - Genetic, environmental, biologic, and psychosocial factors appear to work additively in mental retardation.
      - Although mental retardation may be idiopathic in a number of instances, generally, the more severe the presentation of mental retardation, the more likely the basis for an individuals presentation has been identified (e.g., in 75% of individuals with severe mental retardation and 50% of individuals with mild mental retardation, the basis of such has been identified).

3. **Clinical Features**
   - Clinical features will be dependent on degree/severity of mental retardation and underlying cause.
   - IQ below 70. In infants, a clinical judgment of significantly subaverage age-appropriate intellectual functioning will assist with identification of mental retardation.
   - *Concurrent deficits in age-appropriate adaptive functioning* expected for his or her age and cultural group in at least two of the following areas:
     - Communication.
     - Self-care.
     - Home living.
     - Social/interpersonal skills.
     - Use of community resources.
     - Self-direction.
     - Functional academic skills.
     - Work.
     - Leisure.
     - Health.
     - Safety.
   - Varied physical examination presentations depending on underlying cause.
   - Craniofacial, skeletal, cardiovascular (CV), neurologic, and stature abnormalities may also present as markers in this disorder.
   - Associated psychiatric disorders may be three to four times as common in the retarded population as in the general population.

   DOWN SYNDROME
   - General hypotonia.
   - Oblique palpebral fissures.
   - Abundant neck skin.
   - Small, flattened skull.
   - Slanted eyes and flat nose.
   - High cheekbones.
   - Protruding tongue.
   - Broad, thick hands with short, inward-curving fingers.
   - Single palmar transversal crease.
   - Moro reflex—weak or absent.
   - Language function—weak.
   - Muted affect.

   FRAGILE X SYNDROME
   - Large, long head, and ears.
   - Short stature.
   - Hyperextensible joints.
   - Postpubertal macroorchidism.
   - Intellectual function declines in the pubertal period.
   - High rates of comorbid ADHD.

   PRADER–WILLI SYNDROME
   - Compulsive eating behavior.
   - Hyperphagia.
   - Obesity.
   - Hypogonadism.
   - Small stature.
   - Hypotonia.
   - Small hands and feet.

   CAT'S CRY (CRI-DU-CHAT) SYNDROME
   - Severely retarded.
   - Microcephaly.
   - Low-set ears.
   - Oblique palpebral fissures.
   - Hypertelorism.
   - Micrognathia.

   PHENYLKETONURIA
   - Hyperactive.
   - Erratic, unpredictable behavior—difficult to manage.
   - Eczema.
   - Vomiting.
   - Convulsions.
   - Temper tantrums.
   - Bizarre movements of bodies and upper extremities.
   - Twisting hand movements.
   - Verbal and nonverbal communication is usually severely impaired or nonexistent.
   - Poor coordination.
   - Perceptual difficulties.

4. **Diagnostic Studies**
   - Structured psychiatric interview.
   - Intelligence testing and psychological evaluation.
   - Hearing and speech evaluation.
   - History and physical examination.
   - Clinical observation.
   - Assessment of adaptive functioning (i.e., Vineland Adaptive Behavior Scales).
   - Urine and blood tests to rule out metabolic disorders.
   - Genetic evaluation/karyotyping.
   - Amniocentesis (during pregnancy).
   - Chorionic villi sampling (CVS).

5. **Management**
   PRIMARY, SECONDARY, AND TERTIARY ACTIONS
   - May assist in the prevention, if not alter the course of the disorder, as well as its eventual management.
   - **Primary—Actions to eliminate or reduce the conditions that lead to the development of the disorders associated with mental retardation may include the following:**
     - Genetic counseling.
     - Family counseling.
     - Proper prenatal and postnatal medical care.
     - Immunization.
   - **Secondary—Treatment to shorten the course of the illness:**
     - Early screening for and treatment of metabolic and endocrine disorders (e.g., phenylketonuria [PKU] and hypothyroidism).

- **Tertiary—Treatment to minimize the sequelae or consequent disabilities.**

PSYCHOTHERAPY
- Modified psychiatric treatment for specific disorders based on the child's level of intelligence.
- Individual psychotherapy or parental counseling to deal with developmental or situational crises, or in the treatment of coexisting psychiatric disorders.
- Parents may need assistance in dealing with their grief over having a "defective" child.
- Specific behavioral programs to teach adaptive behaviors and reduce stereotypic behaviors, aggression, and self-injury.

PHARMACOTHERAPY
- Same medications are used for treating psychiatric disorders in children and adolescents with normal IQs (i.e., stimulants for ADHD symptoms) (see Table 5-1).

ENVIRONMENTAL INTERVENTIONS
- Special education programs.
- Specialized infant stimulation and preschool programs.

CLASSIFICATION (IQ)
- Mild mental retardation (MR): IQ 50 to 55–70.
- Moderate MR: IQ 35 to 50–55.
- Severe MR: IQ 20 to 35–40.
- Profound MR: IQ below 20 or 25.

F. Eating Disorders

A. Anorexia Nervosa

1. Definition
- The three essential criteria for anorexia nervosa are self-induced starvation, relentless drive for thinness accompanied by a morbid fear of fatness, and the presence of medical signs and symptoms resulting from starvation.

2. Etiology, Epidemiology, and Comorbidity
- Biologic, social, and psychological factors.
- Midteens, most common age at onset.
- Forty percent of newly diagnosed cases are girls aged 15 to 19, and a significant incidence (i.e., up to 60% of cases) of young women aged 15 to 24.
- Only 30% of these cases are receiving mental health care.
- In the case of bulimia, only 6% are receiving direct treatment.
- Frequently seen in athletes and professions requiring thinness.
- Depression is seen in 65% of cases, and social phobia and obsessive–compulsive disorder (OCD) in 34% and 26%, respectively.
- The majority of individuals with severe eating disorders do not receive adequate care for them, given their initial avoidance of treatment for their conditions.

3. Screening Tools
- **SCOFF Questionnaire:**
  - Do you make yourself **S**ick because you feel uncomfortably full?
  - Do you worry you have lost **C**ontrol over how much you eat?
  - On average, have you lost over **O**ne pound per week during the past 3 months?
  - Do you believe yourself to be **F**at when others say you are too thin?
  - Would you say that **F**ood dominates your life?

4. Clinical Features
- Refusal to maintain body weight at or above a minimally normal weight for height, body mass index (BMI) <17.
- Intense fear of gaining weight even though underweight.
- Disturbance in perception of one's weight and shape and/or denial of the seriousness of current low weight.
- If postmenarchal, the absence of at least three consecutive menstrual cycles.
- May be restricting intake or binge eating/purging, or both. Behaviors include misuse of laxatives, enemas, diuretics, or other medications; excessive exercise; self-induced vomiting; and drinking excessive amounts of water.

5. Diagnostic Studies
- Full psychiatric and physical examination; vital signs (VS) may reveal hypotension and bradycardia, significant skin and hair changes.
- Complete blood count (CBC)—may show leukocytosis, leukopenia, or anemia.
- Electrolytes—hypokalemia.
- Thyroid-stimulating hormone (TSH)—hypothyroidism.
- Electrocardiogram (ECG)—ST segment and T-wave changes.
- Hypercholesterolemia.

6. Treatment
- Hospitalization, depending on patient's medical condition. Generally, inpatient hospitalization is required for <75% below expected body weight. Goal is to medical stabilize.
- **Psychotherapy**—Cognitive behavioral therapy (CBT) and family therapy.
- **Pharmacotherapy**—If underlying depression, treat with selective serotonin-reuptake inhibitors (SSRIs). Cyproheptadine (Periactin) and atypical antipsychotics may increase appetite.

B. Bulimia Nervosa

1. Definition
- Patients have the same fears and body image issues as with anorexia nervosa, but engage in compensatory purging behaviors.

2. **Etiology and Epidemiology**
   - Primarily the same as for anorexia nervosa.
   - May occur in later adolescence.
   - Major difference is that patient may be normal weight or overweight, or have a history of obesity.
3. **Clinical Features**
   - Recurrent episodes of binge eating characterized by eating within a 2-hour period, or eating more than most people would in a similar period, a sense of lack of control over eating during the episode.
   - Behaviors include misuse of laxatives, enemas, diuretics, or other medications; excessive exercise; self-induced vomiting; drinking excessive amounts of water; and fasting. Patients may present with gastrointestinal (GI) complaints of abdominal pain, constipation, or bloating.
   - Behaviors occur at least twice a week for 3 months.
4. **Diagnostic Studies**
   - Full psychiatric and physical examination; VS may reveal hypotension and bradycardia; examination of teeth may reveal pitting or erosion of tooth enamel; calluses may be present on finger used to induce vomiting.
   - Electrolytes—hypokalemia and hypomagnesemia.
   - Serum amylase—hyperamylasemia.
5. **Treatment**
   - **Psychotherapy**—CBT and family therapy.
   - **Pharmacotherapy**—As with anorexia nervosa, treat underlying mood disorders if present. Fluoxetine (Prozac) has been shown to be effective in doses ranging from 60 to 80 mg daily. TCAs have also been effective to reduce binge—purge cycle. These are to be used with caution in view of their increased risk of CV side effects, especially if electrolyte abnormalities are present.

II. Personality Disorders
A. Definition
- Personality disorders are patterns of affect and behavior characterized not only by their deviations from what are considered typical ranges seen within the general population, but especially by their pervasiveness, their enduring features, and their inflexibility if not resilience toward change. Over time, these disorders result in significant distress and psychosocial impairments for the individuals challenged by them, as well as major disruptions in their social, occupational, and other interpersonal relationships. Individuals with these disorders present as major challenges for caregivers and treating providers.

B. Etiology
- Genetic factors may play a role in the etiology and development of such disorders, as well as other psychogenic and environmental factors.

- About 9.1% of the US population (about 1 in 11 people) meet the *DSM-IV* criteria for a personality disorder. Some other recent studies have estimated the percentage between 9.0 and 15.7.

C. Clinical Features
- Inflexible, maladaptive behavior patterns/traits and characteristic responses to life events, which exceed the range of variation, present in most people.
- Results in significant impairments in social, interpersonal, and occupational functioning.
- Manifests fully by late adolescence or early adulthood.
- Influences all aspects of personality including cognition, mood, behavior, and interpersonal style of relating to others.
- Disordered thoughts/behavior must be stable and of long duration; chronic, not just in response to a limited event/stressor.
- Cannot be explained as a result of another adult mental disorder.
- Brain disease, injury, or dysfunction must be excluded as the cause of the disorder.
- Frequently coexists with Axis I conditions and affects their treatment.
- Grouped into three major subtypes/clusters based on predominant symptoms.

D. Diagnostic Studies
- Unless otherwise noted, no specific laboratory test or radiologic examinations are used to make the diagnosis of a personality disorder.
- **Assessment and diagnosis of a personality disorder are made through the use of the following:**
  - Clinical interviews.
  - Self-report inventories (e.g., the Minnesota Multiphasic Personality Inventory (MMPI-2), Personality Diagnostic Questionnaire).
  - Semistructured interviews (e.g., Structured Interview for Diagnosis of Personality Disorders, Personality Disorder Examination, Structured Clinical Interview).
  - Routine history and physical and laboratory tests to rule out any other underlying physiologic disorders (e.g., hyperthyroidism).
  - Various diagnostic studies (e.g., sleep studies, electroencephalograph, or EEG, dexamethasone suppression) have been used to study various disorders, but their clinical use continues to be evaluated.

E. Management
- Psychotherapy with/without pharmacotherapy is the cornerstone of treatment.
- Type of psychotherapy (i.e., psychodynamic, supportive, interpersonal, behavioral, cognitive, dialectical behavior therapy [DBT]) varies according to the disorder and other conditions affecting the patient.

- Pharmacotherapy often focuses on symptom management/relief to allow for better psychotherapeutic/behavioral response.
- **NOTE:** In each subtype of personality disorder that follows, at least three to four of the specific subtype criteria and the general personality disorder clinical features listed previously must be met to make the diagnosis.

CLUSTER A DISORDERS (INCLUDE THOSE WHO APPEAR ODD OR ECCENTRIC)

A. Schizoid Personality Disorder
1. **Definition**
   - The essential characteristic of this disorder is a long pattern of withdrawal, inhibition if not absence of emotional expression, and shyness.
   - Apparent bland and constricted affect.
2. **Etiology**
   - Onset—usually early childhood.
   - Prevalence—not clearly established.
   - Sex ratio—unknown.
3. **Clinical Features**
   - Central characteristic—inability to form relationships or respond to others in a meaningful way, typically resulting in a lifelong pattern of social withdrawal.
   - Appears indifferent to others; lack of response to praise, criticism, or any feelings expressed by others.
   - Often seen by others as eccentric, isolated, or lonely.
   - People with the disorder tend to gravitate toward solitary jobs/activities involving little or no contact with others; many prefer night work to day for this reason.
   - Neither desires nor enjoys close relationships, including being part of a family.
   - Takes pleasure in few, if any, activities.
   - May appear to be cold and aloof.
   - The absence of a clearly diagnosed thought disorder or delusional thinking and a normal capacity to recognize reality and respond appropriately, and an absence of relatives with schizophrenia differentiate it from schizophrenia.
   - May have successful, if isolated, work histories, differentiating it from schizotypal personality disorder and schizophrenia.
4. **Diagnostic Studies**
   - Generally diagnosed through a solid structured psychiatric interview, and possibly additional psychosocial assessment.
5. **Management**
   - **Psychotherapy.**
   - **Pharmacotherapy**—Small doses of antipsychotics, antidepressants, and psychostimulants are effective in some patients (see Table 5-1).
   - It remains unclear what proportion of individuals with this diagnosis will eventually manifest and develop symptoms of schizophrenia.

B. Schizotypal Personality Disorder
1. **Definition**
   - A disorder characterized by patterns of thought and behaviors suggestive of schizophrenia without classic symptoms suggestive of psychosis (e.g., delusions).
   - An acute discomfort with and reduced capacity for close relationships.
2. **Etiology**
   - Three percent of the general population is believed to suffer from this disorder with a greater association evidenced among biologic relatives of patients with schizophrenia.
3. **Clinical Features**
   - Strikingly odd, "obtuse," and/or peculiar behaviors or appearance, even discernible by laypersons.
   - Constricted or inappropriate affect (e.g., laughs inappropriately during conversations).
   - Peculiar notions, ideations, ideas of reference, and illusions.
   - Episodes of derealization.
   - May evidence suspiciousness and/or paranoid ideation.
   - Lack of close friends or confidants other than first-degree relatives.
   - Speech may be distinctive or peculiar; may have meaning only to the person and may need interpretation.
   - Exquisitely sensitive to and aware of the feelings of others, especially negative feelings such as anger.
   - Some involvement in cults, engagement in strange religious practices, or even the occult.
   - Under stress may decompensate and have psychotic symptoms of brief duration.
   - Oddities in their behavior, thinking, perception, and communication, as well as a clear family history of schizophrenia, may differentiate this disorder from individuals with schizoid personality disorder.
   - Absence of psychosis, except rare "fragmented" episodes of psychosis while under stress, differentiates this disorder from schizophrenia, although chronicity of such patterns may suggest that this disorder may be a "precursor personality" of schizophrenia.
4. **Diagnostic Studies**
   - Structured psychiatric interview.
   - Psychological testing may provide additional diagnostic indications as well as assist in differential diagnosis.
5. **Management**
   - **Psychotherapy.**
   - **Pharmacotherapy**—Antipsychotics may be useful in dealing with ideas of reference, illusions,

and other symptoms of the disorder
(see Table 5-1).
- Some patients maintain stable schizotypal personality throughout their lives; marry and work despite the disorder.

C. Paranoid Personality Disorder
1. Definition
- A disorder characterized by suspiciousness, systemized delusions of persecution or grandeur without hallucinations.
- A tendency toward global, excessive, or irrational suspiciousness.

2. Etiology
- 0.5% to 2.5% of the population, with men exhibiting the disorder more frequently than women.
- No familial pattern, although a higher incidence appears in those patients with family members with schizophrenia.

3. Clinical Features
- Long-standing patterns of suspiciousness and mistrust of people in general.
- Begins by early adulthood and appears in a variety of contexts.
- Interprets other people's actions as deliberately demeaning or threatening.
- Refuses responsibility for own feelings and assigns them to others.
- Expects to be exploited or harmed by others in some way.
- Can be affectively restricted, appearing unemotional or, conversely, may exhibit intense and situation-inappropriate affect given an exquisite sensitivity to nuances of potential threat.
- Ideas of reference and logically defended illusions are common.
- Rarely seeks treatment voluntarily; if treatment is requested by family or employer, can "pull themselves together" sufficiently to appear "intact" and not under any apparent distress.
- "Reads" hidden, demeaning, or threatening meanings into benign remarks or events.
- Persistently bears grudges (i.e., is unforgiving of insults, injuries, or slights).
- Perceives attacks on his or her character or reputation not apparent to others, and is quick to react angrily or counterattack.
- May have recurrent suspicions, without justification, regarding fidelity of spouse or sexual partner.
- Differentiated from paranoid schizophrenia by absence of hallucinations or formal thought disorders.
- Differentiated from schizoid personality disorder by absence of interactivity with other people and presence of paranoid ideation.

4. Diagnostic Studies
- Structured psychiatric interview.
- Psychological testing.

5. Management
- **Psychotherapy**—Treatment of choice (1:1); avoid "interpersonal closeness/contact," keep professional.
- **Pharmacotherapy:**
  - Benzodiazepines may be useful in dealing with agitation and anxiety (for very brief periods). Consider addictive potential.
  - Severe agitation/quasi-delusional thinking may be addressed through the use of antipsychotics, such as thioridazine or haloperidol in small doses/brief periods.
- Adequate long-term follow-up studies have not been conducted.
- In general, those with paranoid personality disorder have life-long problems of working and interacting with others.

CLUSTER B DISORDERS (INCLUDE THOSE WHO APPEAR ERRATIC, DRAMATIC, OR OVERIRRATIONAL)
A. ASP Disorder
1. Definition
- A disorder characterized by behaviors deviating sharply from norms, rules, and laws of society. Such behaviors can be hostile or harmful to society.

2. Etiology
- Three percent in men and 1% in women.
- Most common in poor urban areas and among transient residents within these areas and other geographic areas.
- Evidence of conduct disorder with onset is present before 15 years of age.
- Familial pattern—disorder five times more common in first-degree relatives of men with the disorder than in controls.

3. Clinical Features
- Inability to conform to the social norms that govern accepted behavior; repeated infractions of the law and actions leading to arrest may be common (e.g., lying to police if questioned, use of aliases, truancy, running away from home as a child/adolescent, frequent thefts, frequent fights, and substance abuse, drug trafficking).
- A significant feature is a lack of remorse for their inappropriate actions and violation of rules, norms, the rights of others, etc., typically being indifferent or rationalizing their actions. Appear to lack what most consider a "conscience.
- As the disorder progresses, it may be increasingly characterized by the commission of serious antisocial if not criminal acts.
- Such patients can often seem normal, even charming or ingratiating, but underneath, tension, hostility, irritability, and rage are present.

- May appear seductive with opposite sex clinicians and manipulative with same sex clinicians.
- Impulsivity; failure to plan ahead.
- Irritability and aggressiveness.
- Reckless disregard for safety of own self or others.
- Consistent irresponsibility—repeated failure to honor work demands, rules, and financial obligations.
- Exhibit no anxiety or depression—incongruous with their behavior.
- Promiscuity, spouse abuse, child abuse, and drunk driving common in their history—"con men."

4. **Diagnostic Studies**
   - Structured psychiatric interview.
   - Thorough neurologic examination—often shows abnormal electroencephalogram results, soft neurologic signs.
   - History of brain damage in childhood.

5. **Management**
   - **Psychotherapy**—Limits must be established.
   - **Pharmacotherapy**—Used for incapacitating symptoms only.

B. **Borderline Personality Disorder**
   1. **Definition**
      - A disorder characterized by a pervasive pattern of excessive, impulsive behaviors, extreme attitudes, chaotic relationships, chronic anger, suicidal threats, depression, and impaired social and vocational functioning.

   2. **Etiology**
      - One percent to 2% of population, with a preponderance of women exhibiting the disorder (2:1) over men.
      - Diagnosis is usually made before age 40.
      - Prevalence of major depressive disorder, alcohol and other substance abuse disorders, and substance abuse in first-degree relatives of people with borderline personality disorder (BPD).

   3. **Clinical Features**
      - The essential feature of this disorder is a pervasive pattern of instability in relationships, affect, and self-image, accompanied by chronic impulsivity in response to such. As a result, individuals with this disorder frequently present as being in a "state of crisis.
      - Mood swings are common. Short-lived psychotic episodes may be possible, although the symptoms are typically circumscribed, fleeting, or doubtful.
      - Transient, stress-related paranoid ideation or severe dissociative symptoms.
      - May evidence highly unpredictable behavior.
      - Achievements are rarely at the level of their abilities or self-expectations.
      - Recurrent suicidal behavior, gestures, or threats, especially at times of perceived or actual stress.

- Repetitive self-destructive acts (e.g., wrist slashing, self-mutilation) to elicit help from others, express anger, or numb themselves to overwhelming effect. Such self-injury gestures are typically nonsuicidal self-injury (NSSI).
- Tumultuous interpersonal relationships are common markers of this disorder.
- "Cannot tolerate being alone"—may accept strangers as "friends" rather impulsively, with poor judgment, or act promiscuously, placing themselves in precarious if not episodic dangerous situations.
- Frantic efforts to avoid real or imagined abandonment. A sense of abandonment is a persistent feature and complaint associated with this disorder (i.e., "no one understands or cares about me," despite evidence to the contrary from caregivers, family, and friends).
- See people as either "good or bad," nurturant or hateful. Such "splitting" results in idealized versions of what is perceived as "good" and devalued versions of what is "bad.
- Inappropriate, intense anger and/or difficulty controlling anger.
- Often complains of chronic feelings of emptiness, depression, and boredom.
- Lack of consistent sense of identity.
- Markedly and persistently unstable self-image or sense of self.
- Impulsivity in potentially self-damaging areas—spending, sex, substance abuse, reckless driving, and binge eating.

4. **Diagnostic Studies and Differentiation**
   - Psychiatric interview.
   - Psychological testing.
   - Diagnosis is typically made by early adulthood.
   - Biologic studies may aid in diagnosis, but are rarely used clinically.
   - Some sleep studies have shown shortened rapid eye movement (REM) latency and sleep continuity disturbances in individuals with this disorder.
   - Dexamethasone suppression—abnormal test results.
   - Thyrotropin-releasing hormone—abnormal.

5. **Management**
   - **Psychotherapy**—Treatment of choice. Structured and directive treatment is shown to have better results, with firm limit-setting of dramatic and intense behaviors. DBT should be considered as a first-line choice among therapy options.
   - **Pharmacotherapy—To deal with specific personality features that interfere with overall functioning:**
     - Antipsychotics for control of anger, hostility, and brief psychotic episodes.
     - Antidepressants to improve depressed moods.
     - Mood stabilizers may improve global functioning.

- Benzodiazepines for short periods. (Consider addictive potential in use of these medications with this particular personality disorder.)

C. Histrionic Personality Disorder

1. Definition

- A pervasive pattern of excessive emotionality, self-absorption, and attention-seeking behavior. May be characterized by frequent quasi or actual "temper tantrums," efforts to draw attention to oneself (such as by being flirtatious and vain, and overly dramatic).
- May also be characterized by endless verbalizations of their fantasies and experiences.

2. Etiology

- Unknown. Limited data suggest 2% to 3% of population, more frequently diagnosed in women than in men.

3. Clinical Features

- Excitable, emotional, and behave in a colorful, dramatic, extroverted fashion.
- Inability to maintain deep, long-lasting attachments, and develop truly intimate relationships (despite the fact that they may consider relationships to be more intimate than they actually are).
- High degree of attention-seeking behavior—tend to exaggerate their thoughts and feelings and make everything sound more important than it actually is.
- Display temper tantrums, tears, and accusations when not the center of attention or receiving praise or approval.
- Seductive behavior is common, but may have psychosexual dysfunction elements.
- Displays rapidly shifting and shallow expressions of emotions.
- May utilize physical appearance as a way to draw attention to self.
- Style of speech is excessively impressionistic and lacking in detail.
- Can be very suggestible and easily influenced by others or circumstances.
- Typically unaware of, if not confused about, their true feelings and unable to explain their motivations.
- Reality testing becomes impaired under stress.
- Gestures and dramatic punctuation are common in conversations—colorful language, may make frequent slips of the tongue.
- Individuals with this disorder may develop a sensation-seeking pattern, resulting in possible legal difficulties, substance abuse, and promiscuity.

4. Diagnostic Studies

- Structured psychiatric interview. (In interviews, generally cooperative and eager to provide a detailed history.)
- Psychological testing.
- Rule out alcohol or drug use.

5. Management

- **Psychotherapy**—Psychoanalytically oriented psychotherapy (group or person) is the treatment of choice.
- **Pharmacotherapy**—Adjunctive when symptoms are targeted.

D. Narcissistic Personality Disorder

1. Definition

- A disorder that can be characterized as grandiose, often excessive sense of self-importance.
- Arrestment of development at, or regression to, an infantile stage of development.

2. Etiology

- One percent of general population, with a higher risk than normal among children of parents with the same disorder.

3. Clinical Features

- Grandiose sense of self-importance—consider themselves special and expect special treatment.
- Striking sense of entitlement.
- Preoccupied with fantasies of unlimited success, power, brilliance, beauty, or ideal love.
- Believes he or she is "special" and unique and can only be understood by, or should associate with, other special or high-status people (or institutions).
- Seeks and expects excessive admiration.
- May be interpersonally exploitative, taking advantage of others to achieve own ends.
- Typically lacks or unable to express empathy, being unwilling (or unable) to recognize or identify with the feelings of others.
- Often envious of others or believes others are envious of him or her.
- Does not tolerate or manage perceived or actual rejection well and prone to depression.

4. Diagnostic Studies

- Structured psychiatric interview.

5. Management

- **Psychotherapy:**
  - Patients must modify or alleviate their narcissism to make progress—difficult.
  - Chronic and difficult to treat.
  - Aging handled poorly—may be more vulnerable to midlife crises.
- **Pharmacotherapy:**
  - Lithium used in patients who have mood swings.
  - Antidepressants, especially serotonergic drugs, may be useful.

CLUSTER C DISORDERS (INCLUDE THOSE WHO APPEAR ANXIOUS OR FEARFUL)

A. Avoidant Personality Disorder

1. Definition

- A disorder characterized by a pervasive pattern of inhibited social behaviors, exquisite sensitivities to perceived or actual negative evaluations, feelings

of inadequacy and insufficiency, and attendant nervousness regarding personal status and how others perceive the individuals.
- Highlighted by a turning away or withdrawing from relationships because of a fear of humiliation and failure.

2. **Etiology**
   - Although this disorder is thought to be relatively common, with approximately 5% to 10% of the general population evidencing its symptoms, information is not available regarding sex ratio or familial patterns.

3. **Clinical Features**
   - Hypersensitivity to rejection.
   - Reluctance to get involved with people unless certain of being liked.
   - Timidity and shyness.
   - Although may have a great desire for companionship, tend to have difficulty with acquiring and maintaining social relationships, given their expressed need for unusually strong guarantees of uncritical and unconditional acceptance.
   - Sometimes referred to as having an "inferiority complex.
   - When talking with someone, the person expresses uncertainty, shows a lack of self-confidence, and may speak in a self-deprecating manner.
   - Avoids occupational activities that involve significant interpersonal contact because of fear of criticism, disapproval, or rejection.
   - Preoccupied with being criticized or rejected in social situations.
   - Shows restraint within intimate relationships because of fear of being abandoned or ridiculed.
   - Inhibited in new interpersonal situations because of feelings of inadequacy.
   - Views self as socially inept, personally unappealing, or inferior to others.
   - Is unusually reluctant to take personal risks or engage in new activities because he or she fears they may prove embarrassing.
   - Rarely attains much personal advancement or exercises much authority, although eager to please and will take directions from others in authority.
   - Typically has no close friends or confidants; over time, phobic patterns (such as social phobia) and other avoidance patterns may develop and broaden.

4. **Diagnostic Studies**
   - Structured psychiatric interview.

5. **Management**
   - **Psychotherapy:**
     - Individual and group psychotherapy works well in alleviating some of the distress of individuals with this diagnosis.
     - CBT may include social skills training, assertiveness training, and cognitive restructuring to help individuals improve their assessment and appraisal of social events, particularly as they pertain to self-appraisals.
   - **Pharmacotherapy:**
     - Treat anxiety and depression if associated.
     - β-Blockers (e.g., atenolol) to manage autonomic nervous system.
     - Treat hyperactivity if indicated.
     - Serotonergic agents to help rejection sensitivity.

B. Dependent Personality Disorder

1. **Definition**
   - A disorder characterized by a pervasive pattern of dependent/submissive behavior.
   - Usually have a long-standing pathologic relationship with one person on whom they are dependent, rather than on a series of people.

2. **Etiology**
   - A more prevalent appearance of this disorder in women than in men.
   - More common in younger than in older children.
   - People with chronic physical illness in childhood may be most prone to this disorder.
   - Little is known about the cause of dependent personality disorder.

3. **Clinical Features**
   - Pervasive and excessive expressed need to be cared for, nurtured, and emotionally protected.
   - Subordinates own needs to those of others.
   - Allows others to assume responsibility for major areas of their lives.
   - Lacks self-confidence.
   - May experience intense discomfort when alone for more than a brief period.
   - Difficulty making everyday decisions without an excessive amount of advice and reassurance from others.
   - Has difficulty expressing disagreement with others, unrealistically fearing a loss of support or approval.
   - Has difficulty initiating projects or doing things on their own (because of lack of self-confidence in judgment or abilities rather than a lack of motivation or energy).
   - Goes to excessive lengths to obtain nurturance and support from others, to the point of volunteering to do unpleasant things.
   - Urgently seeks another relationship as a source of care and support when a close relationship ends (fear of emotional abandonment).
   - Unrealistically preoccupied with fears of being left to take care of himself or herself.
   - Avoids positions of responsibility and becomes anxious if asked to assume a leadership role.
   - Experiences difficulty in task completion on own accord, but may find it easier to perform these tasks for someone else when directed to do so.

- Relationships are distorted and undermined by their expressed intense attachment needs.
- Pessimism, self-doubt, passivity, and fears of expressing sexual and aggressive feelings typify the behavior of people with dependent personality disorder.
- Tend to have impaired occupational functioning and limited social relationships.
- Many suffer physical or mental abuse because they cannot assert themselves.

4. **Diagnostic Studies**
   - Structured psychiatric interview.
   - Although dependent personality disorder may occur in patients with agoraphobia, it is differentiated from agoraphobia by the high level of overt anxiety or even panic displayed in the latter.

5. **Management**
   - **Psychotherapy:**
     - Insight-oriented therapies.
     - Behavioral therapy, assertiveness training, family therapy, and group therapy have all been used successfully.
   - **Pharmacotherapy:**
     - Used to deal with specific symptoms such as anxiety and depression (common associated features of dependent personality disorder).
     - Imipramine is helpful in patients who experience panic attacks or have high levels of separation anxiety.
     - Benzodiazepines and serotonergic agents also have been useful.
     - Psychostimulants have successfully been used in some cases to treat a patient's depression or withdrawal symptoms.
     - With treatment, prognosis is favorable.

C. Obsessive—Compulsive Personality Disorder

1. **Definition**
   - The defining characteristic of this disorder is an intense preoccupation with effecting orderliness in their lives, expressed perfectionism, and control over both mental thoughts (internal stimuli) and interpersonal (external) events and environments. The disorder itself creates inefficiency and disruption in the lives of individuals by reducing flexibility and undermining true control over events and task conditions.
   - Can be characterized as constriction of the entire personality and affect.

2. **Etiology**
   - Prevalence is unknown, although disorder appears in men more than in women.
   - Diagnosed most often in oldest children.
   - Occurs more frequently in first-degree biologic relatives of people with the disorder than in the general population.
   - Patients often have backgrounds characterized by harsh discipline.

3. **Clinical Features**
   - Characterized by emotional constriction, orderliness, perseverance, stubbornness, and indecisiveness.
   - Pervasive pattern of perfectionism and inflexibility.
   - Preoccupation with orderliness, perfectionism, and mental and interpersonal control at the expense of flexibility, openness, and efficiency.
   - Preoccupation with details, rules, lists, orderliness, neatness, organization, or schedules to the extent that the major point of the activity is lost.
   - Perfectionism demonstrated that interferes with task completion (e.g., inability to complete a project because own overly strict standards are not met).
   - Excessively devoted to work and productivity to the exclusion of leisure activities and friendships.
   - Overly conscientious, scrupulous, and inflexible about matters of morality, ethics, or values (not accounted for by culture or religious identification).
   - Unable to discard worn-out or worthless objects even when they have no sentimental value.
   - Reluctant to delegate tasks or work with others unless others submit to exactly their way of doing things.
   - Adopt a miserly spending style toward both self and others; money is viewed as something to be hoarded for future catastrophes.
   - Show rigidity, stubbornness, and intolerance.
   - Limited interpersonal skills.
   - Formal and serious, and often lacks a sense of humor.
   - May alienate others, given their inflexibility and difficulty with compromise.
   - Eager to please those whom they see as more powerful than themselves, and they carry out these people's wishes in an authoritarian manner.
   - Indecisive and ruminate about making decisions.
   - Lack spontaneity.
   - Diagnosis of personality disorder when significant impairment occurs in their occupational or social effectiveness.
   - May be anxious about not being in control of the patient interview; their answers to questions are unusually detailed.
   - When recurrent obsessions or compulsions are present, OCD is noted on Axis I.

4. **Diagnostic Studies**
   - Structured psychiatric interview.
   - Rule out delusional disorders that may co-occur.

5. **Management**
   - **Psychotherapy:**
     - Unlike those with other personality disorders, those with OCD tend to be aware of the disorder and its negative impact on their lives, and may often seek treatment on their own.

- Do best with nondirective therapy.
- Group therapy can be helpful in facilitating shared experiences and shared skill enhancement.
- Behavioral therapy can be helpful for symptom management and situational control.
- **Pharmacotherapy:**
  - Benzodiazepines can reduce symptoms in patients with severe OCD (short term); unknown whether useful in the personality disorder.
  - Clomipramine and serotonergic agents may be useful if obsessive–compulsive signs and symptoms break through or persist.

III. Mood Disorders

A. Adjustment Disorder

1. Definition

- An emotional reaction to an identifiable stressor (e.g., job loss, physical illness) or event that represents a disproportionate response to what would be expected normally in the general population, resulting in markedly impaired social and occupational functioning.
- Symptoms occur within 3 months of onset of stressor.
- Remission of symptoms occurs within 6 months of termination of the stressor, or of its consequences (i.e., stress reaction diminishes when individuals finds another job after losing the one that resulted in the reaction).
- Reaction is not an exacerbation of some other mental disorder.

2. Etiology

- Acute medical condition is a risk factor in developing adjustment disorder.
- Can occur in adults and children.
- Persons with poor coping skills and inadequate social supports are more prone to develop disorder.

3. Clinical Features

- Symptoms can vary widely—severity does not parallel the intensity of precipitating event.
- May present primarily as anxiety, depression, or mixed features.
- Sadness may be evident.
- Social isolation.
- Difficulty concentrating.
- Preoccupation with the stressful event.
- Sleep disturbance.
- Appetite disturbance.
- Symptoms expected to resolve over time (6 months), but can be associated with severe dysphoria, despondency, and suicidal ideations and attempts.
- Usually do not have same major cognitive deficits as in major depressions (i.e., patients feel bad about their situation, but not themselves).

4. Diagnostic Studies

- Structured psychiatric interview.

5. Management

- Supportive psychotherapy.
- Crisis-oriented psychosocial intervention.
- Short-term, symptom-focused pharmacotherapy (e.g., for insomnia) (see Table 5-1).

B. Major Depression

1. Definition

- Depressed mood + anhedonia – five or more associated symptoms (see Clinical Features below).
- Symptoms occur almost every day, for most of the day for 2 weeks.
- Symptoms represent a change from previous level of functioning.
- Symptoms cause clinically significant distress or impairment in social, occupational, or other important areas of functioning.
- Symptoms are not due to a general medical condition, drug or alcohol abuse, or side effects of prescribed medication.
- Symptoms are not accounted for by bereavement.
- Absence of symptoms of mania or hypomania.
- The differentiation between a major depressive episode and a major depressive disorder is whether there have been (1) repeated episodes, (2) not accounted for by other conditions, and (3) not of a mixed nature (i.e., no manic or hypomanic episodes included).

2. Etiology

- Lifetime prevalence is 15%.
- Ten percent of primary care patients and 15% of medical inpatients, with a 2:1 preponderance of women over men.
- Fifty percent onset between ages 20 and 50 years, although onset can also be observed in childhood and later in life.
- Eighty percent to 90% can be treated effectively.
- Although exact etiology remains unknown, numerous theories may account for its development and course, including:

BIOLOGIC FACTORS

- **Alterations in amine neurotransmitters:**
  - Serotonin.
  - Epinephrine–norepinephrine.
  - Dopamine.
  - Acetylcholine.
  - Histamine.
- **Neuroendocrine dysregulations:**
  - Adrenal axis.
  - Thyroid axis.
  - Growth hormone axis.
  - Genetic factors—Family history of clinical depression.

PSYCHOSOCIAL FACTORS

- Life events or environmental stressors preceding first episode.

- History of family dysfunctional patterns and/or psychopathology.
- Learned helplessness (i.e., sense of powerlessness over conditions and life).
- Limited coping mechanisms.

3. **Clinical Features**
   - Depressed mood.
   - Anhedonia.
   - **At least five of the following for the same 2-week period:**
     - Sleep (insomnia or hypersomnia).
     - Decreased interest.
     - Guilt and decreased self-esteem, worthless feelings.
     - Energy and vegetative symptoms (fatigue and constipation).
     - Concentration (impaired and indecisiveness).
     - Appetite (decreased or increased with weight loss or gain).
     - Psychomotor (retardation or agitation).
     - Suicide (frequent thoughts of death with or without a plan).
     - Somatic complaints (headache, backache, GI complaints, dizziness, numbness, lethargy).
   - Often undiagnosed or misdiagnosed in elderly individuals.

4. **Diagnostic Studies and Differential Diagnosis**
   - Structured psychiatric interview. (Key to diagnosis—careful depression history and mental status examination.)
   - Psychological evaluation and assessment.
   - Complete history and physical examination.
   - Medication review, appropriate laboratory screening tests, or both, to rule out underlying medical conditions (Table 5-2).
   - **Some "bedside measures" used for evaluating depression are as follows:**
     - Beck Depression Inventory.
     - General Health Questionnaire.
   - Need to rule out other causes of major depression.

5. **Management**
   - Treat any underlying medical conditions.
   - Psychotherapy and pharmacotherapy for persistent depressive symptoms.
   - **Pharmacotherapeutic agents:**
     - SSRIs.
       - Add selective norepinephrine reuptake inhibitors (SNRIs)
     - TCA. (Contraindicated in patients with active suicidal ideation.)
     - Monoamine oxidase inhibitors (MAOIs).
     - Benzodiazepines, carbamazepine, valproic acid, and lithium may all be used for the treatment of major depressive disorder if clinically indicated on the basis of patient's presentation; however, they are not first-line medications.
   - Electroconvulsive therapy (ECT) or combination of ECT, psychotherapy, and pharmacotherapy if other measures have been unsuccessful.
   - Medications need to be maintained a minimum of 6 to 12 months or longer after clinical improvement.
   - Current theory recommends lifelong, daily pharmacologic maintenance for those with recurrent depressive episodes.
   - Cessation of psychopharmacologic interventions before 6 months may result in relapse.
   - Patient must be continually assessed for symptoms of mania and hypomania that would change the diagnosis and suicidality.

6. **Suicide and Other Information**
   - Fifteen percent of depressed patients commit suicide.
   - Depressive disorders are associated with 80% of suicidal events.
   - Fifty percent of those with a first major depressive episode have a recurrence.

TABLE 5-2.	Nonpsychiatric Causes of Depression		
Neurologic Disorders	**Endocrine/Metabolic**	**Pharmacologic**	**Other**
All dementias	Cushing syndrome	Benzodiazepines	AIDS
Huntington disease	Addison disease	Barbiturates	Malignancies
Parkinson disease	Thyroid disease	Chloral hydrate	Vitamin deficiencies
Narcolepsy	Parathyroid disorders	Amantadine	Systemic lupus erythematosus
CNS tumors—infections	Diabetes mellitus	Antipsychotics	
CVA, especially left frontal	Renal disease	Bromocriptine	
Neurosyphilis		Levodopa	
Multiple sclerosis		Carbamazepine	
Traumatic brain injury		Diltiazem	
		Ethanol	
		Cocaine or other stimulants	
		Steroids	

AIDS, acquired immune deficiency syndrome; CVA, cerebral vascular accident.

- **Risk factors for recurrence:**
  - Incomplete recovery.
  - Previous recurrences.
  - Strong family history of recurrent affective disorders.
  - History of major depression superimposed on dysthymia.
  - Substance dependence
- **Patients with a depressive disorder should be referred to a psychiatrist in the following situations:**
  - Increased suicidal risk whether verbal or actual gestures, intimations, or patient's lack of response to interventions.
  - Need for hospitalization for worsening of symptoms or evidence of emergent comorbid conditions.
  - Failure of an adequate antidepressant trial.
  - Complicated medical or psychiatric comorbidity.
  - Evaluation for pharmacotherapy.
  - Provision of psychotherapy and pharmacotherapy.

C. Dysthymic Disorder
1. **Definition**
   - Chronically depressed mood (or possibly irritable mood in children or adolescents) for the period of 2 years (1 year in children), with an observed presence of depressed mood for most days.
   - Severity of mood disturbance does not meet criteria for major depression.
   - Periods without depressed mood may have occurred during 2 years, but failed to last more than 2 months.
2. **Etiology**
   - May be a primary disorder in itself.
   - Often secondary to chronic medical problems (e.g., constant pain, cancer) or psychiatric illness (e.g., recurrent major depression, schizophrenia).
3. **Clinical Features**
   - Chronically depressed mood.
   - Low self-esteem.
   - Feelings of inadequacy.
   - Hopelessness.
   - Pessimism.
   - Guilt feelings or brooding over the past.
   - Social withdrawal.
   - Decreased productivity or activity.
   - Low energy.
   - Difficulty with concentration and memory.
   - Irritability or excessive anger.
   - Difficulty making decisions.
   - Generalized loss of interest or pleasure.
   - Greater risk for substance abuse and suicide.
4. **Diagnostic Studies**
   - Structured psychiatric interview.
   - Psychological evaluation and assessment.

5. **Management**
   - **Psychotherapy:**
     - Cognitive therapy.
     - Behavioral therapy.
   - **Pharmacotherapy:**
     - Antidepressants (SSRIs, SNRIs).
     - Patients can progress to develop a major depressive disorder.

D. Bipolar Disorder—Type I
1. **Definition**
   - One or more manic episodes, and sometimes, major depressive episodes. Mania is defined by an abnormally and persistently elevated, expansive, or irritable mood lasting at least 1 week (or less if hospitalization is required).
   - History of depression or hypomania also may be present, but is not essential for the diagnosis—only documentation of manic episode is needed.
   - Symptoms are not due to another mental disorder, substance abuse, medication, or general medical condition (e.g., hyperthyroidism).
   - Mood disturbance is sufficiently severe to cause marked impairment in occupational functioning, social activities, and relationships with others.
   - May necessitate hospitalization to prevent harm to self or others.
   - Psychotic features can be present.
2. **Etiology**
   - May be linked to biologic, genetic, and/or psychosocial factors.
3. **Clinical Features for Mania**
   - **Abnormally and persistently elevated, expansive, or irritable mood plus three (or more) of the following:**
     - Grandiosity/inflated self-esteem.
     - Decreased need for sleep.
     - More talkative than usual, or pressured speech.
     - Flight of ideas or racing thoughts.
     - Distractibility.
     - Increase in goal-directed activity (social behaviors, sexual behaviors, work, or school) or psychomotor agitation.
     - Excessive involvement in pleasurable activities that have a high potential for painful outcome (e.g., unrestrained buying sprees and gambling).
   - Symptoms have been present for at least 1 week or any duration if hospitalization is necessary.
   - Symptoms range from mild to psychotic or delirious.
   - **Mood**—Can be euphoric, irritable, labile, or dysphoric.
   - **Thinking**—Includes racing, disorganized, expansive, or grandiose thoughts.
   - **Behavior**—Can include physical hyperactivity, pressured speech, decreased need for sleep, hypersexuality, increased impulsivity, and risk taking.

4. **Diagnostic Studies**
   - Structured psychiatric interview.
   - Diagnosis is based on history and physical findings. Must rule out other causes of mania or bipolar presentation (Table 5-3).
   - **Laboratory tests:**
     - CBC.
     - Thyroid function tests (TFTs).
     - Urine toxicology screen.
     - Chemistry profile.
     - Hepatic and renal function—blood urea nitrogen (BUN) and creatinine.
     - ECG.
5. **Management**

   ACUTE
   - Maintain a secure environment that prevents flight or self-harm.
   - Evaluate patient for signs of medical disorders, drug intoxication, or side effects of prescribed medication.
   - **Hospitalization and pharmacologic treatment (see Table 5-1):**
     - Lithium.
     - Antipsychotics if psychotic symptoms present or to treat symptoms of mania.
     - Benzodiazepines (e.g., clonazepam, lorazepam) short term for hyperactivity, controlling agitation, decrease anxiety, and improving sleep.
     - In patients with intolerance or unresponsiveness to lithium—valproate or carbamazepine alone or in conjunction with neuroleptic.
   - **NOTE:** Neuroleptics generally result in rapid improvement, but patients with bipolar disorder are at increased risk for neuroleptic malignant syndrome and tardive dyskinesia.

   CHRONIC
   - Preventive treatment with antimanic agents (lithium, valproic acid, carbamazepine).

   - Serum level monitoring to avoid toxicity. More frequently at the beginning of treatment.
   - Therapeutic lithium level range is between 0.5 and 1.5. (Laboratory ranges may differ.)
   - Lithium blood levels are increased by thiazide diuretics, nonsteroidal anti-inflammatory drugs (NSAIDs), neuroleptic agents, and dehydration.
   - Every 6 months assessment of thyrotropin (TSH), BUN, and creatinine.
   - Addition of or replacement with valproic acid or carbamazepine when lithium alone is ineffective.
   - Use of benzodiazepines during periods of sleep deprivation (i.e., times of increased stress) to decrease the risk of manic episodes.
   - Antidepressants may precipitate a manic episode.

   SIGNS AND SYMPTOMS OF LITHIUM TOXICITY
   - Lethargy and fatigue.
   - Ataxia and clumsiness.
   - Weakness.
   - Nausea.
   - Vomiting.
   - Marked tremor.
   - Blurred vision.
   - Confusion.
   - Nystagmus.
   - Increased deep tendon reflexes (DTRs).
   - Mental status change.
   - Seizures.
   - Coma.
   - Cardiac arrhythmias.
   - Lithium toxicity is a medical emergency—needs to be managed in intensive care setting. Treatment includes discontinuing the lithium and treating the dehydration.

   ELECTROCONVULSIVE THERAPY
   - Effective in treating both acute manic and depressive phases of bipolar illness. Generally reserved

TABLE 5-3.	Nonpsychiatric Causes of Secondary Mania		
Metabolic	**Neurologic**	**Pharmacologic**	**Other**
Electrolyte abnormalities	Traumatic brain injury	Amphetamines	Herpes simplex
Thyroid disorders	CNS tumors—infection	Cocaine	AIDS
Adrenal disorders	Seizure disorders	MAOIs	Menses related
Vitamin B_{12} deficiency	Huntington disease	Sedatives	Postpartum
	Neurosyphilis	Hypnotics	
	Multiple sclerosis	Antipsychotics	
	Migraines	Steroids	
	CVA	Excessive thyroxine	
		Isoniazid	
		Disulfiram	
		Cimetidine	

AIDS, acquired immune deficiency syndrome; CVA, cerebral vascular accident.

for situations where standard treatments are not effective.

- **Indications for ECT as primary treatment in bipolar disorder as follows:**
  - Manic delirium.
  - Mania or bipolar depression with neuroleptic malignant syndrome.
  - Psychotic bipolar manic or depressive episodes.
  - Severely compromised health (i.e., serious, continuing suicide attempts).
  - Medical contraindications to mood stabilizers.
  - Lithium must be discontinued before starting ECT because it lowers the seizure threshold.

E. Bipolar Disorder—Type II

1. **Definition**
   - One or more episodes of major depression and hypomania, rather than solely mania.
   - Presence (or history) of one or more major depressive episodes.
   - Presence (or history) of at least one hypomanic episode, but never a manic episode.
   - Symptoms cause clinically significant distress or impairment in social, occupational, or other important areas of functioning.

2. **Etiology**
   - May be linked to biologic, genetic, or psychosocial factors.

3. **Clinical Features**
   - Symptoms of a major depressive disorder together with the clinical features of a hypomanic episode.

   HYPOMANIA SYMPTOMS
   - Distinct period of persistently elevated, expansive, or irritable mood, clearly different from the usual nondepressed mood.
   - **Plus three to four of the following:**
     - Inflated self-esteem or grandiosity.
     - Decreased need for sleep (i.e., feels rested after only 3 hours of sleep).
     - More talkative than usual, or pressured speech.
     - Flight of ideas/thoughts racing.
     - Distractibility.
     - Increase in goal-directed activity, socially, at work, or in school; or sexual or psychomotor agitation.
     - Excessive involvement in pleasurable activities that have a high potential for painful consequences (e.g., unrestrained buying sprees, sexual indiscretions, foolish business investments).
   - Hypomanic symptoms last throughout 4 days.
   - Symptoms are present to a significant degree.
   - Symptoms are associated with an unequivocal change in functioning, uncharacteristic of the person when not symptomatic.
   - Disturbance in mood and change in functioning are observable by others.

- Symptoms of hypomania are not severe enough to cause marked impairment in social or occupational functioning, or require hospitalization. Key in differentiating hypomania from mania.
- No psychotic features.
- Symptoms are not due to another mental illness, substance abuse, medication, treatment, or general medical condition (e.g., hyperthyroidism).

4. **Diagnostic Studies**
   - Diagnosis based on structured psychiatric interview, history, physical examination, and ruling out other conditions that can cause similar symptoms.

5. **Management**
   - Similar to bipolar I pharmacologically. There is a role for lamotrigine (Lamictal) in patients with bipolar II where depression is the predominant feature, keeping in mind the risk of Stevens–Johnson syndrome.
   - Antidepressants may precipitate a manic episode.
   - Medication compliance is a major concern with bipolar disorder. A collaborative relationship between provider and patient is crucial.
   - Suicide is common if untreated.

F. Cyclothymic Disorder

1. **Definition**
   - Symptomatically, a mild form of bipolar II disorder.
   - Characterized by episodes of hypomania and mild depression.
   - Numerous periods of hypomanic symptoms and depressive symptoms exist for at least 2 years (1 year in children and adolescents) and no absence of symptoms for more than 2 months.

2. **Etiology**
   - May be linked to biologic and/or psychosocial factors.
   - **Biologic factors**—30% have positive family histories of bipolar disorder type I.
   - **Psychosocial factors**—trauma/interpersonal loss triggers symptoms.
   - **Onset of symptoms**—insidious; teens or early 20s.

3. **Clinical Features**
   - Symptoms are identical to bipolar II symptoms except less severe in intensity, duration, or both.
   - Changes in mood are irregular and abrupt, and sometimes occur within hours.
   - Episodes of mixed (hypomania and depressive) symptoms with marked irritability are common.
   - Alcohol and substance abuse are common—patients use substances to self-medicate or achieve further stimulation.
   - Often have a history of multiple geographic moves and involvement in religious cults and other subcultures.

- Often not successful in professional and social lives because of this disorder.
4. **Diagnostic Studies**
   - Structured psychiatric interview.
   - Psychological evaluation and assessment.
5. **Management**
   - **Psychotherapy**—CBT assists the patient with regaining control over cognitions and behavioral patterns associated with the disorder.
   - **Pharmacotherapy:**
     - Mood stabilizers.
     - Antidepressants should be used with caution; they pose the same danger of inducing hypomania or manic episodes as in patients with bipolar I and II.
     - Sixty percent respond to lithium.
     - One-third of patients subsequently develop major mood disorders—most often bipolar disorder type II.

IV. Anxiety Disorders

A. Generalized Anxiety Disorder

1. Definition

- Anxiety disorders represent a class of disorders that range from generalized anxiety to posttraumatic disorder to OCDs to a variety of phobias. Psychic emotional and cognitive distress over real or confabulated fears often instigate and/or exacerbate physiologic reactions/conditions, causing additional worries and cyclical emotional processes. Such disorders are among the most commonly diagnosed psychological difficulties in children and adults. Diagnoses are made secondary to observed excessive, uncontrollable worry/distress about multiple life circumstances for a majority of days for 6 months. Anxiety disorders are the most commonly occurring disorders in children, adolescents, and adults.
- Anxiety is typically considered to be a significant excess of worry and reaction over what would be considered warranted or appropriate in given situations.
- Anxiety is difficult to control and often associated with somatic symptoms—fatigue, muscle tension, irritability, difficulty sleeping, and restlessness. These symptoms frequently lead them to multiple other specialists seeking treatment for their somatic complaints.
- Symptoms cause clinically significant distress in social, occupational, or other areas of functioning.

2. Etiology

- May have biologic or psychosocial links.
- Likely familial pattern.
- 2:1 in general population of women over men may present with this disorder, which rises to approximately 60% of more women than men with this disorder over a lifetime (NIMH).
- Fifty percent to 90% of patients often have another coexisting mental disorder.
- Occurrence of several negative life events associated with onset.

3. Clinical Features

- **Anxiety and worry are associated with three or more of the following symptoms:**
  - Restlessness or feeling keyed up/on edge.
  - Easily fatigued.
  - Difficulty concentrating or mind going blank.
  - Irritability.
  - Muscle tension.
  - Sleep disturbance.
- **Other symptoms:**
  - Headaches, dizziness, and tinnitus.
  - Autonomic hyperactivity—shortness of breath, excessive sweating, palpitations, GI symptoms—nausea, vomiting, dysphagia, diarrhea.

4. Diagnostic Studies

- Psychological evaluation and assessment.
- Structured psychiatric interview.

5. Management

- **Psychotherapy:**
  - CBT.
  - Supportive therapy.
  - Insight-oriented therapy.
- **Pharmacotherapy (see Table 5-1):**
  - Antidepressants, primarily SSRIs.
  - Benzodiazepines, used temporarily for <4 weeks while waiting for SSRIs to achieve efficacy. They should be slowly tapered and eventually discontinued altogether.
  - Buspirone.
- Supportive measures.

B. Panic Attack (Not a Codable Disorder)

1. Definition

- A discrete period of intense fear or discomfort, accompanied by at least four (or more) somatic or cognitive symptoms, that develops abruptly and reaches a peak within 10 minutes.
- Can occur in mental disorders other than panic disorder.
- May or may not be associated with any identifiable situational stimulus.

2. Clinical Features

- Presentation—Patients often present at an emergency department (ED) with somatic symptoms and fears that such are suggestive of a heart attack.
- **Intense fear or discomfort plus four or more of the following:**
  - Palpitations, pounding heart, or increased heart rate.
  - Sweating.
  - Trembling or shaking.

- Sensation of shortness of breath or smothering.
- Choking feeling.
- Chest pain or discomfort.
- Nausea or abdominal distress.
- Feeling dizzy, unsteady, lightheaded, or faint.
- Derealization (feelings of unreality) or depersonalization (being detached from oneself).
- Fear of losing control or going crazy.
- Fear of dying (e.g., a heart attack).
- Paresthesias (numbness or tingling).
- Chills or hot flashes.

3. **Diagnostic Studies**
   - Structured psychiatric interview.
   - Detailed history is a critical factor in the evaluation of panic attacks.
   - Focused physical assessment.
   - Disease-specific set of laboratory tests (i.e., TSH, cardiac monitoring).
   - **Common medical disorders that can look like panic attacks:**
     - Hyperthyroidism.
     - Hyperparathyroidism.
     - Pheochromocytoma.
     - Cardiac arrhythmias.
     - Seizure disorders.
     - Medication toxicity (i.e., CNS stimulants, bronchodilators, caffeine).
     - Mitral valve prolapse
     - Pulmonary embolus
     - Hypoglycemia
     - Stimulant use (amphetamines, cocaine, caffeine)
     - Medication withdrawal

4. **Management/Treatment**
   - **Psychotherapy**—CBT is generally viewed as the most effective form of treatment for panic attacks, panic disorder, and agoraphobia. CBT focuses on the thinking patterns and behaviors that are sustaining or triggering the panic attacks and helps individuals review their fears in a more realistic light.
   - **Pharmacotherapy (see Table 5-1):**
     - Benzodiazepines are effective in managing panic attacks.
     - Start with low dose and increase dosage until clearly effective treatment is noted.
     - Refer to psychiatrist for long-term follow-up and care.

C. Panic Disorder, with or without Agoraphobia

1. **Definition**
   - Spontaneous, unexpected occurrence of a number of panic attacks. The *DSM IV-TR* does not specify a minimum number of attacks or a time frame.
   - Occurrence can vary from several attacks in 1 day to a few attacks during a year.

- **At least one of the attacks has been followed by 1 month or more of the following:**
  - Persistent concern about having additional attacks.
  - Worry about the implications of the attack or its consequences (e.g., losing control, having a heart attack, "going crazy").
  - A significant change in behavior related to the attacks.
- Initial attacks must be "uncued" (unexpected) to meet diagnostic criteria.
- Often accompanied by agoraphobia, but also occurs without.

2. **Etiology**
   - May be linked to biologic (drugs, mitral valve prolapse, etc.), genetic, or psychosocial factors.

3. **Epidemiology**
   - Lifetime prevalence is 1.5% to 5.0%.
   - Women are two to three times more prevalent than men.
   - Most commonly develops in young adulthood (mean age: 25), but can occur at any time.

4. **Clinical Features**
   - Symptoms of panic attack.
   - Agoraphobia—anxiety about being in places or situations from which escape may be difficult or in which help may be unavailable, leading to avoidance or marked distress.
   - Associated frequently with major depression, other anxiety disorders, and alcohol and substance dependence.
   - Normal desire to engage in activities, but avoids because of phobias/triggers of panic symptoms; may have personality changes.
   - Frequent use of alcohol or sedative to get rid of anxiety/panic symptoms or prevent occurrence, resulting in substance-abuse problems.

5. **Diagnostic Studies**
   - Structured psychiatric interview.
   - Rule out possible medical causes for panic symptoms.
   - Include detailed physical examination, ECG, chemistry profile, including electrolytes, calcium, magnesium, TFTs, urine toxicology screen, CBC, liver, and renal function tests.
   - Other tests as indicated.
   - Detailed symptom history, medication history, and social history; especially use of caffeine, alcohol, drugs, sedative–hypnotics, nicotine, bronchodilators, CNS stimulants, or withdrawal from CNS depressants.
   - Full psychological evaluation.

6. **Management (see Table 5-1)**
   - Benzodiazepines briefly, to stop panic attacks.
   - Start with low dose and increase dosage as needed until clearly effective.

- Dosage needed may be higher than the range needed for other conditions.
- Reassurance.
- Referral to psychiatrist for further evaluation/treatment.
- SSRIs are first-line treatment. SNRIs and TCAs can be considered second-line treatments. MAOIs have a limited role because of their side effects.

D. Phobia
1. Definition
- Irrational and persistent fear of a specific situation (e.g., elevators, heights), certain activities, or clearly identifiable objects (e.g., spiders).
- Fear out of proportion to the inherent danger.
- Fear cannot be reasoned or explained away.
- People feel no voluntary control of their fears and avoid the situation or object to control the fear.
- Anxiety experienced when in contact or imagined contact with object of fear.
- Patients realize fear is unrealistic.

TYPES OF PHOBIAS
- **Specific phobia:**
  - Animals and insects—dogs, snakes, spiders.
  - Environmental—water, heights, storms.
  - Blood-injury—seeing blood, venipuncture, medical procedures.
  - Situational—closed spaces, flying, bridges, tunnels.
- **Social phobia:**
  - Social interactions—Speaking in public, using public restrooms, speaking to a date, or any activity drawing attention to themselves.
  - Alcohol dependence is common in patients with phobia—may medicate their anxiety with alcohol.
  - Alcohol withdrawal may worsen their anxiety.

2. Etiology
- Unknown—probable biologic, genetic, environmental interactions.
- Genetics—first-degree relatives of people with social phobia are three times more likely to be affected.

3. Clinical Features
- Severe anxiety.
- **Physiologic symptoms secondary to anxiety:**
  - Restlessness.
  - Diarrhea.
  - Dizziness.
  - Palpitations.
  - Excessive sweating.
  - Tremor.
  - Syncope.
  - Tachycardia.
  - Urinary frequency.
- Some patients may engage in risky behaviors in an attempt to overcome the fear (e.g., hang gliding by a person afraid of heights).

4. Diagnostic Studies
- Structured psychiatric interview.
5. Management/Treatment
- Specific phobia—consider exposure therapy, cognitive therapy.
- Social phobia—consider behavioral and cognitive therapy.
- Hypnosis, supportive and family therapy.
- **Pharmacotherapy:**
  - β-Adrenergic receptor antagonists shortly before exposure to stimulus (atenolol 25 to 50 mg or propranolol 20 to 40 mg).
  - SSRIs.
  - Benzodiazepines.
  - Buspirone—May be used as an additive agent with SSRIs.

E. Obsessive—Compulsive Disorder
1. Definition
- An anxiety disorder, manifested by obsessions, compulsions, or both, severe enough to be time consuming (>1 hour per day) or cause marked distress or significant impairment in daily functioning.
- Obsession—recurrent and intrusive thought, feeling, idea, or sensation.
- Compulsion—a conscious, standardized recurring pattern of behavior or thought (e.g., counting, checking, or avoiding).
- Obsessions increase anxiety; carrying out compulsion reduces anxiety.
- Failure to carry out a compulsion increases anxiety.
- Responsive to treatment.
- Symptoms have usually existed for many years before person comes to treatment.
- Symptom onset is generally gradual, but can be abrupt.
- Often have other coexisting disorders—major depressive disorder, social phobia, alcohol use disorders, specific phobia, panic disorder, and eating disorders.

2. Etiology
- Dysregulation of serotonin has been involved in the symptom formation.
- Significant genetic component.
- Biologic, behavioral, psychosocial component.
- Affects 2% to 3% of the population. Fourth most common psychiatric diagnosis.
- Onset at any age—most commonly evident in early adulthood (22 years).
- Childhood—more common in boys than in girls.
- Adulthood—disorder about equal in both.

3. Clinical Features
- Anxiety—central feature.
- Repetitive mental acts or behaviors to reduce anxiety.
- Depressive symptoms.

- **Major symptom patterns listed in order of commonality:**
  - Contamination.
  - Pathologic doubt.
  - Symmetry (precision).
- **Other symptoms:**
  - Religious obsessions.
  - Compulsive hoarding.
  - Trichotillomania (compulsive hairpulling), compulsive nail-biting/skin picking.
- Onset of symptoms for 50% to 70% of patients occurs after a stressful event (e.g., pregnancy, sexual problem, death of a relative).

4. **Diagnostic Studies**
   - Structured psychiatric interview with extensive history (e.g., Yale–Brown Obsessive Compulsive Scale–Y-BOCS) and physical examination to rule out similar conditions: major neurologic disorders—tic disorders, temporal lobe epilepsy, trauma, and postencephalitic complications.
   - **Clinical considerations:**
     - Tourette syndrome—two-thirds of people with Tourette syndrome meet the diagnostic criteria for OCD.
     - Obsessive–compulsive personality disorder does not have the same degree of functional impairment as OCD.
     - Obsessive–compulsive personality disorder is more pervasive and lacks the obsessions, compulsions, rituals, and severe anxiety of OCD.
     - OCD personality traits tend not to disturb the patient, whereas OCD compulsions and obsessions are disturbing and time consuming.

5. **Management/Treatment**
   - Behavior therapy.
   - Family therapy.
   - Group therapy.
   - **Pharmacotherapy (see Table 5-1):**
     - SSRI, first line. TCAs (clomipramine), mood stabilizers, atypical antipsychotics, buspirone, and SNRIs are among the other drugs used if SSRIs are ineffective.
     - Higher doses are often necessary for a beneficial effect.
     - SSRI dosing must be titrated upward over 2 to 3 weeks to avoid GI adverse effects and orthostatic hypotension.
     - Initial therapeutic effects are usually seen after 4 to 6 weeks of treatment; 8 to 16 weeks are needed for maximum therapeutic benefit.
   - Significant proportion of patients seem to relapse if drug therapy is discontinued.
   - **Other clinical considerations:**
     - ECT is used in cases of severely treatment-resistant patients.

- Treatment efficacy for patients with OCD varies greatly from minimal improvement to significant improvement in symptoms.
- One-third of patients with OCD have major depressive disorder.
- Suicide is a risk factor for all patients with OCD.
- **Poor prognostic predictors:**
  - Yielding to compulsions.
  - Childhood onset.
  - Bizarre compulsions.
  - Need for hospitalization.
  - Coexisting major depressive disorder.
  - Delusional beliefs.
  - Presence of a personality disorder.
- **Good prognostic predictors:**
  - Positive social and occupational adjustment.
  - Presence of a precipitating event.
  - Episodic nature of symptoms.

F. **Posttraumatic Stress Disorder**
   1. **Definition**
      - Group of symptoms that develop after the person experiences or witnesses a traumatic event that involves a response of intense fear, helplessness, or horror.
      - Symptoms persist for >1 month.
      - May not manifest until months or years after the traumatic event.
      - **Common situations precipitating posttraumatic stress disorder (PTSD) response are as follows:**
        - Experiences in war, particularly combat.
        - Torture.
        - Natural catastrophes—hurricanes, flooding, earthquakes.
        - Physical or sexual assault (e.g., single or multiple occurrences of trauma).
        - Serious accidents.
   2. **Etiology**
      - By definition, the stressor is the prime causative factor; not everyone experiences the disorder after a traumatic event.
      - Other contributing factors may be individual preexisting biologic and psychosocial factors and events occurring immediately after the trauma.
      - **Predisposing vulnerability factors:**
        - Presence of childhood trauma.
        - Borderline, paranoid, dependent, or ASP disorder traits.
        - Inadequate support system.
        - Genetic—constitutional vulnerability to psychiatric illness.
        - Recent stressful life changes.
        - Perception of an external loss of control rather than an internal one.
        - Recent excessive alcohol intake.

3. **Clinical Features**
   - Recurrent, intrusive, distressing recollections of the event, including images, thoughts, and perceptions.
   - Recurrent, distressing dreams of event—nightmares.
   - Acting or feeling as if the trauma/event were recurring (i.e., hallucination), flashbacks.
   - Intense psychological distress at exposure to internal or external cues that resemble or symbolize an aspect of the traumatic event.
   - Physiologic reactivity distress at exposure to internal or external cues that resemble or symbolize an aspect of the traumatic event.
   - Persistent avoidance of stimuli is associated with the trauma.
   - **Numbing of general responsiveness is not present before the trauma:**
     - Efforts to avoid thoughts, feelings, or conversations associated with the trauma.
     - Efforts to avoid activities, places, or people that arouse recollections of the trauma.
     - Inability to recall an important aspect of the trauma.
     - Markedly diminished interest or participation in significant activities.
     - Feelings of detachment or estrangement from others.
     - Restricted range of affect.
     - Sense of a foreshortened future (does not expect to have a career, marriage, children, or normal life span).
   - **Persistent symptoms of increased arousal are not present before the trauma (two or more of the following):**
     - Difficulty falling or staying asleep.
     - Irritability or outbursts of anger.
     - Difficulty concentrating.
     - Hypervigilance.
     - Exaggerated startle response.
   - **Common feelings are expressed:**
     - Fear of a repetition of the trauma.
     - Fear of sharing the fate of others who died or were injured.
     - Rage at those responsible.
     - Resentment toward those who were not harmed.
     - Remorse over what the person thought or did during the event.
     - Guilt because person survived and others did not.
   - Acute—symptoms lasting < 3 months.
   - Chronic—symptoms lasting 3 months or more.
   - Delayed onset—symptoms do not develop for at least 6 months after a trauma.

4. **Diagnostic Studies**
   - Structured psychiatric interview.

- **Rule out:**
  - Head injury secondary to trauma.
  - Epilepsy.
  - Alcohol use disorders.
  - Other substance-abuse disorders.

5. **Management**
   - May require different types of help at different stages.

   ACUTE
   - Support.
   - Protection/reassurance of safety.
   - Help with decisions and plans.
   - Encouragement to discuss the event.
   - Education about a variety of coping mechanisms (i.e., relaxation, deep-breathing techniques).
   - Education of family members/support persons regarding disorder and how to support patient.
   - Benzodiazepines prn (1 to 7 days) until normal sleep patterns return.
   - Referral to a psychiatrist for additional pharmacotherapy and psychotherapy.

   CHRONIC/DELAYED
   - Support.
   - Education about the disorder and its treatment (pharmacologic and psychotherapeutic).
   - **Pharmacologic treatment (see Table 5-1):**
     - SSRIs are first-line treatment.
     - Eight-week trial—good response, continue for at least 1 year.
     - Other drugs (alternates): SNRIs, TCAs, trazodone, anticonvulsants (carbamazepine, valproate), clonidine, and propranolol.
   - **Psychotherapeutic interventions:**
     - Must be individualized—some patients overwhelmed by reexperiencing traumas.
     - Exposure therapy—eye movement desensitization and reprocessing (EMDR), systematic desensitization. Evidence-based procedures, such as prolonged exposure (PE) therapy and cognitive processing therapy (CPT).
     - Some forms of behavior therapy.
     - Cognitive therapy.
     - Hypnosis.
     - Group therapy and family therapy are also helpful.
   - Hospitalization—when symptoms are particularly severe or when the risk of suicide or other violence is significantly elevated.

G. **Acute Stress Disorder**
   1. **Definition**
      - Acute anxiety symptomatology accompanied by dissociative symptoms brought on by exposure to a traumatic event.
      - **Symptoms:**
        - Occur within 1 month of exposure to an extremely traumatic stressor.

- Last at least 2 days.
- Resolve within 4 weeks. Key in differentiating between this disorder and PTSD.
- Disturbance causes significant distress and impairment in social, occupational, or other areas of functioning *or* prevents person from performing some necessary task such as obtaining medicine or legal assistance or mobilizing personal resources by telling family members about the traumatic experience.

2. **Etiology**

   EXPOSURE TO A TRAUMATIC EVENT
   - **The person experienced, witnessed, or was confronted with an event or events involving:**
     - Actual or threatened death.
     - Serious injury.
     - A threat to the physical integrity of the person or of others.
     - In which the person's response involved intense fear, helplessness, or horror.

3. **Clinical Features**
   - **Either during or immediately after the distressing event, the patient develops at least three of the following dissociative symptoms:**
     - Subjective sense of numbing, detachment, or absence of emotional responsiveness.
     - Decreased awareness of surroundings (being in a daze).
     - Derealization (environment seems unreal or dreamlike).
     - Depersonalization (feeling detached—an outside observer of one's own mental processes or body, or like an automatic machine).
     - Dissociative amnesia (inability to recall an important aspect of the trauma).
   - **Persistent reexperiencing of the traumatic event in one of the following ways:**
     - Recurrent images, thoughts, dreams, illusions, flashbacks, or a sense of realizing the experience.
     - Distress when exposed to reminders of the traumatic event.
     - Marked avoidance of thoughts, feelings, conversations, activity, places, or people that arouse recollections of the trauma.
   - **Marked symptoms of anxiety or increased arousal:**
     - Difficulty sleeping.
     - Irritability.
     - Poor concentration.
     - Hypervigilance.
     - Exaggerated startle response.
     - Motor restlessness.
     - Hard to enjoy activities previously thought pleasurable.
     - Feelings of guilt resuming their usual routine.
     - Hopelessness and despair.

4. **Diagnostic Studies**
   - Structured psychiatric interview.

5. **Management**
   - **Crisis intervention:**
     - Protection.
     - Consolation.
     - Assurance of safety.
   - **Assistance with decisions and plans** (i.e., Greatest help may be the support of those closest as soon as possible; preferably before going to sleep the night after the trauma, talking about what happened with an empathic person or someone who has shared the same or similar experience).
   - **Therapy:**
     - Supportive psychotherapy—focused on working through emotional responses to trauma or stress.
     - Relaxation techniques—for example, progressive muscle relaxation and biofeedback.
     - Group therapy.
     - Benzodiazepines (short term, 1 to 7 days) to assist with sleep until normal sleep patterns return.
     - Persons with acute stress disorder are at increased risk for developing PTSD when not treated.
   - Somatoform disorders, factitious disorder, and malingering
     - Characterized by somatic complaints causing significant impairment without objective physical findings or presence of a significant medical condition to adequately explain the symptoms.

SOMATOFORM DISORDERS
- **Somatization disorder**
  - Symptoms begin before age 30 and last for several years.
  - Four pain symptoms (different systems).
  - Two GI symptoms (other than pain; nausea, vomiting, diarrhea, etc.).
  - One sexual symptom.
  - One pseudoneurologic symptom.
- **Conversion disorder**
  - One or more unintentional symptoms affecting motor or sensory function.
  - Associated with psychological factors preceded by a conflict or other stressor.
- **Hypochondriasis**
  - Preoccupation and fear of having a severe medical illness based on misinterpretation of symptoms in spite of appropriate medical care and reassurance, lasting >6 months.
  - Not delusional in quality or specifically about appearance.
- **Body dysmorphic disorder**
  - Preoccupation with an imagined or excessive physical flaw in appearance.

- **Management/treatment**
  - Medical care should be frequent, preferably by the same provider, addressing specific concerns. Consistency and reassurance are key, always remembering that these patients can develop "real" medical issues.
  - Insight-oriented psychotherapy is appropriate and effective, if patient is willing to participate. Psychopharmacology is only indicated to treat a co-occurring mental illness.
- **Factitious disorders**
  - Intentional physical or psychological symptoms produced by patients to assume the sick role. No objective physical finding explanation for the symptoms.
  - No external motivation.
  - Treatment is focused on good communication among the health care team to avoid unnecessary diagnostic procedures. The patient will rarely agree to psychotherapy.
- **Malingering**
  - Intentional production of false or exaggerated physical or psychological symptoms.
  - Patient has a motive of secondary gain (avoid responsibilities or punishment; to receive free housing, drugs, or monetary compensation; retaliation for perceived loss or injustice).
  - Treatment is essentially to do a thorough evaluation and treat the patient based on objective

data without negative emotions. This will preserve the patient–provider relationship.

V. Psychotic Disorders

A. Psychosis

1. Definition
- A major mental disorder characterized by gross impairment in perception of reality and ability to communicate/interact with others.

2. Etiology
- Multiple causes; can be biologic or emotional in origin (Table 5-4).

3. Clinical Features
- **Common symptoms of psychosis:**
  - Delusions.
  - Hallucinations.
  - Bizarre behavior.
  - Ideas of reference.
  - Paranoia.
  - Disorganized speech.
  - Illogical thinking.
- Psychotic symptoms can occur as part of a primary psychiatric diagnosis (e.g., schizophrenia) or be secondary to multiple medical, neurologic, or substance-abuse disorders.

4. Diagnostic Studies
- Structured psychiatric interview.
- Psychological evaluation and assessment.

TABLE 5-4.	Medical and Neurologic Conditions That Include Psychosis	
Neurologic	**Pharmacologic**	**Others**
Delirium	Amphetamines	AIDS
Dementia	Hallucinogens	Acute intermittent porphyria
CNS tumor—infections	Belladonna	Carbon monoxide poisoning
Huntington disease	Alkaloids	Heavy metal poisoning
Parkinson disease	Cocaine	Systemic levels
Temporal arteritis	Alcohol	Vitamin deficiency (i.e., vitamin B_{12})
Migraine	Barbiturates	Thyroid disorders
Wernicke–Korsakoff syndrome	Benzodiazepines	Adrenal disorders
Neurosyphilis	Steroids	Wilson disease
Herpes encephalitis	Designer drugs (i.e., Ecstasy)	
Sensory deprivation	Ephedrine	
	Antihistamine	
	Cimetidine	
	Digoxin	
	β-Blockers	
	L-DOPA	
	Metronidazole	
	Anticholinergics	
	Thyroid hormone	

AIDS, acquired immune deficiency syndrome; L-DOPA, dopamine.

- **Laboratory studies:**
  - CBC with differential.
  - Serum electrolytes.
  - Fasting blood glucose, lipid profile. (Important to have a baseline due to the role of atypical antipsychotics in treatment.)
- Renal function (BUN/creatinine).
- Calcium.
- Phosphate.
- Liver function tests (LFTs).
- TFTs.
- Rapid plasma reagin (RPR).
- HIV antibody test in high-risk patients.
- Urinalysis.
- Urine toxicology screen—may need to specify specific drugs; routine urine toxicology screens usually monitor for only a limited number of substances.
- ECG.
- Chest X-ray (CXR).
- Head computed tomography (CT) scan or magnetic resonance imaging (MRI).
- Sleep-deprived EEG.
- Blood levels of therapeutic medications—when appropriate.
- Lumbar puncture.

5. **Management**
   - **Pharmacotherapy (see Table 5-1)**—Antipsychotics; typical (haloperidol), atypical (clozapine, olanzapine, risperidone, etc.).
   - Hospitalization (if required).
   - **Therapy:**
     - Supportive therapy.
     - Group therapy.
     - Individual therapy.
     - Behavioral therapy.

B. **Schizophrenia**
   1. **Definition**
      - **A fundamental disturbance of personality characterized by distorted thinking:**
        - Bizarre delusions.
        - Altered perceptions.
        - Inappropriate emotional responses.
      - Onset, time course, and nature of disturbances in emotion, personality, cognition, and motor activity vary widely in patients with schizophrenia.
      - Person's sense of external and internal reality is profoundly distorted.
      - Chronic, relapsing, remitting, debilitating psychotic disorder.
      - Affects every aspect of psychological functioning, including all the ways people think, feel, perceive, decide, view themselves, and relate to others.
      - **Diagnostic requisites**—Symptoms that last a minimum of at least 6 months; 1 month with a minimum of two positive or negative symptoms; deterioration noted in functioning at work, school, and home, or in relationships.

   2. **Etiology**
      - Schizophrenia is a clinical syndrome that probably comprises several disease processes.
      - Exact cause is unknown.
      - Considerable evidence exists that it is a brain disease and neurobiologic in origin.
      - **Leading theories:**
        - Chemical imbalance—level of dopamine.
        - Genetics—biologic relatives of patients with schizophrenia are at greater risk for the disorder.
        - Gestational and birth complications—increased prevalence of winter births; 5% to 15% excess of winter births among people who develop schizophrenia.
        - Statistical association only—not predictive for any person.

   3. **Epidemiology**
      - Most develop symptoms between 17 and 24 years of age, but can develop to age 45.
      - Affects both men and women equally.
      - Men tend to develop earlier (17 to 30 years) and suffer more chronic and severe symptoms.

   4. **Clinical Features**
      - Idiopathic—some patients develop only minimal symptoms; others extreme impairment.
      - Symptoms often vary—patient may appear calm and rational at times, then agitated and incoherent a few hours later.
      - **Typically consists of several stages:**

      PRODROMAL PHASE
      - Usually precedes onset of illness by 1 year.
      - Behavior changes gradually.
      - Begins to withdraw from social interaction.
      - Less attention to personal hygiene/dressing appropriately.
      - Acts peculiarly.
      - Length of phase is extremely variable.

      ACUTE/"ACTIVE" PHASE
      - Development of "positive symptoms" (i.e., abnormal mental activity causing grossly abnormal behavior).
      - Delusions.
      - Hallucinations (auditory most common).
      - Thought-process disorders.
      - Disorganized speaking.
      - Disorganized behavior requiring medical intervention, including hospitalization, typically necessary.

      RESIDUAL PHASE
      - Positive symptoms subside and negative "deficit" symptoms develop (i.e., signs of a deficiency in certain mental functions and absence of normal behaviors).

- Less dramatic than positive symptoms, but can be disabling.

NEGATIVE SYMPTOMS
- Affective flattening.
- Inappropriate affect.
- Apathy.
- Alogia (lack of logic).
- Anhedonia (inability to experience pleasure).
- Impaired attention and concentration signs.
- Impaired capacity in relating to others; may lead to complete withdrawal and avoidance.

TYPES OF SCHIZOPHRENIA
- Form of clinical shorthand for describing the way schizophrenia manifests itself. Categories, primarily descriptive, not clues to origins of disorder or prognosis.

PARANOID TYPE
- Preoccupation with one or more delusions, frequent auditory hallucinations.
- Speech and behavior may appear normal.
- Patients may be anxious, guarded, angry, argumentative, and even violent, although recent studies support that patients with schizophrenia are more likely to be victims of violence rather than perpetrators.
- Exhibit a stiff, formal quality or extreme intensity in interactions with others.
- Can develop later in life.
- Better prognosis regarding employment and independent living than other types.

DISORGANIZED TYPE
- Rambling.
- Incoherent speech.
- Odd/senseless behavior.
- Dampened/inappropriate range of feelings.
- Delusions or hallucinations, if present, are fragmented and disorganized.
- May grimace/giggle inappropriately, behave in a silly or childish way, and withdraw from any social contact.
- Begins in adolescence/young adulthood.
- Lifelong course with significant remissions.

CATATONIC TYPE
- Characterized by abnormalities affecting speech, senses, and movement.
- **Patients may:**
  - Remain in one fixed position.
  - Engage in purposeless movements (e.g., pacing back and forth).
  - Maintain a rigid posture against attempts to be moved.
  - Not speaking or otherwise communicating.
  - Assume bizarre positions.
  - Grimace or gesture in odd ways.
  - Resist or refuse commands.
  - Repeat whatever another person says or does.
  - Lie in a stupor.
  - Sometimes alternate rapidly between extremes of excitement and stupor.
  - Extremely rare type.

UNDIFFERENTIATED TYPE
- Various active symptoms, but no predominant ones.

5. **Diagnostic Studies**
   - Structured psychiatric interview.
   - Psychological evaluation and assessment.
   - Diagnosis by exclusion (does not easily meet criteria for other types).

6. **Management**
   - No known cure.
   - **Psychopharmacology**—Antipsychotics: typical or atypical (see Table 5-1).
   - **Current therapy goals:**
     - Eliminate or reduce symptoms.
     - Minimize often severe side effects of antipsychotic drugs—extrapyramidal symptoms (EPSs), tardive dyskinesia, neuroleptic malignant syndrome, agranulocytosis. Monitor for metabolic syndrome with routine blood work, fasting blood sugar, and lipid profile.
     - Prevent relapse.
     - Socially and occupationally rehabilitate the patient.
   - During acute phase, medical intervention and hospitalization are often needed.
   - People with schizophrenia, especially younger than 55 years, have mortality rates eight times greater than those who do not.
   - **Persons with schizophrenia are at an increased risk for suicide:**
     - Twenty-five percent to 50% of persons with schizophrenia attempt suicide, and 1 in 10 succeeds.
     - Persons often do not express their suicidal intent and act impulsively, making prevention difficult.
   - Aggressive behavior or violence at home is a common problem for parents and other family members of patients with schizophrenia. However, rather than being perpetrators, schizophrenic patients are more commonly victims of violence.
   - Substance abuse, especially alcohol abuse, is common and can exacerbate symptoms.
   - Schizophrenic persons, especially young men, may use drugs or alcohol to relieve anxiety or depression.
   - Sleep disturbances are common.

C. Schizophreniform Disorder
1. **Definition**
   - Identical to schizophrenia, but briefer in duration.
   - Relationship between two conditions is unclear.

2. **Etiology**
   - All symptoms of schizophreniform disorder last 6 months (these include those of the prodromal, active, and residual phases).
   - Persons have a better prognosis than those with schizophrenia.
   - Greater percentage of patients recover completely.
   - **Characteristics of those most likely to recover quickly:**
     - Developed psychotic symptoms quickly (change in behavior within 4 weeks).
     - Confused or disoriented during the psychotic episode.
     - Functioned well before the onset of symptoms.
     - Maintained a normal range and display of emotions rather than blunted feelings.
3. **Clinical Features**
   - Schizophrenia.
4. **Diagnostic Studies**
   - Structured psychiatric interview.
   - **Rule out:**
     - Temporal lobe epilepsy.
     - CNS tumors.
     - Cerebrovascular disease.
     - HIV.
5. **Management**
   - Treatment—same as for schizophrenia including pharmacotherapy (see Table 5-1).
   - Psychosocial care.

D. **Schizoaffective Disorder**
   1. **Definition**
      - Disorder characterized by a combination of symptoms of both schizophrenia and a mood or "affective" disorder (either major depression or bipolar illness).
   2. **Etiology**
      - Less common than schizophrenia.
      - Onset in late adolescence or early adulthood.
      - The combination of a depressive disorder and psychosis greatly increases the risk of suicide.
   3. **Clinical Features**
      - Clinical signs and symptoms of schizophrenia, mania, and depressive disorders.
      - Schizophrenia and mood disorders may be present together or in an alternating sequence.
      - Course may vary from acute exacerbations with remissions or present with a long-term deteriorating course.
   4. **Diagnostic Studies**
      - Structured psychiatric interview.
      - Completed medical examination.
      - Meets criteria for major depression or mania concurrently with the diagnostic criteria seen in schizophrenia.

5. **Management**
   - Treatment should be individualized.
   - Pharmacotherapy is the cornerstone of treatment (see Table 5-1).
   - Occasionally, dysphoric symptoms subside with antidepressant medication alone—if not, add antipsychotic agent to antidepressant. Caution in mania or hypomania.
   - If mania—mood-stabilizing agent (i.e., lithium plus antipsychotic).
   - ECT in some treatment-resistant patients.
   - Psychotherapy may be beneficial for some patients.
   - Long-term outlook is better than for those with schizophrenia.
   - Some improve significantly between episodes of depression or mania.
   - Others suffer chronic residual symptoms and never recover completely or function normally.

E. **Brief Psychotic Disorder**
   1. **Definition**
      - **Sudden onset of at least one (active) positive symptom of psychosis:**
        - Delusions.
        - Hallucinations.
        - Disorganized speech.
        - Grossly disorganized or catatonic behavior.
   2. **Etiology**
      - Symptoms last hours—1 day, but no more than 30 days.
      - Symptoms may appear after an event or series of events that would be extremely stressful to almost anyone in similar circumstances (e.g., combat, a violent attack, or a loved one's death).
   3. **Clinical Features**
      - Onset—late adolescence, early adulthood (late 20s to early 30s).
      - Increased risk in persons with personality disorders.
      - Anyone in a situation with overwhelming stress can develop psychotic symptoms.
      - Can be extremely frightening for affected persons and those around them.
      - May behave bizarrely, screaming and refusing to speak; may repeat nonsense phrases or speak gibberish.
      - Often disoriented and unable to remember recent events.
      - Some become aggressive and suicidal.
   4. **Diagnostic Studies**
      - Structured psychiatric interview.
      - Toxicology screens.
      - Rule out CNS pathology.
      - Rule out cerebrovascular disease.
   5. **Management**
      - Initially, close observation in a safe setting to rule out general medical condition or substance abuse.

- Symptoms may resolve on their own and person recovers quickly.
- **If symptoms persist:**
  - Sedatives or antipsychotics are prescribed (see Table 5-1).
  - Antipsychotics are tapered as soon as symptoms subside.
- Patients then recover fully from psychosis, but some may be troubled by secondary effects (e.g., diminished self-esteem and mild depression) for some time.
- Some patients—symptoms persist, requiring continuing treatment with antipsychotics.
- If symptoms persist for more than 30 days or have increasing severity, diagnosis is changed to schizophreniform or schizophrenia.
- Brief hospitalization may be required—suicide is a concern.

F. Delusional Disorder

1. Definition

- A psychotic disorder whose chief feature is a non-bizarre delusion presents for at least 1 month.
- Several types of delusions—predominant type identified to make the diagnosis.
- Patient has minimal deterioration in personality or function and no other psychopathologic symptoms, and this helps distinguish it from schizophrenia and other psychotic conditions.
- Nonbizarre delusions involve situations that occur in real life (e.g., being followed, poisoned, or deceived by a lover or spouse, having a disease).
- Often do not come to psychiatrist's attention—more often underdiagnosed/misdiagnosed—seen by internists, dermatologists, police, and lawyers.

2. Etiology

- Unknown.
- Paranoid, schizoid, or avoidant personality disorders may increase likelihood.
- Relatively uncommon.
- One percent to 2% of all annual admissions to psychiatric hospitals.
- Average age of onset—35 to 55.
- Slightly more often in women than in men.

3. Clinical Features

- **Main types of delusional disorders:**
  - Grandiose—belief in inflated worth, power, knowledge, identity, or special relationship to a duty or an important famous person.
  - Jealous—belief that one's sexual partner is unfaithful.
  - Persecutory—belief that someone to whom one is close is being treated poorly and unjustly in some way.
  - Somatic—belief that person has some physical defect, disorder, or disease.
  - Erotomanic—belief that person, usually of a higher status, is in love with them (obsession-stalker situation).
  - Mixed—more than one of the above types is present, but no theme is predominant.
  - Unspecified—delusions do not fit into any of the categories.
- Most people look and act more or less normally unless talking about or acting on their delusions.
- Many are angry, hostile, and suspicious.
- Some become reclusive and socially isolated or behave in eccentric ways.
- Most have little or no insight into their problems and refuse to admit anything is wrong with them.
- Sexual problems and depressive symptoms are common complications of delusional disorder.
- Violence is rare but can occur, especially in erotomania.
- Stalker's significant others are more likely to be targets of violence than the fantasy love object.

4. Diagnostic Studies

- Structured psychiatric interview.
- Toxicology screens.
- Rule out CNS pathology.
- Rule out cerebrovascular disease.

5. Management

- Usually do not admit that they have a problem or seek therapy unless forced to by family members or legal action.
- **Pharmacotherapy (see Table 5-1):**
  - Antipsychotic medications (typical or atypical) may decrease delusions and anxiety.
  - Symptoms may not dissipate completely.
  - May relieve somatic delusions.
- **Psychotherapy**—Individual.
  - Brief hospitalization may be required because of risk and safety issues.

VI. Dementia and Delirium

A. Delirium

1. Definition

- A syndrome characterized by the impairment of consciousness and the global impairment of cognitive function that develops over a short period of time (i.e., hours to days). Evidence suggests that this condition can develop in response to a general medical condition, substance intoxication withdrawal, toxicity, or a combination of such factors.

2. Etiology

- **Multiple etiologies may exist, with major causes possibly including:**
  - CNS disease (e.g., epilepsy).
  - Systemic disease, congestive heart failure (CHF), fever, or HIV.
  - Endocrine dysfunction (hypo or hyper).

- Intoxication or withdrawal from pharmacologic or toxic agents, alcohol, or street drugs.
- **Postoperative causes:**
  - Stress of surgery.
  - Postoperative pain.
  - Use of pain medication.
  - Insomnia.
  - Electrolyte imbalance.
  - Infections.
  - Fever.
  - Blood loss.
- **Trauma:**
  - Previous brain injury.
  - Burns.
- Can occur at any age.
- Advanced age is a major risk factor because of metabolic changes in elderly individuals 40% of hospitalized patients older than 65 years have an episode of delirium.
- Patients with a history of prior episodes of delirium are at an increased risk for recurrence under similar conditions.
- Delirium tends to be an underrecognized and underdiagnosed disorder in elderly individuals.

3. **Clinical Features**
   - Sudden onset of symptoms. (**NOTE:** In the absence of any history or psychological dysfunction or other comorbid disorders, the rapid onset of symptomatology should be a major clue in evaluating medical condition and other possible precipitants of this presentation.)
   - Reduced clarity or awareness of the environment.
   - Decreased ability to focus, sustain, or shift attention.
   - Inability to concentrate.
   - Disorganized thinking (not due to other factors or syndromes).
   - May not be able to follow a normal conversation or respond to questions.
   - Lucid periods alternate with symptomatic periods. (**NOTE:** This is another feature that aids in differential diagnosis with dementia or other cognitive disorder.)
   - Abnormal arousal.
   - Disorientation.
   - Rambling, irrelevant, or incoherent speech.
   - Impaired comprehension.
   - Memory impairment (recent memory most affected).
   - Impaired perception—delusions and hallucinations (auditory and visual most common).
   - Most lucid in the morning with symptoms worsening as day progresses.
   - Affective (mood) changes not accounted for by premorbid or comorbid conditions—fear, anger, rage, apathy, dysphoria, euphoria, and combativeness.

- Sleep disturbances—reversal of sleep–wake cycles. Sleep patterns are almost always short and fragmented.
- Exacerbation of symptoms at bedtime (sundowning).
- Associated neurologic symptoms—dysphasia, tremor, asterixis, incoordination, and urinary incontinence. Focal neurologic signs may also be evident.
- **May have a prodromal phase of symptoms:**
  - Anxiety.
  - Drowsiness.
  - Insomnia.
  - Restlessness.
  - Nightmares.
  - Transient hallucinations.

4. **Diagnostic Studies**
   - Structured psychiatric interview.
   - Cognitive evaluation.
   - Face-hand test—used to document cognitive impairment.
   - Physical examination.
   - Neurologic evaluation.
   - Laboratory studies (standard tests).
   - Thyroid profile.
   - **Additional or specific studies based on clinical indicators:**
     - EEG.
     - CT scan or MRI of brain.
     - Blood, urine, and cerebrospinal fluid (CSF) cultures.
     - Vitamin B_{12} and folic acid levels.
     - Lumbar puncture and CSF analysis.
     - Blood and urine toxicology.

5. **Management**
   - Treat the underlying medical cause(s). Resolution of concurrent medical conditions may result in a more rapid resolution of the symptoms associated with delirium.
   - Provide physical, sensory, and environmental support.
   - **Pharmacotherapy:**
     - Transient symptoms of psychosis, if evident, may be treated with antipsychotics, but should be carefully monitored, evaluated for efficacy, and modulated. Evaluation of psychotic symptoms should continue throughout to determine their association with the medical condition instigating the symptomatology.
     - Insomnia—benzodiazepines with short half-lives or hydroxyzine.
   - Symptoms usually recede over a 3- to 7-day period following the identification and removal of causative agent or condition.
   - Some symptoms can take up to 3 weeks to resolve completely.
   - The older the patient and the longer the patient has been delirious, the longer delirium takes to resolve.

- Delirium has a poor prognosis because of the potentially serious underlying medical conditions.

B. Dementia

1. Definition

- A syndrome characterized by increasingly and multiple cognitive impairments affecting memory, language, thinking, emotion, and personality without impairment in consciousness, typically due to multiple etiologies, such as progressive medical conditions, persistent and pervasive effects of long-term substance abuse, and other medical condition/events—for example, multiple cerebrovascular accidents, cerebrovascular disease, and Alzheimer disease (ALZ).
- **Alzheimer dementia**—now more commonly recognized as occurring across a continuum of stages: (a) Alzheimer itself with clear symptoms, (b) mild cognitive impairment (MCI) with mild symptoms, and (c) a "preclinical" stage, when there are no dramatic symptoms, but when recognizable brain changes may already be observed.
- New guidelines suggest and incorporate the use of so-called biomarkers (e.g., such as protein levels in blood or spinal fluid) to diagnose the disease and assess its progress, though the later is used mostly for research purposes at this stage. The new guidelines also make a clearer distinction between Alzheimer dementia and vascular dementia (such as that caused by stroke). Another stage, MCI, can represent an earlier phase of dementia and consists of modest impairments, primarily in memory, which can be a precursor of a more complete Alzheimer presentation later in a person's life.
- The syndrome can represent a meaningful decline in social, environmental, and occupational activities.
- Cognitive changes are not an aspect of normal aging or the result of congenital brain deficits and represent a significant decline from a previous level of functioning.
- Disorder may be progressive or static, permanent or reversible, depending on underlying cause.

2. Etiology

- Multiple causes: more than 50 disorders may result in dementia.
- Thirteen percent of individuals older than 65 years and 50% of individuals older than 85 years will be observed with dementia of the Alzheimer type (most common), with women demonstrating symptomatology more frequently than men.
- ·Fifteen per cent to 30% of all patients have vascular dementia, with a preponderance of men over women in this form of dementia.
- **Other causes:**
  - Hypertension—predisposes to dementia.
  - Parkinson disease.
  - Pick disease.
  - HIV.
  - Drugs, toxins, and alcohol abuse.
  - Intracranial masses.
  - Head injury.
  - Huntington disease.
  - Nutritional disorders.
  - Metabolic disorders.
  - Endocrinopathies.
- Generally considered an illness of elderly people, given their general decline and sometimes dramatic changes in physical status and overall state, as well as other accumulated causes, such as long-term effects of other conditions noted above.
  - Five percent of persons older than 65 years have severe dementia (Alzheimer type).
  - Fifteen percent of persons older than 65 years have mild dementia.
  - Twenty percent of persons older than 80 years have severe dementia.
  - Ten percent to 15% of patients with dementia are treatable because dysfunctional brain tissue may retain capacity for recovery if treatment is timely.

3. Clinical Features

- Usually begins with subtle signs of cognitive dysfunction.
- Gradual onset of symptoms is commonly associated with dementia of the Alzheimer type, vascular dementia, endocrinopathies, brain tumors, and metabolic disorders.
- Signs and symptoms vary greatly depending on the cause, course, and severity, the part of the brain most affected, and on the person's personality before the dementia.
- Memory impairment is an early feature and most prominent characteristic.
- **Early stages of dementia:**
  - Recent memory impairment.
  - Confabulation—language problems.
  - Difficulty in sustaining mental performance.
  - Fatigue.
  - Tendency to fail when a task is different and complex, or requires a shift in problem-solving strategy.
  - Disturbance in orientation.
  - Compromised abstract reasoning.
  - Impaired insight and judgment.
  - Personality changes—apathy, disinterest, labile affect, impaired social skills, exaggerated premorbid personality.
  - Attempts to hide performance and cognitive deficit.
  - Depression, anxiety, excessive orderliness, social withdrawal, and tendency to relate events in minute detail can be characteristic.
  - Sudden outbursts of anger or sarcasm.
  - Paranoia/delusions.

- **Middle—late stages of dementia:**
  - Remote memory loss—confabulation.
  - Mood changes—depression, anxiety, apathy.
  - Personality changes.
  - Emotional lability with no apparent provocation.
  - Loss of orientation.
  - Advanced intellectual impairment.
  - Grossly impaired insight judgment.
  - Perceptual distortion—hallucinations and delusions.
  - Aphasia.
  - Apraxia.
  - Agnosia.
  - Urinary then fecal incontinence.
  - Primitive reflexes may be present on neurologic examination.

4. **Diagnostic Studies**
   - Structured psychiatric interview.
   - Complete medical history from patient and family.
   - Physical examination.
   - Neurologic examination.
   - Neuropsychological testing.
   - Rule out pseudodementia.
   - Detect reversible causes of dementia.
   - EEG, MRI, or CT scan of brain.
   - Laboratory studies (standard tests).
   - Blood and urine toxicology.
   - Thyroid profile.
   - Vitamin B_{12} and folic-acid level.
   - Additional laboratory testing as clinically indicated.
   - HIV testing.
   - Lumbar puncture.
   - ECG.
   - Liver profile.

5. **Management**
   - Treat any underlying causes.
   - **Use all available resources to provide appropriate intervention/care:**
     - Medical.
     - Supportive and educational psychotherapy.
     - Family counseling.
   - Community resources (local support groups for both patient and family/caregivers specific to the type of dementia and stage, such as support groups for caregivers of patients with ALZ).
   - **Pharmacotherapy (see Table 5-1)—treat specific symptom complex including:**
     - Depression.
     - Anxiety.
     - Agitation.
     - Combativeness.
     - Aggression.
     - Insomnia.
     - Perceptual distortion.

- Therapeutics—antipsychotics in low doses (i.e., haloperidol); antidepressants (SSRIs); benzodiazepines, short-acting in small doses.
- **Symptomatic treatment:**
  - Provide a supportive environment.
  - Nutritional.
  - Proper exercise.
  - Recreational and activity therapies.
  - Attention to visual and auditory problems.
  - Treatment of associated medical problems.

VII. Substance-Related Abuse
A. Two Classifications of Substance-Related Disorders
1. **Substance-Use Disorders**
   - Substance abuse.
   - Substance dependence.
2. **Substance-Induced Disorders**
   - Intoxication.
   - Withdrawal.
   - Substance-induced delirium.
   - Substance-induced psychosis.
   - Substance-induced mood disorders.
   - Substance-induced anxiety disorders.
   - Substance-induced dementia.

B. Definitions
1. **Substance Abuse**
   - Characterized by the presence of one or more specific symptoms, indicating the use of a substance has interfered with a person's life and may lead to impairment or distress manifested by one or more symptoms occurring within a 12-month period.
2. **Substance Dependence**
   - Characterized by a maladaptive pattern of substance use, with significant clinical impairment and distress as manifested by three or more of the following occurring within a 12-month period:
     - Continued use of a substance despite significant cognitive and behavioral problems.
     - Loss of control—the person uses more of the substance or for a longer period of time.
     - Persistent desire or unsuccessful efforts to cut down or control use.
     - Spends a majority of time obtaining, using, and recovering from substance abuse.
     - Substance is used to change a mood or feeling.
     - Tolerance.
     - Withdrawal.
     - Giving up or reducing involvement in important social, occupational, or recreational activities because of substance use.
     - Substance use is continued despite knowledge of having a persistent or recurrent physical, psychological, or social problem caused by or worsened by the substance.

C. Etiology
- No definitive etiology is known.
- Genetic, psychodynamic, and neurochemical.

NUMEROUS RISK FACTORS
- Genetics—children of alcoholics are more likely to develop alcoholism.
- More men tend to develop this disorder than women, although this trend has been changing in recent years.
- Family dynamics include a pattern of regular and intense family stress, parenting problems, history of physical or sexual abuse, and permissive attitude toward substance use can be a contributing factor.
- **Environmental dynamics:**
  - Peer group drug use.
  - Poverty.
  - Social isolation.
  - Drug trafficking.
  - Drug accessibility (e.g., physician, physician assistant, pharmacist, nurse).
- **Other psychodynamics/pathology:**
  - Low self-esteem.
  - Poor self-image.
  - Mood disorders.
  - Schizophrenia.
  - Self-medication.
  - Alcohol and nicotine are the most commonly abused substances.
  - Increased prevalence of substance abuse 18 to 22 years of age.
  - Greater risk of substance abuse when onset is before 15 years of age.
  - Recent evidence indicates the use of "gateway drugs" (i.e., alcohol, nicotine, marijuana, inhalants) has increased among children and adolescents.
  - Predictive factors for the progression to substance dependence remain unclear.

D. Epidemiology
- Increased prevalence of substance abuse 18 to 22 years of age.
- Greater risk of substance abuse when onset is before15 years of age.
- Recent evidence indicates the use of "gateway drugs" (i.e., alcohol, nicotine, marijuana, inhalants) has increased among children and adolescents.
- Genetics/psychosocial—children of alcoholics are more likely to develop alcoholism.
- Men > women.
- **Family dynamics:**
  - In general, family stress, parenting problems, history of physical or sexual abuse, and permissive attitude toward substance use can be contributing factors.
- **Environmental dynamics:**
  - Peer group drug use.
  - Poverty.
  - Social isolation.
  - Drug trafficking.
  - Drug accessibility (i.e., physician, physician assistant, pharmacist, nurse).
- **Other psychodynamics/pathology:**
  - Low self-esteem.
  - Poor self-image.
  - Mood disorders (self-medicating).
  - Schizophrenia.
  - Alcohol and nicotine are the most commonly abused substances.
- Predictive factors for the progression to substance dependence remain unclear.

E. Clinical Features
- These features are outlined under the description of the specific substance (see VII).

F. Diagnostic Studies
- Structured psychiatric interview.
- Detailed substance use history.
- Detailed family history.
- Medical history.
- Social history.
- Complete physical examination.
- **Standard laboratory tests:**
  - Blood and urine toxicology screens.
  - HIV testing (intravenous drug use).
  - Liver profile—hepatitis screening.
- Other diagnostic studies based on pertinent physical and historic findings.

G. Management
- **Treatment of substance abuse involves two major goals:**
  - Abstinence.
  - Physical, psychiatric, and psychosocial well-being of the patient.

VIII. Specific Substance-Use and Substance-Induced Disorders

A. Specific Substance-Use Disorder
- Screening tools—CAGE and AUDIT.
- Intoxication or impairment from specific substance.

ALCOHOL INTOXICATION
- **Recent alcohol ingestion accompanied by detoxification:**
  - Withdrawal from the specific substance and the management of associated withdrawal symptoms.
  - Primary use of symptom-specific pharmacotherapy.
  - Support and reassurance.
  - Assessment and treatment of medical complications.
1. **Rehabilitation/Treatment**
   - Inpatient treatment programs.
   - Outpatient treatment programs.
   - Relapse prevention.

- **Self-help groups:**
  - Alcoholics Anonymous (AA).
  - Narcotics Anonymous (NA).
- **Family therapy:**
  - ALANON.
  - ALATEEN.
  - ACOA.
- Individual psychotherapy/group therapy.
- Support and reassurance.
- Assessment and treatment of medical complications.

2. **Pharmacotherapy**
   - Primary use of symptom-specific pharmacotherapy.
     - Disulfiram—provokes severe reaction with ingestion of alcohol.
     - Naltrexone—an opioid antagonist; blocks pleasurable effects of opioids and alcohol.
     - Acamprosate (Campral)—seems to reduce craving of alcohol.
     - Buprenorphine/naloxone (Suboxone)—opioid antagonist/agonist.
     - Methadone—an opioid agonist; is given to replace heroin and suppress withdrawal symptoms.

B. Specific Substance-Induced Disorders

1. **Alcohol Intoxication**
   a. **Recent alcohol ingestion accompanied by:**
      - Maladaptive behaviors.
      - Aggression.
      - Sexual activity.
      - Psychological changes.
      - Impaired judgment.
      - Mood changes.
      - Impaired occupational and social functioning.
      - **One or more of the following symptoms:**
        - Slurred speech.
        - Incoordination.
        - Unsteady gait.
        - Nystagmus.
        - Memory impairment.
        - Stupor of coma.
        - Duration is variable.
        - Blood alcohol level usually more than 0.10%.
   b. **Management**
      - Secure, safe, structured environment.
      - Reassurance.
      - Intramuscular (IM) haloperidol may be useful for controlling assaultiveness.
      - Condition should be differentiated from other causes of abrupt behavioral change.
      - If severe, can lead to respiratory depression, coma, or death.
      - May receive mechanical ventilatory support and monitoring.
      - Attention to patient's acid–base, electrolytes, and temperature.

2. **Alcohol Withdrawal**
   a. **Cessation or reduction of alcohol use that was heavy or prolonged, as well as the presence of the following specific physical and/or psychiatric symptoms:**
      - Autonomic hyperactivity.
      - Tremor.
      - Insomnia.
      - Nausea or vomiting.
      - Transient visual, tactile, or auditory hallucinations.
      - Psychomotor agitation.
      - Anxiety.
      - Seizures.
      - Delirium.
      - Symptoms may last from several hours to several days.
      - These symptoms can lead to delirium tremens, a medical emergency.
      - If delirium is present, it may indicate the presence of other general medical conditions.
   b. **Diagnostic Studies**
      - Structured psychiatric interview.
      - Substance use history.
      - Physical examination.
      - **Rule out:**
        - Lateralizing seizures.
        - Head trauma.
        - CNS pathology.
        - Hepatic failure.
        - Hypoglycemia.
        - Hyponatremia.
        - Hypomagnesemia.
        - Thiamine deficiency and anemias.
        - Blood and urine toxicology screens.
        - Routine laboratory evaluation.
        - LFTs, electrolytes, serum ammonia (if indicated), lipid profile, and CBC.
   c. **Management**
      - Cessation of alcohol use.
      - Provide a calming psychotherapeutic environment with safety precautions, nutritional support, and hydration.
      - Benzodiazepines in titrating doses. Phenobarbital can also be used second line.
      - Diazepam and chlordiazepoxide have a poor IM absorption ratio.
      - Carbamazepine.
      - Clonidine.
      - β-Adrenergic receptor antagonists.
      - Symptomatic treatment of N/V/D, insomnia.
      - Thiamine, folate, magnesium, and other vitamin supplements as indicated.
      - Anticonvulsants if indicated.

3. **Alcohol Intoxication Delirium: Also Known as Delirium Tremens**
   - Delirium tremens (DTs) are one of the most serious alcohol withdrawal symptoms and should always be considered a medical emergency.
   - About 5% of individuals with severe alcohol intoxication will experience DTs. Left untreated, it is estimated that up to 35% of individuals experiencing DTs will die.
   - Withdrawal seizures commonly precede development of alcohol withdrawal delirium, but can occur throughout.
   - Delirium can also appear unheralded.
   - The *essential feature* of the syndrome is delirium that occurs *within 1 week* after cessation or reduction of alcohol intake.
   - **Accompanied by:**
     - Autonomic hyperactivity.
     - Tachycardia.
     - Fever.
     - Diaphoresis.
     - Hypertension.
     - Anxiety and insomnia.
     - Perceptual distortion (visual/tactile hallucinations are common)
     - Fluctuating levels of psychomotor activity.
   - Usually begins in a patient's 30s or 40s after 5 to 15 years of heavy drinking.
   - Can result in significant morbidity and mortality if untreated.
   - **Management:**
     - Cessation of alcohol use.
     - Provide a calming psychotherapeutic environment.
     - Benzodiazepines in titrating doses.
     - May use lorazepam IV if oral route is not available.
     - Antipsychotics may reduce seizure threshold, but may be necessary to treat a superimposed psychosis.
     - Fluids to control dehydration.
     - Skillful verbal support is imperative.
     - Anticonvulsants until seizure etiology is determined.
     - Seclusion is an alternative for combative and uncontrollable patients.
     - High-caloric, high-carbohydrate diet.
     - Thiamine, folate, magnesium, and other vitamin supplements as indicated.

4. **Alcohol-Induced Persisting Amnestic Disorder**
   a. **Wernicke Encephalopathy**
      - **Definition**—An acute neurologic disorder characterized by ataxia, vestibular dysfunction, ocular abnormalities, and confusion.
      - **Etiology**—Caused by thiamine deficiency.
      - **Management:**
        - Reversible with treatment.
        - May clear spontaneously in a few days or weeks or progress into Korsakoff syndrome.
        - Thiamine 100 mg PO two to three times daily for 1 to 2 weeks. May initially use IM.
   b. **Korsakoff Syndrome**
      - **Definition**—A chronic amnestic syndrome characterized by impaired mental functioning including recent memory, anterograde amnesia in an alert and responsive patient. The hallmark is confabulation.
      - **Etiology**—Caused by thiamine deficiency.
      - **Management:**
        - Thiamine 100 mg PO two to three times daily for 3 to 12 months.
        - Twenty percent recovery rate with some improvement in cognitive abilities.

5. **Blackouts**
   a. **Definition**
      - Experience of specific short-term memory impairment with an inability to recall recent events.
      - Similar to episodes of transient global amnesia in that discrete episodes of anterograde amnesia are present.
   b. **Etiology**
      - Blackouts occur in association with alcohol intoxication or severe alcohol abuse.
   c. **Clinical Features**
      - Remote memory is relatively intact.
      - Intellectual functioning is preserved, allowing performance of complicated tasks.
      - The person may appear normal to the casual observer.
   d. **Management**
      - Cessation of alcohol use. Management of withdrawal if indicated. Rehabilitation.

6. **Cocaine Intoxication**
   SYMPTOMS
   - Euphoria.
   - Affective instability.
   - Aggression.
   - Hypervigilance.
   - Impulsive sexual behavior.
   - Impaired judgment.
   - Anxiety.
   - Tension.
   - Anger.
   - Impaired social, occupational, and interpersonal functioning.
   - **With at least two or more of the following physical symptoms:**
     - Tachycardia or bradycardia.
     - Pupillary dilatation.
     - Elevated or lower blood pressure.
     - Perspiration or chills.

- Nausea or vomiting.
- Weight loss.
- Psychomotor agitation.
- Muscular weakness.
- Respiratory depression.
- Chest pain.
- Cardiac arrhythmias.
- Confusion.
- Seizures.
- Dyskinesias.
- Dystonias.
- Coma.

CLINICAL FEATURES

- Cocaine use has numerous adverse effects outside of the diagnostic criteria:
  - Nasal congestion.
  - Inflammation, swelling, bleeding, and ulceration of the nasal mucosa.
  - Perforation of nasal septum.
- IV use of cocaine is associated with local and systemic infections, embolism, and transmission of HIV and hepatitis B and C. Can also be transmitted intranasally if mucosa is compromised.
- Effects are almost immediate.
- Duration is relatively brief.
- Metabolites of cocaine may be present in blood for up to 10 days and in urine for up to 4 days.
- **Major complications of cocaine use:**
  - Cerebral vascular accidents.
  - Nonhemorrhagic cerebral infarction.
  - Hemorrhagic cerebral infarction including subarachnoid, intraparenchymal, and intraventricular.
- Seizures.
- Myocardial infarction.
- Cardiac arrhythmia.
- Cardiomyopathies can develop with long-term use.

DIAGNOSTIC STUDIES

- Structured psychiatric interview.
- Substance use history.
- Extensive physical examination.
- Blood and urine toxicology screens.
- Appropriate laboratory studies.
- ECG.

MANAGEMENT

- Cessation of cocaine use.
- Hospitalization if required.
- Structured, safe, secure environment. Sleep is primary supportive treatment.
- Treat withdrawal symptoms.
- Screen and manage any cardiac or CNS complications.
- Broad treatment approach including social, biologic, and psychological strategies.
- Involvement in support groups, 12-step programs.
- Inpatient or outpatient rehabilitation.

- Individual and family counseling.
- After cessation of cocaine use or acute intoxication, postintoxication depression may occur and may last up to 1 week.
- Pharmacotherapy to reduce craving.
- **Dopaminergic agonists:**
  - Bromocriptine.
  - Amantadine.
- Tricyclics.
- Carbamazepine.
- Off-label use of bupropion, modafinil, and topiramate. Studies are ongoing.

7. **Opiate Withdrawal**
   - Heroin
   - Prescription drugs—morphine, Oxycontin, Dilaudid, fentanyl, Percocet, etc.

a. **Clinical Features**
   - Symptoms develop after discontinuation of drug following a period of heavy use or administration of opioid antagonist.
   - Three or more of the following symptoms: dysphoric mood, nausea/vomiting/diarrhea, muscle aches, lacrimation and/or rhinorrhea, pupillary dilation, piloerection, sweating, yawning, fever, and insomnia.
   - Symptoms cause clinically significant distress in social, occupational, or other important area of functioning.

b. **Treatment**
   - Treat any medical condition—cellulitis, sepsis, subacute bacterial endocarditis, HIV, hepatitis.
   - Psychotherapy/group therapy—treat mood disorders.
   - **Pharmacotherapy:**
     - Symptomatic relief; Phenergan, NSAIDs, clonidine, trazodone, fluids. nutritional support.
     - Suboxone.
     - Methadone.
     - Naltrexone as prophylaxis. Slight chance of overdosing on heroin if relapse occurs.

8. **Nicotine Dependence—Diagnosis**
   - Increasing need and marked tolerance of increased amounts of tobacco products containing nicotine.
   - Marked diminished satisfaction with continued use of the same volume of nicotine products, requiring increased and continued use of greater amounts of the product.
   - The product is taken over larger amounts over time and beyond what was intended ("I'll only smoke one pack, or I'll quit before I become pregnant...").
   - Persistent desire and unsuccessful efforts to decrease or control the amount used.
   - Incorporation of tobacco use into many domains of personal and social functioning.
   - Continuation of usage despite knowledge or awareness of harmful effects and/or negative

impacts on physiologic, psychological, social, and possibly occupational domains of personal functioning.
- **Risk factors:**
  - Genetics.
  - Mental illness.
  - Substance abuse.
- **Possible physiological complications:**
  - Lung cancer and other lung diseases.
  - Heart and circulatory system problems.
  - Additional cancers (e.g., esophageal, laryngeal, throat [pharynx] and mouth, bladder, pancreas, kidney and cervix, and some leukemias).
  - Physical appearance (e.g., changes in structure of skin causing premature aging and wrinkles. Yellowing of teeth, fingers, and fingernails).
  - Possible changes in fertility. Chance of impotence in men.
  - Pregnancy and newborn complications.
  - Cold, flu, and other illnesses. (Smokers are more prone to respiratory infections, such as colds, flu, and bronchitis.)
  - Diabetes (i.e., increase in insulin resistance, possible development of type II diabetes; possible acceleration and progression of extant diabetes process, including progression of complications, such as kidney disease and eye problems).
  - Weakened senses (e.g., alterations in senses of taste and smell, so food is not as appetizing).
  - Family risks. (i.e., Family members of smokers are at a higher risk for lung cancer and heart disease, compared with people who do not live with a smoker.)
- **Nicotine withdrawal—symptoms**
  - Dysphoric or depressed mood.
  - Irritability and anxiety.
  - Difficulty concentrating.
  - Restlessness.
  - Problems falling asleep or frequent waking.
  - Craving for tobacco.
  - Tingling sensations and dizziness.
  - Coughing.
  - Appetite changes.
- **Management/treatment**
  - Nicotine replacement therapy (patches, gum, lozenges, nasal spray, and inhaler).
  - Nonnicotine medications (combinations of medications shown as more effective).
  - Combine a longer-acting medication (e.g., nicotine patch or bupropion [Zyban, Wellbutrin] or varenicline [Chantix])—with a short-acting nicotine replacement product, such as nicotine gum, lozenge, nasal spray, or inhaler).
  - Counseling, support groups, and smoking cessation programs.

SELECTED READINGS

American Psychiatric Association. *Diagnostic and Statistical Manual of Mental Disorders.* 4th ed. Text Revision. Washington, DC: American Psychiatric Association; 2000.

Ebert M, Loosen P, Nurcombe B, eds. *Current Diagnosis & Treatment in Psychiatry.* New York, NY: McGraw-Hill/Appleton & Lange; 2000.

Epocrates Essentials. www.epocrates.com.

Kaplan HI, Sadock BJ, eds. *Synopsis of Psychiatry, Behavioral Sciences, Clinical Psychiatry.* 10th ed. Baltimore, MD: Lippincott Williams & Wilkins; 2007.

Lewis M, ed. *Child and Adolescent Psychiatry: A Comprehensive Textbook.* 3rd ed. Philadelphia, PA: Lippincott Williams & Wilkins; 2002.

Tierney LM, McPhee SJ, Papadakis MA, eds. *Current Medical Diagnosis & Treatment.* Stamford, CT: Appleton & Lange, 2003.

Websites:

National Institute on Child Health and Human Development. http://NICHD.NIH.GOV. Accessed May 15, 2011.

National Institute of Mental Health. http://NIMH.NIH.GOV. Accessed May 20, 2011.

National Institute of Aging. http://NIA.NIH.GOV. Accessed May 2011.

Neurologic Disorders

6

Adrian S. Banning • George S. Bottomley • Judy Nunes

I. Diseases of Peripheral Nerves

A. Complex Regional Pain Syndrome (CRPS, Formerly Reflex Sympathetic Dystrophy)

1. **Disease**
   - Rare extremity disorder.
2. **Etiology**
   - Unknown.
3. **Pathology**
   - Often preceded by trauma, even minor to the area.
   - Severity of symptoms is not related to severity of preceding event or injury.
   - Psychological stress is not considered causative.
   - Symptoms can begin days to weeks after the preceding incident.
4. **Clinical Features**
   - Chronic musculoskeletal disorder. Can present with both localized and diffuse burning pain. Can be accompanied by swelling of the area, dystrophic skin and nail changes of the affected limb, and color and temperature changes of the skin.
   - Limited range of motion of the area is seen as well.
   - Symptoms are not limited to one peripheral nerve distribution area and can involve whole limb area (lower leg) or even anatomical quadrant.
   - Pain is out of proportion to level or severity of stimulation.
   - Symptoms can, but do not always, progress from the involved area being warm, swollen, and sweaty to cool, and then dystrophic.
5. **Diagnostic Studies**
   - Clinical diagnosis, but X-ray or bone scan may be helpful in ruling out differential diagnosis.
6. **Management**
   - No long-term, effective treatment has been proven.
   - Patient education is paramount.
   - Spontaneous remission of symptoms is rare, but can occur in mild cases within several weeks to months. Early mobilization after trauma or surgery lessens the likelihood of development. Two hundred to 1,500 mg of vitamin C appears to reduce the likelihood of CRPS following wrist fracture.
   - Major portion of treatment is exercise and mobilization of the area.
   - Neurontin has been used in treatment as have topical capsaicin and prednisone at 40 mg per day for 2 weeks followed by a taper.
   - IV bisphosphonates, particularly clodronate, may reduce symptoms.

II. Headaches

A. Headaches

1. **General Disease and Pathology**
   - Headaches are classified into two groups:
     - Primary headaches that do not have an underlying pathology related to them (migraines, tension headaches, cluster headaches, etc.).
     - Secondary headaches that are related to an underlying pathology (infection, medication overuse, malignancy).
2. **General Clinical Features to Consider**
   - Red flags (headache warning signs that could indicate secondary headaches):
     - New-onset headaches in patients over 50, those with a history of cancer or with HIV, or those with risk factors for cerebral venous sinus thrombosis.
     - A headache that reaches peak intensity in seconds to minutes ("thunderclap").
     - Any headaches accompanied by fever, neck pain, visual disturbance, or jaw claudication.
     - Any patient with neurologic symptoms (change in cognition, limb or facial weakness, extended aura, etc.) or neurologic abnormalities on physical examination.
     - Although migraine is the most common cause of morning headaches, a headache that wakes one from sleep requires further work-up.
     - Headaches that are brought on by Valsalva or physical exertion or that change with changes in posture.
     - Patients with headache who have any of the above warning signs/features should be referred for specialist assessment.
     - Thunderclap headaches, those suggestive of increased intracranial pressure or those suggestive of infection, need immediate specialist assessment.

- All patients presenting with a headache should have a full cervical examination (inspection for posture, palpation of muscle tone and any muscle or bony prominence tenderness, and full [range of motion] ROM in all directions).
- New-onset headaches or those that are different from what the patient usually experiences should be evaluated through physical examination with blood pressure (BP) and full neurologic exam (including fundoscopic examination).
- Headache diaries or various assessment tools should be used to track headache patterns.

3. **General Diagnostic Studies**
- Magnetic resonance imaging (MRI) should be considered in patients who have a headache that is brought on, not aggravated, by cough, those with unilateral neuralgiform headache attacks with conjunctival injection and tearing (SUNCT), those who present with cluster headaches (see below) or paroxysmal hemicranias.
- Computed tomography (CT) should be considered in patients who have abnormal neurologic examinations of unexplained origin unless MRI is more appropriate.
- CT should also be used within 12 hours from onset in those with thunderclap headaches.
- A lumber puncture with oxyhaemoglobin and bilirubin should be done in patients with thunderclap headaches who have normal CT results.

B. Cluster Headache
1. **Etiology**
- Unknown, may have a positive family history of cluster headaches, associated with smoking and head trauma as well.
2. **Pathology**
- Pathophysiology thought to involve hypothalamic activation and possible vasodilatation and activation of the trigeminovascular system and autonomic features.
3. **Clinical Features**
- Episodic, more common (80% to 90% of patients with cluster headaches) than chronic type (10%).
- Episodic is at least two cluster periods that can last from 7 days to 1 full year and have symptom-free periods in between clusters of at least 1 month.
- In the chronic type, symptom clusters last a year or longer and remission is <1 month.
- Common in middle-aged men, with onset between 20 and 50 years.
- Severe, often excruciating, unilateral, periorbital or temporal sharp and piercing pain.
- The pain is deep, nonthrobbing, and may radiate to the forehead, temple, or cheek; less frequently to the ear, occiput, and neck.

- Duration from 15 minutes to several hours, frequently occur near bedtime often awakening patient from sleep.
- Associated unilateral lacrimation, nasal congestion, and ocular redness; rhinorrhea and Horner syndrome.

4. **Diagnostic Studies**
- MRI to rule out differential diagnosis of severe headache.
- Rule out intracranial hemorrhage, tic douloureux, glaucoma, sinusitis, dental abscess.

5. **Management**
- Prognosis is good and patients tend to respond to abortive measures.
- May spontaneously regress with varying period until next episode.
- Abortive therapy first-line choice is subcutaneous sumatriptan (6 mg).
- Intranasal triptans for those who cannot tolerate subcutaneous.
- Inhalation of 6 to 10 L of 100% O_2 for 15 to 20 minutes.

PREVENTIVE THERAPY
- No current long-duration studies of effective long-term control.
- One hundred and twenty milligram verapamil TID × 2 weeks, prednisone, 10 mg melatonin PO QHS × 2 weeks.
- Surgical options include trigeminal nerve sectioning or injection.
- Reduce stress through relaxation, can use biofeedback, reduce tobacco and alcohol use.

C. Migraine Headache (with Aura and without Aura)
1. **Etiology**
- Presents in patient usually before age 40.
- The lifetime prevalence of migraines is 20% to 25%. About 23 million people in the United States are estimated to have migraines (18% female, 6% male) and over 4 million have at least one attack per month.
- Migraines tend to decrease with age.
2. **Pathology**
- Pathophysiology is polygenetic and multifactorial.
- No longer considered to be caused by vascular dilation and constriction phenomena.
- Thought to be related to primary neuronal dysfunction with activation of trigeminovascular system reflex, cortical spreading depression, and serotonins.
3. **Clinical Features**
- Most common cause of morning headaches.
- Migraine headaches can be preceded by a typical aura in 15% to 33% of patients with migraines.
- Severe, periodic headaches that cause disability.
- Visual symptoms are most common.

- Sensitivity to light as well as sensitivity to noise can occur either during or in between attacks.
- Physical activity may also worsen symptoms.
- Patients have a normal neurologic examination.
- Other premonitory symptoms include fatigue, diminished concentration, sensitivity to light and sound, nausea, and blurred vision.
- Sildenafil may cause migraines.
- Overuse of analgesics can increase chronic pain, particularly migraine.
- Obesity may increase frequency and severity, but not prevalence of migraines.
- Oral contraceptives are not associated with increased risk; however, some resources suggest that women with migraine with aura and those over 35 with migraine without aura should not use combined oral contraceptive pills.
- Current evidence also cannot establish a link between food triggers and migraines.
- Auras are defined as a sensory, visual, or motor disturbance (manifesting singly or together) that precede the headache.
- May include scintillating scotomata, multiple small dots, homonymous visual disturbances, hemisensory disturbance, speech disturbance, and vertigo.
- The headache is usually unilateral and associated with nausea, vomiting, and photophobia.
- Headaches last from several hours to 1 to 2 weeks.
- Last several hours to several days, and can include unilateral pain (sometimes of pulsating nature) of moderate-to-severe intensity.
- Also associated with nausea, vomiting, and photophobia.

4. **Diagnostic Studies**
   - In patients with a clear history of migraine, without red-flag signs or symptoms and who have abnormal neurologic evaluation, neuroimaging is not indicated.

5. **Management**
   - Patients find comfort in lying down in a dark, quiet place.
   - Stress management to reduce the number and severity of migraines.
   - Aspirin 900 mg or Ibuprofen 400 mg is recommended for acute treatment in patients with all severity of migraine.
   - Paracetamol 1,000 mg can be used for acute treatment in mild-to-moderate migraines.
   - Other abortive therapy if simple analgesics have not been effective includes oral triptans, and they should be taken at onset or as soon thereafter as possible.
   - Oral, rectal, or IV antiemetics may be helpful in reducing nausea.
   - Ergotamine is not recommended for use in acute migraine.

- Prophylaxis includes beta blockers. Eighty to 240 mg propranolol per day is the recommended first-line therapy for migraine prophylaxis. Timolol, atenolol, nadolol, and metoprolol can be used as alternatives.
- Antiepileptics may also be beneficial (sodium valproate, gabapentin, and topiramate. Topiramate recently considered pregnancy category D).
- Amitriptyline or venlafaxine can be used as prophylaxis as well.
- SSRIs and botulinum toxin A are not recommended for prophylaxis.
- Note that triptans are contraindicated in patients with various types of heart disease.
- Aspirin is contraindicated in the third trimester of pregnancy.

D. Tension-Type Headaches
  1. **Etiology**
     - Physical manifestation of psychosocial stresses.
     - Associated with depressed state, anxiety.
     - The most common form of headache.
     - Usually begins in middle age and affects women more than men.
  2. **Clinical Features**
     - Episodic.
     - Constricting, bilateral, "band-like distribution," tend to occur later in the day and be associated with anorexia.
     - Recurrent.
     - Pressure-like, squeezing and tightening pain with neck and shoulder tenderness; occasional nausea that occurs 15 days per month for more than 6 months.
     - Tension headache should be considered when a patient has a bilateral, nondisabling headache and has a normal neurologic physical exam.
     - Physical examination may show neck or head musculature contraction.
     - Complete neurologic examination indicated in any new-onset headache, with imaging studies to rule out intracranial abnormalities if indicated.
  3. **Management**
     - Stress management.
     - Aspirin and paracetamol for acute tension headache treatment.
     - Consider tricyclics (amitriptyline 25 to 150 mg at bedtime) for prophylaxis of chronic tension headaches.
     - Botulinum toxin A is not recommended as a prophylaxis of tension headaches.

III. Infectious Disorders
A. Encephalitis
   - Involves inflammatory response of the brain with neurologic dysfunction.

1. **Etiology**
   - Mostly viral, can be bacterial or fungal as well.
   - Herpes simplex encephalitis (HSV) is the most common viral encephalitis; 70% mortality rate if left untreated; type 2 causes neonatal encephalitis; type 1 present in older persons.
   - Arboviruses (epidemic viral encephalitis):
     - Carried by mosquitoes and ticks and tend to be seasonal.
     - Include three viruses causing Western, Eastern, and Venezuelan equine encephalitis; two flaviviruses causing St. Louis and Japanese B encephalitis; and bunyaviruses causing California encephalitis.
     - Leading causes of arbovirus encephalitis in the United States—St. Louis and California encephalitis.
   - Myxovirus (mumps and measles encephalitis):
     - Most common childhood encephalitis.
     - Occasionally occurs in epidemics.
     - Mumps encephalitis: usually mild, seen most in late winter.
   - Measles encephalitis: 15% mortality rate. Number of cases is declining secondary to vaccinations.
   - Cytomegalovirus (CMV): One of the most common causes of encephalitis in the immunosuppressed population.

2. **Pathology**
   - Viral invasion of the brain parenchyma.
   - Meningoencephalitis is seen more often than pure encephalitis.
   - Primary viral invasion of central nervous system (CNS).
   - Infection agents by age:
     - Infants—consider herpes simplex type 2, CMV, rubella, *Listeria monocytogenes, Treponema pallidum,* and *Toxoplasma gondii.*
     - Infants/children—consider influenza virus, Japanese encephalitis virus, eastern equine encephalitis virus, Murray Valley encephalitis.
     - Elderly—consider St. Louis virus, *L. monocytogenes,* West Nile virus, eastern equine encephalitis.

3. **Clinical Features**
   - Presentation is nonspecific, acute, febrile illness.
   - Signs and symptoms based on etiology may include fever, headache, nausea, emesis, photophobia, nuchal rigidity, hepatitis, rash, lymphadenopathy, rash, respiratory complaints, urinary symptoms, retinitis, dementia, cranial nerve defects, cerebellar involvements, and parkinsonism.
   - Ask about recent travel, exposure to animals (dogs, cats, bats, skunks, raccoons, rodents, some primates, sheep, goats, white-tailed deer, birds, horses) or insects (mosquitoes, ticks, sandflies, tsetse flies), recent illness or immunizations, immune status, recreational activities, occupational exposures, and note season of the year.
   - Encephalitis is usually transient and accompanies a systemic viral illness.

4. **Diagnostic Studies**
   - Neuroimaging must be used.
   - MRI is the most sensitive imaging test in the evaluation of encephalitis.
   - CT is an alternative when MRI cannot be done.
   - Cerebrospinal fluid (CSF) analysis is necessary, unless contraindicated, through lumbar puncture (LP) and PCR nucleic acid amplification testing.
   - PCR testing for herpes simplex in all patients with suspected encephalitis.
   - EEG rarely helpful in establishing etiology.
   - Fluorodeoxyglucose positron emission (FDG-PET) tomography or viral cultures of CSF not routinely recommended.
   - Normal glucose shows elevated protein and lymphocytic pleocytosis.
   - Elevated RBCs are seen in herpes encephalitis.
   - Brain biopsy is reserved for patients with focal abnormalities on MRI, who deteriorate clinically despite antiviral therapy and in whom PCR studies are inconclusive.

5. **Management**
   - No definitive treatment in many cases.
   - Acyclovir (10 mg per kg IV every 8 hours in children and adults who have uncompromised renal function, 20 mg per kg for neonates) should be started as soon as possible in all patients with suspected encephalitis while waiting for the results of further testing.
   - Starting treatment for herpes simplex encephalitis as early as possible reduces the likelihood of serious complications or death.
   - CMV: ganciclovir/foscarnet combination.
   - Influenza virus: oseltamivir.
   - For all other types, treat etiologic bacterial, rickettsial, fungal, or ehrlichial agent.
   - Supportive measures including antipyretics, analgesics, anticonvulsants, rest.
   - Watch for syndrome of inappropriate antidiuretic hormone secretion.

B. Meningitis

ACUTE MENINGITIS

1. **Etiology**
   - Medical and neurologic emergency.
   - Estimated 2 to 5 per 100,000 people in the Western world.
   - Permanent neurologic complications in 30% to 50% of illness survivors.
   - Pathogens gain entry through various routes.

2. **Pathology**
   - Spread from contiguous sites of infection (e.g., paranasal sinusitis, mastoiditis, otitis, and osteomyelitis of skull or vertebrae).
   - Direct implantation through LP, penetrating wounds, or surgery.
   - Organism enters intravascular space and choroid plexus, but no opsonization occurs due to low number of WBCs in CSF; inflammatory reaction occurs with lysis of bacteria and release of cell wall components into subarachnoid space and formation of purulent exudates. Meningeal inflammation begins with increased cytokines (interleukins and tumor necrosis factor), amino acids, and free oxygen (O_2) radicals, which then leads to increased permeability of blood–brain barrier, obstruction of CSF flow dynamics, ischemia, and necrosis.
   - Bacterial: Includes both gram-negative and gram-positive organisms.
   - Eighty percent of cases of acute bacterial meningitis (ABM) in immunocompetent infants over 4 weeks of age, children, and adults are caused by *Streptococcus pneumonia* or *Neisseria meningitides*.
   - *Streptococcus pneumonia* is the most common cause of community-acquired ABM.
   - *Listeria monocytogenes* and staph are also common and <10% of cases are caused by gram-negative bacilli like *Escherichia coli, Klebsiella, Entreobacter,* and *Psuedomonas aeruginosa.*
   - The most common causative organisms in ABM in immunocompromised patients are *L. monocytogenes, S. pneumonia,* and *P. aeruginosa.*
   - Nosocomial infections are caused mostly by staph strains.
   - Aseptic meningitis, caused by viruses (Coxsackie viruses, echoviruses, polioviruses, and human enteroviruses 68 to 71 and less commonly herpes simplex virus [HSV] type 2, mumps, and HIV).
   - Fungi occur in malnourished, debilitated, or immunosuppressed patients.
     - Common pathogens include *Cryptococcus, Candida, Fusarium.*
     - Rare pathogens such as *Histoplasma, Coccidioides, Paracoccidioides* infect healthy persons.
   - Tuberculosis (TB), caused by *Mycobacterium tuberculosis,* is seen in malnourished, debilitated, or immunosuppressed persons.

3. **Clinical Features**
   - Most patients have at least two of the following four symptoms: mental status change, fever, headache, and stiff neck.
   - Change in mental status can vary from confusion to coma.
   - Photophobia, nausea, emesis.
   - Late: seizures, stupor, coma, cranial nerve palsies, deafness, focal neurologic signs, and papilledema.
   - Positive Kernig and Brudzinski signs.
   - In infants: irritability, lethargy, seizures, anorexia, bulging fontanelles.
   - May have rash of meningococcemia: diffuse, erythematous maculopapular rash on trunk/extremities/mucous membranes, conjunctiva; becomes petechial.
   - Rapidly evolving rash indicates *N. meningitides* pathogen.

4. **Diagnostic Studies**
   - Obtain blood cultures immediately in suspected meningitis prior to initiating antibiotic therapy.
   - Obtain fast-track neuroimaging, if at all possible, prior to LP if available to look for possible LP contraindications (intracranial mass lesions, midline shift, and obstructive hydrocephalus).
   - LP should be done as soon as possible: CSF examination is essential to diagnosis unless contraindication(s) like papilledema, focal neurologic sign, or coagulopathy is/are present.
   - LP is the most definitive diagnostic study for suspected ABM.
   - CSF profiles differ between the various types of pathogens (Table 6-1).
   - Other testing such as possible latex agglutination antigen tests detect *H. influenzae, S. pneumoniae,* and *Neisseria meningitides.*

5. **Management**
   - Hospitalize as soon as possible (within 90 minutes of presentation to a health care setting, treatment to be commenced within 60 minutes of hospital admission, and begin treatment within 3 hours of presentation to care setting).

TABLE 6–1.	Spinal Fluid Profiles in Acute Meningitis			
Variables	**Pressure**	**WBCs (cells/mm^3)**	**Protein**	**Glucose**
Viral	nl or slight ↑	5–1,000	Slight ↑	nl
Bacterial	↑	1,000–10,000	↑	↓
Chronic/TB	↑	25–500	↑	↓

WBCs, white blood cells; nl, normal; ↑, increase; ↓, decrease; TB, tuberculosis.

- Admission to a neurologic ICU is preferable if possible.
- Hospitalization for observation and prompt administration of appropriate IV antibiotics are essential.
- Bacterial meningitis.
  - IV third generation cephalosporins (cefotaxime or ceftriaxone) are the initial drug of choice in the absence of antibiotic resistance and penicillin (PCN) allergy and can be started empirically.
  - Begin with empiric broad-spectrum antibiotic, then tailor therapy when the organism is identified and its sensitivities are determined.
  - *Listeria monocytogenes*: third generation cephalosporin + amoxicillin.
  - PCN-resistant pneumococcus: vancomycin + third generation cephalosporin.
  - Dexamethasone with or shortly before first administration of antibiotics in *S. pneumonia* or *H. Influenzae*.
  - Suspected *N. meningitides* due to rapidly evolving rash on PE: IV benzyl PCN in the absence of PCN allergy.
  - Common initial antibiotic therapy for ages 2 months to adult:
  - Ceftriaxone, 2 g IV q12h and vancomycin, 10 to 15 mg per kg IV q6h; if over 50 years, add ampicillin 2 g IV q8h.
  - Dexamethasone 0.15 mg per kg IV q6h for 2 to 4 days. Inhibits interleukins and stabilizes the blood–brain barrier, decreases meningeal inflammation.
  - Consider prophylaxis of household occupants, day care workers, teachers with rifampin, ceftriaxone, or ciprofloxacin.
  - Therapy duration: *S. pneumonia*, 10 to 14 days; *N. meningitides*, 3 to 7 days; *H. influenza*, 7 days; *L. monocytogenes*, 14 to 21 days; gram-negative bacilli, 21 days.
- Viral meningitis.
  - Supportive treatment (analgesics for headache, antiemetics for nausea and vomiting).
  - Hospitalization is not required; observation at home by a responsible person is routine.
  - Prognosis is excellent; full recovery in 1 to 2 weeks.
  - Fungal meningitis.
  - Hospitalize for observation and appropriate IV antifungal medication: amphotericin B (lipid complex, liposomal or colloidal dispersion) for several weeks to months, addition of flucytosine may potentiate efficacy.
  - Complications and neurologic sequelae are the same as bacterial meningitis.
  - Mortality rate is 20% to 50%.
- TB meningitis.
  - Initial therapy: rifampin, isoniazid, ethambutol, and pyrazinamide.
  - Specific treatment regimen depends on known regional antibiotic sensitivities and culture information, but duration of therapy is 18 to 24 months.

IV. Movement Disorders
A. Essential Tremor (Familial Tremor, Benign Essential Tremor, Senile Tremor)
1. **Etiology**
   - An uncontrollable (involuntary) tremor at rest involving the head, voice, or hands that worsens with intentional movement.
   - Cause unknown, sometimes an autosomal dominant inheritance.
   - Can begin at any age.
   - Most common of all movement disorders.
2. **Pathology**
   - No associated neurologic disorder.
3. **Clinical Features**
   - Tremor at rest that increases when under emotional stress.
   - On finger-to-nose test, tremor increases as "target" is approached.
   - Typically improves with ingestion of a small amount of alcohol for a short time.
4. **Diagnostic Studies**
   - Physical examination should include evaluation of limb supported at rest, elevated versus gravity, and with goal-directed movements.
   - No CT, MRI, hematologic, or serum abnormalities.
   - Differential diagnosis to include Parkinson, myoclonus, ethyl alcohol (ETOH) withdrawal, drug-induced.
   - Check for thyroid abnormalities, heavy-metal poisoning.
5. **Management**
   - Treatment unnecessary unless causing disability.
   - Stress reduction.
   - Propranolol (60 to 240 mg per day), primidone (starting at 50 mg QD, increasing to 125 mg TID), alprazolam (up to 3 mg QD, divided).
   - Reassure this is not associated with other conditions.
   - Surgical options for refractory cases: deep brain stimulator and unilateral thalamotomy.

B. Huntington Disease
Progressive, fatal movement disorder with dementia and chorea (abnormal movements).
1. **Etiology**
   - Autosomal dominant inherited disorder with a prevalence of 5 per 100,000 people.
   - Onset is usually between ages 30 and 50 and death results between 15 and 20 years later.

2. **Pathology**
   - Abnormal genetic repeat in the Huntington gene, length of repeat may correlate with the speed of progression of the disease.
   - Decreased activity of acetylcholine (ACh) and γ-aminobutyric acid neurons and increased activity of dopaminergic neurons.
3. **Clinical Features**
   - Family history of Huntington disease.
   - Most common initial symptoms are behavior changes like mood changes, irritability, or antisocial changes. Subsequent development of dementia follows. Cognitive/intellectual changes and abnormal or bizarre movements are hallmarks of the illness. The dyskinesia portion can begin as apparent restlessness or fidgeting but progress to full chorea like movements, rigidity, and dystonia.
4. **Diagnostic Studies**
   - Genetic testing.
   - In diagnosed cases, neuroimaging (MRI or CT) can demonstrate cerebral atrophy and caudate nucleus atrophy. Decreased striatal metabolic rate is shown on PET.
5. **Management**
   - There is no cure or way to slow or halt the progression of Huntington disease.
   - Treatments are for symptom reduction only.
   - Tetrabenzine or amantadine can be used for chorea symptoms, 12.5 mg two to three times per day, increasing to 25 mg three times per day.
   - Haloperidol may limit behavioral symptoms or dyskinesias.
   - Clozapine or atypical antipsychotics can also be used for behavioral symptoms.

C. **Parkinson Disease (Paralysis Agitans or Idiopathic Parkinsonism)**
   1. **Etiology**
      - A progressive neurodegenerative disease of unknown etiology.
      - Occurs in all ethnic groups and in men and women equally.
      - Generally begins between 40 and 70 years of age with peak onset in the sixth decade.
   2. **Pathology**
      - Loss of dopamine in the corpus striatum; degeneration of the substantia nigra in the midbrain. Cytoplasmic inclusion bodies in neurons of substantia nigra and locus ceruleus (Lewy bodies).
      - Loss of pigmented cells in the nigra, locus ceruleus, and dorsal motor nucleus of the vagus.
   3. **Clinical Features**
      - Resting tremor—most frequent sign; often unilateral, described as "pill rolling" when it involves the fingers and thumb.
      - Cogwheel rigidity—elicited by passive movement.
      - Bradykinesia—slowness of voluntary movement; difficulty turning in bed, walking, chewing food, rising from chairs, and other activities.
      - Expressionless, unblinking, mask-like face.
      - Decreased postural reflexes—inability of the patient to keep from losing his or her balance when jostled (e.g., when in a crowd).
      - Stooped posture.
      - Festinating gait characterized by involuntary acceleration.
      - Micrographia (small handwriting).
      - Drooling secondary to failure to swallow saliva with normal frequency.
      - Nonmotor clinical features: cognitive dysfunction and dementia, psychosis, hallucinations, mood disorders, fatigue, sleep disturbance, autonomic and olfactory dysfunction.
   4. **Diagnostic Studies**
      - None definitive.
      - Clinical diagnosis based on a constellation of signs and symptoms.
      - Presence of cardinal manifestations: tremor, bradykinesia, rigidity, and gait disturbance.
      - Response to dopaminergic therapy.
      - Differential diagnosis: neurodegenerative disorders, dementia with Lewy bodies, corticobasal degeneration, secondary parkinsonism (drug effect), essential tremor.
   5. **Management**
      - Consider: signs and symptoms, age, stage of disease, degree of functional disability.
      - Options: nonpharmacologic, pharmacologic, and surgical.
      - Nonpharmacologic:
        - Education, support, exercise, nutrition. Keep protein to minimum recommended level and have main protein meal at the end of the day.
        - Maintenance of optimal general health and neuromuscular efficiency with a planned program of exercise and rest.
      - Pharmacologic:
      - Symptomatic treatment:
        - Exogenous levodopa (precursor to dopamine) in combination with peripheral dopa decarboxylase inhibitor. Does not stop progression of disease.
        - Carbidopa/levodopa (Sinemet, Aldomet) starting dose: 25/100/TID.
          - Start low and titrate upward.
          - Short-term side effects: nausea, hypotensive episodes.
          - Long-term side effects: dyskinesias (involuntary movements including restlessness, head-wagging, grimacing, lingual-labial dyskinesia, dystonia), psychiatric (depression, altered sleep patterns, vivid nightmares, auditory and visual hallucinations, paranoia, and frank psychosis),

and fluctuations in motor performance (on–off phenomenon).
  • Due to tolerance and side effects, it is recommended that drug therapy with carbidopa/levodopa be delayed until symptoms significantly affect the patient's life.
  • Dopamine agonists (Parlodel, Mirapex, Requip) direct dopaminergic effect on striatal neurons (bromocriptine, Parlodel, Permax, Mirapex, Requip).
    • Adverse effects: unpredictable sleepiness.
  • Amantadine: antiviral that allows release of dopamine from presynaptic storage sites.
    • Adverse effects: visual hallucinations, skin mottling, nausea.
  • Anticholinergic agents (Artane, Cogentin).
    • Useful for tremor.
    • Adverse effects: dry mouth, blurred vision, urinary retention, confusion.
• Surgical options:
  • Deep brain stimulation, thalamotomy, pallidotomy.

V. Vascular Disorders

A. Cerebral Aneurysm/Intracranial Aneurysm
1. Clinical Features
  • "Berry" or saccular aneurysms.
  • Multiple aneurysms present in 20% of cases.
  • Typically occur anterior to the circle of Willis.
  • Subarachnoid hemorrhage (SAH) is a complication, and the risk of this is increased in "nonwhite," females, those who drink 150 mg of ETOH or more per week, tobacco users, those with hypertension (HTN) or hypercholesterolemia. Older age is also a risk factor for SAH in the presence of an intracranial aneurysm.
  • Can be asymptomatic or have nonspecific symptoms until rupture and result in SAH. After rupture, patient may complain of the classic sudden onset "worst headache of my life" seen in SAH. Focal neurologic deficits are seen depending on the location of the bleed.
  • **Most common initial symptom:**
    • The aneurysm itself may be asymptomatic, but resulting SAH may present with loss of consciousness, headache, nausea, and/or focal neurologic deficits.
2. Diagnostic Studies
  • Angiography is definitive.
  • CT or MRI may not be thorough enough for smaller lesions, especially when surgery is being considered.
3. Management
  • Prompt endovascular/surgical treatment needed for symptomatic aneurysms that have not yet ruptured.

  • Monitor aneurysms smaller than 10 mm with angiograms, consider surgery at size over 10 mm.

B. Intracranial Hemorrhage
1. Disease
  • Intracranial and SAH are subclassifications of hemorrhagic stroke.
2. Etiology/Pathology
  • HTN is usually the cause of a spontaneous intracerebral hemorrhage (ICH) that did not occur from trauma, if the patient does not have evidence of a vascular abnormality like an angioma or aneurysm.
  • Usually occurs in the basal ganglia.
  • Bleeding disorders, tumors, liver disease, alcohol abuse, and anticoagulation therapy can also be causes.
  • Older age and male sex are risk factors.
  • Bleeding occurs into the subarachnoid space usually when due to an AV malformation or aneurysm.
3. Clinical Features
  • Hemorrhages occur suddenly and are accompanied by loss of consciousness in half of patients.
  • Vomiting and headache are common.
  • There can be corresponding focal symptoms depending on the cerebral location of the bleed.
  • Hypertensive etiology hemorrhage is usually accompanied by a rapidly progressive hemiplegia or hemiparesis.
  • Extraoccular movements may be compromised depending on the location of the bleed as well.
  • Look for changes in respiration, ataxia, change in small and reactive pupils, facial weakness.
4. Diagnostic Studies
  • Noncontrast CT is superior to MRI.
  • Look for predisposing factors in lab work.
  • Avoid LP.
5. Management
  • Supportive to symptoms.
  • Intracranial pressure alleviating techniques may be helpful in some cases.
  • Cerebellar hemorrhage requires prompt surgery.

C. Cerebrovascular Accident (CVA, Stroke)
1. Etiology
  • Third leading cause of death in the United States.
  • Classified into several categories depending on whether CVA is caused by a primary ischemic or primary hemorrhagic insult.
  • Ischemia occurs due to reduction in cerebral blood flow with symptoms occurring within 10 seconds due to lack of glycogen in neurons and "energy crisis."
  • Eighty percent of all strokes are ischemic (due to thrombus, emboli, or systemic hypoperfusion) and 20% are hemorrhagic (intracerebral and SAH).
  • Cerebral thrombosis includes lacunar (small vessel, penetrating arteries, atheroma, and

lipohyalinosis) and large vessel thrombosis (atherosclerosis, dissection).

- Cardioembolic source: atrial fibrillation, myocardial infarction (MI), mural thrombus, valvular lesions/prosthesis, anomalies, dilated cardiomyopathy, bacterial endocarditis.
- Hypercoagulable disorders: venous sinus thrombosis (complication of pregnancy, postpartum, sepsis, brain abscess/meningitis), polycythemia, factor V Leiden mutation (protein C, S deficiency, antiphospholipid antibody syndrome, AT III deficiency, OCP, sickle cell disease, homocystinemia).
- Vascular etiologies: fibromuscular dysplasia, temporal arteritis, vasculitis, moyamoya disease.
- Primary hemorrhagic lesions: 20% of patients include ICH (14%), often HTN related (basal ganglia, thalamus, cerebellum, brain stem), amyloid angiopathy (lobar hemorrhage), and SAH (6%).
- Most common cause of SAH is trauma, but if no history of trauma, must rule out intracranial aneurysm.

2. **Pathology**
   - Atherosclerotic damage to aortic arch, carotid bifurcation, or intracranial vessels occurs that produces local thrombus and distal embolism with injury to vascular endothelial cells.
   - Nonmodifiable risk factors: increasing age, male, African American, family history, sickle cell disease, hypercoagulable state.
   - Modifiable risk factors: hypercholesterolemia, HTN, atrial fibrillation, diabetes mellitus (DM), asymptomatic carotid stenosis, transient ischemic attack (TIA), smoking, oral contraceptive use, obesity, alcohol consumption, physical inactivity.

3. **Clinical Features**
   - Ischemic and hemorrhagic stroke: symptoms determined by vascular territory of affected vessel, variable acute or subacute neurologic deficits (e.g., headache, alteration of consciousness, speech disturbance, that is, aphasia or dysarthria, visual deficits, apraxia, agnosia, motor or sensory dysfunction).
   - ICH: abrupt onset of severe headache, hemiplegia, and diminished level of consciousness; may not see these findings if hemorrhage is small.
   - SAH: abrupt onset of headache (worst headache of life), photophobia, nuchal rigidity, Kernig sign, and alteration of consciousness.

4. **Diagnostic Studies**
   - Complete blood count (CBC) to rule out polycythemia; elevated WBCs are present in infective endocarditis, PT, PTT, platelet count, consider syphilis serology, blood cultures, cholesterol profile, ECG/telemetry, chest X-ray (CXR), cardiac echo (transthoracic or transesophageal).
   - Noncontrast CT scan of head is preferable to MRI in acute stages (first 48 hours) as it is faster than MRI and detects intracranial hemorrhage better than MRI in first 48 hours after an acute bleed. Poor detection in posterior fossa stroke, may remain "normal" in initial 12 to 24 hours.
   - MRI/magnetic resonance angiography (MRA). Diffusion-weighted MRI is more sensitive than nondiffusion weighted MRI for visualizing cerebral ischemia.
   - EEG not routinely indicated; useful in distinguishing focal seizure activity from fluctuating symptoms of stroke or TIA.
   - Carotid ultrasound (U/S) identifies occlusion or stenosis of carotid arteries.
   - Cerebral angiography identifies stenosis, thrombosis, aneurysms, arteriovenous malformation (AVM), and other cerebrovascular abnormalities.
   - LP (if no contraindication) if suspicion for SAH and negative CT scan (look for xanthochromia).

5. **Management**
   - Thrombolytics, anticoagulation, antiplatelets, carotid endarterectomy/stent/angioplasty, surgical decompression, medical management, rehabilitation, and secondary prevention.
   - Thrombolytics: recombinant tissue plasminogen activator (rtPA).
   - rtPA most beneficial if within 3 hours of symptoms, no more than 4.5 hours and if no evidence of hemorrhage on CT.
   - Many contraindications to use including recent bleeding or increased risk of bleeding, HTN, systolic >185 mm Hg or diastolic >110 mm Hg.
   - Anticoagulation with warfarin if chronic atrial fibrillation, cardioembolic source, recent MI, valvular disease/prosthetics.
   - Antiplatelet therapy: acetylsalicylic acid, clopidogrel, dipyridamole.
   - Surgical options: ICP monitor, decompression craniotomy with evacuation of hemorrhage, craniectomy and expansion duraplasty if edema/ICP in select cases.
   - Primary and secondary stroke prevention: Evaluate clinical risk profile and manage modifiable risk factors, control HTN, treat hypercholesterolemia, smoking cessation, weight loss, exercise.
   - Supportive therapy: consultation with appropriate rehabilitation services; may include speech, occupational, and physical therapy and social services.

D. Transient Ischemic Attack
1. **Etiology**
   - Characterized by focal ischemic cerebral neurologic deficits, lasting <24 hours (usually minutes to 1 to 2 hours).
   - CVA following TIA most likely in the following 48 hours, CVA after TIA is increased in patients with diabetes or HTN.

- Emboli are most important cause; most common source is carotid or vertebrobasilar circulations.
- Cardiac causes of embolic TIA include atrial fibrillation, rheumatic heart disease, mitral valve disease, cardiac arrhythmia, infective endocarditis, and atrial myxoma.
- Less common causes include fibromuscular dysplasia, meningovascular syphilis, and inflammatory arterial disorders (e.g., giant cell arteritis, systemic lupus erythematosus [SLE], polyarteritis, granulomatous angiitis) and hematologic causes like sickle cell, polycythemia, and syndromes with increased viscosity.
- Crescendo TIAs—occurrence of increasing number and frequency with a high likelihood of evolving to stroke (two or more attacks within 24 hours).

2. **Clinical Features**
- Symptoms vary markedly among patients; however, for a given patient, symptoms tend to be constant.
- Symptoms:
  - Weakness or heaviness of contralateral arm (bear-paw clumsy), leg, or face.
  - Numbness, paresthesias.
  - Slowness of movement.
  - Dysphasia.
  - Monocular visual loss in the eye (amaurosis fugax).
  - Abrupt onset, without warning.
  - Rapid recovery, usually 1 to 2 hours; can be within minutes.
  - One-third of patients with TIAs continue to have attacks without sequelae, one-third experience spontaneous remission, and one-third subsequently suffer brain infarction.

3. **Diagnostic Studies**
- CT scan or MRI of head: excludes small cerebral hemorrhage or tumor that may mimic TIA symptoms; carotid duplex U/S: detects stenosis of internal carotid artery, computed tomography angiography, MRA, or conventional angiography to evaluate carotids and circle of Willis.
- Assess patient for risk factors: CBC, fasting blood glucose, serum cholesterol profile, ECG, echo if suspect cardiac source emboli, blood cultures if endocarditis is suspected, Holter monitor if transient, paroxysmal cardiac arrhythmia is suspected.

4. **Management**
- May warn of imminent stroke, be aggressive.
- Treat or modify controllable risk factors, if atrial fibrillation or cardioembolism, anticoagulants: heparin, follow with warfarin; antiplatelet therapy: aspirin 81 to 325 mg daily; clopidogrel (Plavix) 75 mg daily; carotid endarterectomy; angioplasty; or stenting depending on angiographic findings.

VI. Other Neurologic Disorders

A. Cerebral Palsy

1. **Etiology**
- State of impaired muscle tone, movement, and coordination of various severities in each patient. The conditions are nonprogressive and unresolving.
- However, in some cases, intellectual capacity is normal and those children can lead productive lives of normal span.
- Caused by brain injury or insult either before or during birth or in the perinatal phase. Intrauterine hypoxia is a common cause of insult.

2. **Clinical Features**
- Limb spasticity is common (75% of cases) and carious limbs and combination can be affected. Fine movement deficits and decreased coordination along with involuntary movements are also seen. Sensory and neurologic deficits can also be found.
- Physical examination may reveal limb spasticity, hyperreflexia and microcephaly. Seizure disorders are also possible. Patients with mild forms may improve over time.

3. **Diagnostic Studies**
- MRI may reveal the etiology or the extent of the involved cerebral area.

4. **Management**
- Occupational, physical, and speech therapy.
- Supportive therapy.
- Pharmacologic therapy for seizure control or muscle spasticity possibly needed. Secondary infections such as pneumonia should be prevented.

B. Concussion

1. **Etiology**
- A concussion is actually mild traumatic brain injury (TBI) after blunt or acceleration–deceleration injuries to the head.
- Characterized by a Glasgow Coma Scale (GCS) of 14–15/15, change in mental status or cerebral function after head trauma.

2. **Pathology**
- Mild TBI secondary to trauma.

3. **Clinical Features**
- Can include any of the following physical, cognitive, or behavioral changes or deficits: short- and long-term memory impairment, altered cognitive processing speeds, executive function or difficulty with calculations, fatigue, blurred vision, seizure, dizziness, light-headedness, change in personality, confusion, nausea/vomiting, headache, photophobia, brief loss of consciousness, cognition or memory deficit, change in concentration, vertigo, balance disturbance, anxiety, loneliness, decreased initiative, social problems, tinnitus, or amnesia among other symptoms.

- Diagnosis depends on any alternation in mental processes following a head trauma.
- Depression or changes in social participation or quality of participation can be common.
- Signs and symptoms are often very subtle.
- Symptoms generally resolve for approximately 80% of patients within 6 weeks, but can remain in 30% of patients at the 3-month mark and up to 1 year in 15% of patients.
- Athletes may downplay symptoms to avoid being removed from practice or a game, so consultation to providers trained in concussion evaluation may be helpful.
- Second injury after a concussion can lead to long-term sequelae or death, so initial evaluation and treatment plan must be complete.
- Provider must carefully assess for cognitive or memory symptoms.
- "ABC's and cervical spine should be evaluated.
- General and neurologic exams are important, including a cerebellar exam.
- Some cognitive evaluation should be performed, be it the mini-mental status examination in the ED or a more comprehensive neuropsychological assessment.

4. **Diagnostic Studies**
   - No definitive studies or consistent concussion grading systems.
   - CT is usually negative, even in mild TBI but can be used to look for other results of trauma that may require surgical intervention. CT is not required of all patients.
   - Indications for CT include age over 65 years, loss of consciousness, focal neurologic findings or indication of a basilar skull fracture on exam, GCS <15, two or more episodes of postinjury vomiting, moderate-to-severe headache, history of fall of >4 ft, past medical history (PMH) of coagulopathy.
   - Also CT if a history of loss of consciousness is present and combined with any of the following: any physical findings at neck or above, intoxication, ongoing amnesia, or post-trauma seizures.

5. **Management**
   - No pharmacologic management.
   - A graded return to activity program should be utilized:
     - Patient must remain asymptomatic at each step for at least 24 hours before they can progress onto the next step in the graded activity scale.
     - If injury was not sports related, patient should have no activity until symptom free and must remain so for at least 24 hours, before he/she can progress to light, then moderate, and then normal exercise/activity.
     - If the injury was sports related, the patient must have no activity at all until symptom free and

remain that way for 24 hours before they are allowed to progress to light aerobic activity.
   - After 24 hours of no symptoms with light aerobic activity, patient can progress to noncontact sports-specific training, then from noncontact to full contact, and then to regular game participation.
   - Remember that the patient has to remain symptom free at each stage for at least 24 hours.
   - If they develop symptoms, they must return to the last symptom-free stage. Symptoms remaining after 3 weeks require consultation.
- **Nonpharmacologic/Supportive**
- Patient and a care provider must be carefully educated about warning signs and why and when to return to the emergency department (ED) or for further care including, but not limited to, persistent change in memory or cognition, headache, vomiting, or irritability.
- There is no set amount of time for monitoring post mild TBI.

C. Postconcussion Syndrome
1. **Etiology**
   - Results when symptoms of mild TBI, like headache, judgment, memory or concentration problems, dizziness, irritability, depression, anxiety, sleep disturbance or fatigue, among others, persist unresolved for months to years after the initial injury.
   - Postconcussive *symptoms* include those lasting for 4 weeks or less after an injury.
   - Postconcussive *syndrome,* on the other hand, can be used to indicate symptoms remaining 1 to 3 months after an initial TBI.
2. **Pathology**
   - No relationship to severity of initial symptoms or findings on initial evaluation.
   - Symptoms can be vague and overlap with other pathologies.
3. **Management**
   - Symptom checklists are helpful for diagnosis and follow-up.
   - Treat symptomatically, consultation to concussive specialist or for further neuropsychological testing.

D. Dementia
MILD COGNITIVE IMPAIRMENT (MCI)
1. **Etiology**
   - An interim diagnosis that is the phase between normal aging and dementia that does not affect normal daily function.
   - Amnesic type affects memory and generally leads to Alzheimer disease.
   - Nonamnesic type has cognitive decline in areas other than memory and may also progress to full dementia.

- Twenty-two percent prevalence of cognitive impairment without dementia in adults older than 71 years in the United States.
- Insufficient evidence for screening asymptomatic individuals.

2. **Pathology**
   - Pathogenesis is hippocampal atrophy.
   - Subtypes of MCI can include vascular, neurodegeneration, or dysthymic disorders.
   - Risk factor is genetic presence of apolipoprotein E (APOE) e4 allele.
   - Studies show possible associations with MCI that include APOE with atherosclerosis, DM or peripheral vascular disease; a history of stroke, anticholinergic drug use, DM, smoking, physical fragility, HTN, higher fat content in men (but not women), chronic psychological stress, vitamin D deficiency, and others.
   - Angiotensin-converting enzyme inhibitors, caffeine use, and education level (highest degree obtained) not associated with MCI.

3. **Clinical Features**
   - Decreased olfactory sense may precede development of MCI.
   - Presenting symptoms include forgetfulness, sleep disturbances, anxiety, agitation, irritability, depression, apathy and possibly delusions, hallucinations, or disinhibition. Impairment in cognitive factors would be greater than would be expected for the patient's education level and age.
   - Physical examination: Neurologic examination is usually unremarkable.

4. **Diagnostic Studies**
   - No definitive studies.

5. **Management**
   - Differential: other causes of delirium or dementia, organic, and nonorganic.
   - Many medications can cause cognitive impairment.
   - Treat any underlying causative pathology.

ALZHEIMER DISEASE

1. **Etiology**
   - Unknown.
   - Most common type of dementia (progressive deterioration of cognitive function that results in loss of ability to function at work or in social situations).
   - In the United States, 12.5% of people older than 65 years have Alzheimer disease.
   - Risk factors: genetic presence of APOE e4 allele (chromosome 19), Down syndrome.

2. **Pathology**
   - Extracellular deposition of amyloid-β protein, intracellular neurofibrillary tangles, and loss of neurons.
   - Atrophy of cerebral cortex.

- Most consistent biochemical change is a 50% to 90% reduction in the amount of choline acetyltransferase in the cerebral cortex and hippocampus.
- Profound loss of cholinergic neurons from the hippocampus, neocortex, and nucleus basalis.
- Risk factors: increased age, positive family history.

3. **Clinical Features**
   - Most common initial symptom: slowly increasing memory impairment for newly acquired information with memory for remote events unimpaired and emotional changes including depression, apathy, or forms of agitation or anxiety.
   - Common early symptom: difficulty in word-finding or confusion in following geographic directions.
   - Ask about trouble with activities of daily living (ADLs) such as toileting, feeding, dressing or independent ADLs like balancing a check book, using a cell phone, shopping.
   - Past medical history of head trauma, depression, encephalitis, language or sensory impairment disorders.
   - PE includes BP, neurologic examination and use of cognitive screening tests like mini-mental status examination (MMSE), clock drawing test, or Montreal Cognitive Assessment.
   - Complications include disability of patient and depression among caregivers.
   - Other causes of dementia including vascular dementia, Lewy body disease, Parkinson disease, frontotemporal dementia. Consider thyroid disease, vitamin deficiencies: loss of position and vibratory sense, chronic alcoholism, check B_{12} levels. Neoplasm: metastatic or primary brain tumor, may present as new-onset seizure. Normal pressure hydrocephalus: gait disturbance, urinary incontinence, and dementia.
   - Drug and medication toxicity: history of treatment for psychiatric disturbance, anxiety, insomnia, and seizures.

4. **Diagnostic Studies**
   - Routine Apo E genotyping is not recommended.
   - CSF biomarkers T-tau, P-tau, and positive CSF β-amyloid may indicate developing Alzheimer disease in patients who have MCI.
   - Nondiagnostic, but useful to rule out underlying pathology or evaluate possible differential diagnosis: CBC, electrolytes, calcium, HIV, thyroid panel, B_{12}, folate, glucose, renal studies, liver function tests, ESR, and possibly Lyme titres or neurosyphilis testing, EEG, CXR, urinalysis (U/A).
   - EEG, tomography (CT) scan or MRI scan is performed to rule out vascular disease, subdural hematoma, mass lesions, hydrocephalus, demyelinating disease, and leukodystrophies.

- MRI may demonstrate bilateral hippocampal atrophy.
- Neuropsychological testing may detect subtle cognitive impairment.
- Criteria for the clinical diagnosis of Alzheimer disease based on National Institute on Aging and Alzheimer's Association workgroup recommendations:
  - Progressive deterioration of previous function level and cognitive ability in the absence of other known neurologic or medical problems.
  - Impaired function in usual activities.
  - Diagnosis of cognitive impairment.
  - More than two of the following: changes in personality or behavior impaired ability to retain new information, impaired judgment or reasoning, impaired visuospatial functioning including recognizing familiar objects, faces or places, impaired language skills.
- Median survival is 4 to 6 years after initial diagnosis.

5. **Management**
   - Supportive: consider patient's ability to make decisions, occupational therapy, and support for caregivers as well.
   - Antipsychotics are not recommended for aggression/psychosis in dementia.
   - Environmental modification to support function and nutrition education including driving assessment.
   - Cholinesterase inhibitors may be helpful but not cost effective.
   - Anticholinesterases decrease the hydrolysis of ACh released from the neuron, which results in stimulation of the cholinergic receptor and is thought to improve cognitive performance. Options include rivastigmine, galantamine, and donepezil.
   - Both tacrine and donepezil are hepatotoxic, produce cholinergic side effects, and may exacerbate symptoms related to peptic ulcer and heart disease.
   - Memantine: N-Methyl D-aspartate (NMDA) receptor antagonist.
   - Vitamin E is not shown to prevent Alzheimer disease.
   - Ginkgo biloba and omega-3 fatty acids are not shown to prevent cognitive decline.

E. Delirium

Fluctuating mental status of transient brain dysfunction and disorder of attention with confused consciousness. Delirium differs from dementia in that it is a transient, reversible state, usually related directly to an organic systemic problem like infection, medication, or trauma.

1. **Etiology**
   - Variable and can, but does not have to, coexist with dementia.

2. **Pathology**
   - Variable depending on the causes for the delirium.
3. **Clinical Features**
   - Most common initial symptom: abrupt behavioral or mental status change.
   - Include an abrupt onset of inability to maintain attention and concentration.
   - Short-term memory and recall are also decreased or absent.
   - Patients have decreased orientation and may experience hallucination or other disturbances in perception.
4. **Diagnostic Studies**
   - To rule out infection, head trauma.
5. **Management**
   - Treatment of underlying pathology.
   - Review all medications.

F. Guillain–Barré Syndrome (Acute Idiopathic Polyneuropathy)

- Subacute or acute, progressive polyradiculoneuropathy with progressive weakness and sensory deficits.
- Sensory decline may be less severe than weakness.

1. **Etiology**
   - May follow immunizations, surgery, or recent illnesses.
   - May be immunologically related, but exact pathology is unclear.
   - Association with *Campylobacter jejuni* infection.
   - Subtype Miller Fisher syndrome is characterized by ataxia, areflexia, and opthalmoplegia.
2. **Pathology**
   - Demylenation or axonal degeneration.
3. **Clinical Features**
   - Weakness that generally begins distally and progresses proximally.
   - Symptoms are also generally bilateral.
   - Asymmetric deficits should lead one to consider spinal cord origins.
   - Severity of weakness and distribution varies greatly. Dysthesia and paresthesias are common.
   - Neuropathic and radiculopathic pain is also present in many patients.
   - Can be life-threatening if respiratory muscles involved.
   - Autonomic processes can also be affected and can also be life-threatening including tachycardia, pulmonary irregularities, and hyper/hypotension.
   - Recovery and resolution can take months.
   - Relapse can occur in approximately 3% of cases.
   - Twenty percent of patients have persistent deficit.
4. **Diagnostic Studies**
   - After 2 to 3 weeks, CSF analysis will show markedly increased protein, but otherwise normal cell content.

- Rule out other causes of neuropathies. Heavy metal toxicity, tick-caused paralysis, polio, and botulism can also cause weakness/paralysis.
- Monitor forced vital capacity (FVC) for decline.

5. Management
- Hospitalize until stable.
- Prednisone is contraindicated.
- Intravenous immunoglobulins or plasmaphoresis can be helpful.
- Admit to ICU and consider intubation if FVC declines.
- Avoid atelectasis.

G. Multiple Sclerosis

1. Etiology
- Common neurologic disorder in temperate regions.
- More common presentation in younger adults, of Western European descent, younger than 55 years.
- Genetic association and possibly autoimmune.

2. Pathology
- Demylenation in white matter of the CNS and optic nerves with axonal damage possible.

3. Clinical Features
- Most common initial symptoms include parasthesias, weakness or numbness of a limb, optic neuritis (retrobulbar), urinary symptoms, visual concerns, diplopia, or equilibrium disturbances. Forms include relapsing-remitting, primary progressive and secondary progressive. Diagnosis has to involve various parts of the nervous system being affected at various times.

4. Diagnostic Studies
- No one key definitive diagnostic study.
- MRI more helpful than CT.
- T1 and T2 MRI helpful for demonstrating multiple lesions and in identifying various progressions of the disease.
- MRI shows reduced or permanent demyelination.
- CSF analysis may be helpful.

5. Management
- High-dose steroids may reduce duration of acute exacerbations.
- There is no method to prevent progression.
- Approximately 50% all patients have no lasting deficits 10 years after diagnosis.
- Support groups helpful.
- Beta interferon and subcutaneous glatiramer acetate are also helpful in relapsing–remitting or secondary progressive disease.

H. Myasthenia Gravis

1. Etiology
- Autoimmune disorder.
- Most common disorder of neuromuscular transmission.
- Involves fluctuating weakness in ocular, bulbar, limb, and respiratory muscle.
- Associated with fatigue as weakness increases with exercise of affected muscles and improves with rest.
- Peak age of incidence in women is 20 to 30 years.
- Male incidence peaks in the sixth to seventh decade.

2. Pathology
- Interference of neuromuscular transmission at the postsynaptic site.
- Caused by antibodies to the ACh receptor protein.
- Abnormal hyperplasia or neoplasms of the thymus gland are present in the majority of these patients.

3. Clinical Features
- Usually insidious onset.
- Course of the illness is extremely variable; danger of death is greatest in the first year after diagnosis.
- Fluctuating weakness; repeated or persistent activity of a muscle group exhausts its contractile power, leading to progressive weakness; rest partially restores strength.
- Common presenting features are diplopia, ptosis, weakness of eye closure (present in 90% of cases), bulbar involvement (seen in 80% of patients), difficulty chewing, regurgitation of fluids, dysphagia, low voice volume or nasal speech.
- Disease progresses until muscle weakness is noted in the limbs, neck and respiratory muscles (results in diminished vital capacity).
- Deep tendon reflexes are seldom altered.
- Smooth and cardiac muscles are not involved.
- Pupils respond normally to light and accommodation.
- Associated disorders include SLE, rheumatoid arthritis, and thymic tumors in approximately 10% of patients with myasthenia (predominately older males) and thyrotoxicosis in about 5% of patients with myasthenia.

4. Diagnostic Studies
- Clinical diagnosis: Sustained activity that results in weakness and contractility that improves with rest are virtually diagnostic (e.g., increasing droop of eyelid while looking at the ceiling or diplopia when fixating in lateral or vertical gaze for 2 to 3 minutes).
- Thyroid function studies.
- CXR and CT of mediastinum: rule out thymoma.
- Serum anticholinergic (anti-ACh) receptor antibody levels for binding, blocking, or modulating types (radioimmunoassay method most accurate and most widely used); 15% of patients with myasthenia gravis may be seronegative.
- May also test for muscle receptor specific tyrosine kinase antibodies.
- Electrodiagnostic studies: repetitive nerve stimulation studies and single fiber EMG.
- Tensilon (edrophonium anticholinesterases inhibitor) test may help establish diagnosis. Initially 2 mg IV is given (dosage is repeated to 10 mg); if

objective abatement of muscle weakness is determined within 1 to 2 minutes, myasthenia gravis is highly likely.

- Neostigmine 1.5 mg IM should improve myasthenic weakness in 10 to 15 minutes.
- Ice pack test in patients with ptosis: place ice pack on eyelids to cool muscles for 1 minute, test for ptosis.

5. **Management**
- Anticholinesterase agents: pyridostigmine 15 to 90 mg q6h and 180 mg of a long-acting preparation at bedtime.
- Neostigmine 15 mg before excessive physical activity or meals.
- Observe for cholinergic crisis: nausea, vomiting, pallor, sweating, salivation, colic, diarrhea, meiosis, bradycardia.
- Intermittent eye-patching to eliminate diplopia.
- Rapid immunomodulating agents.
- Plasmapheresis or plasma exchange—temporary measure, used for managing acute exacerbations or in preparation for thymectomy.
- Chronic immunomodulating and immunosuppressive agents.
- Corticosteroids for moderate-to-severe symptoms refractory to cholinesterase inhibitors (CEIs). Hospitalization and careful observation for respiratory difficulty is advisable.
- Immunosuppressants: azathioprine, 2 to 3 mg/kg/day, or cyclosporin, 5 mg/kg/day, in patient with severe generalized weakness.
- Surgical thymectomy: improvement in 75% to 80% of patients. Controversial in patients without pre-existing thymoma, but recommended in patients 18 (postpuberal) to 50, especially in those not responding to other therapy.
- Myasthenic crisis: rapid and severe deterioration with respiratory failure and quadriparesis. Requires plasma exchange and ventilator management.

I. Seizure Disorders
- Seizure: a paroxysmal event due to abnormal, excessive hypersynchronous discharges from an aggregate of cortical neurons.
- Epilepsy: recurrent, unpredictable, and unprovoked seizures due to a chronic, underlying process.

1. **Etiology**
- May result from primary CNS dysfunction, underlying metabolic derangement, or systemic disease.
- Febrile seizures of childhood, idiopathic (most common), head trauma, stroke, vascular malformations, SAH, mass lesions, meningitis, brain abscess, encephalitis.
- Hypoglycemia, hyponatremia, hypocalcemia, hyperosmolar state, uremia, hepatic encephalopathy,

drug overdose, drug withdrawal (alcohol most common), hyperthermia.

2. **Pathology**
- Sudden, excessive, and disorderly electrical discharge of CNS neurons.
- Initiation phase: High-frequency action potentials lead to longer depolarization of neuronal membrane and influx of extracellular calcium, opening of sodium channels.
- Propagation phase: Nearby excitatory neurons are recruited with loss of inhibitory neurons and changes in the amount and conductance of neurotransmitters and ion channels.

3. **Clinical Features**

PARTIAL (FOCAL) SEIZURES
- Simple partial seizures: Consciousness is preserved; common auras include an epigastric rising sensation, feelings of fear, detachment, and déjà vu.

TYPES OF SIMPLE PARTIAL SEIZURES
- Motor: focal twitching of extremity.
- Somatosensory: hallucinations, flashing lights, paresthesias.
- Autonomic: pallor, flushing, sweating, piloerection, rising epigastric sensation, vomiting.
- Dysphasia, distortion of memory, forced thinking, fear, hallucinations, feelings of déjà vu.
- Complex partial seizures: focal seizure activity with transient impairment of consciousness (illusions, hallucinations, dyscognitive states).
- Motor: focal rhythmic twitching of extremity, the involved area may enlarge through the recruitment of more neurons and result in "Jacksonian march" (increased motor deficit).
- In postictal state a focal deficit such as hemiparesis (Todd paralysis) may persist (up to 36 hours).
- Usually begin with aura.
- Typical behaviors are automatisms (e.g., lip-smacking, chewing, and repeated swallowing).
- Most common type of adult seizures; formerly known as psychomotor or temporal lobe seizures.
- Partial seizures with secondary generalization:
  - Activity spreads to involve both hemispheres and usually involves tonic–clonic activity.
- Generalized seizures: All are characterized by abrupt loss of consciousness with no detectable focal onset:
  - Absence seizures—(petit mal) sudden, brief loss of consciousness without loss of postural control, typically begin in childhood with episodes of staring or "daydreaming," minimal motor manifestations (e.g., eyelid twitching), 60% spontaneously remit.
  - Myoclonic seizures—brief jerks involving part or all of the body.
  - Clonic—rhythmic jerking of the body.

- Tonic—brief attacks of stiffness (usually extensor spasms) in part or all of the body.
- Atonic—losses of postural tone (drop attacks) resulting in falls.
- Tonic–clonic—(grand mal) bilateral tonic extension of trunk and limbs (tonic phase), followed by loud vocalization (cry) and synchronous muscle jerking (clonic phase); urinary incontinence, cyanosis, and tongue-biting are common.
  - Differential diagnosis:
    - Syncope.
    - Psychological disorders (pseudoseizures).
    - Migraine.
    - TIA.
    - Sleep disorders.
    - Movement disorders.
    - Metabolic disturbance.

4. Diagnostic Studies
- MRI is study of choice for detection of epileptogenic lesions.
- EEG is the most important laboratory test for diagnosis, although may be normal or nonspecific.

5. Management
- Treat underlying condition that causes or contributes to seizure activity: correct metabolic disturbance (hyponatremia, hypoxemia, hypo/hyperkalemia), resect tumor, arteriovenous malformations, treat infection (brain abscess).
- Avoid precipitating factors like sleep deprivation, alcohol intake, stress.
- Antiepileptic drugs (AEDs):
  - Therapeutic drug monitoring should be used to determine compliance and minimize toxicity.
  - Follow serum drug levels, liver function tests, CBC.
  - Start low and titrate dose upward until seizures are controlled or dose-related side effects occur (abnormal liver functions, nausea, emesis, vertigo, neutropenia, sedation, rash, gingival hyperplasia [Dilantin]).
- If poorly controlled, add second agent and wean first.
- Patient education is crucial.
- Psychosocial issues to consider with AED therapy:
  - Noncompliance (50%).
  - Social implications include loss of independence (driving restrictions dependent on state law), unemployment, restrict alcohol intake, risk of seizure-related injury, sudden death.
- Generalized tonic–clonic seizures: carbamazepine, phenytoin, valproic acid, Lamictal, phenobarbital, primidone, Keppra.
- Partial seizures: carbamazepine, Neurontin. With/without secondary generalization: valproic acid, Lamictal, Topamax, Lamictal, phenobarbital, Neurontin.
- Absence seizures: valproic acid, ethosuximide, Lamictal.
- Myoclonic seizures: valproic acid, Dilantin, primidone, Topamax.
- Moderation in diet, exercise, and alcohol intake.
- Surgical treatment options if medically refractory: cortical resection, hemispherectomy, corpus callosotomy, vagal nerve stimulator.

J. Status Epilepticus
- True medical emergency.
- Most common neurologic emergency.
- Continuous seizure activity or frequent seizures without interictal return to baseline clinical state of greater than 15 to 20 minutes duration.

1. Etiology
- AED withdrawal or noncompliance, metabolic disturbance, drug toxicity, CNS infection, tumors, head trauma, SAH, withdrawal of alcohol, baclofen, benzodiazepines, barbiturates.

2. Treatment
- Airway and oxygen, consider intubation.
- Rapid neurologic assessment.
- Draw chemistry profile and tox screen while establishing venous access.
- Give thiamine and amp of D50.
- Lorazepam 0.02 to 0.03 mg per kg, Valium 0.1 to 0.3 mg per kg, or Versed 0.2 mg per kg.
- Close monitoring of hemodynamics.
- Load with Dilantin, rate not to exceed 50 mg per minute, risk of arrhythmias and hypotension.
- Continuous ECG and monitoring BP, oxygenation/ventilation.
- If persistent activity at 30 to 60 minutes, add Dilantin 5 to 10 mg per kg, phenobarbital 50 to 100 mg per minute to max of 25 mg per kg.
- If >60 minutes, pentobarbital 5 to 15 mg per kg load or propofol.

K. Syncope
1. Etiology
- Abrupt transient loss of consciousness and postural tone (syncope) followed by rapid and complete recovery.
- Lightheadedness, loss of strength, and other symptoms that characterize an impending or incomplete fainting spell (presyncope).
- Reduction in cerebral blood flow (the most common type of syncope). Includes vasodepressor syncope (rapid drop in BP and slowing of heartbeat often precipitated by fear, pain, and anxiety). Other causes include reduced blood volume, cardiac arrhythmias, and orthostatic hypotension.
- Impaired cerebral metabolism (anoxia, hypoglycemia, acidosis, drug intoxication, acute alcoholism, hyperventilation, and associated respiratory alkalosis).

2. **Pathology**
   - A small number of patients have a primary neurologic or cerebrovascular cause that includes transient brain stem ischemia (e.g., vertebrobasilar migraine or ischemia) or subclavian steal.
3. **Clinical Features**
   - Sensations of lightheadedness; sudden, brief loss of consciousness and decreased muscle tone, dizziness, weakness, temperature change, or decreased motor power may be a prelude to the full episode.
   - More apt to occur in standing position.
   - Focal neurologic symptoms associated with syncope suggest an underlying disorder such as TIA or epilepsy.
   - Can be present immediately before or after the syncopal episode.
4. **Diagnostic Studies**
   - Complete history: number of episodes, associated symptoms, prodrome, position, preceding events, duration, recovery, age, medications, comorbidities, temporal relationship to eating.
   - Physical examination: orthostatic BP, Valsalva maneuvers, complete neurologic examination.
   - ECG, ambulatory electrocardiograph 24 to 48 hours, cardiac Echo, EEG, CT, carotid U/S, brain natriuretic peptide, exercise test.
   - In more extreme cases, tilt table or electrophysiologic study (EPS).
   - EEG or ambulatory ECG is diagnostic in 5% to 10% of cases. If symptoms develop while being monitored and no ECG changes occur, rhythm disturbance is eliminated as possibility.
   - Ambulatory EEG if seizure disorder is suspected.
5. **Management**
   - Dependent on etiology.

L. Gilles de la Tourette Syndrome (Tourette Disorder)

Series of motor or phonetic tics or repetitious behaviors.

1. **Etiology**
   - Onset usually in childhood between the ages of 2 and 15.
   - Commonly diagnosed as psychiatric disorders initially.
   - Can be a presentation of Wilson disease.
2. **Pathology**
   - Autosomal dominant features with variable penetration.
3. **Clinical Features**
   - Often associated with obsessive-compulsive symptoms as well.
   - Patients have tic-like movements of the face, head, and neck, including blinking, shrugging, head thrusting, sniffling. Verbal or phonetic tics can include grunts, barks, throat-clearing, obscene words, repeating others' speech, repeating words or phrases or imitating others.
   - Tics can include self-harmful behaviors like pulling hair, biting lips or tongue.
   - Diagnosis can be clinical and is often missed initially.
4. **Management**
   - Social embarrassment and other social implications are possible and should be considered in treatment.
   - Refer all patients with suspected Tourette syndrome to appropriate specialists.
   - Symptomatic: haloperidol or other antipsychotics or dopamine blocking medicines used.

SELECTED REFERENCES

Adams RD, Victor M, eds. *Principles of Neurology*. 7th ed. New York, NY: McGraw-Hill Companies Inc; 2001.

Aminoff MJ, Kerchner GA. Nervous system disorders. In: McPhee SJ, Papadakis MA, Rabow MW, eds. *Current Medical Diagnosis & Treatment*. 50th ed. New York, NY: McGraw-Hill Companies Inc; 2011:927–994.

Biller J, ed. *Practical Neurology*. 1st ed. Philadelphia, PA: Lippincott-Raven; 1997.

Carlini ME, Shandera WX. Infectious diseases: viral & rickettsial. In: Tierney LM Jr, McPhee SJ, Papadakis MA, eds. *Current Medical Diagnosis & Treatment*. 38th ed. Stamford, CT: Appleton & Lange; 1999:1255–1290.

Chaudhuri A, Martin PM, Kennedy PGE, et al. EFNS guideline on the management of community-acquired bacterial meningitis: report of an EFNS Task Force on acute bacterial meningitis in older children and adults. *Eur J Neurol*. 2008;15:649–659.

Complex regional pain syndrome. Headache. DynaMed. http://dynaweb.ebscohost.com. Accessed June 16, 2011.

Dehn RW, ed. *Moser's Primary Care for Physician Assistants*. 1st ed. New York, NY: McGraw-Hill Companies Inc; 1999:511–520.

Diagnosis and management of headache in adults. A national clinical guideline. National Guideline Clearing House. Agency for Healthcare Research and Quality. U.S. Department of Health and Human Services. http://www.guideline.gov/content.aspx?id=13446&search=headache. Accessed July 11, 2011.

Ferri F. *Ferri's Clinical Advisor, 2004*. Philadelphia, PA: Mosby; 2004:334.

Moe PG, Benke TA, Bernard TJ, et al. Neurologic & muscular disorders. In: Hay WJ, Levin MJ, Sondheimer JM, et al, eds. *Current Diagnosis and Treatment: Pediatrics*. 19th ed. New York, NY: McGraw-Hill Companies Inc; 2009:673–749.

Petit JM. *Primary Neurologic Care*. St Louis, MO: Mosby; 2001:35–41.

Seidel HM, Ball JW, Dains JE, et al. Neurologic system. In: *Mobsy's Guide to Physical Examination*. 4th ed. St Louis, MO: Mosby; 1999:755–804.

Tunkel AR, Glaser CA, Bloch KC, et al. The management of encephalitis: clinical practice guidelines by the Infectious Disease Society of America. *Clin Infect Dis*. 2008;47:303–327.

Wright DW, Merck LH. Head trauma in adults and children. In: Tintinalli JE, Stapczynski JS, Cline DM, et al, eds. *Tintinalli's Emergency Medicine: A Comprehensive Study Guide*. 7th ed. New York, NY: McGraw-Hill Companies Inc; 2011:chap 254. http://www.accessmedicine.com/content.aspx?aID=6388784. Accessed October 17, 2011.

Zaidat OO, Lerner AJ. *The Little Black Book of Neurology*. 4th ed. St Louis, MO: Mosby; 2002.

Musculoskeletal Disorders

Patrick C. Auth • Jennifer Hixon • Robert D. Howard

I. Infections

A. Acute Osteomyelitis

1. **Etiology**
   - Bone marrow infection caused by blood-borne pathogens.
   - Commonly affects children (boys more than girls).
   - Be aware with intravenous (IV) drug user.

2. **Pathology**
   - May be triggered by trauma or obvious primary focus of infection (e.g., boil and sore throat); usually seeding is hematogenous, anaerobic, or aerobic infections.
   - *Staphylococcus aureus*—most common offender.
   - Group A streptococci—common in children.
   - Group B streptococci and *Escherichia coli*—neonates.
   - *Haemophilus influenzae* bone infections have almost completely been eliminated with recent immunizations.
   - *S. aureus*, *Pseudomonas aeruginosa*, *Serratia*, and *Candida albicans* bone infections are common with injection drug use.
   - After an open fracture or open reduction with internal fixation—*S. aureus*, *P. aeruginosa*, and coliforms.
   - Patients with sickle cell anemia—*Salmonella*.
   - *P. aeruginosa* is associated with puncture wounds of the foot.
   - *Pasteurella multocida* infection commonly follows cat bites.

3. **Clinical Features**
   - Patient identified by refusal to bear weight or move extremity.
   - Acute onset with high fever, chills, malaise, and sometimes soft-tissue abscess.
   - Early radiographic changes include soft-tissue swelling, followed by periosteal evaluation, demineralization (10 days to 2 weeks later), sequestra (dead bone with surrounding granulation tissue), and periosteal new bone growth later; cannot rely on early radiographic changes to confirm diagnosis.
   - Bone scan shows focal increased activity.
   - Magnetic resonance imaging (MRI) shows changes in bone and bone marrow, usually before plain radiographs.
   - Computed tomography (CT) scan shows a radiolucent area in cancellous bone and signs of periosteal elevation—limited role in acute osteomyelitis.
   - Elevated white blood cell (WBC) count and erythrocyte sedimentation rate (ESR); blood cultures are usually positive.
   - C-reactive protein (CRP) is the most sensitive monitor for the course of infection.

4. **Management**
   - Identification of the organism(s).
   - Aspiration is helpful for antibiotic choice.
   - IV antibiotics followed by a course of oral antibiotics after temperature has normalized (total 6 weeks or until ESR and CRP return to normal).
   - Limb should be immobilized.
   - Indications for surgery—drainage of abscess; debridement of tissue; refractory patients.

B. Chronic Osteomyelitis

1. **Etiology**
   - May result from inappropriate treatment of acute osteomyelitis, trauma to bone, hematogenous spread, soft-tissue spread, or complication of surgery.
   - Infected host may be immunocompromised (e.g., immunosuppressed, diabetic, and IV drug abuse).

2. **Pathology**
   - *S. aureus* anaerobes are frequent offending organisms.
   - In IV drug users—*P. aeruginosa*.
   - Skin and soft tissue are often involved; fistulous tracts develop into epidermoid carcinoma.
   - Periods of quiescence followed by acute exacerbations.

3. **Clinical Features**
   - Patient presentation is characterized by flares of infection with associated pain, swelling, and pus formation—alternating with periods of quiescence.
   - Radiographs demonstrate abnormal bone texture with thickening, diffuse cavity formation.

- Sequestrum appears as localized mass of bone, denser than its surroundings.
- Nuclear medicine studies disclose activity of disease.
- CT scan—excellent for detection of sequestra, cortical destruction, soft-tissue abscesses, and sinus tracts.
- Operative sampling of deep specimens from multiple foci is the most accurate means of identifying the pathologic organism.
- WBC may show moderate leukocytosis.
- ESR is usually elevated; positive blood cultures.

4. **Management**
- Combination of IV antibiotics based on deep cultures, surgical debridement, bone grafting, stabilization, soft-tissue coverage (flaps), and amputations.
- Empiric therapy is not indicated in chronic osteomyelitis.
- Refractory patients may require surgical intervention.

II. Inflammatory Disorders

A. Rheumatoid Arthritis (RA)
1. **Etiology**
   - The most common form of inflammatory arthritis.
   - Affects women more than men.
   - Peak age of onset, 25 to 55 years of age.
2. **Pathology**
   - Most likely related to cellular-mediated immune response (T cell); incites inflammatory response initially against soft tissues and later against cartilage and bone, and this leads to joint destruction.
3. **Clinical Features**
   - Insidious onset of morning stiffness, fatigue, low-grade fever, and polyarthritis.
   - Most commonly, hands and feet are affected early.
   - Involvement of knees, elbows, shoulders, ankles, and neck is also common.
   - Chronic swelling, thickening of metacarpophalangeal (MCP) joint and proximal interphalangeal (PIP) joint, and the pannus ingrowth gradually denude articular cartilage and lead to chondrocyte death.
   - Range of motion (ROM) is limited, and ulnar deviation of the MCP joint is present.
   - Interosseous atrophy and rheumatoid nodules of the bony prominences.
   - Hand deformities—swan-neck deformity and boutonniere deformity.
   - There may be systemic involvement of other organ systems—for example, lung, heart, skin, eye, gastrointestinal (GI), and genitourinary system.
   - Sjögren syndrome—associated with RA. Symptoms include decreased salivary and lacrimal gland secretion; dryness affects conjunctiva, cornea, mouth.
   - Felty syndrome—RA with splenomegaly and leukopenia.
   - Still disease—acute-onset RA with fever, rash, splenomegaly, and lymphadenopathy.

4. **Diagnostic Studies**
   - Laboratory studies may show elevated ESR and CRP, positive rheumatoid titer, and presence of anti-cyclic citrullinated protein antibodies; hypochromic, normocytic anemia is usually present.
   - Radiographs include periarticular erosions and osteopenia of the hand (i.e., MCPs, PIPs), joints, wrist (i.e., carpal bones), cervical spine (C-spine) (Figure 7-1).

5. **Management**
   - Treatment goal—controlling synovitis and pain, maintaining joint function, preventing deformities.
   - Drug therapy— disease-modifying antirheumatic drugs (DMARDs) started once diagnosis is confirmed and adjusted with the goal of suppressing disease activity. Synthetic DMARDs: methotrexate, sulfasalazine, leflunomide, antimalarials, and minocycline. Biologic DMARDs: tumor necrosis factor (TNF) inhibitors, abatacept, rituximab, and tocilizumab. Nonsteroidal anti-inflammatory drugs (NSAIDs) provide symptomatic relief and should be used in conjunction with DMARDs; low-dose corticosteroids produce prompt anti-inflammatory effect, but multiple side effects limit their long-term use.

FIGURE 7-1. **RA of the hands and wrists.** Note the involvement of the wrist joints, MCP joints, and IP joints. (From Daffner RH, ed. *Clinical Radiology: The Essentials.* 2nd ed. Baltimore, MD: Lippincott Williams & Wilkins; 1999:436, with permission.)

- Artificial tears—used to treat dryness of eyes.
- Physical and occupational therapies may be used to improve patient's function.
- Exercise to preserve joint motion, muscular strength, and endurance. ROM exercise needs to be done once a day.
- Weight loss for overweight patients to reduce the wear and teat placed on arthritic joints of the lower extremities.
- Splints and braces can be used on affected joints to prevent destruction.
- Synovectomy adjunct to medical therapy.
- When joint pain and swelling interfere with function and joints do not respond to conservative therapy, total joint replacement may be indicated.

B. Reiter Syndrome (Reactive Arthritis)

1. **Definition**
   - Common features including oligoarticular arthritis, mouth ulcers, conjunctivitis, urethritis, or cervicitis (can't pee, can't see, and can't climb a tree).
2. **Etiology**
   - Most patients develop within days or weeks of either dysenteric or sexually transmitted disease (occurs most commonly in young men).
   - *Chlamydia trachomatis*—usual causative organism of postvenereal variety.
   - Need to determine whether *Ureaplasma* is causative organism.
   - Dysenteric form following enteric bacterial infection (e.g., *Shigella, Salmonella, Yersinia,* and *Campylobacter*).
3. **Pathology**
   - Epidemiologically similar to other reactive arthritis syndromes, characterized by sterile inflammation of joints from infections originating at nonarticular sites.
4. **Clinical Features**
   - Fever, malaise, anorexia, and weight loss.
   - Buccal ulceration or balanitis (it is possible for only two features to be present).
   - Uveitis.
   - Arthritis—most commonly asymmetric and frequently involves large weight-bearing joints (usually knee, ankle, and foot).
   - Can appear seriously ill (fever, rigors, tachycardia, and exquisitely tender joints).
   - Mucocutaneous symptoms can include balanitis, stomatitis, and keratoderma blennorrhagica (hyperkeratotic skin lesions of palms, soles, and around nails).
   - Most symptoms disappear within days to weeks.
5. **Diagnostic Studies**

   BLOOD
   - Human leukocyte antigen B27 (HLA-B27)—positive in 60% to 80% of patients in non-human immunodeficiency virus related Reiter syndrome.
   - WBC—10,000 to 20,000 with neutrophilic leukocytosis.
   - Elevated ESR, moderate normochromic anemia.
   - Hypergammaglobulinemia.

   SYNOVIAL FLUID
   - WBC 1,000 to 8,000 cells per mm_3.
   - Bacterial culture negative.
   - Collaborative tests—culture or serology positive for *C. trachomatis* or stools positive for *Salmonella, Shigella, Yersinia,* and *Campylobacter* support the diagnosis.

   IMAGING-X-RAY
   - Periosteal proliferation, thickening, spurs, erosions at articular margins, residual joint destruction, syndesmophytes (spine), sacroiliitis.
6. **Management**
   - Treatment—symptomatic.
   - No treatment is necessary for conjunctivitis; iritis may require treatment.
   - Treatment is unnecessary for mucocutaneous lesions.
   - NSAIDs—mainstay of therapy.
   - Patients who do not respond to NSAIDs may respond to sulfasalazine or to methotrexate.
   - Physical therapy during recovery phase.
   - Prompt treatment of precipitating processes reduces the chance of developing Reiter syndrome.

C. Septic Arthritis

1. **Etiology**
   - May be hematogenous (e.g., secondary to upper respiratory infection and impetigo), contiguous spread from an adjacent infection, or through direct inoculation (e.g., puncture wound).
   - Also may develop as a complication of a diagnostic or therapeutic procedure.
   - Most commonly affects knee, hip, shoulder, and ankle; also can affect other joints.
   - Most commonly affects in infants hips.
   - Predominantly monoarticular (90%).
   - Medical emergency because delay in treatment may lead to joint destruction.
2. **Pathology**
   - *S. aureus* is the most common cause of nongonococcal septic arthritis, accounting for about 50% of all cases.
   - Methicillin-resistant *S. aureus* (MRSA) and group B streptococcus have become increasingly frequent causes of septic arthritis.
   - In newborns and infants up to 3 months of age, the most common causative organisms are *S. aureus* and group B *Streptococcus*.
   - In infants and children (3 months to 14 years), the most common causative organisms are *S. aureus, Streptococcus pyogenes, Streptococcus pneumoniae,* and *H. influenzae*, decreased with vaccination.

- In sexually active adults ages 15 to 40 with acute monoarticular septic arthritis, the most common causative organisms are *Neisseria gonorrhoeae*, *S. aureus*, streptococci, and aerobic gram-negative bacilli (uncommon).
- In sexually active adults ages 40 and older with acute monoarticular septic arthritis, the most common causative organisms are *N. gonorrhoeae* and *S. aureus*.

3. **Clinical Features**
   - Failure to use involved joint, swelling, tenderness, and localized warmth.
   - Sudden onset of monoarticular arthritis should be considered septic until proven otherwise.
   - Fever occurs at some point in 90% of patients.
   - Patient also resists passive movement of joint.
   - Toddler may refuse to walk if lower extremity is involved.
   - Constitutional signs are helpful in suggesting an infection, but not pathognomonic.

4. **Diagnostic Studies**
   - Diagnosis—confirmed by direct arthrocentesis with synovial fluid analysis, culture.
   - Obtain aerobic and anaerobic cultures.
   - Definitive diagnosis requires the demonstration of causative bacteria on Gram stain, by culture, or by using both.
   - Complete blood counts (CBCs) and ESR also should be checked.
   - Plain radiographs—usually normal early, but provide baseline evaluative tool for subsequent study of joint changes.
   - Later examination shows joint space narrowing, destruction without appropriate treatment.
   - Certain gas-producing organisms (e.g., *E. coli* anaerobes) may generate articular gas.
   - MRI and CT scans are sensitive in detecting fluid in joints that are not accessible to physical examination (e.g., the hip), and Ultrasound (U/S) can also be used; need to image joints especially the hip to confirm there is an effusion
   - Radionuclide imaging techniques may aid the diagnosis of septic arthritis in joints difficult to aspirate.

5. **Management**
   - Treatment must be initiated before available culture results.
   - Begin with broad-spectrum antibiotic; may require change based on Gram stain, and vancomycin should be used whenever MRSA is likely.
   - Length of parenteral therapy is usually 10 days to 6 weeks.
   - CBC and blood cultures should be monitored routinely.
   - Consider open drainage if loculation is suspected.
   - Joint rest encouraged until inflammation subsides, then physical therapy may be introduced slowly.

D. Psoriatic Arthritis
1. **Etiology**
   - 1:1 male:female ratio.
   - Onset—40 to 50 years of age.
   - Affects approximately 5% to 20% of patients with psoriasis.
   - Psoriasis precedes onset of arthritis in 80% of patients.
   - More common in patients with severe skin disease than those with mild skin findings.

2. **Pathology**
   - Emerges long after or commensurate with cutaneous psoriasis.

3. **Clinical Features**
   - Forms of psoriatic arthropathy include psoriatic nail disease and distal interphalangeal (DIP) involvement, asymmetric oligoarthropathy, symmetric polyarthropathy, arthritis mutilans, and psoriatic spondylitis.
   - Insidious onset, usually peripheral arthritis asymmetric, with "sausage" appearance of fingers and toes.
   - Joint swelling, tenderness, warmth, and decreased ROM.
   - Nail changes include pitting, traverse ridging, onycholysis, keratosis, yellowing, and destruction of nails.
   - Sacroiliac joint involvement is common.
   - May be associated with ankylosing spondylitis.
   - Dry erythematous papular skin lesions, conjunctivitis.

4. **Diagnostic Studies**
   - Serum rheumatoid factor (RF) negative.
   - Elevated ESR.
   - Elevated uric acids.
   - HLA-B27 present—spondylitis.
   - Radiographic findings include osteolysis, DIP pencil-in-cup deformity, lack of osteoporosis, bony ankylosis, asymmetric sacroiliitis, and atypical syndesmophytes.

5. **Management**
   - Treat symptomatically.
   - Encourage exercise to maintain strength and flexibility.
   - Treatment of skin lesions may be accompanied by improvement in peripheral articular symptoms.
   - NSAIDs are usually sufficient for mild cases; methotrexate is the drug of choice for patients who do not respond to NSAIDs; cases that are refractory to methotrexate usually respond to the addition of TNF inhibitors.
   - Other agents that may benefit are cyclosporine, retinoic acid derivatives, and psoralen plus ultraviolet.
   - Corticosteroids are not as effective in psoriatic arthritis compared with other forms of

inflammatory arthritis and may precipitate pustular psoriasis during tapers; antimalarials may exacerbate psoriasis.

E. Systemic Lupus Erythematosus

1. Etiology

- Chronic inflammatory autoimmune disease of unknown origin that affects multiple organs.
- Affects women more than men, mainly young women.
- Higher prevalence in African Americans, Hispanics, Asians, and Native Americans than Caucasian women.
- Greatest cluster between 20 and 40 years of age.

2. Pathology

- Clinical manifestations thought to be secondary to trapping of antigen–antibody complexes in the capillaries of visceral structures, leading to inflammation and tissue damage, and affecting multiple organs.
- B-cell hyperactivity with overproduction of auto-antibodies is present.

3. Clinical Features (Table 7-1)

- Course and severity of systemic lupus erythematosus (SLE) varies widely—fever, anorexia, malaise, weight loss, skin lesions, oral ulcers, eye pain, and arthritic pain.
- Malar (butterfly) rash, discoid rash, photosensitivity, arthritis, serositis, oral/nasopharyngeal ulcer,

TABLE 7-1.	Clinical Features of SLE	
Organ System	**ARA Criteria for Classification of SLE**	**Other Features**
Constitutional		Fever, malaise, anorexia, weight loss
Cutaneous	1. Malar rash	Alopecia
	2. Discoid rash	Raynaud phenomenon
	3. Photosensitivity	Other rashes: subacute cutaneous LE, urticaria, bullous lesions
	4. Oral/nasopharyngeal ulcers	Vasculitis
		Panniculitis (lupus profundus)
Musculoskeletal	5. Nonerosive arthritis	Arthralgia/myalgia
		Myositis
		Ligamentous laxity
		AVN of bone
Cardiopulmonary	6. Pleuritis	Pleural effusions
		Pericarditis myocarditis
		Pneumonitis
		Verrucous endocarditis (Libman–Sacks syndrome)
		Interstitial fibrosis
		Pulmonary hypertension
Renal	7. Proteinuria (>500 mg/dL)	Nephrotic syndrome
	Urinary cellular casts	Renal insufficiency
		Renal failure
Neurologic	8. Psychosis	Organic brain syndrome
	Seizure	Cranial neuropathies
		Peripheral neuropathies
		Cerebellar signs
GI		Serositis
		Ascites
		Vasculitis (bleeding/perforation)
		Pancreatitis
		Elevated levels of liver enzymes

(Continued)

TABLE 7-1.	**Clinical Features of SLE (Continued)**	
Organ System	**ARA Criteria for Classification of SLE**	**Other Features**
Hematologic	9. Hemolytic anemia	Anemia of chronic disease
	Leukopenia (<4,000/mL)	Lupus anticoagulant
	Lymphopenia (<1,500/mL)	Thrombosis
	Thrombocytopenia (<100,000/mL)	Splenomegaly
		Lymphadenopathy
Other systems		Sicca complex
		Conjunctivitis/episcleritis
Laboratory	10. ANA	Lupus band test on skin biopsy
	11. Anti-dsDNA	Anticardiolipin antibody
	Anti-Sm antigen	Lupus anticoagulant
	False-positive VDRL	Hypocomplementemia
	LE preparation	

ARA, American Rheumatism Association (now The American College of Rheumatology).
From Kimberly RP. Lupus erythematosus: systemic and local forms. In: Kelley WN, ed. *Textbook of Internal Medicine.* 1st ed. Philadelphia, PA: JB Lippincott Company; 1989:287, with permission.

pleuritis, pericarditis, nephritis, psychosis, and seizures.
- Joint involvement—most common feature, affecting 75% of patients with SLE.
- Joints commonly involved are PIPs, MCPs, carpus bones, knees, and ankle.

4. **Diagnostic Studies**
- Serum RF usually positive.
- Positive antinuclear antibodies (ANAs), sensitive but not specific for SLE.
- Positive antibodies to double-stranded deoxyribonucleic acid (anti-dsDNA) antibody and to anti-Smith (anti-Sm), specific but not sensitive for SLE.
- False-positive Venereal Disease Research Laboratory (VDRL) test.
- CBC may disclose hemolytic anemia, leukopenia, lymphopenia, or thrombocytopenia.

5. **Management**
- Goal of treatment is to suppress disease manifestation while minimizing the cumulative toxicity of treatment.
- Supportive treatment; avoidance of, or protection from, ultraviolet light.
- Early intervention when infection occurs with acute flares of SLE.
- Avoid physical, emotional stress.
- Treatment—symptomatic, local steroids or antimalarial drugs for cutaneous manifestations, NSAIDs for arthritic symptoms.
- Immunosuppressive agents such as cyclophosphamide, chlorambucil, and azathioprine are used in cases resistant to corticosteroids.

F. **Ankylosing Spondylitis**
1. **Etiology**
- Usually affects males more than females.
- Onset—usually 15 to 30 years of age.
2. **Pathology**
- Chronic inflammatory disease of joints in axial skeletal and sacroiliac joints.
3. **Clinical Features**
- Onset—usually gradual, with intermittent periods of diffuse low back pain, profound morning stiffness.
- Patients cannot put their head down flat while lying in supine.
- Symptoms advance in a cephalad direction, back motion becomes restricted.
- May result in fixed cervical, thoracic, or lumbar hyperkyphosis and restriction of chest expansion.
- May have painless effusions of larger joints and chin-on-chest deformity.
- Uveitis.
- Often associated with heart disease and pulmonary fibrosis.
- Extraskeletal manifestations: aortitis, colitis, arachnoiditis, amyloidosis, and sarcoidosis.
4. **Diagnostic Studies**
- Elevated ESR, histocompatibility antigen, HLA-B27 usually positive.
- Test for RF is usually negative.
- Earliest radiographic changes are in sacroiliac joints showing subchorial erosion of the sacroiliac joints.

- Later changes of spine show squaring and generalized demineralization of vertebral bodies and progressive ankylosis.
- The term *bamboo spine* is used to describe these late findings (Figure 7-2).

5. **Management**
  - Goal—preserve motion.
  - NSAIDs, rest, and physiotherapy to maintain joint movement are helpful to control inflammation.
  - For patients whose symptoms are refractory to NSAIDs, TNF inhibitors, such as etanercept, adalimumab, and infliximab, are alternatives.
  - If deformity progresses quickly, mobilization may be necessary.
  - Osteotomy.

G. Bursitis
1. **Etiology**
  - Inflammation of synovium-like cellular membrane overlying bony prominences.
2. **Pathology**
  - Inflammation may be secondary to trauma, infection, or arthritic conditions (e.g., gout, RA, and osteoarthritis).
  - Normal structure allows skin, tendon, and muscle to slide over each other.
  - As a result of the trauma, infection, or inflammation, fluid accumulates in bursa.

FIGURE 7-2. Radiograph of the pelvis in advanced ankylosing spondylitis. Both sacroiliac joints have undergone bony fusion, and prior sacroiliac sclerosis and erosions are now gone. Bilateral syndesmophytes bridge intervertebral disks at multiple lumbar levels, and there is marked osteopenia. (From Humes DH, ed. *Kelley's Essentials of Internal Medicine.* 2nd ed. Philadelphia, PA: Lippincott Williams & Wilkins; 2001:360, with permission.)

- Fibrinous loose bodies, adhesions, or fibrosis may occur in bursa.
3. **Clinical Features**
  - Usually begins abruptly with focal soft-tissue swelling.
  - May be painful or nonpainful, and crepitus over a bony prominence.
  - Active and passive ROM limited.
  - Common locations include subdeltoid, olecranon, ischial, trochanteric, semimembranosus-gastrocnemius, prepatellar bursa.
4. **Diagnostic Studies**
  - Radiographs for the evaluation of bony prominence disclose soft-tissue calcifications.
5. **Management**
  - Bursitis caused by trauma responds to rest, immobilization, NSAIDs, and local corticosteroid injections.
  - Avoid repetitive motions.
  - Prevent recurrence with use of protective padding, elbow and knee pads.
  - Treatment of underlying collagen vascular disease or crystalline arthritis controls bursitis.
  - Bursitis due to infection requires aspiration to identify elevated WBCs, crystals, and bacteria.
  - Olecranon and prepatellar bursae most be drained.
  - Most common sites affected—olecranon, prepatellar bursa.
  - Most common cause of septic bursitis—*S. aureus.*

H. Adhesive Capsulitis (Frozen Shoulder)
1. **Etiology**
  - Specific etiology is unknown.
  - There may be an inflammatory component that leads to stiffness in shoulder.
  - Has been observed in the presence of subacromial impingement as well as C-spine degenerative disease, acromioclavicular (AC) arthritis, post-traumatic bursitis, and inflammatory synovitis of shoulder.
  - Most resistant form of adhesive capsulitis can occur with certain medical conditions—most common, diabetes mellitus (DM).
  - Has tendency to occur during fifth to sixth decades and appears to affect women more than men.
2. **Pathology**
  - Pain and stiffness in glenohumeral joint that cannot be explained on the basis of joint incongruity.
  - Typically lasts 18 to 24 months.
3. **Clinical Features**
  - Three clinical phases: (1) painful phase with gradual onset of diffuse pain; (2) phase of progressive stiffness with decreased ROM, affecting activities of daily living; (3) thawing phase with gradual return of motion.

- Usually, no precipitating cause is specifically remembered, although it is not unusual to get a history of trauma to the shoulder.
- There usually is generalized aching of the shoulder leading to stiffness.
- Patient voluntarily restricts the motion of the affected shoulder, leading to more stiffness.
- The more stiffness, the more pain, and thus a cycle ensues.
- Pain—often worse at night.
- Patient progressively becomes disabled functionally.
- Hallmark objective finding on clinical examination is that of restriction of passive ROM in comparison with unaffected side.

4. **Diagnostic Studies**
   - No studies are diagnostic of adhesive capsulitis, although plain film radiographs should be completed to assess for the presence of underlying pathology (i.e., subacromial impingement, rotator cuff tear, calcific tendinitis, and malignancy) that may be causal.
5. **Management**
   - Mainstay of treatment—rehabilitation program designed to improve ROM in shoulder, decrease stiffness, increase strength, which includes passive as well as active stretching of restricted planes of motion.
   - Exercises should be performed in therapy office and at home.
   - Anti-inflammatory and pain medications.
   - Refractory patients may benefit from closed manipulation of shoulder under general anesthesia and arthroscopic release.
   - If high risk of fracture to humerus exists, such as would be the case in osteopenic patient, rare consideration may be given for open release of adhesions to restore motion to shoulder.

I. Rotator Cuff Tendinitis
1. **Etiology**
   - Usually develops between adolescence and 40 years of age.
   - Common in athletes and laborers with repeated overhead motions.
2. **Pathology**
   - Tendons of rotator cuff are supraspinatus, infraspinatus, teres minor, subscapularis.
   - Supraspinatus tendon is the most common rotator cuff tendon to develop tendinitis.
   - Rotator cuff tendinitis results from impingement syndrome and is characterized by pain with overhead activity.
3. **Clinical Features**
   - Reproducible pain by abduction and internal rotator of upper extremity.
   - Pain over deltoid.
- Positive supraspinatus test—pain with abduction against resistance.
- Positive impingement sign—wincing of patient with forward flexion of upper extremity.

4. **Diagnostic Studies**
   - Usually normal radiographs.
5. **Management**
   - Ice for first 24 to 48 hours.
   - Shoulder pendulum and wall-climbing exercise.
   - Discontinue aggravating activity, especially overhead use of upper extremities.
   - NSAIDs, physical therapy.
   - Chronic tendinitis—local corticosteroid injections.

J. de Quervain Tenosynovitis
1. **Etiology**
   - Repetitive motion disorder due to pinch, wrist/thumb flexion and can occur with racket sports, golfers; there is history of no direct trauma.
   - Most common in 30- to 50-year-old women engaged in repetitive actions.
2. **Pathology**
   - Stenosing tenosynovitis affects abductor pollicis longus (APL) and extensor pollicis brevis (EPB).
3. **Clinical Features**
   - Pain (APL and EPB) at site; increased with gripping and extending thumb.
   - Tenderness of first dorsal compartment and radial styloid.
   - Positive Finkelstein test—fist with thumb across palmar surface of hand as ulnar deviated by the examiner.
   - Pain distal to styloid process of radius indicative of de Quervain disease.
4. **Diagnostic Studies**
   - Usually normal radiographs.
5. **Management**
   - Immobilization (i.e., splinting) of thumb, keeping the interphalangeal (IP) joint free.
   - NSAID, phonophoresis, activity modification.
   - If symptoms persist, additional therapy of local corticosteroid injections warranted and, occasionally, surgical release of first compartment.
   - Surgery complications include injury to the sensory branch of the radial nerve or failure to decompress the EPB.

K. Lateral Epicondylitis (Tennis Elbow)
1. **Etiology**
   - Can be the result of overuse injuries, poor technique in racket sports, or wrist weakness resulting in forced extension of wrist (e.g., tennis players making backhand strokes and people knitting).
2. **Pathology**
   - Degeneration or inflammation at extensor muscle group origin, principally in extensor carpi radialis brevis; rubs and rolls over lateral epicondyle and radial head.

- Pulling of extensor origin, resulting in microtears at the peristernal insertion.

3. Clinical Features
- Localized tenderness of lateral epicondyle, exacerbated by resisted wrist extension, pronation of forearm, and gripping activities.

4. Diagnostic Studies
- Usually normal radiographs.

5. Management
- Avoidance of painful activity.
- Rest, ice applications, NSAIDs.
- Physical therapy—for example, stretching, strengthening, U/S, and electrical stimulation—is helpful in reducing symptoms and permitting return to function.
- Lateral epicondylitis—tennis elbow strap designed to decentralize the area of stress.
- Equipment modifications may be helpful (flexible racket, larger grip).
- Neutral wrist position is maintained by wrist brace.
- Corticosteroid injections may be added if conservative measures are unsuccessful.
- Surgical (release of the common extensor origin and/or debridement of the pathologic tissue) options are reserved for severe refractory patients.

L. Medial Epicondylitis (Golfer's Elbow)

1. Etiology
- Less common and more difficult to treat than lateral epicondylitis.
- Overuse of flexor forearm muscles stresses and inflames tendinous insertion at medial epicondyle.
- Seen in certain manual activities, household activities, golfers.

2. Pathology
- Inflammation of affected area at pronator teres-flexor carpi radialis interface.

3. Clinical Features
- Tenderness is localized to the region of medial epicondyle.
- Reproduced by forcefully extending elbow against resistance with forearm supinated and wrist dorsiflexed.
- Medical epicondyle pain is worse with pulling activities and elbow flexion.

4. Diagnostic Studies
- Usually normal radiographs.

5. Management
- See II. K. 5.

M. Lumbosacral Sprain and Strain

1. Etiology
- Cause—acute or chronic muscle tendon or ligamentous strain, lumbar disk herniation, degenerative changes of spine, or osteoporosis.
- History of twisting or lifting.
- Predisposing factors include repetitive movements of lifting, pushing, pulling, or bending; sedentary lifestyle; obesity; poor posture; stress; loss of flexibility.

2. Pathology
- Tearing of muscle fibers or distal ligamentous attachments of the paraspinal muscles.
- Most often at iliac crest or lower lumbar/upper sacral region.

3. Clinical Features
- Discloses tense, hard, paraspinal, paravertebral muscle spasms of the lumbosacral spine.
- Possible absence of normal lordotic curve, presence of a list, or both.
- Decreased ROM of the lumbosacral spine.
- Absence of neurologic involvement (pain radiating below the knee and ankle reflex changes).

4. Diagnostic Studies
- Baseline radiographs are not indicated; if obtained, may be normal or show degenerative joint or reverse lordotic curve.
- The Agency for Healthcare Research and Quality guidelines for obtaining radiographs are summarized in Table 7-2.
- MRI, CT scan not necessary for initial evaluation—indicated when symptoms persist with neurologic involvement.

5. Management
- Brief bed rest; more than a day or 2 in bed is usually counterproductive.
- Begin walking as soon as possible; do as much normal activity as possible.
- Ice massage to muscle spasm for first 48 hours, followed by moist heat the following day.
- Analgesics or NSAIDs; muscle relaxers for the first several days may be helpful.
- Strengthening of paravertebral muscles with William McKenzie flexion extension exercises.

TABLE 7-2.   AHRQ Criteria for Lumbar Radiographs in Patients with Acute Low Back Pain

Possible fracture: major trauma, minor trauma in patients >50 y, long-term corticosteroid use, osteoporosis, >70 y

Possible tumor or infection: >50 y, <y, history of cancer, constitutional symptoms, recent bacterial infection, injection drug use, immunosuppression, supine pain, nocturnal pain

From the Agency for Healthcare Research and Quality. http://www.ahrq.gov/, with permission.

- Education regarding proper lifting technique, proper body mechanics, and weight loss if patient is obese.

N. Cervical Sprain and Strain
1. Etiology
- Overuse of musculature of posterior neck and shoulders as a result of unbalanced force exerted on area.
- Commonly seen after sudden turning of neck.
- Acceleration or "whiplash": acceleration flexion-extension neck injury—result of sudden, abrupt movement of head such as motor vehicle accident (MVA), sporting activity, assaults, accidental fall.
- Torticollis (stiff neck) occurs predominantly after excessive exposure to cold or activities requiring unusual or prolonged rotation or twisting of neck musculature.

2. Pathology
- Result of tearing of musculature and supporting structures of neck.
- Neck muscles respond to overuse by tightening into protective spasm to prevent further disruption.

3. Clinical Features
- May include pain increased with movement, discomfort, and tightness in posterior neck, visual symptoms, dizziness, tinnitus, and headache, tension-like, beginning in occiput region.
- Referred pain to interscapular area and shoulder.
- Palpable muscle spasms, unilateral or bilateral of the sternocleidomastoid, trapezium, or paraspinal muscles; muscle trigger points can be localized.
- Decreased ROM of the neck.
- Neurologic examination is often normal.

4. Diagnostic Studies
- C-spine radiographs—not needed routinely for uncomplicated diagnosis; indicated if symptoms continue past time of improvement; or to rule out at the time of injury, joint subluxation, fracture, avulsion fracture, congenital anomalies, or OA.
- Most common radiographic findings—straightening of normal lordotic curve indicates acute muscle spasm.
- MRI—indicated for disk herniation, detection of cord abnormalities.
- Bone scan—indicated for osseous involvement.
- CT scan—indicated for spinal stenosis, nerve root compression.

5. Management
- NSAIDs, analgesics, muscle relaxants.
- Ice for 24 hours, then alternate with heat.
- Use of collar may be helpful in acute phase of injury; long-term use is not recommended.
- Decreased activity for 24 to 48 hours; then, as tolerated, physical therapy (i.e., ROM exercises, ultrasonography, and deep massage) is useful if

symptoms persist or increase 48 to 72 hours after initial examination.
- Patients with paresthesia, muscle weakness, loss of reflexes, sensory loss, or evidence of bony injury require immediate stabilization with rigid cervical collar; additional studies: MRI and neurologic consult.

O. Fibromyalgia
1. Definition
- A clinical syndrome characterized by diffuse pain, extreme fatigue, stiffness, painful tender points, and sleep disturbance.
- American College of Rheumatology defined two criteria for diagnosing fibromyalgia in 1990: (1) history of widespread pain and (2) pain in at least 11 of 18 tender point sites on digital palpation with force of 4 kg.

2. Etiology
- Thought to be a disorder in restorative stage 4 sleep.
- Fibromyalgia affects middle-aged women commonly, but can also affect either gender of any age.
- The third most common rheumatic disorder, after OA and RA.

3. Pathology
- Muscle biopsy may show type II muscle fiber atrophy, moth-eaten appearance of type I fibers, or ragged red fibers, all of which suggest subclinical injury to muscle, thought to be caused by chronic muscle tension or chronic hypoxia.
- Muscles at tender points show decreased oxygenation, evidence of abnormal energy metabolism.
- As yet, none of these findings occur consistently enough to be useful as diagnostic test.

4. Clinical Features
- Patients frequently are unable to localize their pain.
- Patients feel worst in the morning; fatigue is a major component of disorder.
- Symptoms are worsened by physical and psychological factors (e.g., cold, noise, and stress).
- There may be complaints of numbness and tingling, often mistaken for nerve entrapment syndrome.
- No physical findings suggest inflammation (e.g., painful, swollen joints).
- Upon careful questioning, patients almost uniformly report frequently waking at night; detailed sleep pattern history is important in the diagnosis of fibromyalgia.
- There may be symptoms of depression and hypochondriasis, although no evidence exists that fibromyalgia patients as a group are different psychologically from other patients with chronic pain.

5. Diagnostic Studies
- No radiographic findings of fibromyalgia have been established.

- Laboratory studies—normal except in disclosing diseases such as hypothyroidism and DM, which can mimic fibromyalgia.
6. **Management**
   - Goals of therapy—provide education as to how sleep deprivation can decrease pain threshold and lead to more sleep deprivation.
   - Pharmacotherapy is used to help patients reestablish normal sleep pattern.
   - Tricyclics—for sleep.
   - Fibromyalgia involves serotonin deficiency; serotonin reuptake inhibitors may benefit patients.
   - Analgesics may be used for nighttime pain.
   - Physical therapy should be geared toward conditioning exercise program.
   - Aerobic exercises are aimed at increasing cardiovascular work, which improves stage 4 sleep.
   - Swimming—exercise of choice because of relaxing effect of water on muscles.
   - Biofeedback may be helpful in controlling stress.

III. Inherited or Developmental Disorders

A. Scoliosis
1. **Definition**
   - Lateral curvature of spine of >10°, usually thoracic or lumbar, associated with rotation of vertebrae.
   - Curve may be convex to right or left.
   - Rotation of vertebral column around its axis occurs and may cause rib-cage deformity.
   - May be associated with kyphosis (humpback) or lordosis (swayback).
   - Most common type—idiopathic (80% of patients), usually begins about ages 8 to 10; more common in girls than in boys (4:1 to 5:1); classically asymptomatic.
   - Most patients have a family history.
2. **Etiology**

   STRUCTURAL SCOLIOSIS
   - Idiopathic.
   - Congenital defects of spine.

- Paralytic or musculoskeletal (due to polio, cerebral palsy, muscular dystrophy).
- May be related to hormonal factors (melatonin), brain stem, or proprioception disorder.

FUNCTIONAL SCOLIOSIS
- Poor posture.
- Uneven leg length.

CLASSIFICATION OF SCOLIOSIS BY CAUSE (Table 7-3)
3. **Clinical Features**
   - Patients are often referred from school screening.
   - Forward bending test—most sensitive clinical test for scoliosis because it brings into profile rotation of ribs and vertebrae.
   - While standing behind the patient, ask the patient to bend forward with arms hanging free, feet together, knees straight.
   - Examine for the elevation of rib cage on one side and the depression on the other.
   - In the lumbar spine, examine for the elevation of paravertebral muscle mass on one side.
   - There may be visible pelvic obliquity with patient standing erect.
   - Presence of café au lait spots, skin tags, or axillary freckles is suggestive of neurofibromatosis.
   - Presence of hairy patches or dimples over the spine is suggestive of spinal dysraphism.
4. **Diagnostic Studies**
   - Obtain anteroposterior (AP), lateral radiographs to measure curve.
   - Preferable to use film size at least 14 in × 17 in.
   - Cobb angle—measure of curve magnitude.
   - MRI or myelograms with CT scanning indicated for noted structural abnormalities on plain films, excessive kyphosis, juvenile onset. Rapid curve progression, neurologic signs/symptoms, associated symptoms, and left thoracic/thoracolumbar curves.
5. **Management**
   - Most idiopathic curves do not progress to the point of requiring treatment.
   - Treatment options include observation, bracing, and surgery.

TABLE 7-3.	Classification of Scoliosis by Cause

- Idiopathic scoliosis: infantile (younger than 3 y), juvenile (from 3 to 10 y of age), adolescent (from 10 y of age to skeletal maturity)
- Neuromuscular scoliosis: neuropathic (e.g., cerebral palsy, spinal cord trauma, poliomyelitis, and muscular dystrophy)
- Congenital scoliosis: failure of formation, failure of segmentation
- Neurofibromatosis
- Connective tissue scoliosis: Marfan syndrome, Ehler–Danlos syndrome
- Osteochondrodystrophy: diastrophic dwarfism
- Metabolic scoliosis: secondary to nerve root irritation, postural

Adapted from Hu SS, Tribus CB, Tay BK, et al. Disorders, diseases, and injuries of the spine. In: Skinner HB, ed. *CURRENT Diagnosis and Treatment in Orthopedics*. 4th ed. New York, NY: McGraw-Hill; 2006:chap 5. http://www.accessmedicine.com/content.aspx?aID = 2319334. Accessed February 6, 2012, with permission.

- Exercise and electrical stimulation have shown little effect on the normal history of curve progression.
- Curve observation—indicated while child is growing.
- Bracing—reserved for children and some adolescent patients with progressive curves in the 20° to 40° range; however, bracing is not always effective, even with a well-made brace and good compliance.
- Surgery to fuse involved vertebrae—appropriate for progressive curves of more than 50°.
- Pseudoarthrosis of fusion or paralysis can occur following surgery.
- Surgery complication is a neurologic deficit not present preoperatively.

B. Spinal Stenosis

1. Etiology
- Narrowing of spinal canal or neural foramina produces nerve root compression, root ischemia, variable back, and leg pain.
- Central stenosis produces compression of the thecal sac.
- Usually affects men twice as often as women.
- More common in late middle age.
- Lateral stenosis produces compression of the individual nerve roots.
- Impingement of nerve roots lateral to the thecal sac as they pass through the lateral recess and into the neural foramen.
- Nerve root compression can occur at more than one level.
- Seen more frequently in combination with central stenosis.
- Can appear as an isolated entity involving middle-aged or young adults with symptoms of radicular pain unrelieved by rest and without tension signs.

2. Pathology
- Acquired stenosis—most common type; usually degenerative, resulting in loss of disk volume; increased pressure on apophyseal joints; and hypertrophy of soft tissue and bony structures, resulting in decrease in the diameter of spinal canal.
- Can be congenital, idiopathic, or developmental.

3. Clinical Features
- Insidious back pain that increases with time and extremity paresthesia with ambulation and extension, relieved by lying supine or with flexion of spine.
- Complaints of lower-extremity pain, numbness, "giving way."
- Possible pain and sensitivity loss over one or more dermatomes.
- ROM of spine discloses pain with extension.
- Normal pulses.
- May have neurologic findings.

4. Diagnostic Studies
- Radiographs disclose disk degeneration, facet hypertrophy, flattening of lordotic curve, subluxation.
- Plain CT scan, postmyelo-CT scan, and MRI—standard imaging modalities to assess nerve root entrapment.
- Bone scan or MRI may be helpful to rule out malignancy.
- Electromyogram (EMG) may be used to assess nerve root involvement, but sensitivity is variable and depends on examiner.

5. Management
- Majority of patients can be treated nonsurgically.
- Discourage activities that cause pain.
- Rest, physical therapy (i.e., flexion-based exercises), NSAIDs, weight reduction, back exercises, exercise program.
- Spinal or facet joint corticosteroid injection for refractory pain.
- Surgery is indicated for patients with positive studies, persistent pain, and alteration in activities of daily living.

C. Developmental Dysplasia of the Hip

- Previously called *congenital hip dysplasia.*
- "Screening for DDH: the U.S. Preventive Task Force concluded that there is insufficient evidence to recommend routine screening for developmental dysplasia of the hip in infants as a means to prevent adverse outcomes.
- Potential harms from screening include examiner-induced hip pathology caused by vigorous provocative testing, elevated risk for certain cancers from increased radiation exposure from followup radiographic tests, parental psychosocial issues from the diagnosis and therapy, and false positives results leading to unnecessary and potentially harmful followup and intervention." http://www.uspreventiveservicestaskforce.org/uspstf06/hip-dysp/hipdysrs.htm.

1. Etiology
- Unknown.
- Ethnic, genetic factors probably have a role.
- Increased incidence in North American Indians and first-born Caucasian children.
- Almost nonexistent in Chinese and African American infants.
- About 60% of children with developmental dysplasia of the hip (DDH) are firstborn.
- Eighty percent of DDH occurs in girls.
- Left is more common than the right.
- Positive family history.
- Other predisposing factors include conditions that limit fetal movement in uterus (e.g., oligohydramnios, intrauterine torticollis, and breech fetal positioning).

2. **Pathology**
   - Any hip in which normal relation between acetabulum and femoral head is altered.
   - By 11 weeks of gestation, hip joint is fully formed.
   - At birth, femoral head is firmly seated within acetabulum and held there by surface tension of synovial fluid.
   - In hips with dysplasia, fit is lost and head can be displaced easily from acetabulum.
   - Pathologic specimens show varying degrees of hip joint malformation from mild capsular laxity to severe acetabular, femoral head, and neck malformations.
   - Congenital hip dysplasia—refers to hip that may be provoked to subluxate or dislocate (regarding degree of contact between acetabulum and femoral head) but can be reduced into acetabulum.
   - Congenital hip dislocation—condition where no contact exists between the femoral head and acetabulum, and femoral head is not reducible.

3. **Clinical Features**
   - Most patients are detectable at birth.
   - Despite screening examinations, some patients are missed.
   - Diagnostic test for DDH—caused by femoral head gliding in and out of acetabulum over a ridge of abnormal acetabular cartilage:
     - Ortolani test is performed with infant positioned supine and hips and knees flexed at 90°; middle finger placed over greater trochanter, whereas thumb is placed over lesser trochanter bilaterally; hips are abducted slowly with pressure over greater trochanter bilaterally. Palpable sensation (typically, a click or clunk) indicates reduction of dislocated or subluxed hip.
     - Ortolani sign decreases markedly after 1 to 2 months of age.
     - Barlow sign is performed with infant positioned supine with the legs facing the examiner; hips flexed at 90°, knees fully flexed, each hip evaluated individually; examiner's other hand stabilizes the opposite femur and pelvis; examiner places thumb medially over the lesser trochanter and index finger laterally over the greater trochanter; examiner presses thumb backward and outward. Examiner feels for the movement of the head of the femur laterally against resistance as it slips out onto the posterior lip; examiner then, with the index finger, presses the greater trochanter head forward and inward. Examiner feels for a sudden movement of the femoral head inward as it returns to the hip socket. Movement in both directions is positive for Barlow sign, indicative of dislocatable hip.
   - Three phases are recognized commonly: (1) dislocated (Ortolani-positive, early, Ortolani-negative, late, when femoral head cannot be reduced); (2) dislocatable (Barlow-positive); and (3) capable of being subluxed (Barlow-suggestive).
   - In older children, secondary adaptive changes may be evident to include waddling gait, asymmetry of the gluteal, thigh, labial folds.
   - There may be apparent shortening of affected leg.

4. **Diagnostic Studies**
   - Radiographs and U/S are not needed when clinical examination is negative.
   - U/S—good adjunct in an infant whose femoral head has not started to ossify.
   - Normal radiographs do not rule out the possibility of DDH.

5. **Management**
   - Goal—contains femoral head within acetabulum, thereby stimulating growth and deepening of acetabulum and development of joint stability.
   - An abduction brace—usually sufficient for newborns and infants; should be continued until acetabular development and joint stability have occurred.
   - Closed manipulation of joint under general anesthesia may be necessary in refractory patients, and open reduction is reserved for patients who fail to maintain closed reduction.
   - Physical examination discloses mild-to-moderate restriction of hip motion.
   - Abduction can be particularly limited, easily noticeable if both legs are spread at the same time; this maneuver prevents pelvis from tilting.

D. **Legg–Calvé–Perthes Disease**
   1. **Etiology**
      - Idiopathic osteonecrosis of femoral head in children.
      - Thought to be related to interruption of blood flow to femoral epiphysis; femoral head has tentative blood flow.
      - Typically affects children between 4 and 10 years of age.
      - Four times more common in boys than in girls.
      - Unilateral in 90% of patients.
      - Increased incidence with a positive family history, low birth weight, and abnormal birth presentation.
      - Uncommon in African Americans.
   2. **Pathology**
      - After bone dies and loses structural integrity, articular surface of femoral head may collapse, leading to deformity and arthritis.
      - Self-limiting disease with revascularization usually occurs within 2 years.
      - Patients presenting with a bone age of 6 years have a poor prognosis.
   3. **Clinical Features**
      - Presenting complaint—limping for several weeks.

- Pain, often knee pain, effusion from synovitis, remember that hip pain is often referred to the knee.
- Limp worsens by day's end, related to activity.
- Complaints of pain usually involve aching into groin or proximal thigh.

4. **Diagnostic Studies**
- AP, frog-leg lateral radiographs of pelvis show increased density of femoral head as an early sign; gross deformity in patients with advanced disease.
- Radiographs may be negative at first, due to initial softening of the femoral head which is sufficient to cause symptoms, but insufficient to change the radiographic appearance of the femoral head.
- In the initial stage of the disease (1 to 3 months), the capital femoral epiphysis fails to grow because of the lack of the blood supply. The hip radiograph demonstrates widening of the cartilage space of the affected hip and a small size ossific nucleus of the femoral head, followed by a subchondral stress fracture line in the femoral head. As the disease progresses, the femoral head becomes more radiopaque and calcification of the necrotic marrow occurs, with resultant crushing of the avascular trabeculae in the dome of the epiphysis.
- If plain radiographs are normal, MRI (very sensitive) or bone scan is an excellent diagnostic tool.

5. **Management**
- No current interventions accelerate the process of revascularization.
- Observation—typically indicated for children younger than 6 years who do not exhibit significant subluxation and maintain at least 40° to 45° of abduction.
- NSAIDs help decrease pain and inflammation in patients without allergy or sensitivity to these medications.
- More significant treatment includes bracing with bed rest to "contain" femoral head within acetabulum and minimize flattening.
- Before initiating treatment, motion must be regained; bed rest and traction are commonly required.
- Osteotomy and other surgery are reserved for older children; best performed by pediatric orthopedic surgeon.

E. Pes Planus (Flatfoot)

1. **Etiology**
- Unknown.
- May be acquired (congenital), result of trauma, tendon degeneration, or arthritis.
- Between 3 and 5 years of age, normal longitudinal arch develops in most children.
- Estimated that by age 10, only 4% of population has pes planus.
- Always bilaterally.

2. **Pathology**
- Loss of support for arch and subsequent acquired flatfoot deformity.
- Characterized as either flexible or rigid (tarsal coalition).
- Flexible—most common form in children.

3. **Clinical Features**
- Loss of longitudinal arch on weight-bearing.
- Heel becomes more valgus and forefoot abducted.
- When child is not weight-bearing or is standing on tiptoes, arch is recreated.
- ROM is usually normal, but secondary contracture of Achilles tendon may develop in older children or adults.
- Flexible flatfoot—usually painless.
- If pain is present, it does not usually develop until patient is adolescent or adult.
- Aching occurs along plantar aspect of midfoot.
- There may be some aching into leg.

4. **Diagnostic Studies**
- Radiographs is not usually necessary in asymptomatic children.
- Standing lateral radiographs of foot show loss of longitudinal arch.
- On standing AP view, there may be lateral shift (subluxation) of navicular on the head of talus.

5. **Management**
- Conservative management for congenital flatfoot deformities.
- Modifications to shoe and orthotic devices have not been proved to alter natural development of longitudinal arch.
- A longitudinal arch support may benefit the patient, not necessary for the asymptomatic flexible flatfoot.
- For symptomatic flexible flatfoot, a semirigid longitudinal arch support and Achilles stretching exercise may be of some benefit.
- Parents and other family members may expect varied treatment, although they should be educated that in the past, treatment modalities were offered without any scientific basis.
- In symptomatic patients, acetaminophen, local heat, and massage may be used.
- If fatigue symptoms or activity-related discomfort persists, shoe modifications provide support.

F. Osgood–Schlatter Disease

1. **Etiology**
- 5:1 incidence in active adolescents (11 to 15 years of age) versus more sedentary; 2:1 to 3:1 greater incidence in boys.
- Onset of the disease during early adolescence coincides with the development of the secondary ossification.

2. **Pathology**
- Osteochondritis of the tibial tuberosity.

- Results from repetitive injury or small avulsion injuries at the bone–tendon junction where the patellar tendon inserts into the secondary ossification center of the tibial tuberosity.
- Can occur unilaterally or bilaterally.

3. Clinical Features
- Pain exacerbated by running, jumping, and kneeling activities.
- Some report pain after prolonged sitting with knees flexed.
- Tenderness and swelling at insertion of the patellar tendon into the tibial tubercle.
- Motion is typically unrestricted.
- Patellofemoral joint is stable.

4. Diagnostic Studies
- In acute phase of initial episode, radiographs usually show soft-tissue swelling.
- In more chronic patients, small spicules of heterotopic ossification may be seen anterior to the tibial tuberosity, with local prominence.

5. Management
- Ice after sports, NSAIDs, quadriceps stretching, and use of a protective knee pad for those who have pain with kneeling.
- Temporary cessation of provocative activity and, occasionally, immobilization are indicated for more recalcitrant symptoms.
- Return to full training for athletes can average 6 to 7 months.
- Surgery is considered for patients symptomatic after growth is completed.

IV. Degenerative Disorders

A. Osteoarthritis (Degenerative Joint Disease, DJD)
1. Etiology
- Most common form of arthritis.
- Eighty percent of adults 65 years of age and older demonstrate radiographic changes of OA.
- Younger than 45 years, the disease is more prevalent in men.
- Older than 55 years, the disease is more prevalent in women.

2. Pathology
- Joints undergo degenerative changes including subchondral bony sclerosis and loss of articular cartilage.
- OA is the result of failed attempt of chondrocytes to repair damaged cartilage; characterized by increased water content, alterations in proteoglycans, collagen abnormalities, and binding of proteoglycans to hyaluronic acid.
- OA can be primary from an intrinsic defect or secondary from a trauma, infection, or congenital disorders.

3. Clinical Features
- Common sites involved are hand: DIP, PIP.

- Other sites involved are wrist, hip, knee (most common joint affected), and cervical/lumbar spine.
- Onset—insidious, usually pain and stiffness after exercise or use of joint.
- Pattern of involvement—multiple joints; however, often initially with single joint involvement.
- Slowly progressive disease.
- Classic hand deformities—Heberden nodes, hard and painless nodules of dorsolateral aspects of DIP joint secondary to bony overgrowth; Bouchard nodes, hard and painless nodules on PIP.

4. Diagnostic Studies
- Radiographic characteristic—osteophytes and "joint space" narrowing, subchondral cysts from microfractures/bone repair.
- Hand: DIP, PIP, the MCP, and carpometacarpal joints of the thumb.
- Foot: evidence of hallux valgus at first metatarsophalangeal (MTP).
- Hip: superolateral involvement (Figure 7-3).
- Knee: asymmetric involvement.
- MRI—reserved for preoperative evaluation and management.

5. Management
- Treatment begins with supportive measures (i.e., activity modification and cane), NSAIDs, glucosamine chondroitin, capsaicin topical skin cream, and application of heat.

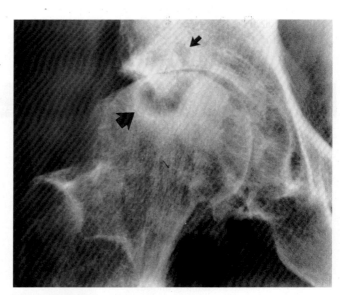

FIGURE 7-3. **OA of the hip**. There is narrowing of the hip joint, particularly superiorly. Large degenerative synovial cysts (geodes) are present in both the femoral head *(large arrow)* and the acetabulum *(small arrow)*. Note the osteophyte formation in both the acetabulum and the femoral head. (From Daffner RH, ed. *Clinical Radiology: The Essentials*. 2nd ed. Baltimore, MD: Lippincott Williams & Wilkins; 1999:438, with permission.)

- Modalities may include physical therapy or acupuncture.
- Intra-articular corticosteroid injection.
- Intra-articular viscosupplement injection.
- Surgical procedures ranging from arthroscopic debridement to arthroscopic total joint arthroplasties may be useful and advance patients resistant to nonoperative treatment.

B. Disk Herniation/Herniated Nucleus Pulposus

1. **Etiology**
   - Usually a disease of young and middle-aged adults because disk nucleus desiccates and is less likely to herniate in older patients.

2. **Pathology**
   - Disk degeneration with aging includes loss of water content and annular tears.
   - Molecular changes in disk with aging alter structural properties of disk and annulus fibrosis that contains the disk.
   - Most often involves L4–L5 disk, followed closely by L5–S1 in the lumbar spine.
   - Lumbar central prolapse may precipitate cauda equina compression syndrome—a medical emergency presenting with bilateral buttock or bladder dysfunction, saddle anesthesia, and lower-extremity motor sensory dysfunction, which require emergency treatment with surgical decompression of neural elements to prevent permanent dysfunction.

3. **Clinical Features (Table 7-4)**
   - May present with low back pain with radiation below knee and sciatica involving lower nerve root at that level (leg pain more than back pain). In the cervical spine, presentation may be neck pain with radicular paresthesia from nerve root involvement.

- Self-protected gait; localized tenderness, spasm of affected area; decreased spine flexion; increased pain with Valsalva maneuvers (i.e., coughing, sneezing, and bowel movements); diminished or absent reflexes; diminished sensation in dermatome pattern; with positive tension signs.
- Lumbar—positive straight leg raising and sitting nerve root test, positive contralateral straight-leg-raising test specific herniated nucleus pulposus.
- Occupational risks such as jobs that require lifting, prolonged standing, or repetitive lifting need to be assessed.
- Note Waddell and nonorganic physical signs for inappropriate symptoms.

4. **Diagnostic Studies**
   - Radiography may demonstrate disk space narrowing and rule out other pathologic evidence, and should be deferred for 6 weeks.
   - CT myelography demonstrates cord and nerve root compression.
   - MRI is superior for identifying cord pathology and neural tumors.
   - EMG demonstrates findings 3 weeks after nerve root pressure, although it rarely provides more information than good physical examination. This may be used for preoperative evaluation and management.

5. **Management**
   - Limited activity, short-term bed rest (2 days) with support underneath knees and neck, NSAIDs, ice, progressive ambulation, and mobilization with back rehabilitation successful in returning most patients to normal function.
   - Early intervention with physical therapy may be helpful for symptomatic relief.

TABLE 7-4.	Neurologic Syndromes Produced by Lumbar Disk Protrusion		
	L5	**S1**	**L4 (Less Common)**
Disk protrusion	Lateral protrusion at L4–L5	Lateral protrusion at L5–S1; central protrusion at L4–L5	L3–L4
Sensory disturbances	Pain and paresthesia in the region of the hip, groin, posterolateral thigh, and dorsal surface of foot, especially between first and second toes	Pain and paresthesia in midgluteal region, posterior part of thigh, calf, outer plantar surface of foot to fourth and fifth toes	Pain in anterior thigh
Weakness	Dorsiflexors of foot or extensor of big toe; walking on heels is more difficult than walking on toes	Flexor muscles of toes and foot, abductors of toes, hamstring muscles; walking on toes is more difficult than on heels	
Reflex loss	Usually none, although ankle jerk may be diminished	Loss or decrease of ankle jerk	Loss of knee jerk
Methods for diagnosis	CT; MRI; myelography; EMG of paraspinal muscles (wait 3 weeks after initial injury)	See L5 syndrome; MRI especially good; loss of asymmetry of H-reflex	See L5 syndrome

From Paty DW, Beall SS. Neurology. In: Kelley WN, ed. *Essentials of Internal Medicine.* 1st ed. Philadelphia, PA: JB Lippincott Company; 1994:724, with permission.

- Aerobic conditioning, proper lifting education, and body mechanics are important factors in avoiding missed work days and returning patients to work.
- If patients fail to improve with 6 weeks of conservative treatment, further diagnostic studies are indicated (e.g., bone scan to rule out spinal tumors or infection).
- Lumbar epidural steroids may be helpful in patients with predominantly sciatica.
- Patients with positive studies, neurologic findings, tension signs, without mitigating psychosocial factors are the best candidates for surgical discectomy.

V. Trauma

A. Fractures

CLASSIFICATION CONSIDERATIONS
- Direction of fracture line—oblique, transverse, spiral.
- Condition of bone—comminuted, impacted, segmented, pathologic, stress, avulsion, incomplete.
- Condition of soft tissue—open/closed fracture.
- Deformity—displacement, angulation, rotation, shortening.

CLAVICLE FRACTURES
1. **Etiology**
   - Most common fracture in children, with majority in middle one-third of the clavicle twice as common in males than in females.
   - Clavicle fractures of adolescents and adults result from moderate- or high-energy traumatic impacts (i.e., MVA and sports injury).
   - Clavicle fractures in children younger than 2 years suspect abuse.
2. **Mechanism of Injury**
   - Fall on outstretched hand and shoulder.
   - Fall onto shoulder.
   - Direct trauma to clavicle.
3. **Clinical Features**
   - Pain with ROM, deformity, tenderness, and swelling of shoulder.
   - Patient may hold arm against chest to protect against motion.
   - Crepitus at fracture site.
   - Evaluate carefully for neurovascular (NV) injury, pneumothorax, and hemothorax.
   - Fractures at the lateral one-third may be associated with disruption of the coracoclavicular ligament.
   - Fractures at the medial one-third need to be evaluated for chest injury.
4. **Diagnostic Studies**
   - AP and 45° cephalic tilt view.
   - Ultrasonography may be substituted for plain radiography in an urgent/emergent setting.

5. **Management**
   - Middle third clavicle fractures—arm sling for 4 to 6 weeks for adults.
   - Indications for orthopedic consult include NV compromise, distal and proximal clavicle fractures.
   - Indications for acute operative management include displaced fractures with compromise of skin, open fractures, and vascular injuries.
6. **Complications**
   - Rare.
   - Must closely evaluate for other associated injuries.

HUMERUS: MIDSHAFT HUMERUS FRACTURES
1. **Etiology**
   - Most humeral shaft fractures occur as a result of direct injuries, including falls, direct blow to arm, MVAs, and gunshot wounds.
   - Common site of pathologic fracture from metastatic breast cancer.
2. **Mechanism of Injury**
   - Direct blow or bending force applied to midhumerus.
   - Caused by fall onto arm or elbow or violent muscle contraction; suspect physical abuse in children with long spiral fractures.
3. **Clinical Features**
   - Cardinal signs of fracture: pain, swelling, deformity, crepitation.
   - Shortening of upper extremity.
   - Careful NV evaluation.
   - Weak or absent dorsiflexion of wrist or decreased sensation on back of hand suggests injury to the radial nerve.
   - Evaluate for compartment syndrome.
4. **Diagnostic Studies**
   - Two radiographs of humerus taken at 90° to each other.
   - Include radiographs of shoulder and elbow.
5. **Management**
   - Uncomplicated fractures—coaptation splints, upper-arm sling and swathe, orthopedic referral 3 to 5 days. Surgical reduction depends on the type of fracture, displacement, and patient compliance, which may include plating or intramedullary rods.
   - Emergent referral with NV deficit, open fractures, or spiral fractures; radial nerve injury, nonunion, brachial artery and vein.
6. **Complications**
   - Radial nerve injury can occur.

ELBOW: RADIAL HEAD AND NECK FRACTURES
1. **Etiology**
   - Relatively common injury; present in nearly 20% of all elbow injuries. Radial head fracture is most common in adults, whereas radial neck fracture is most common in children.

2. **Mechanism of Injury**
   - Commonly occurs as a result of direct fall on out-stretched arm with arm in pronation which forces radial head into capitellum.
3. **Clinical Features**
   - Swelling of lateral elbow.
   - Limited ROM, especially with forearm rotation, elbow extension.
   - Pain increased with passive supination and pronation ROM.
   - Point tenderness of radial head.
   - Careful NV evaluation is imperative, with attention to brachial artery and median nerve function.
4. **Diagnostic Studies**
   - AP, lateral, oblique radiographs of elbow.
   - Radiographs may be normal.
   - Positive fat pad sign (sail sign)—sail-shaped lucency in front of joint, indicative of intra-articular hemarthrosis, may be only clue to nondisplaced radial head fracture (Figure 7-4).
5. **Management**
   - Acute treatment—long arm splint, elbow at 90°, follow-up with orthopedist.
   - Definitive treatment, nondisplaced fractures—casting with sling for comfort, active ROM exercises, analgesics.
   - Immediate orthopedic consult for open or closed reduction for fracture dislocations, restricted ROM, and severe comminution. Closed reduction can result in long-term stiffness and decreased ROM.

6. **Complications**
   - Minimal limitation of elbow extension and forearm rotation; chronic pain.

FOREARM: FRACTURES OF SHAFT OF RADIUS (GALEAZZI FRACTURES)

1. **Etiology**
   - Radial shaft fracture at the junction of middle and distal thirds of radius.
   - Complicated by subluxation or dislocation at distal radioulnar joint (DRUJ).
2. **Mechanism of Injury**
   - Fall on extended, pronated wrist or direct blow to dorsolateral aspect of wrist.
3. **Clinical Features**
   - Pain, swelling, deformity of wrist.
   - Tenderness of wrist and DRUJ.
   - Distal ulna head displaced posteriorly.
   - Anterior interosseous nerve palsy may occur, which results in loss of pinch.
4. **Diagnostic Studies**
   - Radiographs to include entire length of radius and ulna, wrist, elbow.
   - AP, lateral radiographs.
   - Findings suggestive of DRUJ disruption—widening of DRUJ on AP view, fracture of base ulnar styloid, dislocation of radius, shortening of radius beyond 5 mm relative to distal ulna.
   - CT scanning is indicated to evaluate the DRUJ disruption for preoperative evaluation and management.

FIGURE 7-4. **Elbow fat pad. A:** Lateral radiograph shows elevation of the anterior *(large arrow)* and posterior *(curved arrow)* fat pads in patient with a subtle fracture of the distal humerus. **B:** Lateral radiograph of the opposite shows the normal position and appearance of the anterior fat pad *(arrow)*. The posterior fat pad is never visible under normal circumstances. (From Daffner RH, ed. *Clinical Radiology: The Essentials.* 2nd ed. Baltimore, MD: Lippincott Williams & Wilkins; 1999:459, with permission.)

5. **Management**
   - Well-molded sugar-tong splint, referral to ortho-pedic surgeon for next day.
   - Open reduction internal fixation (ORIF).
6. **Complications**
   - Dorsal angulation of radial fracture.
   - Subluxation of DRUJ.
   - Compartment syndrome.

NIGHTSTICK FRACTURES—ISOLATED FRACTURE OF THE ULNA

1. **Etiology**
   - Results from direct trauma, common in MVAs, block a punch or blow.
2. **Mechanism of Injury**
   - Direct blow to the shaft of the ulna by hard object such as bat, stick, golf ball.
   - Occasionally caused by fall with direct contact to the ulna shaft.
3. **Clinical Features**
   - Point tenderness/pain, specific swelling at fracture site.
   - Pain at fracture site with elbow or wrist ROM.
   - Detectable deformity if displacement has occurred.
   - With displacement of >50% or angulation of >10°, can suspect associated wrist or elbow injury.
4. **Diagnostic Studies**
   - AP, lateral, and oblique views of the shaft of the ulna.
   - Consider additional studies of elbow and wrist if angulation or displacement has occurred.
5. **Management**
   - Nondisplaced fracture acute phase—long arm cast or functional bracing.
   - Displaced/angulated—long arm splint with orthopedic surgical referral for ORIF.

FOREARM: MONTEGGIA FRACTURE

1. **Etiology**
   - Fracture of proximal third of ulna with anterior dislocation of radial head.
2. **Mechanism of Injury**
   - Fall on outstretched, extended, pronated elbow.
   - Direct blow to posterior aspect of the proximal ulna.
3. **Clinical Features**
   - Pain at elbow.
   - Radial head is palpated in antecubital fossa; forearm is shortened.
   - Radial nerve neurapraxia is common.
   - Patients may demonstrate loss of thumb extension, or paresthesias to dorsum of thumb, second and third fingers.
4. **Diagnostic Studies**
   - Radiographs to include entire length of radius and ulna, wrist, elbow.
   - AP, lateral radiographs.

5. **Management**
   - Double sugar-tong splint, promptly referred to orthopedic surgeon.
   - ORIF; pediatric patients may only require closed reduction and immobilization.
6. **Complications**
   - Neuropraxia of radial nerve.
   - Compartment syndrome.
   - Nonunion.

WRIST: COLLES FRACTURE

1. **Etiology**
   - Sixty percent to 70% of Colles fractures occur among postmenopausal women.
   - Ten percent to 15% occur in younger patients from violent injuries.
   - Fracture of lower-end of radius with posterior displacement of distal fragment.
   - Smith fracture—fracture of lower radius with anterior displacement.
   - Occurs in younger adults from accidents on bicycles, motorcycles.
2. **Mechanism of Injury**
   - Fall on outstretched hand with wrist in extension.
3. **Clinical Features**
   - Pain, swelling, tenderness, ecchymosis dorsum of wrist.
   - "Silver fork deformity" or "dinner fork deformity" due to displacement.
   - Limited ROM.
   - Palmar paresthesias due to tension or pressure on the median nerve.
   - Evaluate median nerve function, capillary refill.
4. **Diagnostic Studies**
   - AP, lateral, oblique radiographs of wrist.
   - CT Scanning may be used preoperatively for evaluation and management planning.
   - Examine radiographs for associated fractures (i.e., ulnar styloid, scaphoid, and lunate), scapholunate dissociation.
5. **Management**
   - Acute treatment—double sugar-tong or volar splint, wrist 15° in palmar flexion and ulnar deviation, forearm neutral position, elbow 90°.
   - Referral to orthopedic follow-up.
   - Indications for orthopedic consult—intra-articular extension, severe comminution, inability to maintain reduction, progressive symptoms of median nerve injury, open fractures.
6. **Complications**
   - Malunion.
   - Joint stiffness.
   - Median nerve compression.
   - Extensor pollicis longus tendon rupture.

WRIST: SCAPHOID FRACTURES

1. **Etiology**
   - Commonly occurs due to fall during athletic activities.
2. **Mechanism of Injury**
   - Fall on an extended wrist, outstretched hand.
3. **Clinical Features**
   - Radial side wrist pain, classically in anatomic snuffbox.
   - Anatomic snuffbox tenderness positive or negative must be written on all charts of patients with hand injuries.
   - Concavity of snuffbox may be obscured because of slight swelling.
   - High index of suspicion is necessary to avoid complications that would delay recognition and treatment.
4. **Diagnostic Studies**
   - PA, lateral, right, and left obliques; PA views of clenched fist in radial and ulnar deviation.
   - Negative radiographs do not exclude scaphoid fracture.
   - Examine radiographs for signs of ligament disruption and scapholunate dissociation.
   - Repeat radiographs in 2 weeks may disclose fracture.
   - If radiographs remain negative, bone scan, CT, tomogram, or MRI is indicated.
5. **Management**
   - Thumb spica splint for suspected, nondisplaced scaphoid fractures or for navicular tenderness even with negative radiography.
   - Orthopedic consult for displaced fractures and nondisplaced proximal scaphoid fractures due to increased incidence of poor healing, nonunion, early signs of avascular necrosis (AVN).
6. **Complications**
   - Fractures of middle and proximal portion of scaphoid prone to AVN and nonunion, due to vascular anatomy.

HAND: METACARPAL NECK FRACTURES

1. **Etiology**
   - Fracture of fifth metacarpal, most commonly known as boxer's fracture, followed by fourth and second metacarpal.
   - Least common in first metacarpal.
2. **Mechanism of Injury**
   - Direct impact on metacarpal head with hand in clenched fist position.
   - Palmar displacement of metacarpal head.
3. **Clinical Features**
   - Careful inspection of skin over MCP for laceration caused by a tooth, especially if a history of striking a person in the mouth.
   - Ensure no rotational deformity is present.
   - MCP depressed.
   - MCP joint tender, swollen, decreased ROM.

4. **Diagnostic Studies**
   - Lateral radiograph to measure angle of displacement.
   - AP, oblique views.
5. **Management**
   - Lacerations over MCP joint; treat aggressively as human bite.
   - Fourth and fifth metacarpal neck fractures with 20° to 40° angulation, without rotational deformity—ulnar gutter splint (wrist, 15° to 30° extension; MCP, 70° to 90°; PIP/DIP, 5° to 10°).
   - Second and third metacarpal neck fractures usually require open reduction and fixation.
   - Rotational malalignment, multiple fractures, and open fractures require orthopedic consultation.
6. **Complications**
   - Prominent metacarpal head in palm (affects grip).
   - Loss of reduction.
   - Rotational malunion.

HAND: MALLET FINGER FRACTURES (AVULSION FRACTURES)

1. **Etiology**
   - Forced flexion of fingertip against actively extended digit.
   - Occurs in sports (e.g., catching a ball) and minor incidents (e.g., putting on socks, washing laundry, and making beds).
2. **Mechanism of Injury**
   - Avulsion of extensor tendon from base of distal phalanx.
3. **Clinical Features**
   - Pain, swelling, tenderness of DIP joint.
   - Inability to extend distal phalanx.
4. **Diagnostic Studies**
   - AP, lateral, oblique radiographic views of digit.
5. **Management**
   - Extension splinting of DIP joint for 6+ weeks.
   - Indications for pinning include displaced (>2 mm) fragment or avulsions involving >30% of articular surface of distal phalanx.
6. **Complications**
   - Mallet finger deformity.

GAMEKEEPER/SKIER'S THUMB

1. **Etiology**
   - Injury to the ulnar collateral ligament (UCL) of the thumb, causing instability of the MCP joint.
2. **Mechanism of Injury**
   - Forced abduction of the thumb usually from a fall.
3. **Clinical Features**
   - Pain, swelling, and point tenderness at the ulnar aspect of the MCP joint.
   - Valgus stress may reveal unstable MCP joint.
   - Weakness in pinch strength.
4. **Diagnostic Studies**
   - Plain radiograph AP and lateral, stress X-rays may be used for preoperative evaluation and management.

5. **Management**
   - Partial UCL tears should be immobilized in a thumb spica splint or cast for up to 4 weeks.
   - Complete rupture requires surgical repair and bracing.

SUBUNGUAL HEMATOMA

1. **Etiology**
   - Bleeding and increased pressure under nail.
2. **Mechanism of Injury**
   - Direct trauma to nail.
3. **Clinical Features**
   - Evidence of bleeding under the nail.
   - Increasing pain that increases with dependency.
4. **Diagnostic Studies**
   - Plain radiograph to rule out fracture to be done before evacuation of hematoma.
5. **Management**
   - Mild hematoma may be treated conservatively with ice and elevation.
   - Moderate to severe symptoms require evacuation of nail bed.

HIP FRACTURES: FEMORAL NECK FRACTURES

1. **Etiology**
   - Common in elderly persons, who have decreased bone mass and increased frequency of falls.
   - More common in women than in men.
2. **Mechanism of Injury**
   - Minor or indirect trauma in elderly patients, especially those with osteoporosis.
   - Younger patients' femoral neck fractures due to high impact major trauma (i.e., MVA).
3. **Clinical Features**
   - Hip pain; leg may be slightly shortened and externally rotated.
   - Evaluate NV status.
4. **Diagnostic Studies**
   - AP with hip maximally internally rotated and lateral view of hip.
5. **Management**
   - Orthopedic consult.
   - Operative treatment most often needed.
6. **Complications**
   - Incidence of AVN of femoral head and nonunion increased because of compromise of blood supply to femoral head after fracture, infection, emboli, nonunion.

INTERTROCHANTERIC FRACTURES

1. **Etiology**
   - Fracture between the greater and the lesser trochanters of the femur.
   - Common in elderly with osteoporosis.
2. **Mechanism of Injury**
   - Associated with fall, MVA, or direct impact.
   - May have twisting mechanism of the lower extremity.

3. **Clinical Features**
   - Pain and inability to weight bear on affected side.
   - Extremity usually held in external rotation.
4. **Diagnostic Studies**
   - Plain radiograph with AP and cross table lateral view of the hip and full length view of the femur.
5. **Management**
   - Orthopedic consult with open reduction and internal fixation is required unless medically unstable.
6. **Complications**
   - Nonunion.
   - Medical instability due to prolonged bed rest and immobility.

SUBTROCHANTERIC FRACTURE

1. **Etiology**
   - Common in elderly with osteoporosis.
   - Occurs in younger patients with high energy impact trauma (MVA).
   - Femur fracture just inferior to the lesser trochanter.
2. **Mechanism of Injury**
   - Falls, trauma, MVA, gunshot wounds.
3. **Clinical Features**
   - Pain, swelling, and deformity present.
   - Lower extremity shortening may be present.
   - ROM is extremely limited.
4. **Diagnostic studies**
   - AP radiographs of the femur with cross table lateral.
5. **Management**
   - Orthopedic evaluation for open reduction and internal fixation.
6. **Complications**
   - Nonunion.
   - Shortening of extremity.

HIP DISLOCATION

1. **Etiology**
   - Uncommon injury occurring with high impact trauma such as MVA football injury, skiing injury.
   - Most hip dislocations are posterior.
2. **Mechanism of Injury**
   - Direct trauma forces femoral head from acetabulum.
3. **Clinical Features**
   - Severe lower extremity pain with loss of ROM and weight-bearing.
   - Posterior dislocation—lower extremity shortened, internally rotated and adducted.
   - Anterior dislocation—externally rotated, but may be extended or flexed.
4. **Diagnostic Studies**
   - AP, cross table lateral, and oblique radiographs of the pelvis prior to reduction.
   - CT or MRI indicates postreduction for associated injury.

5. **Management**
   - Orthopedic consultation.
   - Urgent closed reduction with sedation.
   - Open reduction may be required if closed reduction is unsuccessful.
6. **Complications**
   - AVN, associated injuries, OA.

PELVIS: FRACTURE

Acetabulum

1. **Etiology**
   - Commonly occurs in younger patients from high impact trauma (MVA).
2. **Mechanism of Injury**
   - High impact trauma such as MVA or fall/jump from height.
   - Fractures are identified and classified by the exact location of the fracture line(s).
3. **Clinical Features**
   - Acetabular fractures most often occur with associated injuries to lower extremity, abdominal and neurologic injury.
   - Lower extremity may be positioned as to the position of the hip joint.
4. **Diagnostic Studies**
   - AP radiograph of the pelvis, with lateral and oblique.
   - CT scanning may be necessary to identify associated injuries and preoperative evaluation and management planning.
5. **Management**
   - Medical stabilization and preoperative preparation.
   - Orthopedic referral for open reduction and internal fixation.
6. **Complications**
   - Infection, deep vein thrombosis (DVT), sciatic nerve damage, vascular injury.

PATHOLOGIC FRACTURES

1. **Etiology**
   - Fracture from minimal infarct to weakened bone from medical condition.
   - May be a result of tumor, infection, and genetic disorder.
2. **Mechanism of Injury**
   - Minor fall, trauma, or axial load.
   - Occurs at the area of cortex weakness.
3. **Clinical Features**
   - Pain, swelling, and deformity at fracture site.
   - Sudden loss of use where fracture has occurred.
4. **Diagnostic Studies**
   - Plain radiography may identify the fracture site.
   - CT/MRI scanning may be required for preoperative evaluation and management planning.
5. **Management**
   - Medical evaluation and stabilization.
   - Orthopedic consult for the evaluation of healing potential and recovery.

6. **Complications**
   - Nonunion.
   - Recurrence.

PATELLA FRACTURE

1. **Etiology**
   - Commonly occurs in younger patients from direct blow or trauma.
   - More common in women than in men.
2. **Mechanism of Injury**
   - Fall with direct trauma, impact with dashboard in MVA.
3. **Clinical Features**
   - Pain, swelling, deformity.
   - Limited knee extension with pain.
4. **Diagnostic Studies**
   - AP, lateral, and merchant view of the knee.
5. **Management**
   - Immobilization for nondisplaced fractures 4 to 6 weeks.
   - Open reduction and internal fixation for displaced fractures.
6. **Complications**
   - Infection if skin abrasion is present.
   - Nonunion.
   - Loss of ROM secondary to prolonged immobilization.

PILON FRACTURE (ALSO CALLED TIBIAL PLANFOND FRACTURE)

1. **Etiology**
   - Fracture of the distal tibia from impact with the talus.
   - Interrupts the joint space of the ankle joint.
2. **Mechanism of Action**
   - Injury occurs from forceful axial load to high impact trauma such as MVA.
3. **Clinical Features**
   - Severe pain, rapid swelling, and deformity.
4. **Diagnostic Studies**
   - Plain radiographs with AP, lateral, and mortise view.
   - CT scanning for preoperative evaluation and management planning.
5. **Management**
   - Medical stabilization.
   - Surgical stabilization is required. Technique varies with associated injuries.
6. **Complications**
   - Soft-tissue injuries.
   - Infection, osteomyelitis.
   - AVN.

TIBIA/FIBULA FRACTURES

1. **Etiology**
   - Occurs from impact direct trauma.
   - Tibia fracture is the most common long bone fracture.
   - Tibia fractures may occur in shaft, plateau, distal malleolus.

- Fibula fractures may occur shaft, head, distal malleolus.
2. **Mechanism of Injury**
   - Occur from fall, athletic trauma.
   - High impact—MVA, gunshot wounds.
3. **Clinical Features**
   - Pain, deformity, unable to weight bear if tibial fracture.
   - Isolated fibula fracture may allow weight-bearing.
   - Plateau fractures may have effusion at the knee.
4. **Diagnostic Studies**
   - Plain radiographs include AP, lateral of entire shaft.
   - CT scanning in tibial plateau fractures because they are easy to miss.
5. **Management**
   - Medical stabilization.
   - Antibiotic prophylaxis if open fracture.
   - Orthopedic referral.
   - Immobilization with variable weight-bearing status for nondisplaced fractures.
   - Displaced fractures may require open reduction and fixation.
6. **Complications**
   - Nonunion distal tibia is a common area for a nonunion.
   - Infection, osteomyelitis.
   - Loss of ROM secondary to prolonged immobilization.

PEDIATRIC FRACTURES
1. Distal radius fractures—occurs from fall on outstretched hand; see fracture management and Salter-Harris classification of pediatric fractures.
2. Supracondylar fractures of the humerus—occurs from fall on outstretched hand, very common, usually extrarticular.
3. Tillaux fractures—fracture of the tibial epiphysis from fall or athletic injury.
4. Torus fractures—fracture of one side of the cortex causing "buckle" in the bone shaft.
5. Triplane fractures—fracture that occurs through physis, epiphysis, and metaphysis, resulting in closure and failure of growth plate.

SALTER–HARRIS CLASSIFICATION FRACTURES
1. **Etiology**
   - Fractures involving the physis—the cartilaginous epiphyseal plate near the ends of the long bones of growing children.
2. **Pathology**
   - **Five types:**
     - Type I: fracture of growth plate.
     - Type II: fracture of growth plate with fracture of metaphysis.
     - Type III: fracture of growth plate and portion of epiphysis.

- Type IV: single fracture through growth plate, metaphysis, and epiphysis.
- Type V: nothing fractured, crushing injury to growth plate.
3. **Clinical Features**
   - Potential for growth disturbances is least for type I and increases with each type; the worst prognosis is associated with type V fractures.
   - Swelling, tenderness in the region of the physis.
4. **Diagnostic Studies**
   - Radiographs.
5. **Management**
   - Immobilization.
   - Refer to orthopedist for follow-up.
   - Gentle reduction attempted initially for type I and II fractures usually requiring general anesthesia.
   - Type III and IV fractures usually require open reduction to align the growth plate correctly.
   - Type V fractures have a high complication rate because they are not identified early.

SPINE COMPRESSION FRACTURES
1. **Etiology**
   - Burst fracture—occurs in young people usually from jump/fall from height.
   - Lumbar compression fractures—occur in the elderly from osteoporosis, tumor, or systemic illness.
   - Pathologic fracture—compression fracture secondary to tumor, malignancy.
2. **Mechanism of Injury**
   - Burst—axial load in fall from height transferred through the spine.
   - Compression—soft cortex fails with time and degeneration.
3. **Clinical Features**
   - Pain and point tenderness at level of fracture.
   - May develop neurologic symptoms if nerve compression occurs.
4. **Diagnostic Studies**
   - AP and lateral plain radiograph.
   - CT scanning may be necessary for complete visualization of fracture.
   - MRI should be ordered if neurologic symptoms develop.
   - CT-guided biopsy if malignancy is suspected.
5. **Management**
   - Orthopedic consult.
   - Neurosurgical consult if neuro symptoms and signs occur.
   - Kyphoplasty/vertebroplasty may be attempted.
   - Analgesics for pain control.
   - Bracing and rehabilitation services.

STRESS FRACTURES
1. **Etiology**
   - Consistent overloading of bone that eventually weakens the periosteum to failure.

- Common in athletes such as runners, gymnasts.
- Also occurs in the military because of excessive marching.

2. **Mechanism of Injury**
   - Pattern of overuse, without single traumatic injury.
   - Sudden onset of vigorous activity without appropriate training or preparation.

3. **Clinical Features**
   - Tenderness of affected area at the end of activity early on, then advancing to pain during entire activity and at rest.
   - History may include change of sport, surface used in training, change of shoes, sudden onset of repetitive activity.
   - Areas most common: metatarsals, midshaft of the tibia, midshaft of the femur, humerus.
   - Adolescents are predisposed because of weaker bone, increase in formal activities, and ignoring of pain symptoms.

4. **Diagnostic Studies**
   - AP/lateral X-ray may disclose cortical fracture line.
   - If negative, repeat in 2 weeks, looking for a periosteal reaction of bone healing.
   - Bone scanning with technetium will disclose stress fractures and stress reactions within 10 days of the injury.
   - MR testing can be done, but is not cost-effective unless suspicious of tumor.

5. **Management**
   - Discontinue the causative activity and adjust training regimen.
   - Rest phase should be 4 to 6 weeks.
   - Occasionally, a splinting device is necessary for comfort, such as a Reece-orthopedic shoe or removable walking cast.
   - Exercise may continue using non-weight-bearing activity such as swimming, which may promote healing if fracture is of a weight-bearing bone.
   - Prevention of reoccurrence should include proper footwear, gait analysis, appropriate rehabilitation, and consistent training surface.

6. **Complications**
   - Surgical intervention is rarely required.
   - Recurrence is common.

B. Dislocations

ELBOW

1. **Etiology**
   - Disassociation of ulna to humerus and then to elbow.
   - Most common dislocation in children.

2. **Mechanism of Injury**
   - Fall on outstretched hand.
   - Usually, hyperextension injury.

3. **Clinical Features**
   - Moderate to severe pain, with obvious deformity.

- NV compromise may occur (brachial artery, median, ulnar, and radial nerve).
- Associated with supracondylar and radial head fractures.

4. **Diagnostic Studies**
   - X-ray AP/lateral.
   - CT scanning may be required to determine occult fracture.

5. **Management**
   - Reduction should be accomplished as soon as possible—usually under sedation.
   - X-ray pre- and postreduction.
   - Document NV status pre- and postreduction.
   - Stable reduction can be splinted in 90° of flexion for 7 to 10 days, followed by progressive ROM.
   - Open treatment is indicated for persistent instability, intra-articular fragments, medial epicondylar fractures, and coronoid process fractures.

6. **Complications**
   - NV injury.
   - Associated fractures.

SHOULDER GLENOHUMERAL DISLOCATION

1. **Etiology**
   - Most common dislocated joint in adults.
   - Anterior (majority) or posterior displacement of the humeral head from the glenoid fossa. Inferior, superior, and intrathoracic dislocations are rare and are associated with significant trauma.

2. **Mechanism of Injury**
   - Anterior—forced external rotation and abduction of arm, most common shoulder dislocation.
     - Example: direct blow to arm while throwing.
   - Posterior—rare (<5%), humeral head drops below glenoid fossa.
     - Example: occurs with severe muscle constriction such as seizure and electrocution.

3. **Clinical Features**
   - Acute pain, deformity, and loss of arm movement.
   - First-time dislocation traumatic to soft tissue.
   - Recurrence is common.
   - Check NV status—axillary nerve injury may occur.

4. **Diagnostic Studies**
   - Plain radiographs with AP/lateral/Y (scapular) views pre- and postreduction.

5. **Management**
   - Reduction with sedation.
   - Document NV status pre- and postreduction.
   - Sling plus swathe for 4 weeks in young patients and 2 weeks in elderly persons, then rehabilitation.
   - Recurrent dislocations can require surgical correction.

6. **Complications**
   - NV injury—axillary nerve.
   - Recurring injury.
   - Associated soft-tissue injury.

PATELLA

1. **Etiology**
   - Displacement of patella from the femoral condyles.
2. **Mechanism of Injury**
   - Usually occurs from a twisting injury to the extended knee.
   - More common in women.
   - Occurs with strong muscle contraction of quadriceps in full extension.
3. **Clinical Features**
   - Pain with obvious deformity and knee effusion.
   - NV compromise is rare.
4. **Diagnostic Studies**
   - AP/lateral plain radiographs with sunrise view—pre- and postreduction.
5. **Management**
   - Reduction with sedation.
   - Immobilization in extension for 3 weeks.
   - Rehabilitation referral.

KNEE DISLOCATION

1. **Etiology**
   - Uncommon injury, associated with direct trauma.
2. **Mechanism of Injury**
   - Direct impact to knee joint with associated injury.
   - Occurs from MVA, fall, athletic injuries.
3. **Clinical Features**
   - Severe pain and deformity.
   - Weight-bearing not possible.
   - NV status should be carefully examined.
4. **Diagnostic Studies**
   - Plain radiograph pre- and postreduction.
   - Ultrasonography to evaluate vascular status.
   - CT angiography to evaluate arterial status, even if there is spontaneous reduction.
5. **Management**
   - Orthopedic referral.
   - Urgent reduction and splinting.
   - Evaluation and monitoring of NV status.

ANKLE DISLOCATION

1. **Etiology**
   - Occurs with major trauma or injury.
   - Rarely it does not include fracture because of complex ankle anatomy.
2. **Mechanism of Injury**
   - Major trauma such as MVA or high velocity athletic injury.
3. **Clinical Features**
   - Pain, edema, deformity, and non-weight-bearing.
   - Dislocation may be anterior, posterior (most common), lateral, or superior.
   - NV status must be evaluated.
4. **Diagnostic Studies**
   - Plain radiographs AP, lateral.
   - Pre- and postreduction films.
   - CT scanning may be used for preoperative evaluation and management planning.

5. **Management**
   - Orthopedic referral.
   - Urgent reduction.
   - Surgical repair likely requires open reduction and internal fixation.

FOOT DISLOCATION

1. **Etiology**
   - Uncommon and occur from trauma or athletic injury.
   - More common in men than in women.
   - Usually occurs in the Lisfranc (between the midfoot and the forefoot) joint.
2. **Mechanism of Injury**
   - High impact trauma, athletic injuries.
3. **Diagnostic Studies**
   - Plain radiographs including AP, lateral, and oblique.
   - CT scanning for the evaluation of associated fractures.
   - MRI for tendinous/ligamentous associated injuries.
4. **Clinical Features**
   - Pain, edema, and deformity.
   - NV status must be evaluated.
5. **Management**
   - Orthopedic referral.
   - Urgent reduction with pre- and postradiographs.
   - Commonly require surgical reduction.

C. **AC Subluxation (Shoulder Separation)**
   1. **Etiology**
      - Typically due to fall onto the tip of the shoulder with arm tucked into side or onto the outstretched hand.
   2. **Pathology**
      - **Six types**—regarding degree of AC displacement:
        - Type I: sprain of AC ligaments.
        - Type II: AC joint disruption.
        - Type III: disruption of coracoclavicular ligament with 25% to 100% increase of coracoclavicular space compared with normal side.
        - Type IV: posterior displacement of distal clavicle into or through trapezius.
        - Type V: detachment of deltoid and trapezius muscle from distal half of clavicle; coracoacromial space 100% to 300% greater than in normal shoulder.
        - Type VI: decrease of coracoclavicular space with clavicle inferior to acromion and coracoid.
   3. **Clinical Features**
      - Pain over the joint.
      - Lifting arm—painful if not impossible.
      - Obvious deformity with type III and higher, examining patient with shirt removed.
      - Patient has difficulty or inability to raise arm at shoulder.

4. **Diagnostic Studies**
   - AP radiograph of both shoulders with and without 10-lb weights placed in patient's hands, which tend to increase the degree of separation in affected shoulder, such that it is more apparent in comparison with uninjured side, as well as ipsilateral views without weights.
   - Attention must be given to ruling out differential pathology (e.g., fracture of acromion and clavicle, as well as rotator cuff tear).

5. **Management**
   - Types I, II, and III may be treated with the use of sling for 1 to 3 weeks.
   - As pain diminishes, initiate protected ROM protocol, with the use of ice and NSAIDs.
   - Progress to strengthening, rehabilitation over time.
   - In types IV and V, closed reduction may be attempted; however, types V and VI typically require open surgical reduction with repair of disrupted ligaments.

D. Rotator Cuff Tear

1. **Etiology**
   - Multifactorial to include fatigue failure of cuff tissue (e.g., repetitive overhead use); mechanical failure associated with subacromial impingement; normal aging; intrinsic etiology such as hypovascularity and tendinopathy.
   - Most tears begin at supraspinatus tendon on greater humeral tuberosity.
   - As tears enlarge, they extend posteriorly to involve infraspinatus and teres minor or anteriorly to involve subscapularis.
   - Most common cause of shoulder pain in patients older than 40 years.
   - Traumatic event initiates symptoms in half of patients.
   - Appears to affect men and women equally and involves dominant and nondominant arms.

2. **Pathology**
   - Investigation of vascular anatomy of rotator cuff has demonstrated dearth of vascularity involving insertion of supraspinatus at greater tuberosity.
   - Critical area because most cuff tears originate here.
   - Also suggested that hypovascularity of tendon may contribute to poor repair potential after tear has occurred.
   - Tear may spread due to increased tension on remaining intact fibers, with resulting sequential failure.

3. **Clinical Features**
   - Most common symptom—pain, usually associated with mild-to-moderate dysfunction and some limitation of ROM.
   - Night pain is common due to inability to sleep on involved side.

- More significant tears of supraspinatus involve pain and loss of motion with respect to abduction, forward elevation, and internal rotation.
- There usually is weakness (due to both reduction of intact muscle fibers and painful inhibition), particularly involving abduction.
- There may be visible muscle atrophy of infraspinatus and supraspinatus fossa.

4. **Diagnostic Studies**
   - MRI can be sensitive and specific for partial- and full-thickness tears.
   - Sonography can evaluate a tear and biceps tendon.
   - Plain film radiography is not specific or sensitive for full-thickness tears, although stress views may accentuate humeral head migration.
   - Greater tuberosity sclerosis, spurring, cyst formation, along with subacromial spurring, associated with chronic rotator cuff disease and may be evident on plain film radiography.

5. **Management**
   - Based on the level of pain, dysfunction, and anatomy of the tear.
   - Conservative—rehabilitation, NSAIDs, corticosteroid intra-articular injection, ROM preservation.
   - Surgical intervention—patients who remain symptomatic can benefit from arthroscopic debridement, bursectomy, and acromioplasty, with or without distal clavicle resection.

E. Subacromial Impingement Syndrome

1. **Etiology**
   - Any pathologic process that decreases space between the rather rigid coracoacromial arch and greater tuberosity of supraspinatus insertion may result in mechanical squeezing of rotator cuff and bursa between these two hard surfaces.
   - Patients are typically older than 40 years.

2. **Pathology**
   - Morphologic alterations in anterior acromion (e.g., spurring) or changes in rigidity of coracoacromial ligament may result in decreased pliability of these structures, which may begin to compress rotator cuff as arm is brought up into forward elevation.
   - Theorists have questioned whether the presence of subacromial impingement is primary or contributing factor in the formation of rotator cuff tears.

3. **Clinical Features**
   - Patients usually have history of pain, particularly with use of arm above chest or shoulder level.
   - In early stages, pain occurs with activity and resolves at rest.
   - With disease progression, patients attempt to rest affected arm at their side with resulting stiffness, possibly leading to adhesive capsulitis.
   - Pain eventually occurs even at rest.

- In all stages, pain may be reported to radiate into the deltoid, as well as back into the scapula and lateral to the base of the neck.
- A positive impingement sign can be demonstrated in early stages of impingement, in which pain is reproduced as arm is brought into full forward elevation, causing coracoacromial arch to contact greater tuberosity.
- Pain with abduction and internal rotation of affected arm.
- Diffuse tenderness to palpation as well as painful inhibition to strength testing also may be present.
- Relief of pain with subacromial space injection of Xylocaine diagnostic of subacromial impingement syndrome.

4. **Diagnostic Studies**
   - Plain radiographs often demonstrate signs of mechanical impingement (e.g., sclerosis, spur formation, and cystic changes) in area of supraspinatus insertion of greater tuberosity.
   - These changes are usually demonstrable on AP view.
   - Lateral view may show encroachment of subacromial spur.
   - MRI demonstrates bone changes, as well as any associated rotator cuff deterioration, cuff tears, and changes in subacromial bursa.

5. **Management**
   - Goals of therapy—restore and maintain ROM, reduce inflammation of soft tissues, strengthen supporting musculature.
   - Subacromial injection of corticosteroid plays a role in patients who do not experience relief with oral anti-inflammatory medications.
   - Patients who fail conservative therapy may be candidates for surgical treatment of impingement lesions.
   - Surgical options include resection of coracoacromial ligament, anterior acromioplasty, distal clavicle excision, and bursectomy.

F. Thoracic Outlet Syndrome

1. **Etiology**
   - Idiopathic etiology, but is associated with heavy loading of brachial plexus and overuse injuries.
   - Has occurred in the presence of congenital abnormalities (e.g., a cervical rib, abnormally long transverse process of seventh cervical vertebra, and anomalous fibromuscular band in thoracic outlet).
   - Posttraumatic fibrosis of scalene muscles also has been implicated.
   - Poor posture with slumping shoulders may contribute.
   - Women 20 to 50 years of age are most commonly affected.

2. **Pathology**
   - Compression of structures (e.g., brachial plexus and subclavian artery or vein) because they exit a narrow space between superior shoulder girdle and first rib.
   - These structures may be affected individually or in combination.

3. **Clinical Features**
   - Symptoms consistent with nerve compression are most common, including paresthesias of arm, forearm, and ulnar side of hand.
   - There can be pain involving upper arm, shoulder, and neck.
   - Other complaints include headaches, weakness, and loss of coordination.
   - Symptoms of vascular compression can include swelling and discoloration of arm.
   - The Adson sign and the Wright test are useful in assessing vascular compression.
   - Occasionally, there can be emboli of arteries and thrombosis of subclavian vein.

4. **Diagnostic Studies**
   - AP and lateral radiographs of C-spine identify cervical rib or abnormally long transverse process.
   - Views of lung help rule out an apical lung tumor or infection.
   - Ultimately, no gold standard diagnostic tool for the presence of thoracic outlet syndrome; however, MRI, electrodiagnostic evaluation with evoked potentials, and U/S can be helpful in ruling out alternative diagnoses.
   - Color flow duplex scanning for vascular evaluation.
   - Arteriography is useful in assessing compression of the axillary artery.

5. **Management**
   - Because diagnosis is both clinical and controversial, most patients are treated nonsurgically.
   - Physical therapy programs stress muscle strengthening and postural education.
   - Avoidance of strenuous physical activity, heavy load to area (backpack), prolonged overhead tasks.
   - Function must be optimized because possible sequelae include frozen shoulder, complex regional pain syndrome (reflex sympathetic dystrophy [RSD]), and brachial plexus injury.
   - NSAIDs, muscle relaxants, and transcutaneous electrical nerve stimulation (TENS) units can help decrease the severity of symptoms.
   - Surgical resection of cervical rib may be considered in refractory patients; however, complication rate is high and success rate variable.

G. Subluxation of the Radial Head (Nursemaid's Elbow)

1. **Etiology**
   - Most common elbow injury in young children.
   - Parent or older sibling lifts, swings, or pulls a child when forearm is pronated and elbow extended.

2. **Pathology**
   - Radial head pulled in distal direction and becomes loaded or wedged in annular ligament.
3. **Clinical Features**
   - Immediately after injury, child cries, but initial pain subsides quickly.
   - Thereafter, child is reluctant to use arm, but otherwise does not appear in great distress.
   - There typically is tenderness over radial head as well as resistance of attempted supination; however, there is no swelling at the elbow.
4. **Diagnostic Studies**
   - Radiographs are usually normal; used to rule out other injuries, if history is uncertain or examination is equivocal.
5. **Management**
   - Closed manipulation to reduce injury; should only be performed by providers familiar with the treatment of this type.
   - Immobilization—unnecessary unless delay occurs from time of injury until radial head has been reduced or unless the child does not move the arm after a couple attempts of reduction; in this patient, sling may be used with expectation that normal function of arm returns in a few days.

   APOPHYSITIS OF THE HIP AND PELVIS
1. **Etiology**
   - Overuse injury to the growth plate in adolescent patients.
   - Occurs from tendinous attachment at apophysis, causing irritation at the site of attachment.
2. **Mechanism of Injury**
   - Overactivity/overuse of muscles surrounding the pelvis and hip.
3. **Clinical Features**
   - Dull pain at the site of inflammation.
   - May be slight swelling, no deformity.
4. **Diagnostic Studies**
   - Plain radiograph is only indicated if symptoms persist.
5. **Management**
   - Rest, ice, and flexibility exercises.
   - Avoidance of overuse activities.
   - Physical therapy for flexibility routine for return to athletics.

H. Osteochondritis Dissecans
1. **Definition**
   - Condition in which segment of articulating and underlying subchondral bone becomes separated from surrounding bone.
   - Typically involves the knee.
2. **Etiology**
   - Trauma—possibly result of focal insufficiency in end-arterial blood supply leading to necrosis.
   - Primarily affects children younger than 12 years of age and young adults.

- Males more than females, 3:1.
3. **Pathology**
   - Primary change in bone.
   - Loss of subchondral bone support leads to degenerative cartilage changes: softening, fibromatous, fissuring.
4. **Clinical Features**
   - Intermittent joint pain, clicking, swelling, locking, stiffness.
   - May be asymptomatic until fragment detaches, then experience locking or giving way in the knee.
   - Focal tenderness over involved part of joint.
   - May have effusion, atrophy of supporting musculature, crepitus, decreased ROM.
5. **Diagnostic Studies**

   IMAGING
   - Plain radiographs, AP, lateral, and "tunnel" view; first study to confirm diagnosis.
   - Appears as well-demarcated fragment of bone surrounded by radiolucent zone.
   - If separated, fragment may be seen elsewhere in joint and defect is present in articular surface.

   MRI
   - Useful to delineate bony lesion.
   - Difficult to assess and identify the status of overlying articular cartilage.
   - Healing progression is difficult to follow.

   CT SCAN
   - Provides architectural description of lesion.
   - Essentially replaced by MRI.

   ARTHROSCOPY
   - Definitive procedure to assess underlying cartilage and for definitive treatment.
6. **Management**
   - Non-weight-bearing immobilization with intermittent maintenance of ROM.
   - Follow closely 12 weeks for healing; fragment displacement may occur, for which arthroscopy is indicated.
   - Should be followed initially every 6 to 8 weeks with serial radiographs to check for healing and possible displacement.
   - Expect healing in 3 months.
   - In 1 year, radiographs usually show no residual abnormality.
   - NSAIDs can help with discomfort and inflammation.
   - Most lesions heal without surgical intervention.
   - On occasion, early surgical intervention is needed.
   - Orthopedic consultation is recommended.

I. Chondromalacia (Patellofemoral Syndrome)
1. **Etiology**
   - Typically idiopathic, although other causes include cumulative trauma, patellar instability,

patellar malalignment, synovitis, increased patellar compression, and primary OA.

- May result from weakness of quadriceps mechanism, particularly involving vastus medialis obliquus (VMO).
- Affects women more than men.
- In the absence of trauma, condition is often bilateral.

2. Pathology

- Refers to softening or fissuring of articular surface of patellofemoral joint.
- Outcome—OA of patellofemoral joint.

3. Clinical Features

- Usually anterior knee pain in area where patellar articulation is worse.
- Increased pain with prolonged sitting as well as jumping, climbing, and squatting.
- There may be history of knee giving way.
- Positive apprehension test—whereby patient becomes apprehensive if examiner attempts to move patella medially or laterally with knee extended.
- Pain is also increased with hyperflexion of knee.
- Comparative thigh circumference may show atrophy of affected side involving VMO.

4. Diagnostic Studies

- Plain radiograph evaluation includes AP, lateral, patellar (Merchant) views; last view is helpful in ruling out malalignment and arthritis of patella.

5. Management

- Begin strengthening of VMO, flexibility program.
- Weight loss is recommended to decrease stress on the patellofemoral joint.
- Short-term NSAID use.
- Use of elastic knee sleeve for patellar stabilization.
- Sleeve may incorporate doughnut for purposes of improving tracking of patella within femoral sulcus.

ILIOTIBIAL BAND SYNDROME

1. Etiology

- Lateral knee pain from inflammation of iliotibial band (ITB) bursa.
- Occurs with continuous running/movement.
- Most common cause of knee pain in runners.

2. Mechanism of Injury

- Occurs from lack of flexibility of the ITB.

3. Clinical Features

- Pain during onset of running, then resolves.
- Point tender over lateral condyle.
- Pain occurs with stair climbing and running downhill.
- Ober test causes pain and resistance to adduction.

4. Diagnostic Studies

- No imaging is necessary.

5. Management

- Physical therapy for flexibility regime.
- NSAIDs for anti-inflammatory effect.

- Resistant symptoms may respond to corticosteroid injection.

J. Posterior Cruciate Ligament Injury (Knee)

1. Etiology

- Patient reports fall onto flexed knee or sustained an anterior force to bent knee (dashboard injury).
- Can occur alone, but typically occurs in association with tear(s) of anterior cruciate ligament (ACL), collateral ligament, or meniscus.

2. Pathology

- Believed to be the most important of knee ligaments because it provides 95% of total resistance to posterior translation at all angles of flexion.

3. Clinical Features

- Bruising anteriorly, especially on anteromedial aspect of proximal tibia; should alert to possible posterior soft-tissue injury.
- Large effusion is commonly present and persists for several days following injury.
- Tests classically indicative of posterior cruciate ligament (PCL) tear include posterior drawer and posterior pivot shift tests.
- There may be visible posterior sag (subluxation) of tibia.

4. Diagnostic Studies

- Arthrocentesis can be performed in acute phase to relieve pressure and generally returns blood; if fat globules are present, associated fracture is likely.
- AP, lateral, Merchant (patellar) radiographs are usually negative; however, "tunnel" view is best to view intercondylar notch to identify occasional bony avulsion.
- MRI will demonstrate acute and chronic injury, as well as combination injury to ACL and meniscus.

5. Management

- Depends on patient age, degree and age of injury, involvement of other structures.
- Initial treatment includes rest, ice, compression, and elevation (RICE), along with knee immobilizer, crutches, and short-term NSAIDs.
- Additional treatment includes physical therapy to regain ROM and establish quadriceps dominance because it helps compensate for lost function of PCL.
- Need for surgical reconstruction of PCL based on response to conservative treatment.

K. ACL Injury (Knee)

1. Etiology

- Seventy percent of ACL injuries occur during sporting events.
- Decelerating, twisting, cutting, or jumping injury associated with a "pop" or giving-away episode.

2. Pathology

- Three bands of ACL—primary restraint of anterior translation of tibia regarding the femur.
- Most commonly, tear is interstitial, irreparable.

3. Clinical Features
- Large effusion is commonly present.
- Anterior drawer test is often positive (knee flexed to 90°); however, the Lachman test (knee flexed 15° to 20°) is more sensitive and is easier to perform immediately after injury.
- Pivot shift test is also helpful.
- These tests show laxity in ACL such that tibia displaces anteriorly.

4. Diagnostic Studies
- Arthrocentesis can be performed in acute phase to relieve pressure and generally returns blood; if fat globules are present, associated fracture is likely.
- AP, lateral, Merchant (patellar) radiographs—usually negative, although they may show avulsion of either tibial attachment of ACL or lateral capsular margin of tibia (Segond fracture).
- MRI will demonstrate and diagnose acute and chronic injury, as well as combination injury to ACL and meniscus.

5. Management
- Depends on patient age, degree and age of injury, as well as involvement of other structures.
- Initial treatment includes RICE, knee immobilizer, crutches, and NSAIDs.
- Additional treatment can range from physical therapy and bracing to surgical reconstruction of ligament and repair of associated tissues.
- Despite treatment, some patients have residual ACL laxity, necessitating bracing to stabilize knee for the performance of certain activities.
- Chronic ACL laxity may predispose traumatic extension of injury, as well as injury to associated structures.

L. Collateral Ligament Injury (Knee)
1. Etiology
- Typically traumatic.
- Medial collateral ligament (MCL) tears commonly result from valgus force without rotation.
- Less common lateral collateral ligament (LCL) injury—result of pure varus producing force to knee.
- These injuries can occur alone or associated with meniscal, ACL, or PCL tear.

2. Pathology
- Partial or complete tear of primary, medial, or lateral stabilizer of knee.
- Examination disclosing joint space opening of <5 mm considered a grade I tear of involved ligament, whereas opening of <10 mm considered a grade III (complete) tear.
- Grade II tear falls between these two extremes.

3. Clinical Features
- Localized swelling, pain, ecchymosis, stiffness of involved side (medial or lateral).
- History may develop an ability to have continued with ambulation and participation with athletics following acute injury.

- MCL may be tender anywhere between medial femoral condyle insertion and its tibial insertion.
- LCL may be tender anywhere from lateral femoral condyle insertion to fibular head insertion.
- Knee examined in 25° of flexion to relax posterior capsule, while varus and then valgus force is applied by palm of examining hand to involved knee.

4. Diagnostic Studies
- Plain film X-rays, although typically negative, may show avulsion from femoral origin of MCL or fibular insertion of LCL.
- MRI may be used for preoperative evaluation and management planning.

5. Management
- Treatment of all grades of MCL tears is usually conservative because potential for MCL healing is great.
- RICE coupled with crutches and short-term NSAIDs is usually adequate for MCL tears, as well as grades I and II LCL tears.
- Grade III LCL tears invariably involve tear to posterolateral capsular complex; best treated surgically to avoid late healing instability.
- For grades II and III MCL injuries, use of hinged knee brace with gradual return to full weight-bearing over a 4-week period.
- Rehabilitation includes early ROM, quadriceps strengthening exercises.

M. Meniscal Tear (Knee)
1. Etiology
- Results from trauma or degenerative change; however, may report history of minimal or no trauma.
- Ligamentous instability can predispose meniscal tears.

2. Pathology
- Meniscus fibrocartilage serves to increase knee stability and joint congruency, and improve nutrition and lubrication of articular cartilage.
- Tears can be partial thickness or complex.

3. Clinical Features
- Patient complains of joint line pain, catching, popping, locking.
- There may be effusion evident as well as thigh wasting.
- Compression testing (e.g., Apley and McMurray) may elicit pain.

4. Diagnostic Studies
- Obtain AP, lateral, notch, patellar views to provide overall assessment of joint congruity, degree of joint space narrowing, or DJD.
- MRI is the diagnostic procedure of choice in determining both presence and degree of tear.

5. Management
- Conservative care consists of activity modification, NSAIDs, rehabilitation.

- Failure of conservative care arthroscopy is indicated.
- Partial-thickness tears, as well as stable vertical or oblique tears <5 mm long, can be left alone.

N. Ankle Sprains

1. **Etiology**
   - Falls, twisting injuries, MVAs.
   - May be classified as grade I, II, or III.
   - Grades I and II—incomplete tears and differ in severity; grade III—complete dissolution of ligamentous connection.
   - Sprains (ligament tears) must be differentiated from strains (muscle-tendon unit tears), although often difficult.
   - Patients may report that they felt a "pop," followed by immediate pain, swelling, and inability to walk.

2. **Pathology**
   - Collateral ligaments (anterior talofibular, calcaneofibular) are injured 85% of the time, as would be consistent with inversion injury.
   - Differential diagnosis includes peroneal tendon tear or subluxation, neurapraxia of superficial and deep peroneal nerve, sprain of subtalar joint, fracture of base of fifth metatarsal or talar dome, avulsion fracture of calcareous or talus, or injury to calcaneocuboid joint.
   - Injury to syndesmosis, thick ligaments connecting distal fibula and tibia, occurs in 5% of ankle sprains.
   - Less common eversion injuries involve deltoid ligaments.

3. **Clinical Features**
   - Pain on palpation of injured ligaments helps determine specific structures involved, although tenderness may be more diffuse, to include side opposite area of subjective complaint.
   - There may also be swelling, ecchymosis.
   - There may be reduction in joint mobility from swelling, painful inhibition.
   - Drawer testing may disclose joint instability or laxity.
   - Question patient for history of ankle sprains because symptoms from acute injury may be superimposed on chronic ankle instability.
   - Gait may be antalgic, favoring affected side.

4. **Diagnostic Studies**
   - Radiographs of ankle are indicated if tenderness or crepitus is present over malleoli, ankle joint, syndesmosis, or other bony structures.
   - MRI, CT scan, and CT arthrography are helpful in ruling out ligamentous disruption, occult fracture in refractory patients.

5. **Management**
   - Three phases of treatment that can last 2 weeks for minor injuries and up to 8 weeks or longer for more complicated injuries.

PHASE 1
- Consists of NSAIDs, ice compression, elevation.
- Brace or air stirrup can provide limitation of inversion/eversion, as well as promote soft-tissue healing.

PHASE 2
- Begins when patient can bear weight without increased pain.
- Continue use of stirrup or brace.
- Begin exercise to increase ROM and strength.

PHASE 3
- Usually begins 4 to 6 weeks after injury.
- Begin functional conditioning with proprioceptive, endurance, agility training.

ACHILLES TENDON RUPTURE

1. **Etiology**
   - Most common of the Achilles tendon disorders.
   - Seventy-five percent of ruptures occur during sports-related activities (i.e., basketball, racket sports, soccer, and softball).
   - Common in patients between 30 and 50 years old.

2. **Pathology**
   - Mechanism of injury is mechanical overload from an eccentric contraction of the gastrocsoleus.

3. **Clinical Features**
   - History of sudden, sharp pain in calf.
   - Sudden pain in the heel after attempting pushing-off movement.
   - Accompanied by an audible pop.
   - Ankle plantar flexion is markedly weak or absent.
   - Positive Thompson test (patient prone and affected knee bent 90°, squeezing the calf causes plantar flexion of the foot if the foot or the Achilles tendon is intact or partially torn, but not if there is complete rupture of the tendon).

4. **Diagnostic Studies**
   - MRI will demonstrate full thickness tear and location of fragments.

5. **Management**
   - Surgical repair allows for early ROM.
   - Closed management usually consists of long leg casting in slight plantar flexion with gradual dorsiflexion.

PLANTAR FASCIITIS

1. **Etiology**
   - Most common cause of heel pain.
   - Inflammation and/or irritation of the plantar fascia from repetitive strain injury.

2. **Mechanism of Injury**
   - Running injury, poor footwear, hard surface with prolonged activity.
   - May have history of increase in activity.

3. **Clinical Features**
   - Heel pain most severe with first few steps upon awakening then decreases.
   - Pain then increases after prolonged use.

4. **Diagnostic Studies**
   - Plain radiograph may reveal calcaneal spur.
5. **Management**
   - Physical therapy for stretching of the plantar fascia.
   - Night splint, orthotics, taping arch support for athletic events.

O. **Spondylolysis**
1. **Etiology**
   - Defect in pars interarticularis.
   - Most common form of low back pain in children, adolescents.
2. **Pathology**
   - Defect in pars due to fatigue fracture from repetitive hyperextension (i.e., gymnasts and football lineman), in which there is a hereditary predisposition, congenital, trauma, or is associated with disk degeneration.
   - Usually affects L5 on S1 or L4 on L5.
3. **Clinical Features**
   - Appears late in childhood or early adult life with low back pain, often with sciatica and occasionally with neurologic loss in lower extremity.
   - Palpation of lumbar spine may disclose definite step in line of spinous process.
4. **Diagnostic Studies**
   - Plain lateral and oblique radiographs of spine show defect in the "neck" of "Scottie dog," in which "Scottie dog" becomes decapitated; the "head" of the dog is formed by articular process, and the "eye" is the pedicle.
   - Bone scan shows increased uptake at the pars interarticularis.
5. **Management**
   - Treatment aimed at symptomatic relief to include activity restriction, flexion exercise, strengthening exercises (i.e., back and abdomen), and bracing.
   - Bracing or casting advocated for acute lesions.
   - Surgery is indicated if conservative measures are not effective.

SPONDYLOLISTHESIS (Table 7-5)
1. **Etiology**
   - Forward slippage of one vertebra on another.
   - Isthmic spondylolisthesis is most common.

- Presents during the preadolescent growth, between the ages 10 and 15 years.
2. **Pathology**
   - Spondylolisthesis can be classified into six types (see Table 7-5).
3. **Clinical Features**
   - May be asymptomatic or may present with back and leg pain.
   - Rarely present with radicular pain or bowel or bladder dysfunction.
   - Young patients may have Phalen–Dickson sign: tight hamstrings, and a knee-bent, hips-flexed gait.
   - Palpation may disclose a step-off secondary to a prominent spinous process.
4. **Diagnostic Studies**
   - Radiographic examination will show a defect on the lateral view; percentage of slippage is measured on this view.
   - Oblique radiographs will demonstrate the "broken neck" on the "Scottie dog."
   - Bone scans are useful for identifying stress fractures.
5. **Management**
   - Low-grade spondylolisthesis (grade I or II) can be managed with conservative measures, such as restriction of aggravating activity, bracing, and physical therapy.
   - Surgical intervention is reserved for patients who fail to respond to conservative measure or if there is a progression in the slippage.

VI. Other Disorders

A. **Scleroderma (Systemic Sclerosis)**
1. **Etiology**
   - Cause unknown—autoimmunity, fibroblast dysregulation, and occupational exposure (i.e., trichloroethylene, silica dust, and polyvinyl chloride) have been implicated.
   - Systemic sclerosis occurs in between 4 and 12 patients per million population per year.
   - Four times more common in women than in men.
   - Present in all racial groups and geographic areas.
   - Disease onset is highest between 25 and 50 years of age.
   - Raynaud phenomenon—initial complaint in 60% to 70% of patients.

TABLE 7-5.	Classification of Spondylolisthesis		
Class	**Type**	**Age**	**Pathology/Other**
I	Congenital	Child	Congenital dysplasia of S1 superior facet
II	Isthmic	5–50	Predisposition leading to elongation/fracture of pars (L5–S1)
III	Degenerative	Older	Facet arthrosis leading to subluxation (L4–L5)
IV	Traumatic	Young	Acute fracture/other than pars
V	Pathologic	Any	Incompetence of bony elements
VI	Postsurgical	Adult	Excessive restriction of neural arches/facets

2. **Pathology**
   - Characterized by thickening and fibrosis of skin (scleroderma) and internal organs (heart, lungs, kidneys, GI tract).
   - Skin thickening due to accumulation of collagen in lower dermis.
   - Fixation and immobility of skin caused by replacement of subcutaneous tissue with fibrous band.
3. **Clinical Features**
   - Variable in extent and progression.
   - **Two principal syndromes of prognostic and therapeutic importance (Table 7-6):**
     - Diffuse scleroderma—at risk for rapidly progressing, widespread skin involvement and early development of complement of internal organ abnormalities.
     - Limited scleroderma, slowly progressive skin changes—restricted to fingers, hands, and face, and may have extended course of illness before visceral abnormalities. This group has CREST syndrome variant of scleroderma (subcutaneous calcinosis, Raynaud phenomenon, esophageal dysmotility, sclerodactyly, telangiectasia).
   - Common findings include subcutaneous edema, fever, and malaise. Skin becomes thickened and hidebound, with loss of normal folds, telangiectasia, pigmentation, and depigmentation.
   - Dysphagia, hypomotility of GI tract, pulmonary fibrosis, pericarditis, myocardial fibrosis.
4. **Diagnostic Studies**
   - Nonspecific serologic abnormalities are common.
   - ANAs positive.
   - RF positive.
   - Moderate elevations of ESR; hypergammaglobulinemia, proteinuria, and cylindruria appear with renal involvement.
5. **Management**
   - Treatment—symptomatic and supportive.
   - Goal—reduction of tissue fibrosis; interferon-γ, photoactivated methoxypsoralen, experimental anti-mast cell drugs, methotrexate, carboprostacyclin, and D-penicillamine are the agents tried or under investigation.
   - Glucocorticoids are useful in inflammatory muscle disease and active interstitial lung inflammation.
   - Occupational and vocational therapy to maintain hand function.

B. **Complex Regional Pain Syndrome**
   - Formerly called reflex sympathetic dystrophy.
   - Other synonyms for RSD are still in use—sympathetically maintained pain, shoulder-hand syndrome, Sudeck atrophy, minor dystrophy.
1. **Etiology**
   - Unknown.
   - Bone or soft-tissue injury commonly precipitates RSD.
   - Nerve-injured patients are particularly susceptible.
   - Injury may be trivial in nature.
   - Thirty percent of patients have no injury.
2. **Pathology**
   - Autonomic nervous system (ANS) dysfunction.
3. **Clinical Features**
   - More commonly affects upper extremity, but can occur in lower extremity.

TABLE 7-6.	An Approach to Classification of Systemic Sclerosis	
Characteristics of Disease	**Diffuse Scleroderma**	**Limited Scleroderma**
Onset of Raynaud phenomenon	<2 y before other symptoms	>2 y before other symptoms
Initial symptoms	Finger edema Arthralgia Raynaud phenomenon Visceral complaint	Raynaud phenomenon (>90%)
Tendon friction rubs	60%	<1%
Extent of skin involvement	Acral and trunk	Acral only
Pace of skin involvement	Rapid in first 2 y	Minimal
Visceral involvement[a]		
GI	90% early	70% early
Lung	70% early	60% late
Heart	50% early	50% late
Kidney	25% early	Rare
Anticentromere antibody	<50%	60%–70%
Antitopoisomerase 1 antibody	30%–40%	<5%

[a]Type of visceral involvement, total percentage risk, peak incidence of onset (early = first 3 y; late = after 3 y).
From Hume HD, ed. *Kelley's Essentials of Internal Medicine.* 2nd ed. Philadelphia, PA: Lippincott Williams & Wilkins; 2001:373, with permission.

- **Three stages:**
  - Stage 1—can last up to 3 months. Hallmark is pain out of proportion to original injury. ANS symptoms can include swelling of affected extremity, increased sweating, change in skin color from red to cyanotic, temperature changes, increased hair growth, and nail growth.
  - Stage 2—occurs after 3 to 4 months and marked by loss of skin lines, change in skin appearance to that of pale and waxy, joint stiffness, brittle nails, muscle spasms, and persistent pain.
  - Stage 3—occurs after 8 to 9 months, when irreversible changes occur. Extremity becomes atrophic with loss of muscle and skin, permanent joint contractures, loss of motion, and persistent pain that becomes severe.
- Serious consequences include loss of function of affected extremity.
- Psychiatric problems include anxiety, depression, and potential for suicide.

4. **Diagnostic Studies**
- Plain film radiographs, obtained in any stage, may show spotty areas of osteoporosis or demineralization in bones of affected extremity.
- Bone scans may show increased uptake in the limb, usually distal to the point of injury.

5. **Management**
- Sympathetic anesthetic blocks can be diagnostic, therapeutic.
- If block results in pain relief, series of three to six blocks over a 2- to 3-week period is indicated.
- Immediately after each block, ROM and stress-loading programs are begun, usually under direction of physical or occupational therapist.
- Physical and/or occupational therapy is helpful in maintaining motion and decreasing pain.
- Oral steroids, NSAIDs, and tricyclic antidepressants can decrease pain and allow patient to sleep, but do not alter the course of disease.
- TENS is a useful adjunct in control of pain, and may obviate need for stronger narcotic pain medication.
- Biofeedback may assist patient in controlling autonomic functions of body that regulate sweating, skin temperature, and blood flow.

C. Pronator Syndrome
1. **Etiology**
- Source of compression includes fascial bands, tumors, ganglions, the anconeus epitrochlearis, cubitus valgus, bony spurs, and a medical epicondyle nonunion.

2. **Pathology**
- Median nerve compressed in the proximal forearm by one or more of the following structures: ligament of Struthers, lacertus fibrosus, pronator teres muscle, or proximal fibrous arch on the undersurface of the flexor digitorum superficialis muscle.

3. **Clinical Features**
- More severe pain in the volar forearm than in the wrist or hand.
- Pain increases with activity.
- Paresthesias may resemble carpal tunnel syndrome.
- Sensory and motor deficits similar to carpal tunnel syndrome.
- Dysesthesia may include distribution of the palmar cutaneous nerve.
- Tinel sign is positive at the forearm, not at the wrist.
- Phalen maneuver will not provoke symptoms, usually no night pain.
- Resisted forearm pronation with elbow extended reproduces pain.

4. **Diagnostic Studies**
- EMG and a nerve conduction velocity study are helpful to confirm diagnosis.

5. **Management**
- Splinting for 3 to 6 months.
- NSAIDs.
- Surgical treatment for global decompression of all potential sites of compression yields a variable treatment.

D. Ulnar Neuropathy (Cubital Tunnel Syndrome)
1. **Etiology**
- Source of compression includes fascial bands, tumors, ganglions, the anconeus epitrochlearis, cubitus valgus, bony spurs, and a medical epicondyle nonunion.

2. **Pathology**
- The region that the ulnar nerve is most commonly compressed is at the cubital tunnel along the medial elbow.

3. **Clinical Features**
- Paresthesia and numbness involving the ring and little fingers.
- Symptoms may be aggravated by full flexion of the elbow and may awaken the person from sleeping with the elbows flexed.
- Patients may have clumsiness and lack of dexterity.
- Positive Tinel sign at the elbow.
- Positive Froment sign: as the patient tries to hold a piece of paper placed between the thumb and the index finger, the IP joint flexes in an attempt to substitute flexor pollicis longus activity for lost adductor pollicis strength.

4. **Diagnostic Studies**
- EMG.

5. **Management**
- Conservative treatment: elbow pads to protect the ulnar nerve from trauma.
- Splint holding the elbow at 45° of flexion.
- Surgical decompression of the ulnar nerve.

E. Carpal Tunnel Syndrome

1. Etiology
- Disorder is often seen with a history of repetitive use of hands, prolonged use of vibratory tools.
- Also may occur in pregnancy, amyloidosis, flexor tenosynovitis, endocrine disorders (DM and hypothyroidism), tumors within the carpal tunnel, and may follow injuries of wrists.

2. Pathology
- Compression of median nerve within carpal canal that rests under transverse carpal ligament (nerve entrapment).

3. Clinical Features
- Onset is usually insidious and decreased hand strength.
- History of weakness, clumsiness in the hand, paresthesia in the median nerve distribution.
- Paresthesia in the median nerve distribution increased with use and awakes patient from sleep.
- Positive Tinel test—tap over palmar surface of wrist, pain in median nerve distribution.
- Positive Phalen test—flex wrist for 30 to 60 seconds, paresthesia radiating to median nerve distribution.
- Positive compression test—compress carpal canal for 30 seconds, paresthesia of median nerve distribution. Decreased sensation and two-point discrimination of median nerve. Muscle weakness or atrophy of thenar eminence is late finding.

4. Diagnostic Studies
- Nerve conduction studies (EMG) are useful in locating lesion of median nerve.

5. Management
- Immobilization of wrist (i.e., splinting, worn by patient to hold wrist in neutral position) particularly while sleeping.
- Modify activity to reduce repetitive use, NSAIDs.
- Persistent symptoms require additional therapy of local corticosteroid injections.
- Relative indication for surgery—constant sensory loss, failure of nonoperative treatment, thenar atrophy.

RADIAL TUNNEL

1. Etiology
- Compression of the radial nerve throughout the arm in the extensor/supinator muscle mass.
- Paresthesias in the radial nerve distribution may occur.

2. Mechanism of Injury
- May be history of humeral fracture, overuse.

3. Clinical Features
- Paresthesia in the radial nerve distribution.
- May be weakness associated with grip.

4. Diagnostic Studies
- Radiograph and MRI may be necessary to identify fracture or lesion causing compression.

- EMG study will determine location and severity of compression.

5. Management
- Conservative care including immobilization and NSAIDs.
- Surgical decompression is indicated if conservative care fails.

TARSAL TUNNEL

1. Etiology
- Compression of the tibial nerve in the medial aspect of the ankle.

2. Mechanism of Injury
- May occur with a history of prior ankle or foot trauma, body mechanics dysfunction.
- Occasionally, nerve is compressed by tumor or growth.

3. Clinical Features
- Pain, paresthesia at the medial aspect of the ankle which increases with eversion.
- Positive Tinel sign at the medial ankle.
- Abnormal sensory exam.

4. Diagnostic Studies
- EMG study will confirm location and severity of compression.
- MRI may be indicated to evaluate for tumor or growth causing compression.

5. Management
- Corticosteroid examination into the tunnel.
- Night splint may improve symptoms.
- Surgical excision of tumor or growth, or decompression of nerve may be indicated if conservative care fails.

F. Ganglion Cyst

1. Etiology
- Most common soft-tissue tumor of the hand, occurring in the hand and wrist.
- Usually dorsal carpal ganglion and located over scapholunate ligament, but can be volar.

2. Pathology
- Thought to be the result of outpouching of wrist capsule and contains fluid similar to joint fluid.
- Origin (stalk) from wrist joint.

3. Clinical Features
- Lesions—soft, mobile, nontender.
- Cyst may transilluminate.

4. Management
- Reassure patient.
- Most ganglia require no treatment.
- Aspiration with large-bore (16G or 19G) needle is helpful to confirm diagnosis; surgical excision if it recurs and is symptomatic or if concern is present regarding exact nature of mass.

POPLITEAL (BAKER) CYST

1. Etiology
- A cyst in the posterior aspect of the knee due to intra-articular pathology in the knee.

2. **Mechanism of Injury**
   - Most popliteal cysts are a result of a meniscal tear that causes an irritant to the posterior joint capsule that causes the cyst.
3. **Clinical Features**
   - Patients may identify a fullness and palpate the cyst in the popliteal space.
   - Cyst is generally nonpainful.
   - Cystic fluid may leak into the calf causing calf tightness and/or pain.
4. **Diagnostic Studies**
   - Sonography will confirm popliteal cyst and rule out DVT.
   - MRI testing may be necessary to determine intra-articular pathology.
5. **Management**
   - Aspiration and intra-articular corticosteroid injection.
   - Immobilization, rest, and compression for a brief period may contribute to the success of the steroid injection.
   - Surgical excision may be required if conservative treatment fails.

G. **Dupuytren Contracture**
   1. **Etiology**
      - Usually seen in men between ages 40 and 60 years.
      - Genetic predisposition.
      - Associated with epilepsy, alcoholism, diabetes, cirrhosis, and tuberculosis.
   2. **Pathology**
      - Disease represents pathologic change in preexisting normal fascia.
      - Proliferative fibrodysplasia of subcutaneous palmar connective tissue can lead to contractures because of nodules and cords that develop progressively.
      - Cause unknown.
   3. **Clinical Features**
      - Nodules are often painful when first noticed.
      - Ring and little finger are most often involved.
      - Thumb web space can also be involved.
      - Pathognomonic sign—nodule located at distal palmar crease or over proximal phalanx of finger.
      - Flexion contracture—most frequently an MCP joint; can affect PIP joint; rarely, DIP joint.
      - Other areas involved include dorsum of PIP joints, dorsum of penis (Peyronie disease), plantar fascia (lederhosen disease).
   4. **Management**
      - Nonsurgical treatments (e.g., vitamin E, steroids, and allopurinol) are not of proven value.
      - Surgery is indicated for contractures of 30° of MCP or PIP joints.

H. **Charcot Joint (Diabetic Foot, Neuropathic Foot)**
   1. **Etiology**
      - Peripheral neuropathy resulting from DM, peripheral vascular disease, or other disease states.
      - Because of lack of sensation and impaired tissue nutrition, repetitive intrinsic/extrinsic trauma leads to fractures of surrounding bony anatomy.
   2. **Pathology**
      - Joints damaged and ultimately disintegrated by multiple nonhealing fractures.
      - Usually occurs in midfoot, although other joints can be involved, from ankle to MTP joints.
   3. **Clinical Features**
      - Advanced changes typically alert patient; include swelling, pain, redness, and alteration in the shape of the foot.
      - Associated changes may include skin breakdown and discharge, leading to the formation of painless ulcer.
   4. **Diagnostic Studies**
      - Plain film radiographs disclose evidence of fracture and associated changes, although they may be read as normal with early Charcot's patients with swelling and pain.
      - Difficult to differentiate Charcot's changes with osteomyelitis, although as a rule, osteomyelitis develops in an adult patient with diabetes only if overlying skin has been violated.
   5. **Management**
      - Relative rest to include non-weight-bearing and stabilization (e.g., bracing and casting).
      - In advanced patients, surgical resection of bony prominences or arthrodesis may be necessary.
      - Multidisciplinary consult is often necessary to treat associated disease entity involvement.

I. **Gout**
   1. **Etiology**
      - Ninety percent of patients with primary gout are men older than 30 years.
      - Onset is usually postmenopausal for women.
      - May be precipitated by rapid fluctuations in serum urate levels from food and alcohol excess, surgery, diuretics, or uricosuric drugs.
   2. **Pathology**
      - Disorder of metabolism, causing hyperuricemia, leading to monosodium urate (MSU) crystal deposition in joints.
   3. **Clinical Features**
      - Sudden onset, frequently nocturnal pain.
      - Involved joint swollen, exquisitely tender; overlying skin tense, warm, and dusky red.
      - MTP joint of great toe is most susceptible.
      - Feet, ankles, and knees are commonly affected.
      - Distribution of the arthritis is usually asymmetric.

- Tophi (crystal deposition) present in ear helix, eyelid, olecranon, and Achilles are usually in chronic form.

4. **Diagnostic Studies**
   - Radiographs disclose "punched-out" periarticular effusions, radiolucent urate tophi, and soft-tissue tophus.
   - Elevated serum acid level (>7.5 mg per dL).
   - During attack, ESR and WBC count are frequently elevated.
   - Joint fluid analysis shows MSU crystals (thin, tapered intracellular crystals), strongly negative birefringence.

5. **Management**
   - Initial treatment with indomethacin.
   - Allopurinol is used to lower serum uric acid levels in hyperuricemic patients with chronic gout.
   - Colchicine is used for prophylaxis following recurrent attacks.
   - Corticosteroids are reserved for patients with acute gout and those unable to take NSAIDs.
   - Restrict diets high in purine (e.g., kidney, liver, and sweet breads).
   - Avoid food or alcohol that precipitates attack.

J. Pseudogout (Chondrocalcinosis)

1. **Etiology**
   - Often seen in persons older than 60 years.
   - May be familial.
   - May be associated with metabolic disorders (e.g., hyperparathyroidism, Wilson disease, DM, hyperthyroidism, and gout).

2. **Pathology**
   - Deposition of calcium phosphate crystals in articular cartilage.
   - Crystals are shed into the joint, and this leads to phagocytosis and enzyme release by leukocytes.

3. **Clinical Features**
   - Acute or recurrent and rarely chronic arthritis.
   - Usually involves large joints (e.g., knees and wrists).

4. **Diagnostic Studies**
   - Radiographs disclose calcification of cartilaginous structures and signs of DJD.
   - Normal serum urate levels.
   - Identification of calcium pyrophosphate crystals in joint aspirates is diagnostic of pseudogout.

5. **Management**
   - Treat primary disease.
   - NSAIDs.
   - Colchicine PO is effective for prophylaxis.
   - Joint aspiration.
   - Intra-articular injection of triamcinolone.
   - Significant joint destruction—surgical treatment indicated.

K. Bunion—Hallux Valgus

1. **Etiology**
   - Bunion is a bursa over an unduly prominent first metatarsal.
   - Exostosis (excess bone) on the metatarsal.
   - Intrinsic factors include pes planus, metatarsus primus varus, RA, and connective tissue disease.
   - Most common cause is poorly fitted shoes.

2. **Pathology**
   - Hallux valgus deformity consists of the great toe in a valgus position.

3. **Clinical Features**
   - Medial eminence pain of the first metatarsal.
   - Medial head deviation of the head of the first metatarsal.
   - Bursa thickening.

4. **Diagnostic Studies**
   - Radiographs, weight-bearing AP, lateral, and oblique.

5. **Management**
   - Soft felt pad.
   - Comfortable, wide-laced shoes.
   - Surgical management is recommended for painful deformity.

HAMMER TOE

1. **Etiology**
   - Flexion deformity of the PIP joint of the toe with hyperextension of the MTP and DIP.

2. **Mechanism of Injury**
   - Idiopathic, but associated with second toe longer than first, poor footwear.

3. **Clinical Features**
   - Obvious deformity with pain at PIP from constant contact with shoe.
   - Callous formation may occur at PIP.

4. **Diagnostic Studies**
   - Weight-bearing AP and lateral radiograph of the foot.

5. **Management**
   - Conservative care includes bracing or strapping.
   - Surgical correction of the deformity is based on flexible or fixed deformity.

INTERDIGITAL NEUROMA

1. **Etiology**
   - Compression of the common digital nerve.
   - Most common site between third and fourth metatarsal heads.

2. **Mechanism of Injury**
   - Compression occurs from overuse, poor fitting shoes, degenerative disease.

3. **Clinical Features**
   - Pain and point tenderness in the area of the neuroma.
   - Pain is sharp and burning typical of nerve pain.

4. **Diagnostic Studies**
   - MRI is the only study that can isolate the neuroma, but is used in preoperative evaluation and planning.

SELECTED REFERENCES

Browner BD, Levine AM, Jupiter JB, et al, eds. *Skeletal Trauma*. Vols 1 and 2. 3rd ed. Philadelphia, PA: WB Saunders; 2009.

Bucholz RW, Berrey BH, Birch JG, et al. *Orthopaedic Decision Making*. 2nd ed. St Louis, MO: Mosby; 1996.

Coleman R, Reiland A. Orthopedic emergencies. In: Humphries RL, Stone C, eds. *CURRENT Diagnosis and Treatment Emergency Medicine*. 7th ed. New York, NY: McGraw-Hill; 2011:chap 28. http://www.accessmedicine.com/content.aspx?aID=55750959. Accessed January 21, 2012.

Daffner RH, ed. *Clinical Radiology: The Essentials*. 2nd ed. Baltimore, MD: Lippincott Williams & Wilkins; 1999:405–493.

Dambro MR, ed. *Griffith's 5-Minute Clinical Consult*. 20th ed. Baltimore, MD: Lippincott Williams & Wilkins; 2012.

Dandy DH, Edwards DJ, eds. *Essential Orthopedics and Trauma*. 5th ed. Philadelphia, PA: Elsevier Science; 2009.

Eiff PM, Hath RL, Calmbach WL, eds. *Fracture Management for Primary Care*. 1st ed. Philadelphia, PA: WB Saunders; 1998.

Feliciano DV, Moore EE, Mattox KL, eds. *Trauma*. 6th ed. Stamford, CT: Appleton & Lange; 2008.

Goljan EF, ed. *Pathology*. 1st ed. Philadelphia, PA: WB Saunders; 1998.

Goroll AH, May LA, Mulley AG, eds. *Primary Care Medicine Office Evaluation and Management of the Adult Patient*. 3rd ed. Philadelphia, PA: Lippincott-Raven; 1995.

Hahn BH. Systemic lupus erythematosus. In: Longo DL, Fauci AS, Kasper DL, et al, eds. *Harrison's Principles of Internal Medicine*. 18th ed. New York, NY: McGraw-Hill; 2012:chap 319. http://www.accessmedicine.com/content.aspx?aID=9136499. Accessed January 21, 2012.

Hughes SPF, Porter RW. *Textbook of Orthopaedics and Fractures*. 1st ed. New York, NY: Oxford University Press; 1997.

Kelley WN, ed. *Textbook of Internal Medicine*. 3rd ed. Philadelphia, PA: Lippincott-Raven; 1998.

Kimberly RP. Lupus erythematosus: systemic and local forms. In: Kelley WN, ed. *Textbook of Internal Medicine*. 1st ed. Philadelphia, PA: JB Lippincott; 1989:286–290.

Langford CA, Gilliland BC. Periarticular disorders of the extremities. In: Longo DL, Fauci AS, Kasper DL, et al, eds. *Harrison's Principles of Internal Medicine*. 18th ed. New York, NY: McGraw-Hill; 2012:chap 337. http://www.accessmedicine.com/content.aspx?aID=9139675. Accessed January 21, 2012.

Mengel MB, Schwiefert LP, eds. *Ambulatory Medicine*. 5th ed. Stamford, CT: Appleton & Lange; 2005.

Menkes JS. Initial evaluation and management of orthopedic injuries. In: Tintinalli JE, Stapczynski JS, Cline DM, et al, eds. *Tintinalli's Emergency Medicine: A Comprehensive Study Guide*. 7th ed. New York, NY: McGraw-Hill; 2011:chap 264. http://www.accessmedicine.com/content.aspx?aID=6390597. Accessed January 21, 2012.

Miller MD, ed. *Review of Orthopaedics*. 5th ed. Philadelphia, PA: WB Saunders; 2008.

Newell KA. Common fractures and dislocations. In: Moser RL, ed. *Primary Care for Physician Assistants*. 1st ed. New York, NY: McGraw-Hill; 1998:353–357.

Paty DW, Beall SS. Neurology. In: Kelly WN, ed. *Essentials of Internal Medicine*. 1st ed. Philadelphia, PA: JB Lippincott; 1994:673–750.

Puffer JC. *Sports Medicine*. New York, NY: McGraw-Hill; 2003.

Shah A, Clair EW. Rheumatoid arthritis. In: Longo DL, Fauci AS, Kasper DL, et al, eds. *Harrison's Principles of Internal Medicine*. 18th ed. New York, NY: McGraw-Hill; 2012:chap 321. http://www.accessmedicine.com/content.aspx?aID=9136970. Accessed January 21, 2012.

Skihhner HB. *Current Diagnosis and Treatment in Orthopedics*. 4th ed. New York, NY: Lange Medical Books/McGraw-Hill; 2006.

Snider RK, Greene WB, Johnson TR, et al. *Essentials of Musculoskeletal Care*. 2nd ed. Rosemont, IL: American Academy of Orthopaedic Surgeons; 2006.

Tierney LM Jr, McPhee SJ, Papadakis MA, eds. *Current Medical Diagnosis and Treatment*. 51st ed. Norwalk, CT: Appleton & Lange; 2012.

Tintinalli JE, Ruiz E, Krome RL, eds. *Emergency Medicine: A Comprehensive Study Guide*. 5th ed. New York, NY: McGraw-Hill; 2010.

Weinstein SL, Buckwalter JA, eds. *Turek's Orthopaedics Principles and Their Application*. 5th ed. Philadelphia, PA: JB Lippincott; 1994.

Wilson SC, Skinner HB. Orthopedic infections. In: Skinner HB, ed. *CURRENT Diagnosis and Treatment in Orthopedics*. 4th ed. New York, NY: McGraw-Hill; 2006:chap 8. http://www.accessmedicine.com/content.aspx?aID=2321297. Accessed January 21, 2012.

Skin Disorders

8

Naveed Ahmed

I. Metabolic Skin Disorders

A. Seborrhea

1. **Etiology**
   - Not clearly defined.
2. **Pathology**
   - Precise pathology not known, but skin rash occurs in areas of high sebaceous gland concentration and activity such as the scalp, face, and body folds.
   - Histopathologic studies show a nonspecific inflammatory reaction in the dermis, spongiosis, and dilated follicular openings with neutrophils.
   - The role of *Pityrosporum ovale*, a skin commensal, in the pathogenesis of seborrhea is not clear, although some patients show improvement with antifungal preparations.
3. **Clinical Features**
   - Seborrhea (Figure 8-1) occurs in infants and adults; adult men are more affected than women.
   - Pattern of involvement in infants includes scalp (cradle cap), flexural areas, and perioral region with erythematous plaques with fine, white scales to thick, yellow-brown, waxy plates of scales.
   - Areas of involvement in adults are scalp, eyebrows, eyelashes, beard, and mustache, as well as nasolabial folds, postauricular sulci, trunk, and intertriginous regions of groin.
   - Pruritus, itching, burning sensations may occur in adults.
4. **Diagnostic Studies**
   - Not typically performed; diagnosis based on clinical findings.
5. **Management**
   - Selenium sulfide shampoos, 2% ketoconazole shampoo, or ketoconazole cream.
   - Sodium sulfacetamide 10% sulfur, 5% lotion/cream.
   - Ciclopirox 1% shampoo.
   - Severe cases may require oral antifungal therapy. (Patients with serum and crust are treated with oral antistaphylococcal antibiotics.)
   - Corticosteroid (CS) preparations for inflammation may be used with close monitoring for skin atrophy.

B. Psoriasis

1. **Etiology**
   - Hereditary disorder affecting men and women equally, and triggered by factors such as stress, physical trauma, medications (including systemic and class I topical CSs), and occasionally, acute streptococcal infections.
2. **Pathology**
   - Epidermal cells are produced at an accelerated rate due to a T-cell-mediated alteration in the cellular kinetics of keratinocytes causing the cell cycle to be significantly shortened (10 times faster than normal), and their maturation to be abnormal.
   - T-cell activation and proliferation lead to production of cytokines interleukin-2, tumor necrosis factor-α (TNF-α), interferon-γ. Under the influence of cytokines, inflammation and hyperproliferation of the epidermal keratinocytes occur.
3. **Clinical Features**
   - Lesions of psoriasis are variable in distribution, arrangement, shape, and type.
   - Five variants are plaque, pustular, guttate, inverse, and erythrodermoid.
   - Plaque lesions (Figure 8-2) are the most common type of lesions—oval to round, erythematous plaques with distinct borders and covered with silvery-white, thick scale on scalp, elbows, forearms,

FIGURE 8-1. **Seborrheic dermatitis**. (Courtesy of Smith Kline & French Laboratories.)

FIGURE 8-2. **Psoriasis**. (From Hall JC, ed. *Sauer's Manual of Skin Diseases*. 10th ed. Philadelphia, PA: Lippincott Williams & Wilkins; 2010, with permission.)

hands, knees, feet, and lumbosacral region. Auspitz phenomenon occurs with removal of scale.

- Nails are pitted in about 25% of patients with psoriasis; oil spots—yellow-to-brown discolorations under nail bed are pathognomonic for psoriasis.
- **Less common lesions of psoriasis:**
  - Pustular—deep, sterile, yellow pustules that evolve into red macules on palms and soles occurring as exacerbations and remissions for years.
  - Guttate—small, erythematous papules with fine scale occurring as discrete lesions and confluent plaques; can occur after streptococcal infection.
  - Inverse—occur in axillary or inguinal regions and lack characteristic scale.
  - Erythrodermoid—generalized, involving most of the skin; patient is acutely ill in a hypermetabolic state typically requiring hospitalization.

4. **Diagnostic Studies**
   - Skin biopsy demonstrates pathophysiology of increased mitosis in keratinocytes and endothelial cells, and inflammatory cells in the dermis and epidermis.
   - Acitretin. Advantage: Effective for palmar-plantar-pustular, erythrodermic, and pustular types of psoriasis better, effective; helps arthritis. Disadvantage: Teratogenic; may be as effective as monotherapy for plaque psoriasis. Classification: *Acitretin* 0.5 mg per kg are also effective, as are systemic methotrexate (MTX) and CS therapy.

- **Dermatologic agents:** Retinoids and antipsoriatic agents.
- **Pharmacokinetics:** Acitretin is administered orally. Oral absorption of acitretin is optimal when administered with food, therefore, in clinical studies, acitretin was given with food. Following administration of a single 50-mg oral dose to 18 healthy subjects, maximum plasma concentrations ranged from 196 to 728 ng per mL.

5. **Management**
   - **Categories of therapeutics used to treat psoriasis:**
     - Topical preparations—tar-based medications, anthralin, and high-potency CSs are first-line therapy for plaque-type psoriasis; vitamin D analogs (calcipotriene) and retinoids (vitamin A analogs), tazarotene are alternatives to topical CSs without risks for skin atrophy.
     - Phototherapy—with ultraviolet B (UVB) light or photochemotherapy with psoralen ultraviolet A-range light treatment.
     - Antimetabolites—MTX.
     - Immunosuppressives—cyclosporin A.
     - Biologics—immunomodulators, such as alefacept, that interfere with T-cell activation and block costimulatory molecules; and efalizumab, a monoclonal immunoglobulin G antibody that blocks T-cell binding.

C. Pityriasis Rosea

1. **Etiology**
   - Unknown etiology; possibly related to viral syndrome occurring before the onset of skin lesions as reported by about 20% of patients.

2. **Pathology**
   - Unknown mechanism causes eruption of solitary erythematous plaque followed by generalized erythematous rash within 1 to 2 weeks of original lesion; typically, all lesions resolve spontaneously within 6 to 12 weeks.
   - Disorder occurs more frequently in spring and fall seasons.

3. **Clinical Features**
   - Single, oval, pink-red plaque with a collarette scale on the advancing border, measuring 2 to 5 cm, usually erupts on trunk; "herald patch."
   - Multiple, smaller oval lesions appear on the trunk, upper arms, and thighs with their long axes along the lines of cleavage producing a classic "Christmas tree" pattern (Figure 8-3).
   - Pruritus accompanies lesions in most patients.

4. **Diagnostic Studies**
   - Diagnostic studies are not required.
   - Diagnosis is based on clinical findings.

5. **Management**
   - Lesions of pityriasis rosea resolve spontaneously without therapy.

FIGURE 8-3. Pityriasis rosea. (Courtesy of Syntex Laboratories, Inc.)

- Pruritus may necessitate therapy for patient comfort—oral antihistamines, emollients, and low-potency CSs are sufficient for most patients.
- Oral erythromycin stearate 250 mg four times daily (for adults) for 2 weeks effectively controls eruption.
- Rarely, severe pruritus occurs, requiring either systemic CSs or UVB therapy.

D. Apocrine and Sebaceous Gland Disorders

ACNE VULGARIS

1. **Etiology**
   - Most common chronic skin disease of adolescents and young adults.
   - Tends to be more severe in males than in females.
   - Stress, environmental, and genetic factors contribute to the development of acne.
2. **Pathology**
   - Complex process of hormonal influence on pilosebaceous units interacting with bacteria *Propionibacterium acnes*.
   - Androgens stimulate sebaceous glands to produce increased quantities of sebum, and bacteria secrete lipase to convert lipids to fatty acids; both the sebum and fatty acids cause inflammatory response in the pilosebaceous unit.
   - Hyperkeratinization occurs in the lining of follicle causing follicular plugging.
   - Comedones (whiteheads and blackheads) are formed.
   - Papules, pustules, nodules, and scarring develop as a result of follicular rupture and complement activation inducing an inflammatory response.
3. **Clinical Features**
   - Lesions of acne vulgaris are noninflammatory (comedones) and inflammatory (papules, pustules, and fluctuant nodules) classically on the face, neck, thorax, buttocks, and upper arms.
   - Severe forms of acne have inflammatory cysts, and sinus tracts, abscesses, and scarring.
4. **Diagnostic Studies**
   - Diagnostic studies are not necessary to diagnose acne vulgaris.

- Hormone studies—dehydroepiandrosterone sulfate, free testosterone, follicle-stimulating hormone, and luteinizing hormone levels—may be useful to rule out polycystic ovary syndrome as an underlying cause of severe, persistent acne in a hirsute female.

5. **Management**
   - Comedolytics—topical tretinoin.
   - Sebum suppressive medications—antiandrogens such as spironolactone, oral contraceptives; systemic isotretinoin. Potential side effects and teratogenic risks from systemic isotretinoin require additional monitoring of liver function, triglyceride levels, and prevention of pregnancy throughout therapy.
   - Anti-inflammatories, including benzoyl peroxide; topical and systemic antibiotics (i.e., topical erythromycin or clindamycin, oral tetracyclines or erythromycin); intralesional triamcinolone acetonide.
   - Therapies for disfigurement caused by acne lesions include dermabrasion, chemical peels, carbon dioxide (CO_2) laser resurfacing, scar revision, injection with collagen or fat, and soft-tissue augmentation.

ROSACEA

1. **Etiology**
   - Unclear etiology; persistent vasomotor instability may be an underlying factor leading to permanent vasodilation and lesion formation.
   - Predominantly affects women of Celtic origins between the ages of 30 and 50.
   - History of facial flushing in the presence of increased temperature or with alcohol consumption.
2. **Pathology**
   - Increased reactivity of facial capillaries to heat and other stimuli cause flushing and, later, development of telangiectases.
   - Perifollicular inflammation and dilated capillaries give rise to papule, pustule, and nodule formation.

- Demodex mite present in increased numbers in facial skin of persons with rosacea, but a direct cause and effect has not been demonstrated in pathogenesis of rosacea.

3. **Clinical Features**
   - Symmetric erythema of face, telangiectases, papules, small pustules, and central facial edema characterize rosacea (Figure 8-4).
   - Comedones are absent in rosacea.
   - Rhinophyma and metophyma occur.
   - Chronic conjunctivitis, blepharitis, and episcleritis cause characteristic red eyes.
   - Rosacea keratitis can lead to corneal ulceration.

4. **Diagnostic Studies**
   - Skin biopsy may be helpful for staging of rosacea.

5. **Management**
   - Topical metronidazole, sulfacetamide plus sulfur lotion, clindamycin, or erythromycin.
   - Systemic tetracycline, doxycycline, erythromycin, or minocycline.
   - Bactrium DS or metronidazole used for resistance cases. (Resistant cases can be treated with 100 to 200 mg per day of minocycline or with 200 mg of metronidazole twice daily.)
   - Isotretinoin is useful for severe and/or granulomatous rosacea.
   - Clonidine to reduce facial flushing.
   - Avoidance of factors provocative of facial flushing—hot beverages, alcohol, sunlight, and spicy foods.
   - Avert paradoxical exacerbations of existing telangiectasias, papules, and pustules by abstaining from use of potent topical fluorinated steroids on face.

HIDRADENITIS SUPPURATIVA

1. **Etiology**
   - Etiology unknown but can be associated with severe acne and pilonidal sinuses.
   - Predisposing factors include obesity, apocrine duct obstruction, and a family history of acne, hidradenitis suppurativa.

FIGURE 8-4. **Rosacea.** (Courtesy of Hoechst-Roussel Pharmaceuticals, Inc.)

2. **Pathology**
   - Previous theory of duct obstruction, dilation, and resultant inflammatory changes is questionable in the presence of histopathologic findings of multiple sinuses of follicular origin and epithelium-lined cysts.
   - Initial occlusion of the follicle with keratinous material may be followed by cystic alteration of the hair follicle and involvement of the apocrine gland.
   - Bacterial infection facilitates extension of the disease with sinus tract formation and scarring.

3. **Clinical Features**
   - Commonly affects the axillary, inguinal, and perianal regions.
   - Women have higher incidence of axillary involvement; men prone to anogenital involvement.
   - Lesions include double blackheads; tender, inflammatory nodules/abscesses; sinus tracts; scarring in the form of band or bridge fibrosis, keloids, and contractures.
   - Purulent drainage from abscesses, sinus tracts, or both.

4. **Diagnostic Studies**
   - No specific studies necessary for diagnosis of hidradenitis suppurativa.
   - Bacterial cultures of exudate from lesions may guide antibiotic therapy.

5. **Management**
   - Weight loss helps to reduce activity.
   - Smoking cessation.
   - **Abscesses should be managed aggressively—incision and drainage of fluctuant masses and intralesional injection of all nodules/abscesses with triamcinolone acetonide.**
   - Systemic antibiotic therapy (tetracycline derivative, cephalosporin, clindamycin, ciprofloxacin, doxycycline, minocycline) based on culture and sensitivity report.
   - Isotretinoin may be useful early in the disease.
   - Surgical management of recurrent hidradenitis with fibrosis and sinus tract formation.
   - Antiandrogens (oral contraceptives, spironolactone), oral CSs, cyclosporine, and CO_2 laser vaporization are other therapeutic options.
   - TNF-α blockers.

E. Hypersensitivity Reactions

ATOPY/ECZEMA

1. **Etiology**
   - Typically, disorder begins in childhood.
   - Hereditary predisposition to atopic dermatitis (Figure 8-5) with slight predominance in males.
   - Trigger factors for the development of atopic dermatitis include allergens and contact irritants such as wool, nickel, fragrances, latex; cold, dry climate; stress; foods.

FIGURE 8-5. Atopic dermatitis. (Courtesy of Geigy Pharmaceuticals.)

2. Pathology
- Altered immune reactions occur in genetically predisposed persons when exposed to trigger factor(s):
  - Increased T-cell activation.
  - Abnormal cell-mediated immunity.
  - Overproduction of immunoglobulin E (IgE).

3. Clinical Features
- Pruritus is a hallmark of atopic dermatitis causing "itch–scratch" cycle.
- Acute lesions are erythematous, edematous papules/plaques with poorly defined borders; scaling may or may not be present. Oozing and crusting of lesions, and secondary bacterial infection occur. Excoriations are common.
- Chronic lesions are characterized by lichenification and painful fissures, or nummular configuration (Figure 8-6).
- Other manifestations of atopy may be present—conjunctival and pharyngeal irritation/itching, rhinorrhea, edema, and discoloration of nasal mucosa, Dennie–Morgan sign.

4. Diagnostic Studies
- Serum IgE levels are increased.
- Radioallergosorbent test may be performed, but is of limited value in the management of patients.
- Viral culture for herpes simplex virus (HSV) to differentiate HSV infection from crusting atopic dermatitis.

FIGURE 8-6. **Nummular eczema.** (Courtesy of Johnson & Johnson.)

5. **Management**
   - Avoidance of triggers and elimination of scratching are essential to management.
   - Application of topical, nonsteroidal immunomodulators such as pimecrolimus or tacrolimus.
   - Use of leukotriene inhibitors and/or cyclosporine to interrupt/suppress aberrant T-cell activity.
   - Acute lesions require wet dressings; topical or systemic antibiotics (e.g., cephalexin, dicloxacillin) for *Staphylococcus aureus* infection; topical CSs; oral antihistamines for pruritus.
   - Chronic lesions necessitate daily hydration of skin with unscented bath oils and application of unscented emollients or mentholated lotions; oral antihistamines for pruritus; topical CSs or tar-based ointments for inflammation; and cyclic administration of erythromycin or other antistaphylococcal regimen to control staphylococcal colonization.

URTICARIA/ANGIOEDEMA

1. **Etiology**
   - IgE or complement-mediated edema of the dermis and/or subcutaneous tissues.
   - Urticaria may be caused by antigens from foods, drugs, insect bites; physical or environmental stimuli such as exposure to sunlight or cold, pressure/vibrations, exercise; infectious etiology such as viral hepatitis and infectious mononucleosis.
   - Idiopathic (40% of all patients) and hereditary causes of urticaria also exist.

2. **Pathology**
   - Mast cells are stimulated to degranulate by IgE or complement activation.
   - Histamines cause vasodilation of venules and resultant edema of dermis and subcutaneous tissues.

3. **Clinical Features**
   - Typical urticarial lesions are blanchable, pink, edematous papules or plaques that may be oval, linear, or bizarre in pattern—the lesions may coalesce.
   - Acute lesions of urticaria typically resolve within 24 hours.
   - Angioedema is a painless, deeper form of urticaria classically affecting the eyelids, lips, tongue, hands, feet, and genitals; the larynx and gastrointestinal (GI) tracts are affected less commonly—anaphylaxis can occur with IgE-mediated reactions.

4. **Diagnostic Studies**
   - Urticaria and angioedema are diagnosed on clinical findings.
   - Persistent urticaria and hereditary angioedema may require diagnostic studies.

5. **Management**
   - Identify and eliminate causative factors when possible.
   - Oral antihistamines are the mainstay of therapy for acute episodes of urticaria.

CUTANEOUS DRUG REACTIONS

1. **Etiology**
   - Medications administered topically, enterally, or parenterally induce changes in skin and mucous membranes.
   - Most cutaneous drug reactions are hypersensitivity-immune responses (types I to IV); nonimmunologic drug reactions also can occur.
   - Most cutaneous drug reactions are self-limiting if the offending medication is discontinued; life-threatening reactions can be unpredictable.

2. **Pathology**
   - **Immune response to drug causes hypersensitivity reactions I to IV:**
     - Type I—IgE-mediated urticaria and angioedema.
     - Type II—cytotoxic reactions (drug, in combination with cytotoxic antibodies, causes lysis of cells).
     - Type III—drug-induced vasculitis and serum sickness (deposition of immune complexes in small vessels).
     - Type IV—morbilliform reactions (Figure 8-7) (cell-mediated immune reaction).
   - Nonimmunologic, cutaneous drug reaction—genetic inability to detoxify or acetylate certain medications, particularly anticonvulsants and sulfonamides.

3. **Clinical Features**
   - Exanthematous or morbilliform rashes are the most common skin eruption from drug reaction characterized by generalized distribution of bright red macules and papules that coalesce to form plaques; rash typically begins 2 to 3 days from the onset of medication use. Antibiotics, nonsteroidal anti-inflammatory drugs (NSAIDs), allopurinol, and thiazide diuretics are frequently the cause of the skin eruption.
   - Urticarial (IgE-mediated) lesions are the second most common form of cutaneous drug reactions, occurring usually within minutes to hours of drug administration. Urticarial lesions are edematous, erythematous wheals and plaques that blanch and

FIGURE 8-7. **Cutaneous drug reaction.** (From Hall JC, ed. *Sauer's Manual of Skin Diseases.* 10th ed. Philadelphia, PA: Lippincott Williams & Wilkins; 2010, with permission.)

disappear within 24 hours after offending medication is stopped. Antibiotics, NSAIDs, opiates, and radiocontrast media are the most common offending agents.

- Erythema multiforme (EM) is the third most common cutaneous drug rash depicted as discrete, erythematous macules, papules, and plaques on the distal extremities and face. Iris or target lesion may not be present in drug-induced EM. Most frequently, sulfonamides, penicillins, phenobarbitals, and hydantoins are the cause of the reaction.
- Less common forms of drug reactions are acneiform, eczematous, exfoliative, fixed, photosensitivity, and vasculitic.
- Fever, abdominal and joint pains may accompany cutaneous drug reactions.

4. **Diagnostic Studies**
- Diagnosis is usually made from clinical findings.

5. **Management**
- Discontinuation of causative medication.
- Oral antihistamine for exanthematous drug eruption.
- Drug-induced urticaria/angioedema, use systemic CSs, antihistamines.
- EM minor drug reactions require symptomatic therapy.

F. **Skin Manifestations of Internal Diseases**
- Many systemic diseases manifest through the skin.
- Several lesions with their characteristics, locations, and disease associations are described in Table 8-1.

TABLE 8-1.   Skin Manifestations of Internal Diseases

Lesion	Characteristics	Location	Associated Disease/Medication Use or Exposure
Acanthosis nigrans	Diffuse velvety, thickening, and hyperpigmentation	Axillae and body folds	Adenocarcinoma of GI or GU tract Endocrine disorders
Erythema nodosum	Tender, indurated nodules in subcutaneous fat	Lower legs most frequent location; knees, arms	Poststreptococcal infection, oral contraceptives, sulfonamides
Hellotrope	Reddish-purple hue with edema	Eyelids and periorbital region	Dermatomyositis
Livedo reticularis	Mottled blue discoloration of skin in netlike pattern	Arms, legs, buttocks	Vascular disorders SLE
Myxedema	Edematous, doughy induration of skin	Generalized	Hypothyroidism
Necrobiosis lipoidica	Distinct, waxy, multicolored (pink, yellow, tan) plaque, late ulceration with pain	Shin	DM
Periungual telangiectasia	Erythema and telangiectases, thrombosis of capillary loops	Periungual	Dermatomyositis SLE
Vitiligo	White macules or plaques caused by destruction of melanocytes	Around eyes, mouth, elbows, digits, knees, low back, genital region	Thyroid disease Addison disease DM Pernicious anemia

GU, genitourinary; SLE, systemic lupus erythematosus.

II. Skin Tumors

- Neoplasms of the skin are classified by tissue type and as benign—not causing harm—or malignant—harmful; characterized by anaplasia, invasion, and metastasis.
- Common benign and malignant skin tumors are summarized in Table 8-2 and pictured in Figures 8-8 to 8-11.

III. Viral Infections of the Skin

A. Herpes Simplex Infections

1. **Etiology**
   - HSV type 1 (HSV-1—primary agent of nongenital infections) and HSV type 2.
   - Extragenital types: labialis, gingivostomatitis, whitlow, gladiatorum, eczema, herpeticum.
   - Urogenital and neonatal infections.

2. **Pathology**
   - Transmission by way of direct skin-to-skin or skin-to-mucosa contact.
   - Virus penetrates epidermal cells, reproduces, lyses infected cells, and causes intraepidermal lesions and local inflammation.
   - Virus migrates to autonomic and/or sensory ganglia and lies dormant awaiting reactivation.
   - Neonatal transmission from HSV-infected mother to infant during vaginal delivery.

3. **Clinical Features**
   - Primary infection has incubation period of 2 to 20 days; symptomatic primary infection with fever, headache, malaise, myalgia, and regional lymphadenopathy is relatively uncommon. Children with primary HSV infection tend to present with gingivostomatitis, whereas young women with primary HSV infection tend to present with herpetic vulvovaginitis.

TABLE 8-2. Skin Tumors

Tumor	Etiology	Characteristics	Location	Management
Benign				
Hemangioma	Proliferation of endothelial cells that develop at birth	Red to purple vascular nodule or plaque	Primarily head and neck	Resolve spontaneously by age 5
Lipoma	Composed of fat cells; some contain connective tissue	Soft, mobile, round or lobulated subcutaneous tumors	Neck, trunk, and extremities	Excision
Epidermal cyst (sebaceous cyst)	Invagination of epidermis into dermis with subsequent detachment from epidermis	Soft, mobile dermal to subcutaneous nodule; not tender until rupture occurs	Face, neck, ears, scalp, upper trunk	Spontaneous rupture is common
Seborrheic keratosis	Hereditary; lesions appear after age 30	Tan to brown or black macules, papules, nodules with a waxy and "warty" look	Face, trunk, upper extremities	Cryotherapy for irritated lesions only
Skin tag (acrochordon)	Lesions occur in obese persons and in pregnancy	Pedunculated, soft, fleshy, skin colored, round to oval tumors	Neck, axillae, groin	Electrodesiccation
Malignant				
Basal cell carcinoma (most common skin cancer in United States)	Chronic exposure to UVB light	Shiny, pink to red nodule, may have "rodent" ulceration with rolled border, telangiectasia	Face—medial and lateral canthi, nasolabial folds; head; neck; trunk in men	Low potential for metastasis
Melanoma	Genetic predisposition, sunlight exposure	"ABCDE" (**a**symmetry, irregular **b**orders, multi**c**olored, **d**iameter >6 mm, **e**levated surface	All areas of skin containing melanocytes	High potential for metastasis; risk of metastasis dependent on depth of lesion at excision
Squamous cell carcinoma	Chronic exposure to UVB light; HPV infection; environmental toxin exposure	Variable appearance from small, scaling erythematous plaque to fungating mass	Any skin or mucous membrane surface can be affected	Potential for metastasis via hematogenous and lymphatic channels exists

HPV, human papillomavirus.

FIGURE 8-8. Seborrheic keratoses. (From Hall JC, ed. *Sauer's Manual of Skin Diseases.* 10th ed. Philadelphia, PA: Lippincott Williams & Wilkins; 2010, with permission.)

FIGURE 8-9. Basal cell carcinoma. (Courtesy of Texas Pharmacal.)

FIGURE 8-10. Malignant melanoma. (Courtesy of Syntex Laboratories, Inc.)

FIGURE 8-11. Squamous cell carcinoma. (Courtesy of Westwood Pharmaceuticals.)

- Recurrent HSV classically displays a prodrome (in 24 hours preceding lesion outbreak) of burning, itching, tingling; systemic symptoms are not usually present.
- Characteristic skin lesions (Figure 8-12) are painful vesicles on erythematous base, evolving into pustules and, finally, erosions that may be moist or crusted. Mucosal vesicles quickly become painful erosions; gingiva involved with edema, tenderness, and purplish discoloration.
- Recurrent HSV infections tend to have fewer lesions than primary outbreak. Recurrences of genital herpes are more frequent than herpes labialis, and are precipitated by body stressors, UVB exposure.
- Immunocompromised patients are at high risk for HSV reactivation and may require antiviral prophylaxis.
4. **Diagnostic Studies**
   - HSV viral culture, antigen detection tests, HSV antibody titers.

FIGURE 8-12. Herpes simplex. (Courtesy of Dermik Laboratories, Inc.)

- Tzanck smear of vesicle fluid positive for herpes virus (not specific to simplex or zoster) when multinucleated giant cells observed.

5. **Management**
   - Skin-to-skin contact should be avoided during outbreak of cutaneous HSV infection.
   - Acyclovir 5% ointment. Apply six times daily for 7 days. Approved for initial genital herpes and limited mucocutaneous HSV infections in immunocompromised individuals.
   - Penciclovir 1% cream. Apply q2h while awake for recurrent orolabial infection in immunocompetent individuals.
   - For severe disease caused by proven or suspected acyclovir-resistant strains, hospitalization should be considered. Foscarnet, 40 mg per kg of body weight, q8h until clinical resolution is attained. Appears to be the best available treatment.
   - Childbearing-aged women who have genital herpes should inform health care providers who care for them during pregnancy about HSV infection.
   - Episodic antiviral therapy during recurrent episodes might shorten the duration of lesions.
   - Suppressive antiviral therapy can ameliorate or prevent recurrent outbreaks and asymptomatic transmission.
   - The safety of systemic acyclovir and valacyclovir therapy in pregnant women has not been established. Current findings do not indicate an increased risk for major birth defects after acyclovir treatment. The first clinical episode of genital herpes during pregnancy may be treated with oral acyclovir. Acyclovir treatment near term might reduce the rate of abdominal deliveries among women who have frequently recurring or newly acquired genital herpes by decreasing the incidence of active lesions. Routine administration of acyclovir to pregnant women who have history of recurrent genital herpes is not recommended by most clinicians.
   - Analgesic use is dependent on the extent and severity of individual patients.
   - Cool compresses. Extensive erosions on the vulva and penis may be treated with cool water, silver nitrate 0.5%, or Burrow's compresses applied for 20 minutes several times daily. This effective local therapy reduces edema and inflammation, macerates and debrides crust and purulent material, and relieves pain. The legs may be supported with pillows under the knees to expose the inflamed tissues and promote drying.
   - *Herpetic facial paralysis:* Reactivation of geniculate ganglion infection implicated in pathogenesis of idiopathic facial palsy (Bell palsy). HSV-1 shedding detected in 40% of cases. Inflammation plays a major role in pathogenesis; glucocorticoids may be effective.
   - **Herpes zoster pain management:** Early control of pain with narcotic analgesics is indicated; failure to manage pain can result in failure to sleep, fatigue, and depression. Best to begin with more potent analgesics and then reduce potency as pain lessens.
   - Condom use is suggested for all sexual encounters because sexual transmission of HSV has been documented during periods without obvious lesions (asymptomatic viral shedding).
   - Consider testing for HIV and syphilis in patients with primary HSV genital infection.

B. Herpes Zoster Infection
   1. **Etiology**
      - Varicella zoster virus (VZV) reactivation from latency in sensory and autonomic ganglia of patients with prior primary VZV infection.
   2. **Pathology**
      - Replication of VZV occurs in ganglia when cellular and humoral immunity wane with increasing age; immunosuppression from chemotherapy, HIV disease; malignancy; and after radiotherapy (5% of all VZV reactivation occurs in children <15 years of age). Reactivated VZV travels down the sensory nerve causing itching, burning, and pain in area where lesions appear.
   3. **Clinical Features**
      - Prodrome of neuralgia, paresthesia in the area of involved dermatome before eruption of lesions. Few patients have constitutional symptoms of headache, malaise, and fever.
      - Active-stage lesions (Figure 8-13) appear as erythematous papules evolving into grouped and/or confluent vesicles filled with clear fluid, changing to pustules, and finally red-brown crusting lesions occurring in unilateral, dermatomal pattern. Thorax affected most frequently (>50%), followed by trigeminal, lumbosacral, and cervical areas (10% to 20% each). Multi-dermatomal (contiguous or noncontiguous) and recurrent eruptions occur in HIV-infected persons. Ophthalmic zoster may cause serious complications—ophthalmologist should always be consulted.
      - Chronic stage of postherpetic neuralgia (PHN) persists for weeks to years. Nerve damage from inflammation and scarring may cause nerves to misfire resulting in burning, lancinating, shooting pain after lesions resolve.
   4. **Diagnostic Studies**
      - Diagnostic testing is generally not necessary. Viral culture to rule out HSV may be useful in select patients.

FIGURE 8-13. **Herpes zoster.** (Courtesy of Drs. J. Rico and N. Prose, Owen/Galderma.)

- Tzanck smears are nonspecific, and do not differentiate herpes zoster from herpes simplex.
5. **Management**
   - Prevention—VZV vaccine can increase immunity, and oral antiviral agents can reduce the incidence of reactivation of VZV.
   - Immunization—VZV vaccine may boost humoral and cell-mediated immunity and decrease the incidence of zoster in populations with declining VZV-specific immunity.
   - Penciclovir 500 mg PO tid for 7 days, 77% bioavailable. Reduce dose in individuals with diminished renal function.
   - **Active herpes zoster requires the following:**
     - Antiviral agents (acyclovir, valacyclovir, famciclovir as first-line agents; foscarnet for resistant VZV, and combination of acyclovir with recombinant α-2-interferon for the prevention of disseminated zoster in immunosuppressed patients).
     - Aggressive pain management with narcotic analgesics, if necessary.
     - Moist dressing application to affected area(s).
     - Chronic PHN requires pain management by way of topicals (lidocaine gel, capsaicin cream), transcutaneous electrical nerve stimulation, nerve block; oral tricyclic antidepressants, and/or analgesics.

C. Molluscum Contagiosum

1. **Etiology**
   - Caused by poxvirus, molluscum contagiosum virus (MCV-1 and MCV-2), transmitted by skin-to-skin contact. Occurs primarily in children, sexually active adults, and HIV-infected persons.

2. **Pathology**
   - Self-limited viral infection of epidermis in which infected keratinocytes have increased turnover rate as they migrate toward the superficial epidermis.
   - The incubation period for the virus is 3 weeks to 3 months from initial exposure to virus.
3. **Clinical Features**
   - Lesions are small, discrete, umbilicated, dome-shaped papules, and range in color from pearly white to skin tone (Figure 8-14).
   - There may be a single lesion or multiple lesions present on face, trunk, extremities, and/or genital region (HIV-infected patients tend to have larger lesions occurring over wider body distribution; lesions in immunocompromised patients tend to be resistant even to aggressive therapy).
   - Lesions typically resolve spontaneously in 3 to 6 months without scarring.
   - Autoinoculation occurs frequently causing the lesions to occur for 6 months to 3 years from the onset of initial lesions.
4. **Diagnostic Studies**
   - Molluscum bodies (inclusion bodies) are visible on the examination of lesion biopsy.
   - Diagnostic studies are not necessary to make diagnosis.
5. **Management**
   - Avoid skin-to-skin contact with individuals who have mollusca. HIV-infected individuals with mollusca in the beard area should be advised to minimize shaving facial hair or grow a beard.
   - Immunocompetent patients do not require therapy unless lesions are in the area of frequent irritation/trauma, or autoinoculation is persistent.
   - Therapeutic interventions include curettage, cryosurgery, electrodesiccation, and topical retinoic acid.

FIGURE 8-14. **Molluscum contagiosum.** (Courtesy of Drs. J. Rico and N. Prose, Owen/Galderma.)

D. Human Papillomavirus (HPV) Infections

1. **Etiology**
   - HPV is a papovavirus causing cutaneous and mucosal infections in humans.
   - Common cutaneous HPV infections are common warts, plantar warts (Figure 8-15), and flat warts (verruca vulgaris/plantaris/plana, respectively).
   - Cutaneous transmission occurs by way of direct contact of virus at point of small epidermal defect.
   - Mucosal HPV infections cause genital warts (condylomata acuminata), cervical dysplasia/carcinoma, and intraepithelial neoplasia of anogenital region.

2. **Pathology**

   CUTANEOUS
   - Several HPV types infect keratinized skin causing slow-growing, benign epithelial hyperplasia.
   - The HPV replicates within the differentiated cells of the epidermis causing excessive proliferation and retention of the stratum corneum. This process, in turn, causes papule formation.

3. **Clinical Features**
   - Clinical presentation—varies with the type of HPV causing infection, in addition to the location and size of the lesion(s). Viral warts tend to be asymptomatic, but may cause discomfort or tenderness depending on the location and size of the lesion.
   - Verruca vulgaris and plantaris—firm, hyperkeratotic papules measuring between 1 and 10 mm with red-to-brown punctations (thrombosed capillary loops are pathognomonic for warts). Borders may be rounded to irregular with vegetations and clefts.
   - Verruca plana—numerous, discrete, small, flat, flesh-colored papules measuring 1 to 5 mm in diameter and 1 to 2 mm in height, typically on face, hands, shins.

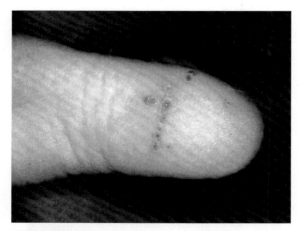

FIGURE 8-15. Plantar warts. (Courtesy of Reed & Carnrick Pharmaceuticals.)

   - Condylomata acuminata—tiny papules evolve into soft, fleshy, cauliflower-like lesions, skin colored to pink or red, occurring in clusters in the genital regions and oropharynx. Lesions persist for months to years; may resolve spontaneously, remain unchanged, or grow if not treated. Increased risk of cervical dysplasia/carcinoma.

4. **Diagnostic Studies**
   - Cutaneous HPV lesions are diagnosed based on clinical characteristics.
   - Mucosal HPV lesions also are diagnosed clinically, but they may require acetic acid testing for whitening (nonspecific finding), or biopsy.
   - Testing for sexually transmitted infections (HIV, syphilis) should be considered for patients with genital HPV lesions; anoscopy or proctoscopy may be necessary. Periodic Papanicolaou (Pap) smear testing of women for cervical carcinoma is essential after detection of HPV infection.

5. **Management**
   - Apart from the avoidance of contact with infectious lesions, no effective methods for the prevention of HPV infections are available at present. Barrier methods of contraception may be helpful in preventing transmission of condyloma acuminatum and other anogenital HPV-associated diseases. Vaccines consisting of virus-like particles (VLPs) can prevent papillomavirus disease in animal models. One study of an HPV-16 VLP vaccine in uninfected women has shown protection from cervical infection with the homologous virus. More extensive clinical trials of these preparations are likely to demonstrate reductions in the rates of cervical HPV disease.
   - Most warts resolve spontaneously within 2 years in immunocompetent patients.
   - **Verruca vulgaris and plantaris therapies include the following:**
     - Topicals—over-the-counter (OTC) salicylic acid preps and plasters.
     - Cryotherapy, electrocautery, CO_2 laser surgery, hyperthermic immersion, intralesional bleomycin.
     - Verruca plana—tretinoin cream; topical 5-fluorouracil for recalcitrant flat warts.
     - Condylomata acuminata—therapies are similar to those used for common warts.
     - Patient-applied topicals:
       - External genital warts: Podofilox 0.5% solution or gel, twice daily for 3 days, followed by 4 days with no therapy, for a total of 4 weeks.
       - Imiquimod 5% cream: once daily at bedtime, three times weekly for up to 16 weeks.
       - Cryotherapy, electrocautery; CO_2 laser, interferon, and topical 5-fluorouracil are

reserved for use on recalcitrant condylomata acuminata.

- Condom use to prevent HPV transmission and Pap smears to screen for cervical dysplasia are essential adjunctive therapies in the management of condylomata acuminata.
- The Gardasil vaccine has minimal side effects. The main adverse effects of the vaccine are pain, swelling, and erythema at the injection site. A small number of subjects may experience a low-grade fever. Adverse events are not more common in women who are already infected with a vaccine HPV serotype. Gardasil appears to have no influence on pregnancy rates or associated diseases, and birth defects are not increased.
- Nearly every woman receiving the Gardasil vaccine generates type-specific antibody, and levels of antibody remain high for at least 3 years. In FUTURE II, 68% of the subjects maintained high levels of antibody to HPV 18 at 3 years, but the incidence of HPV disease did not increase as a consequence of falling antibody levels.

E. Viral Exanthems
- Exanthems—cutaneous expression of a primary systemic infection caused by viruses, bacteria (including *Rickettsia*), and parasites.
- Summary of common viral exanthems is shown in Table 8-3.

IV. Bacterial Infections of the Skin

A. Impetigo
1. Etiology
- *S. aureus* and/or group A β-hemolytic *Streptococcus pyogenes* (GABHS) cause epidermal infection.
- Age of onset.
  - Primary infections more common in children. Secondary infections, any age. Bullous impetigo: neonates, especially; children <5 years.

2. Pathology
- Minor tears in skin act as a portal of entry for common skin flora, or skin flora secondarily infect skin traumatized by other dermatoses.

3. Clinical Features
NONBULLOUS
- Small vesicles/pustules form erosions covered by honey-colored crusts.
- Occurs on face, neck, arms, legs, buttocks.

BULLOUS
- Vesicles and bullae with clear-to-turbid fluid rupture to form shallow erosions with gray-to-hemorrhagic crusts.
- Lesions develop on face, hands, trunk, and intertriginous areas.

4. Diagnostic Studies
- Not performed routinely.
- Culture grows *S. aureus* and/or *S. pyogenes* Group A.
- Gram stain of lesion—gram-positive cocci in clusters or tetrads (*Staphylococcus*) or in chains (*Streptococcus*) with polymorphonuclear neutrophils.

5. Management
- Daily bath with benzoyl peroxide wash (bar).
- Check family members for signs of impetigo. Use ethanol or isopropyl gel for hands and/or involved sites.
- Two percent mupirocin ointment TID for 10 days has been shown to be as effective as oral antibiotics.
- Amoxicillin with clavulanate, dicloxacillin, clarithromycin, azithromycin for *S. aureus* or mixed infections.
- Penicillin VK, erythromycin, cephalexin for GABHS.

B. Cellulitis and Necrotizing Cellulitis
1. Etiology
- *S. aureus* and GABHS most common in adults.
- *Haemophilus influenzae*, GABHS, and *S. aureus* are the most common in children.
- Multiple other gram-positive and gram-negative organisms, as well as fungi, may be the causative organism.

2. Pathology
- Organisms enter the skin through small breaks in the epidermis, infecting the dermal and subcutaneous tissues.
- Virulent organisms may disseminate by way of blood or lymphatics.

3. Clinical Features
- Erythematous, edematous, tender area of variable size, with increased temperature and irregular but distinct borders (Figure 8-16).
- Commonly occurs on lower extremities of adults, whereas lesions caused by *H. influenzae* in children occur most frequently on face and neck. Extremital lesions in children tend to be caused by *S. aureus*.
- Lesions of necrotizing cellulitis/fasciitis change rapidly from tender induration to necrotic tissue.
- **Risk factors for development of cellulitis include the following:**
  - Immunosuppression from diabetes, HIV, malignancy, cirrhosis.
  - Trauma to skin from injection drug use, bites, burns, lacerations, abrasions, surgical incisions.
  - Skin disorders/dermatoses, lymphedema, peripheral vascular disease.

TABLE 8-3. Viral Exanthems

Exanthem	Rash Characteristics	Pattern/Progression	Incubation, Season, and Transmission	Etiologic Agent	Therapies	Complications
Rubeola (measles)	Erythematous maculo papular rash; often slightly hemorrhagic; as rash fades in same pattern it appeared, desquamation and tan yellow discoloration occur; these resolve within 7–10 days	Rash begins faintly at hairline, lateral upper neck, rapidly spreading across face, neck, arms, and upper chest in first 24 hours; spreads next to back, abdomen, thighs in second 24 hours; feet involved by third day	9–12-day incubation Spring Transmission via inhalation of aerosolized respiratory droplets Prodromal phase with fever, coryza, and Koplik's spots	Measles virus (paramyxovirus)	Prevention by immunization with live attenuated measles vaccine; antipyretics for high fever, adequate fluids, bed rest for acute infection; treatment of complications as appropriate	Encephalitis, pneumonia, otitis media, thrombocytopenia; DIC in rare cases
Rubella (German measles)	Pink macular, popular rash; confluent on trunk; no scaling or residual pigmentary changes	Rash begins on forehead/face and moves interiorly to trunk and extremities on first day; rash fades within 3 days	14–21-day incubation Spring Transmission via inhalation of airborne respiratory droplets	Rubella virus (togavirus)	Prevention by immunization with attenuated live rubella virus	Congenital rubella syndrome if exposure occurs in first trimester of pregnancy without adequate maternal immunization
Varicella zoster (chickenpox)	Intensely pruritic, erythematous papules evolve rapidly into vesicles (dewdrops on rose petal); vesicles umbilicate and form pustules with creamy white exudate; red-brown crusts form; crusts resolve in 1–3 weeks	Within 8–12-hour period first crop of lesions appear and evolve; lesions first occur on face/scalp; next lesions appear on extremities and trunk with all stages (papules to crusts) of lesions present at same time	10–21-day incubation Winter and spring Transmission via airborne droplets and from direct contact with uncrusted lesions	VZV (herpesvirus)	Immunization now available; acute infection treat pruritus with lotions and antihistamines; oral acyclovir decreases severity of infection; bacterial superinfections treat with antibiotics	Bacterial superinfection of lesions with S. aureus, S. pyogenes group A may most common complication in children <5 years; varicella encephalitis, Reye's syndrome, and pneumonia complicate varicella in older patients
Roseola infantum (exanthema subitum)	Small, blanchable, pink mascules and papules that may be discrete or confluent	Rash appears on neck and trunk suddenly after 3–4 days of high fever in otherwise healthy child	5–15-day incubation	Herpesvirus type 6 and type 7	Symptomatic	Rare sequelae
Erythema infectiosum (fifth disease)	Slapped cheeks—edematous, erythematous confluent plaques of malar region; reticulated, lacy erythematous macules on neck, trunk, and extensor surfaces of extremities	Facial plaques occur first, fading over 1–4 days; rash appears on neck, trunk, extensor extremities lasting 5–9 days; lesions may recur for weeks to months	4–14 days Late winter, early spring Transmission via droplet aerosol	Parvovirus B19	Symptomatic	Unusual
Hand-foot-mouth disease	Multiple small pink to red, linear, discrete macules on hands, feet, and buccal mucosa, hard palate, and tongue; vesicles have clear fluid	Macules evolve into vesicles rapidly; oral vesicles become painful erosions causing refusal to eat in young children	3–6 days Warm months in temperate climates Transmission via oral-oral or oral-fecal routes	Coxsackie virus A16	Topical dyclonine or lidocaine solution for oral lesions; symptomatic	Sequelae rare; Coxsackie virus infection implicated in aseptic meningitis, myocarditis, and spontaneous abortion

DIC, disseminated intravascular coagulation.

FIGURE 8-16. **Streptococcal cellulitis (erysipelas).** (Courtesy of Burroughs Wellcome Company.)

4. **Diagnostic Studies**
   - Common forms of cellulitis may not require extensive diagnostic testing.
   - Cultures for bacteria or fungi from lesion, exudates, or biopsy specimen for atypical cases of cellulitis.
   - Gram stain; potassium hydroxide (KOH) prep for fungi.
   - Skin biopsy may be useful to differentiate noninfectious causes of tender, erythematous, edematous skin lesions from infectious causes.
   - Skin biopsy necessary to confirm the diagnosis of necrotizing cellulitis/fasciitis.

5. **Management**
   - Amoxicillin with clavulanate, dicloxacillin, clarithromycin, azithromycin for penicillinase-producing organisms.
   - Penicillin VK, erythromycin, cephalexin if organism is not penicillinase producing.
   - Cephalosporin recommended for *H. influenzae* infections.
   - Treatment of necrotizing cellulitis/fasciitis caused by *S. aureus* and GABHS organisms requires nafcillin, oxacillin, or cefazolin IV.
   - Surgical exploration and debridement, and histopathologic examination of tissues required for necrotizing infections of soft tissues.

C. Folliculitis, Furuncle, Carbuncle

1. **Etiology**
   - Bacterial causes—*S. aureus*, most common cause; *Pseudomonas aeruginosa*, "hot tub folliculitis."
   - Fungal causes—*Candida*, dermatophytes.
   - Others—syphilis, herpes simplex.

2. **Pathology**
   - Occlusion of skin with hair follicles, from clothing, prosthetic devices, and natural skin folds predisposes to infectious folliculitis.
   - Shaving, plucking, and waxing of hair are additional means of inciting folliculitis.
   - Infections of the upper portions of the hair follicle can progress to deeper infections such as furuncles (deep nodule or abscess) or a carbuncle (confluent, interconnecting abscesses involving several hair follicles).

3. **Clinical Features**
   - Bacterial folliculitis—lesions are singular or clustered, small papules, or pustules with surrounding erythema.
   - Bacterial furuncle—a tender nodule (1 to 2 cm) with a central plug of necrotic material above a fluctuant abscess, and the surrounding area of cellulitis.
   - Bacterial carbuncle (Figure 8-17)—larger and more painful than furuncle, involving many interlocking furuncles/abscesses and openings draining pus. Cellulitis surrounds the carbuncle as evidenced by erythema and induration of the area.
   - Hematogenous spread of the localized infection is possible causing bacteremia and distant metastatic foci of infection.

4. **Diagnostic Studies**
   - Folliculitis may require Gram stain and culture for bacteria; KOH prep or culture for fungi.
   - Gram stain and culture of exudate from furuncle, carbuncle.
   - Blood cultures may be necessary in febrile patients.

5. **Management**
   - Bacterial folliculitis—treatment, mupirocin ointment or systemic therapy with dicloxacillin, cephalexin for *S. aureus*.
   - Hot tub folliculitis—no therapy necessary; lesions resolve spontaneously in most patients. Recalcitrant lesions may be treated with ciprofloxacin.

FIGURE 8-17. **Carbuncle.** (From Abner Kurtin. Folia Dermatologica, No. 2, Geigy Pharmaceuticals, with permission.)

- Furuncle/carbuncle—treatment includes heat to the affected area to promote drainage.
- Incision and drainage are the therapy of choice in healthy persons.
- Systemic antibiotics should be given to immuno-compromised patients.
- Prevention of recurrent lesions by decreasing carrier state of *S. aureus* with nasal application of mupirocin ointment and use of antibiotic soaps.

D. Skin Manifestations of Systemic Bacterial Infections (Table 8-4; Figures 8-18 to 8-20)

V. Mycotic Infections of the Skin, Hair, and Nails

A. Dermatophytoses
1. **Etiology**
   - *Microsporum, Trichophyton,* and *Epidermophyton* species commonly transmitted as fomites from other people; from contact with pets such as dogs and cats; and autoinfection from one area of dermatophyte infection to another body region.
2. **Pathology**
   - Dermatophytes infect the keratinized tissues—stratum corneum, hair, and nails by digesting keratin.
   - Factors facilitating dermatophyte infection include increased skin moisture from humidity, occlusive clothing/gear, sweating; chronic dermatoses such as atopy; altered immunity from CS use, chemotherapeutics, HIV, and diabetes mellitus (DM); and decreased circulation to distal extremities as in chronic arterial insufficiency.
3. **Clinical Features**
   - Areas affected by dermatophytes and classic lesions:

   HAIR
   - Tinea capitis findings range from annular, scaling lesions, and broken hair shafts to inflammatory pustules and scarring alopecia.
   - Tinea barbae lesions are papules and pustules of the hair follicles easily confused with *Staphylococcus* folliculitis and acne vulgaris.

   NAILS
   - Onychomycosis—inclusive term for nail infections caused by all forms of fungi—dermatophytes (tinea unguium), molds, and yeasts; occurs most commonly on great toe with findings ranging from opaque, thickened, and cracked nails to subungual hyperkeratosis and onycholysis. Progresses to other nails if not treated with systemic antifungals.

   EPIDERMIS (Figure 8-21)
   - Tinea faciale/manuum/corporis/cruris/pedis lesions are erythematous plaques with clearly defined borders, scaling, cracking, and vesicles. Bullae and erosions occur on the hands and feet as well.
4. **Diagnostic Studies**
   - Direct microscopy of skin/nail/hair scrapings with KOH prep for fungal elements.
   - Wood's lamp examination for green fluorescence of *Microsporum species*.
   - Fungal cultures may be obtained, but require 4 to 6 weeks for the growth of organisms.
5. **Management**

   PREVENTION
   - Apply powder containing imidazoles or tolnaftate to areas prone to fungal infection after bathing.

   HAIR AND NAILS
   - For infections of keratinized skin: use if lesions are extensive or if infection has failed to respond to topical preparations, such as griseofulvin for hair infections; itraconazole or terbinafine for nail infections.
   - Be aware of drug–drug interactions and hepato-toxicities with systemic antifungal therapies.
   - Extensive fungal infections of the hair and scalp may require surgical drainage of pus, antibiotic therapy, or both, for secondary bacterial infections.

   EPIDERMIS
   - Topical antifungals are adequate for superficial epidermal dermatophyte infections.
   - Systemic therapies should be considered for recalcitrant infections.

B. Tinea Versicolor (Figure 8-22)
1. **Etiology**
   - *Malassezia furfur* (previously known as *P. ovale, P. orbiculare*)
   - Lipophilic yeast that normally resides in the keratin of skin and hair follicles of individuals at puberty and beyond.
   - An opportunistic organism, causing pityriasis versicolor and *Malassezia* folliculitis; it is implicated in the pathogenesis of seborrheic dermatitis.
   - *Malassezia* infections are not contagious.
   - Overgrowth of resident cutaneous flora occurs under certain favorable conditions.
2. **Pathology**
   - Lipophilic yeast (normal skin flora) present in bodily areas with increased sebaceous activity.
   - Infection occurs more frequently in summer with excess heat and humidity.
   - Risk of overproliferation of resident flora increased in Cushing disease, CS therapy, immunosuppression, oral contraceptives, pregnancy, malnutrition, and burns.
3. **Clinical Features**
   - Multiple, well-delineated round to oval macules of various colors (white to hues of brown) and size

TABLE 8-4. Skin Manifestations of Systemic Bacterial Infections

Disease	Causative Organism	Pathophysiology	Skin Rash	Management	Sequelae/Prognosis
Rocky Mountain spotted fever	*Rickettsia rickettsii* **Rickettsia**	*Dermacentor variabilis* (dog) and *andersoni* (wood tick) transmit *R. rickettsii* to human through bite	Characteristic rash of small blanching, pinking macules begins on wrist and ankles spreading to the palms and soles; within a day, rash spreads proximally on the extremities, the trunk, and face; lesions become hemorrhagic within 4–5 days	Doxycycline Tetracycline (Alternative: chloramphenicol)	DIC can occur as does death from delayed/incorrect diagnosis; sequelae include multiple types of neurologic deficits
Meningococcemia	*Neisseria meningitides* **Gram-negative diplococci**	Bacterial invasion (meningococcal) of endothelial cells and neutrophils causes damage and necrosis of vessel walls; skin infarction, edema, and RBC leakage cause skin lesions; endotoxin from meningococci causes hypotension	Small, irregular pink to purple macules, papules, and petechiae over entire body; purpura, ecchymoses, and areas of black-gray necrosis appear in fulminant meningococcemia	Penicillin G or ceftriaxone Chloramphenicol for penicillin allergic contract prophylaxis: rifampin, ceftriaxone, ciprofloxacin for adults	Acute infection fatal if not treated Early treatment in acute infection has >90% recovery rate Cranial nerve deficits can persist Adrenal hemorrhage (Friderichsen–Waterhouse) and purpura fulminans at presentation have high mortality
Gonococcemia	*Neisseria gonorrhoeae* **Gram-negative diplococci**	Immune complex formation and deposition from hematogenous dissemination of untreated mucosal *N. gonorrhoeae* infection cause hemorrhagic and painful skin lesions	Erythematous macules become painful pustules with central hemorrhage and/or necrosis in the acral areas—primarily on fingers, small joins of hands; may be in web spaces, on feet	Ceftriaxone IM Cefixime Quinolones (not approved for use in pregnancy, lactation, or for persons ≤ 17 years of age)	Dissemination of gonococcus to joins, tendons, liver, and endocardium can occur; untreated endocarditis can be fatal; skin/joint lesions typically resolve gradually
Scarlet fever	*S. pyogenes* group A **Gram-positive cocci** (GABHS)	Exotoxin produced by GABHS from infection of pharynx, tonsils, or skin causes exanthem, petechiae	Fine, erythematous rash on trunk; punctate lesions evolve into confluent scarlatiniform rash; Pastia's lines; desquamation occurs after 4–5 days as exanthem disappears	Penicillin Erythromycin Azithromycin Cephalosporins	Nonsuppurative: acute glomerulonephritis, rheumatic fever, erythema nodosum *Suppurative:* local extension of infection—peritonsillar abscess, acute sinusitis, suppurative cervical lymphadenopathy

(Continued)

TABLE 8-4. **Skin Manifestations of Systemic Bacterial Infections** *(Continued)*

Disease	Causative Organism	Pathophysiology	Skin Rash	Management	Sequelae/Prognosis
Toxic shock syndrome	*S. aureus* **Gram-positive cocci** MTSS—tampon use associated NMTSS—deep abscesses, surgical wound, postpartum infections, osteomyelitis	Toxin (TSST-1) from *S. aureus* absorbed through mucous membranes or wound causing systemic illness of fever, erythroderma, hypotension, and multiorgan failure	Sunburn type rash of diffuse macular erythema, and erythema of mucous membranes (conjunctival, oral, vaginal); ulcérations may occur on mucosal surfaces; palmar and plantar epidermal desquamation occurs 7–14 days after onset of skin rash	Critical care admission for organ failure Antistaphylococcal therapy: IV nafcillin, oxacillin cefazolin Find and treat source of local *S. aureus* if NMTSS	NMTSS has higher mortality than MTSS MTSS has high incidence of recurrence in untreated cases; risk can be greatly reduced with judicious use of tampons (lowest absorbency left in place for short time frames—4–6 hours) and antibiotic therapy
Lyme disease	*Borrelia burgdorferi* **Spirochete**	*Ixodidscapularis and pacifica* (deer) ticks transmit *B. burgdorferi* after biting and feeding on human (>18-hour contact)	Erythema migrans lesion occurs at bite site in 75% of patients with Lyme disease; lesion is erythematous macule or papule, which enlarges to plaque with central clearing over several days	Doxycycline, Amoxicillin, Ceftriaxone IM Avoid known habits habitats of *I. scapularis* and *I. pacificus* (United States) Wear long pants and long-sleeved shirts, tucking pants into socks Apply tick repellents containing W-diethyl-m-toluamide ("DEET") to clothing and exposed skin Check regularly for ticks and promptly remove any attached ticks Acaricides containing permethrin kill ticks on contact and can provide further protection when applied to clothing After a recognized tick bite, the risk of infection with *B. burgdorferi* is low and antibiotic prophylaxis is not routinely indicated Therapy with amoxicillin or doxycycline for 10 days may be given to prevent Lyme disease in the following circumstances:	Neurologic manifestations of meningoencephalitis, cranial nerve palsies, sensory/motor deficits, mental status changes occur Cardiac abnormalities of AV block, left ventricular dysfunction, and pericarditis are transient Arthritides of single to multiple joints—most commonly the knee—occur in 60% of untreated cases

Disease	Organism / Diagnosis	Description	Clinical Features		Treatment	Notes
				Tick engorged (feeding for >24 h), *Ixodes* nymph from a hyperendemic area, pregnancy, immunocompromised status, follow up difficult, or patient anxious Temperature of >38° C may represent human granulocytic ehrlichiosis or babesiosis transmitted with tick bite Immunization for prophylaxis of LB is now available for those at high risk of infection with the Lyme vaccine LYMErix. It contains recombinant outer-surface protein A Mycotic infections of the skin, hair, and nails		
Syphilis	*Treponema pallidum* **spirochete** Positive fluorescent treponemal antibodies (**FTA**) on darkfield microscopy	Sexually transmitted bacterial infection; primary lesion occurs at site of inoculation; infection becomes systemic shortly after inoculation; organism may remain latent for decades	*Primary*—chancre (small papule becomes painless ulceration with raised border) *Secondary*—erythematous maculopapular rash diffusely over body; condylomata lata; patchy hair loss *Tertiary*—gumma; annular nodules		*Primary and secondary syphilis*—benzathine penicillin 2.4 million units IM *Late latent syphilis*—benzathine penicillin 2.4 million units IM/week for three consecutive weeks *Neurosyphilis*—penicillin G IV or procaine penicillin IM with probenecid of 10–14 days	Untreated primary syphilis may progress to secondary syphilis, and eventually to tertiary syphilis; late complications include endocarditis and neurosyphilis; syphilis can be transmitted to the fetus in utero; fetal outcomes vary from mild congenital syphilis infection to stillbirth dependent on factors ranging from duration of infection to host resistance

AV, atrioventricular; DIC, disseminated intravascular coagulation; IM, intramuscular; IV, intravenous; MTSS, menstrual toxic shock syndrome; NMTSS, nonmenstrual toxic shock syndrome; RBC, red blood cell.

FIGURE 8-18. **Primary syphilis.** (Courtesy of the Upjohn Company.)

(1 to 30 cm) distributed over the upper trunk, neck, upper arms, axillae, abdomen, groin, and thighs with fine scale visible on scraping.

- Lesions are typically asymptomatic; they may be hypopigmented or hyperpigmented.

4. **Diagnostic Studies**
   - Direct microscopy of scale mixed with KOH shows classic "spaghetti and meatball" configuration of fungal hyphae and spores.
   - Wood's lamp examination for yellow-green fluorescence of scales.

5. **Management**
   - Once-weekly application of ketoconazole 2% shampoo (Nizoral), applied as a lotion to the neck, trunk, and proximal extremities 5 to 10 minutes before showering, may help prevent recurrences.
   - Selenium sulfide suspension 2.5%. When applied for 10 minutes every day for seven consecutive days, the suspension (available as Selsun or in

FIGURE 8-20. **Secondary syphilis (condylomata lata).** (Courtesy of J. E. Moore and the Upjohn Company.)

generic forms) resulted in an 87% cure rate at a 2-week follow-up evaluation. Blood and urine levels determined during this study showed that no significant absorption of selenium took place. The suspension is applied to the entire skin surface from the lower posterior scalp area to the thighs.

FIGURE 8-19. **Secondary syphilis.** (Courtesy of K.U.M.C.)

FIGURE 8-21. **Tinea corporis.** (From Hall JC, ed. *Sauer's Manual of Skin Diseases*. 10th ed. Philadelphia, PA: Lippincott Williams & Wilkins; 2010, with permission.)

FIGURE 8-22. **Tinea versicolor.** (Courtesy of K.U.M.C. and Sandoz Pharmaceuticals.)

Another commonly recommended schedule is to apply the lotion and wash it off within 24 hours. This is repeated once each week for a total of 4 weeks. There are many suggested variations of this treatment schedule. Wash the scalp with the lotion at the same time.

- Terbinafine solution (Lamisil solution 1% spray bottle). Application of the spray to the affected areas twice a day for 1 week is effective. Lamisil spray is available as an OTC product.
- Miconazole, ketoconazole, clotrimazole, econazole, or ciclopirox olamine is applied to the entire affected area one or two times a day for 2 to 4 weeks. The creams are odorless and nongreasy but expensive.

C. Candida

MUCOSAL

1. Etiology
- *Candida albicans* and other *Candida species*.

2. Pathology
- Suppression of immunity, systemic antibiotic therapy, or both, cause the overgrowth of *Candida* organisms of the normal flora resulting in oral and/or vulvovaginal candidiasis. Severe immunocompromise of HIV disease and chemotherapy may lead to deep candidiasis of the esophagus and tracheobronchial tree, as well as invasive candidiasis and fungemia.

3. Clinical Features
- Candidal lesions are white plaques on an erythematous surface that bleeds when the lesions are gently dislodged.

- Vaginal discharge is white, thick, curd-like, typically occurring in the week before the onset of menses.
- Mucosal and deep candidal infections are clinical markers and defining criteria in HIV disease.

4. Diagnostic Studies
- KOH prep visualized by direct microscopy for pseudohyphae and budding yeasts.

5. Management
- Topical antifungal therapy with itraconazole solution, clotrimazole troche for oropharyngeal candidiasis; patients with HIV disease respond to topical therapy, but tend to have recurrences and eventually require systemic prophylactic therapy.
- Uncomplicated candidal vulvovaginitis may be treated with a single dose oral fluconazole, or 3 to 7 days of therapy with imidazoles (e.g., terconazole and miconazole).

CUTANEOUS

1. Etiology
- *Candida albicans*.

2. Pathology
- *Candida albicans* superficially infects moist, warm skin, macerated and occluded, such as intertriginous areas, genital regions, and web spaces (Figure 8-23).
- Risk factors for developing cutaneous candidiasis include occupations requiring frequent hand wetting or immersing in water, use of occlusive clothing/diapers, obese stature, immobility, and CS therapy.

3. Clinical Features
- Erythematous papules and pustules coalesce forming plaque of erythema with fine scale at visually distinct margin of lesion; erosions and edema of affected area are common.

FIGURE 8-23. **Candidiasis.** (Courtesy of Smith Kline & French Laboratories.)

- Satellite lesions are characteristic of cutaneous candidiasis.
4. **Diagnostic Studies**
   - KOH preparation of lesion scraping visualized under direct microscopy for budding yeasts and pseudohyphae.
5. **Management**
   - Topical nystatin cream or imidazole creams.
   - Prevention of lesions by keeping skin dry, frequent diaper changes, and use of cotton undergarments and nonocclusive clothing; using powder with antifungal such as miconazole; decreasing *C. albicans* colonization by washing with benzoyl peroxide soap.
   - Castellani paint brings almost immediate relief of symptoms (i.e., candidal paronychia).

FIGURE 8-24. **Scabies.** (Courtesy of Hoechst-Roussel Pharmaceuticals.)

VI. Parasitic Infestations of Skin and Hair

A. Scabies
1. **Etiology**
   - *Sarcoptes scabiei*, an ectoparasite, is the etiologic agent of scabies.
     - Transmission: Usually spread by skin-to-skin contact; fomites.
2. **Pathology**
   - The scabies mite, *S. scabiei*, is transmitted by skin-to-skin contact, or from clothing or bedding infested with the mite. (The mite is able to survive more than 2 days while off human skin where it normally feeds and multiplies.) The female mite burrows into the skin to lay eggs, feed, and defecate leaving scybala (fecal particles) to incite a hypersensitivity reaction in the host; the mites can exist for months to years.
   - Pruritus and dermatitis develop from sensitization to *S. scabiei* within 1 month of initial infestation. Subsequent infestations cause immediate pruritus.
   - Persons living in institutionalized facilities are at high risk for scabies infestation.
3. **Clinical Features**
   - Intense pruritus with minimal skin findings is a classic presentation of scabies.
   - Mite burrows (5 mm to several cm in length) occur in areas where stratum corneum is thin such as finger webs, wrists, genital region, inframammary ridge, buttocks (Figure 8-24).
   - Crusted lesions containing high concentrations of mites are more likely to occur in immunocompromised patients.
   - Smooth nodules measuring 5 to 20 mm may be part of the clinical picture in a small minority of patients (<10%).

- Secondary lesions from scratching and rubbing, and bacterial infection, are common, as are urticaria and eczematous dermatitis at sites of infestation.
4. **Diagnostic Studies**
   - Direct visualization of mite, eggs, and scybala under microscope from a skin scraping of burrow, flexor aspects of wrists, and penis. A drop of mineral oil is placed over a burrow, and the burrow is scraped off with a no. 15 scalpel blade and placed on a microscope slide.
5. **Management**
   - Choice of scabicide based on effectiveness, potential toxicity, cost, extent of secondary eczematization, and age of patient.
   - Permethrin is effective and safe but costs more than lindane.
   - Lindane is effective in most areas of the world, but resistance has been reported. Seizures have occurred when lindane was applied after a bath or used by patients with extensive dermatitis. Aplastic anemia after lindane use was also reported. No controlled studies have confirmed that two applications are better than one. Clean clothing should be put on afterwards. Clothing and bedding are decontaminated by machine washing at 60° C. Pruritus can persist for up to 1 to 2 weeks after the end of effective therapy. After that time, cause of persistent itching should be investigated.
   - **Recommended regimens:**
     - Permethrin 5% cream applied to all areas of the body from the neck down. Wash off 8 to 12 hours after application. Adverse events are very low. Permethrin (Elimite cream, Acticin cream) is a synthetic pyrethrin that demonstrates extremely low mammalian toxicity. It is the drug of choice for the treatment of scabies in

children and adults of all ages. Several studies show that it is more effective than lindane. A diminished sensitivity to permethrin has been documented. One application is said to be effective but a second treatment 1 week after the first application is now a standard practice. The OTC permethrin preparation (Nix) is lower in strength (1%) and ineffective against scabies. Unlike lindane, permethrin undergoes insignificant absorption (2%), after which it is rapidly degraded.

- Lindane (γ-benzene hexachloride) 1% lotion or cream applied thinly to all areas of the body from the neck down; wash off thoroughly after 8 hours. **NOTE:** Lindane should not be used after a bath or shower, and it should not be used by persons with extensive dermatitis, pregnant or lactating women, and children younger than 2 years. Mite resistance to lindane has developed in North, Central, and South America and Asia. Low cost makes lindane a key alternative in many countries.
- Lindane is available as a cream, shampoo, and lotion. Lotion dispensed from bulk containers may not be agitated; therefore, the concentration of lindane may be inadequate. Reports of lindane resistance have appeared. A second treatment 1 week after the first application is standard practice. A follow-up examination at 2 to 4 weeks is recommended. Approximately 10% of lindane is absorbed through intact skin. Lindane accumulates in fat and binds to brain tissue. Pruritus may persist for weeks. Additional, unprescribed applications, without documented evidence of persistent infestation, may be dangerous. Lindane should be avoided in children younger than 2 years, pregnant or nursing women, and patients with HIV or AIDS. Children with severe, underlying, cutaneous disease may be at greater risk for toxicity. This is also true for premature, emaciated, or malnourished children and those with a history of seizure disorders.
- **Alternative regimens:**
  - Crotamiton 10% cream applied thinly to the entire body from the neck down, nightly for two consecutive nights. Wash off 24 hours after second application.
  - Crotamiton (Eurax lotion). A study of children with scabies showed an 89% cure rate after 4 weeks with permethrin 5% cream (Elimite) and a 60% cure rate with crotamiton cream. The toxicity of crotamiton is unknown. Reported cure rates for once-a-day application for 5 days range from 50% to 100%.

- Sulfur 2% to 10% in petrolatum applied to skin for 2 to 3 days. Sulfur has been used to treat scabies for more than 150 years. The pharmacist mixes 6% (5% to 10% range) precipitated sulfur in petrolatum or a cold cream base. The compound is applied to the entire body below the neck once each day for 3 days. The patient is instructed to bathe 24 hours after each application. Sulfur applied in this manner is highly effective, but these preparations are messy, have an unpleasant odor, stain, and cause dryness. Sulfur in petrolatum was thought to be safer than lindane for treating infants, but the safety of topical sulfur has never been established.
- Benzyl benzoate 10% and 25% lotions. Several regimens are recommended. Swabbing only once; two applications separated by 10 minutes, or two applications within a 24 hour or 1 week interval. Twenty-four hours after application, preparation should be washed off and clothes and bedding changed. The compound is an irritant and can induce pruritic irritant dermatitis, especially on face and genitalia.
- Benzyl benzoate with sulfiram. Several regimens are recommended, swabbing only once.
- Esdepallethrine 0.63%.
- Malathion 0.5% lotion.
- Sulfiram 25% lotion. Can mimic effect of disulfiram. No alcoholic drinks should be consumed for at least 48 hours.
- Ivermectin 0.8% lotion.
- Systemic ivermectin.
- Ivermectin 200 μg per kg PO. Single dose reported to be very effective for common as well as crusted scabies. To be repeated in 15 to 30 days. Average adult dose is 15 mg. Two to three doses, separated by 1 to 2 weeks, usually required for heavy infestation or in immunocompromised individuals. May effectively eradicate epidemic or endemic scabies in institutions such as nursing homes, hospitals, and refugee camps. Not approved by the U.S. Food and Drug Administration or European Drug Agency.
- For infants, young children, pregnant/lactating women, permethrin or crotamiton regimens or precipitated sulfur ointment should be used with application to all body areas. Lindane and ivermectin should not be used.
- All clothing, bedding, towels must be washed and/or dried using heat, and have no contact with body for minimum of 72 hours.
- Fingernails should be trimmed and scabicidal lotion left under nails to eradicate mites—reapply lotion after hand washing.
- Sexual partners within last month should be examined and treated.

B. Pediculosis Capitis, Corporis, Pubis

1. **Etiology**
   - Lice infestations in humans are caused by ectoparasites.
     - Head lice—*Pediculus humanus* var. *capitis*.
     - Body lice—*P. humanus corporis*.
     - Pubic lice—*Phthirus pubis* (Figure 8-25).

2. **Pathology**
   - All three lice are transmitted by person-to-person contact or by fomites such as hats, headsets, clothing, and bedding. Body and pubic lice require direct physical contact, whereas head lice are transmitted more frequently by way of fomites.

3. **Clinical Features**
   - Pruritus in affected area is the most common presenting symptom.
   - Lice and nits (small, white, oval-shaped capsules firmly attached to hair shaft at exit point of hair follicle) are visible on gross examination.
   - Excoriations, secondary bacterial infections, or both, may be present.
   - Papular urticaria at site of lice bites may be present.
   - Eyelashes may be infested with *P. pubis* in prepubertal patient, or infrequently, *P. humanus capitis*.
   - Body lice live in clothing (near seams) and bedding; they infest human host only for feeding.

4. **Diagnostic Studies**
   - Diagnostic studies are not necessary for the diagnosis of lice infestation; the diagnosis is clinical based on observation of lice/nits.

5. **Management**
   - Topically applied insecticides. Ideally, should have 100% activity against louse and egg. Malathion kills all lice after 5 minutes of exposure and >95%

FIGURE 8-25. **Pediculosis pubis.** (Courtesy of Dr. J. Boley.)

of eggs fail to hatch after 10 minutes of exposure. Synthetic pyrethroids, synergized pyrethrins, and Malathion are the most efficacious and safe. Lotion preparations are preferred. Creams, foams, and gels are also available.

- **Recommended regimen:**
  - Permethrin. Synthetic pyrethroid. OTC 1% products: Nix. 5% product: Elimite is prescription. Product applied to infested area(s) and washed off after 10 minutes. Not totally ovicidal. Has residual activity in that the incubation period of louse eggs is 6 to 10 days. Should be reapplied in 7 to 14 days.
  - Pyrethrin and piperonyl butoxide. Pyrethrins derived from extract of chrysanthemums. Products: RID mousse, RID shampoo, A-200, R and C, Pronta, Clear Lice System.
  - Malathion 0.5% in 78% isopropyl alcohol (Ovide). Applied to involved site for 8 to 12 hours; binds to hair providing residual protection. Indicated in lindane-resistant cases. Should not be used in children younger than 6 months.

- **Alternative regimen:**
  - Pyrethrins with piperonyl butoxide applied to scalp and washed off after 10 minutes.
  - Lindane 1% shampoo applied for 4 minutes and then thoroughly washed off. Not recommended for pregnant or lactating women. Not totally ovicidal and lacks residual activity in that the incubation period of louse eggs is 6 to 10 days. The agents should be reapplied in 7 to 14 days. Retreatment may be necessary if live lice are found or eggs are observed at the hair–skin junction.
  - Ivermectin 0.8% lotion or shampoo.

- **Systemic therapy:** Oral ivermectin 200 μg per kg. Repeat on Day 10 to kill emerging nymphs.
- Acquired resistance to insecticides occurs worldwide mainly to pyrethrins and pyrethroids, but also to Malathion. If resistance is suspected, an alternative agent should be used. Other alternatives include newer insecticides and oral ivermectin in cases of resistance to both pyrethroids and Malathion.
- Head lice—comb hair with fine toothed-comb to remove nits after lotion application.
- Body lice—discard infested clothing or treat with 1% Malathion powder or 10% dichlorodiphenyl-trichloroethane powder (nits viable in clothing for 1 month).
- Pubic lice—treat sexual partner(s); bedding and clothing need to be decontaminated by washing, drying, or both, with heat and removal from body contact for at least 72 hours; eyelashes should be coated with petroleum jelly or occlusive ophthalmic ointment two or three times per day for 10 days.

SELECTED REFERENCES

Behrman RE, Kliegman RM, Jenson HB, eds. *Nelson's Textbook of Pediatrics*. 19th ed. Philadelphia, PA: WB Saunders; 2011.

Braunwald E, Fauci AS, Kasper DL, Hauser SL, Longo DL, Jameson JL, eds. *Harrison's Principles of Internal Medicine*. 17th ed. New York, NY: McGraw-Hill; 2008.

Fitzpatrick TB, Johnson RA, Wolff K, Suurmond D, eds. *Color Atlas and Synopsis of Clinical Dermatology: Common and Serious Diseases*. 6th ed. New York, NY: McGraw-Hill; 2009.

Gilbert DN, Sande MA, Moellering RC, eds. *The Sanford Guide to Antimicrobial Therapy 2003*. 41st ed. Dallas, TX: Antimicrobial Therapy; 2011.

Habif TP, ed. *Clinical Dermatology: A Color Guide to Diagnosis and Therapy*. 4th ed. St. Louis, MO: Mosby; 2004.

Hall JC, ed. *Sauer's Manual of Skin Diseases*. 10th ed. Philadelphia, PA: Lippincott Williams & Wilkins; 2010.

Leonardi CL, Papp KA, Pariser DM. Recent developments in t-cell specific biological therapy for the treatment of psoriasis.

9

Endocrine Disorders

Ellen D. Feld • Daniela Cheles-Livingston • Ann McDonough Madden

I. Pituitary Disorders

A. Anterior Pituitary

1. Pituitary Tumors

a. Etiology

- Several cell types comprise the pituitary gland; each cell type may give rise to pituitary adenomas.
- Clinical consequences are associated commonly with hypersecretion of one of pituitary gland's products or by compression of nearby anatomic structures.
- Pituitary tumors also can be "nonfunctioning," secreting biologically inactive hormones.

b. Pathology

- Formerly classified as chromophobic, eosinophilic, and basophilic; usually benign neoplasms.
- **Six types have been defined, according to secretory characteristics:**
  - Prolactin secreting (prolactinomas are the most common secretory pituitary tumors).
  - Growth hormone (GH) secreting.
  - Adrenocorticotropic hormone (ACTH) secreting.
  - Melanocyte-stimulating hormone (MSH) secreting.
  - Thyroid-stimulating hormone (TSH) secreting; follicle-stimulating hormone (FSH)/luteinizing hormone (LH) secreting—all rare.
- Anterior pituitary anatomic features with clinical consequences: relationship with the hypothalamus, which secretes the releasing factors, location in the sella turcica, below the optic chiasm.
- Mass effects of pituitary tumors cause disruption in the optic chiasm with typical visual field defect—bitemporal hemianopsia.

c. Clinical Features

- Manifestations—headache, typical visual field defect, and cranial nerve III palsy.
- **Hormonal abnormalities are characterized by specific effects:**
  - Excess prolactin—symptoms of hypogonadism and infertility.
  - Oligomenorrhea, amenorrhea, or galactorrhea is more common in women; decreased libido and impotence in men.
  - Excess GH results in acromegaly in adults and gigantism in children and also produces clinical findings of diabetes mellitus (DM) or glucose intolerance.
  - Excess ACTH—Cushing disease and pigmentation due to association of increased MSH.
  - Excess TSH—rare tumors.
  - Excess gonadotropins—rare tumors.

d. Diagnostic Studies

- Endocrinologic studies—to determine the type(s) of pituitary hormone(s) hypersecreted.
- Hypersecretion of prolactin—increased prolactin level.
- ACTH hypersecretion (see Chapter 16, II. B. 1.).
- Excess GH—diagnosed by association with increased insulin-like growth factor I levels and glucose suppression test.
- Primary hypersecretion of TSH is rare, accompanied by increased T_3 and T_4; secondary hypersecretion of TSH, due to hypothyroidism, is common.
- LH and FSH hypersecretion (secondary) occurs in primary gonadal failure accompanied by low gonadal hormone concentrations; primary hypersecretion of LH and FSH is rare.
- Visual field testing and neurologic testing if mass effect is considered.
- Magnetic resonance imaging (MRI) has become the study of choice in the evaluation of sellar lesions.

e. Management

- For prolactinomas, dopamine agonist (bromocriptine) as pharmacologic therapy has partially replaced the need for surgery.
- Surgery is a preferred treatment for all pituitary tumors, except prolactinoma.
- Ketoconazole is beneficial in surgically untreatable cases of Cushing disease.

2. Hypopituitarism

a. Etiology

- Hypopituitarism results from either anterior pituitary destruction or deficient hypothalamic regulatory function.
- Can be caused by congenital (rare) or acquired lesions, such as tumors, infiltrative disorders, trauma, vascular lesions (Sheehan syndrome

caused by postpartum pituitary infarction), postsurgery, or radiation therapy.

b. Pathology
- Hypopituitarism is often slow appearing, and may result in single or multiple hormone deficiencies.
- GH deficiency has the strongest impact when it appears in childhood.

c. Clinical Features
- GH deficiency—during infancy and childhood manifests as growth retardation, short stature (dwarfism with normal mental development), and fasting hypoglycemia. Adults with GH deficiency have mild to moderate central obesity, increased systolic blood pressure, increased low-density lipoprotein (LDL) cholesterol, and reduced cardiac output as well as reduced muscle and bone mass, reduced physical and mental energy, impaired concentration and memory, and depression.
- TSH deficiency—results in secondary thyroid gland hypofunction. Fatigue, weakness, weight change, and hyperlipidemia. In infants: dwarfism with delayed mental development—cretinism (see II. A. 3.).
- Gonadotropin deficiency—during childhood manifests as delayed puberty and causes failure of epiphyseal closure; the resulting clinical picture is that of tall adolescents with eunuchoid features. Adult features: amenorrhea, loss of secondary sexual characters, infertility, decreased libido, and impotence.
- ACTH deficiency (see V. A. 4.).
- Prolactin deficiency—failure of lactation.

d. Diagnostic Studies
- Imaging: MRI studies.
- GH deficiency: no established "gold standard" test. Evaluation—levodopa test should be performed for patients with known hypothalamopituitary disease, cranial irradiation, or childhood onset of GH deficiency.
- TSH deficiency: low TSH with low T_4 and T_3.
- ACTH deficiency (see V. A. 4.).
- Gonadotropin deficiency can be evaluated by concurrent measurement of serum gonadotropins and gonadal hormone production.

e. Management
- TSH and ACTH deficiencies require thyroid hormone and corticosteroids replacement, respectively.
- In GH deficiency—hormone replacement, important in children and adults who are symptomatic or have severe deficiency.
- For FSH and LH deficiencies—replacement with end-organ hormones: estrogen, progesterone, and testosterone.

B. Posterior Pituitary
1. Diabetes Insipidus
a. Etiology
- Diabetes insipidus (DI) is caused by the deficiency of the peptide arginine vasopressin (AVP), also called antidiuretic hormone (ADH).
- **Causes of DI can be categorized as:**
  - Central/neurogenic deficiency of AVP owing to autoimmune destruction of AVP secreting cells, pituitary neoplasms, trauma, surgery, infections, and infiltrative sarcoid granuloma.
  - Nephrogenic—less common, caused by intrinsic renal disease, abnormal receptors sensitivity.
  - Other causes—sickle cell anemia and long-term lithium therapy.

b. Pathology
- Cause of central DI is AVP absence.
- Nephrogenic DI is caused by the loss of renal sensitivity to AVP.
- Regardless of the cause, patients produce large volumes of dilute urine.

c. Clinical Features
- Polyuria (up to 20 L per day), polydipsia, nocturia, intense thirst, with craving for ice water.
- Children may have enuresis.
- If water intake is limited, hypovolemia and dehydration with hypotension and vascular collapse develop rapidly.
- Associated manifestations of anterior pituitary or hypothalamic defects may be present.

d. Diagnostic Studies
- **No single diagnostic lab test**
  - Twenty-four-hour urine collection for volume (< 2 L per day rules out DI) and creatinine (to ensure accurate collection).
  - Serum for osmolality, glucose, potassium (hypokalemia causes polyuria), sodium, and uric acid.
  - Urinalysis—low specific gravity, but is otherwise normal, no glucosuria.
  - Serum osmolality is greater than urine osmolality.
  - Hypernatremia if access to water is restricted or if hypothalamic thirst center is damaged.
  - In nephrogenic DI, serum vasopressin is high during modest fluid restriction.
  - Hyperuricemia implicates central DI.
  - Dehydration test followed by "Vasopressin challenge test" to differentiate between neurogenic and nephrogenic causes; in central DI, urine osmolality increases above plasma osmolality, whereas in nephrogenic DI, urine osmolality barely shows an increase.
- MRI of brain to evaluate hypophysis/hypothalamus.

e. **Management**
- Neurogenic DI can be treated with vasopressin analog desmopressin acetate (DDAVP), aqueous vasopressin subcutaneously and intranasally.
- Treatment of nephrogenic DI is difficult; mainly, salt restriction and thiazide diuretics.

2. **Syndrome of Inappropriate Antidiuretic Hormone Secretion**
   a. **Etiology**
   - Excess ADH produces hypotonic, euvolemic hyponatremia.
   - The most common causes of syndrome of inappropriate antidiuretic hormone (SIADH): stroke, meningitis, central nervous system (CNS) tumors.
   - Other causes: ectopic ADH—small cell lung cancer, drugs.

   b. **Pathology**
   - ADH is inappropriately high for plasma osmolality. Consequence: water retention leading to hyponatremia and decreased plasma osmolality.
   - Important to distinguish SIADH from adreno-cortical insufficiency and hypervolemic hyponatremia syndromes: congestive heart failure (CHF), nephrotic syndrome, renal insufficiency.

   c. **Clinical Features**
   Symptoms are usually seen with serum sodium levels <120 mEq per L.
   - Patients with mild or slowly developing hyponatremia may have no symptoms.
   - Weakness, anorexia, nausea with or without vomiting, headaches, irritability, muscle cramps, lethargy, confusion, seizures, coma, and, eventually, death.
   - Despite water retention, patients with SIADH have *no* edema.
   - In the brain, if extracellular fluid is low in sodium, osmosis occurs, leading to fluid shift into intracellular spaces and cellular edema; mentation changes may be difficult to distinguish from the brain metastasis.

   d. **Diagnostic Studies**
   - Diagnosis *cannot* be made in the presence of renal, adrenal, pituitary, and thyroid disorders and diuretic treatment because all of them can alter free-water clearance.
   - Serum Na^+ concentration <130 mEq per L (<130 mmol per L).
   - Decreased serum osmolality (<280 mOsm per kg) with inappropriately increased urine osmolality (>150 mOsm per kg).
   - Low blood urea nitrogen (<10 mg per dL) and hypouricemia (<4 mg per dL) are not only dilutional, but result from increased urea and uric acid clearances in response to the volume-expanded state.

e. **Management**
- Mainstay of therapy, water restriction (500 to 1,000 mL per day) and adequate sodium in the diet.
- If sodium is between 125 and 134, fluid restriction allows homeostasis to occur.
- If due to chronic disease or age, or if patient is unable to restrict fluids, treat with demeclocycline, a tetracycline derivative, which inhibits ADH at renal tubular level.
- Furosemide, combined with saline, for symptomatic hyponatremia can lead to balance through increased excretion of free water.
- Only in life-threatening circumstances, hypertonic (3% saline) infusion may be necessary. Infuse along with diuretics, to avoid pulmonary edema secondary to fluid overload. Do not correct hyponatremia too rapidly because of the risk of contraction of the brain cells resulting in demyelination.

II. Thyroid Disorders

A. Hypothyroidism

1. **Etiology**
   - Primary: in United States—Hashimoto thyroiditis (autoimmune), idiopathic atrophy, antithyroid medications, lithium, excessive iodine in susceptible people, and iatrogenic (postthyroidectomy/postradioiodine ablation). Worldwide—iodine deficiency.
   - Secondary/tertiary: owing to pituitary/hypothalamic disorders.

2. **Pathology**
   - Primary hypothyroidism results in TSH elevation (lack of negative feedback); serum free thyroxine levels are usually reduced.
   - Less commonly, secondary hypothyroidism characterized by decreased serum TSH and free thyroxine.

3. **Clinical Features**
   - **Symptoms:**
     - Lethargy and fatigue.
     - Intolerance to cold.
     - Impaired memory and decreased cognitive function.
     - Constipation.
     - Weight gain.
     - Decreased libido and fertility, irregular anovulatory cycles and menorrhagia.
     - Depression.
   - **Physical examination:**
     - Coarse, dry skin; atrophy of dermis; brittleness of nails; thinning of lateral eyebrows; nonpitting peripheral edema; facial puffiness.
     - Thyroid gland may be enlarged, decreased in size, or absent (e.g., postthyroidectomy).
     - Muscle strength is decreased; deep tendon reflexes are delayed.

- Slow, hoarse speech.
- Hypothermia (in severe forms).
- Bradycardia, cardiomegaly and diastolic hypertension.
- Myxedema—most severe presentation.
- Subclinical hypothyroidism—subtle and difficult to recognize without high level of clinical suspicion.
- Congenital hypothyroidism—associated with severe mental and motor retardation (cretinism).

4. Diagnostic Studies
- Decreased total T_4 and, especially, decreased free T_4.
- Elevated TSH by radioimmunoassay (except in secondary hypothyroidism).
- Subclinical hypothyroidism—increased TSH and normal T_3 and T_4.
- Hashimoto thyroiditis—high titers of antibodies against thyroperoxidase and thyroglobulin.
- Other tests: increased cholesterol.

5. Management
- Thyroid hormone replacement—mainstay of management. Monitor TSH levels at 6-week intervals after starting/changing doses. Slow, small, increasing dosages for patients with cardiovascular risks.
- Elderly patients and those with angina, myocardial infarction, or CHF must be monitored carefully for adverse reactions as metabolism increases, or not treated at all until cardiovascular status is stabilized.
- Anticoagulants, insulin, and oral hypoglycemics may need to be decreased. Oral cholestyramine may increase T_4 requirements.

B. Thyroiditis
- Group of disorders associated with inflammation of the thyroid gland; most of them associated with hypothyroidism.

1. Hashimoto Thyroiditis (Chronic Lymphocytic Thyroiditis)
a. Etiology
- Most common form of thyroiditis and hypothyroidism.
- Autoimmune etiology.
- Occurs six times more commonly in women than in men.
b. Pathology
- Immune-mediated destruction of thyroid parenchyma.
- Hashimoto thyroiditis can be associated with other autoimmune diseases (adrenal insufficiency, vitiligo).
c. Clinical Features
- Patients may be euthyroid or hypothyroid.
- Thyroid gland may be symmetrically, diffusely enlarged, firm, or rubbery, and is usually nontender; surface is irregular or nodular.
- Complication: slow progression to hypothyroidism.

d. Diagnostic Studies
- Thyroid function tests (TFTs) disclose hypothyroidism.
- Antithyroid antibodies are present.
e. Management
- Thyroid hormone replacement (shrinks gland even in euthyroid patients).

2. Painful Subacute Thyroiditis (de Quervain Thyroiditis)
a. Etiology
- Probably viral, may be preceded by upper respiratory infection.
b. Pathology
- Thyroid enlargement and inflammation.
- Self-limited disease; presents with thyrotoxicosis in early stage, followed by several months of hypothyroidism.
- Young and middle aged women are most commonly affected.
c. Clinical Features
- Gland is moderately enlarged, exquisitely tender, and firm; one or both lobes may be affected.
- Pain in the thyroid region radiating to the jaw or the ear.
- Fever, sweating, heat intolerance, malaise, and myalgias.
- No ophthalmopathy.
- Thyrotoxicosis develops in 50% of patients and lasts several weeks.
- Subsequent hypothyroidism lasts 4 to 6 months.
d. Diagnostic Studies
- Lymphocytosis and elevated erythrocyte sedimentation rate (ESR).
- T_3 or T_4 levels are elevated initially and may fall later.
- Low thyroid radioiodine uptake (RAIU).
e. Management
- Acute illness subsides in 3 to 8 weeks.
- Aspirin or other nonsteroidal anti-inflammatory drugs (NSAIDs).
- Initial stage—β-blockers; antithyroid medication is not effective.
- Longer, hypofunctional stage—hormone replacement.

3. Painless Thyroiditis (Silent, Postpartum)
a. Etiology
- Characterized by thyrotoxic phase, then hypothyroid phase; occurs in women with euthyroid Hashimoto thyroiditis. About 50% of the patients eventually develop permanent hypothyroidism.
b. Pathology
- Enlargement, followed by atrophy.
c. Clinical Features
- Thyrotoxic phase typically lasts 2 to 6 weeks, followed by hypothyroid phase.
- Malaise, fatigue, and weight loss.
- Nontender thyroid enlargement.

   d. **Diagnostic Studies**
- TFTs can be normal; or mild hyperfunction initially, followed by hypofunction.
- ESR is normal or slightly elevated.

   e. **Management**
- Most patients need no treatment because of short duration and mild manifestations of the initial phase. Antithyroid medication is not effective.
- Second stage, the hypofunctional one—thyroid replacement therapy.

C. Hyperthyroidism (Thyrotoxicosis)

1. **Etiology**
- Graves disease—the most common cause of hyperthyroidism in the United States.
- Autoimmune—hyperthyroidism is caused by TSH receptor–stimulating antibodies.
- Female: male ratio, 6:1.
- **Additional causes of hyperthyroidism:**
  - Toxic multinodular goiter (Plummer disease).
  - Solitary hyperfunctioning nodule.
  - Early stage of subacute thyroiditis (de Quervain).
  - Exogenous thyroid hormone.
  - Rarely, secondary hyperthyroidism due to pituitary tumor secreting TSH.

2. **Pathology**
- Normally, the thyroid gland secretes thyroxine (T_4) and triiodothyronine (T_3) under pituitary TSH stimulation, which in turn is stimulated by thyrotropin-releasing hormone (TRH) from the hypothalamus. The secretion of TRH and TSH is controlled by negative feedback from free thyroid T_4 and T_3.
- In hyperthyroidism, the production of thyroid hormones is unregulated or autonomous.
- Graves disease is caused by a thyroid-stimulating immunoglobulin.
- Another way to classify and understand hyperthyroidism is to evaluate the gland's activity, directly, by radioimmunoassay. When the thyroid's production and secretion activities are high (Graves disease, toxic goiter, solitary "hot" nodule), the RAIU is elevated. In subacute thyroiditis, RAIU is low; the gland is not actively producing hormone and the excess T_4 is due to the leakage of hormone caused by the inflammatory process. With exogenous thyroid hormone, RAIU also is low.

3. **Clinical Features**
- **Symptoms:**
  - Anxiety, irritability, restlessness, difficulty concentrating, insomnia, emotional lability, and tremor.
  - Weight loss despite increase in appetite; loose stools.
  - Dyspnea and palpitations.
  - Patients with underlying cardiovascular disease may develop angina and heart failure.
  - Increased sweating and heat intolerance.
  - Fatigue and weakness.
  - Excessive lacrimation and diplopia.
  - In elderly individuals, thyrotoxicosis can be asymptomatic; also, it may present only with atrial fibrillation, or as apathetic hyperthyroidism.
- **Physical examination:**
  - Hyperactivity, rapid speech, and anxious appearance.
  - Skin moist, warm, smooth; hair often fine in texture, alopecia may occur; pretibial myxedema.
  - Eye findings: retraction of upper lid (lid lag), exophthalmos (in Graves only), eye irritation; all may be asymmetric.
  - Fine tremor of tongue.
  - Hyperactive deep tendon reflexes, proximal muscle weakness.
  - Thyroid gland is usually enlarged (goiter); however, goiter may not be apparent in elderly patients or if thyroid gland is substernal. Absence of goiter does not rule out hyperthyroidism.
- **Characteristics of goiter vary with etiology:**
  - Graves disease: symmetrically enlarged, soft or firm, with smooth surface, possibly slight tenderness, venous hum, arterial bruit, or palpable thrill.
  - Toxic multinodular goiter: the gland may be larger than in Graves, asymmetric, firm, and irregular, with two or more discrete nodules.
  - Subacute thyroiditis: gland is moderately enlarged, tender, and asymmetric.
  - Absence of goiter suggests possibility of exogenous thyroid hormone.

4. **Diagnostic Studies**
- Increased serum thyroid hormones (T_3, T_4, or both), increased free T_4 and T_3 (free T_3 is a better indicator of hyperthyroidism than free T_4).
- In conditions with increased serum estrogen (pregnancy, estrogen therapy, acute hepatic process), thyroid-binding globulin is increased, possibly resulting in high serum T_4 or T_3; however, free thyroid hormone levels will be normal.
- TSH is suppressed.
- RAIU is elevated or low (see II. C. 2.).
- In Graves disease—TSH receptor antibodies and antimicrosomal antibodies are elevated.

5. **Management**
- **Medical treatment:**
  - Good response in patients with increased RAIU.
  - Propylthiouracil (PTU) and methimazole. Methimazole is generally preferred (less likely to cause hepatic necrosis). However, PTU is preferred in pregnant women because of methimazole association with fetal anomalies.
  - For symptom relief: β-adrenergic blockers (to decrease catecholamine effect).

- Radioactive iodine therapy (ablative): the treatment of choice in nonpregnant adults. Also safe in adolescents.
  - **Surgical treatment:**
    - Indicated for patients not responding to medical therapy, having contraindication to radioactive iodine (pregnancy), or not willing to take medication; also, for patients with large goiters and local symptoms (compression).

D. Thyroid Storm
1. **Etiology**
   - Uncommon form of thyrotoxicosis, life-threatening emergency.
   - Generally, precipitating factor is major stress or illness (e.g., surgery, infection, delivery, or trauma).
   - Mortality rate is high.
2. **Pathology**
   - Graves disease, multinodular goiter, or solitary hyperfunctioning nodule.
3. **Clinical Features**
   - Exaggerated signs and symptoms of thyrotoxicosis, including high fever, delirium, nausea, vomiting, dehydration, tremulousness, and anxiety.
   - Cardiovascular manifestations include atrial fibrillation with rapid ventricular response, hypotension, and death.
4. **Diagnostic Studies**
   - Highly elevated serum T_3 and T_4.
   - Electrocardiogram (ECG) may show sinus tachycardia, atrial fibrillation, or flutter.
5. **Management**
   - Aggressive approach using antithyroid medical therapy (methimazole or PTU).
   - Oral or intravenous (IV) sodium iodide to decrease thyroid hormone release.
   - Propranolol to block the peripheral cardiovascular effects of excess thyroid hormone.
   - Glucocorticoids to inhibit peripheral conversion of T_4 to T_3.
   - Supportive therapy and treatment of underlying illness.

E. Thyroid Nodules
1. **Etiology**
   - Common, increasing prevalence with increasing age.
   - Nodularity may be caused by any number of thyroid disorders, as well as some nonthyroid conditions.
   - Must consider cancer in 10% to 20% of cases.
2. **Pathology**
   - Adenomas, cysts, colloid nodules (the most common nodules), localized thyroiditis, and cancer (mostly papillary and follicular carcinoma).
3. **Clinical Features**
   - Most nodules, regardless of pathology, are asymptomatic; symptoms may arise from the compression of surrounding structures; may range from sensation of pressure to dysphagia.
   - Signs and symptoms of hyperthyroidism or hypothyroidism may occur.
   - Characteristics vary: smooth, firm, irregular, sharply outlined, discrete, multinodular, and usually painless.
   - Suspect cancer if rapid growth, fixed in place, with no movement on swallowing; other risk factors: prior head and neck irradiation, male gender, and extremes of age.
4. **Diagnostic Studies**
   - TSH, free T_4, to assess thyroid function.
   - Fine-needle aspiration cytology—the best method to assess for malignancy.
   - Ultrasound—baseline and follow-up.
   - CT scanning is helpful for larger nodules/multinodular goiters to assess for tracheal compression and local extension.
5. **Management**
   - Most important—exclude malignancy.
   - Treatment according to specific diagnosis, patient's age, presence or absence of symptoms, and suspicion of cancer.
   - For malignancy: surgery followed by thyroid radioiodine ablation.

III. Parathyroid Disorders

A. Primary Hyperparathyroidism
1. **Etiology**
   - Mostly adenoma of parathyroid glands, less frequently diffuse hyperplasia.
   - Occurs in some patients as part of multiple endocrine neoplasia (MEN) and in 20% of patients taking lithium.
2. **Pathology**
   - Parathyroid hormone (PTH) is oversecreted because of diminished inhibitory feedback from a reduced number of calcium-sensing receptors.
   - Excess PTH results in hypercalcemia directly (bone and renal action) and indirectly, by stimulating the synthesis of 1,25-dihydroxy-vitamin D.
   - By contrast, secondary hyperparathyroidism is caused by calcium and vitamin D deficiency (for renal causes see IV, C.) or by skeletal resistance to PTH action.
3. **Clinical Features**
   - Hypercalcemia (see Chapter 10, XX. C. 3.).
4. **Diagnostic Studies**
   - Serum calcium (total and/or ionized) elevated; also, increased urinary calcium.
   - Serum phosphorus decreased.
   - PTH (radioimmunoassay) elevated.
   - 1,25-Dihydroxy-vitamin D elevated.
   - Renal imaging may show renal stones.
   - Bone radiography—osteopenia.

5. **Management**
   - Treatment of hypercalcemia (see Chapter 10, XXI. C. 5.).
   - Criteria for surgical removal of the parathyroid gland or glands: symptomatic hypercalcemia, younger age, high level of hypercalcemia, osteoporosis, and kidney stones.

B. Hypoparathyroidism

1. **Etiology**
   - Follows parathyroid or thyroid surgery.
   - Can be autoimmune or induced by hypomagnesemia.
2. **Pathology**
   - Reduced PTH secretion results in hypocalcemia (decreased mobilization from bone, reduced renal reabsorption, and diminished 1,25-dihydroxy-vitamin D activation).
   - Pseudohypoparathyroidism—PTH level elevated, but tissues are resistant to its effect.
3. **Clinical Features**
   - Hypocalcemia (see Chapter 10, XXI. B. 3.).
4. **Diagnostic Studies**
   - Hypocalcemia (corrected for albumin), hyperphosphatemia, and low PTH level—diagnostic triad.
   - If magnesium is low, it indicates a reversible hypoparathyroidism.
5. **Management**
   - Treatment of hypocalcemia (see Chapter 10, XXI. B. 5.).

IV. Metabolic Bone Disorders

A. Osteoporosis

1. **Etiology**
   - Osteoporosis may be primary (postmenopausal and senile) or secondary, following a chronic disease.
   - Causes of secondary osteoporosis—hypogonadism in both genders, Cushing syndrome, thyrotoxicosis, hyperparathyroidism, immobilization, malignancy, multiple myeloma, DM, liver disease, celiac disease, heparin therapy, and anticonvulsant treatment.
   - Risk factors for postmenopausal osteoporosis—thin body habitus, Caucasian or Asian race, smoking, heavy alcohol use, low calcium and vitamin D diets, and physical inactivity.
2. **Pathology**
   - Osteoporosis is characterized by bone mass reduction in both mineral component and protein matrix.
   - Primary postmenopausal osteoporosis—mostly trabecular bone loss; results in vertebral compression fractures and fractures of the distal wrist.
   - Primary senile osteoporosis—age related, affecting both men and women—characterized by trabecular and cortical bone loss; increased risk of hip fractures.

3. **Clinical Features**
   - Usually asymptomatic; first symptom can be a fracture, back pain, or deformity.
   - Vertebral, hip, and distal radius (Colles) fractures (may occur with no trauma).
   - When spine compression occurs (mostly upper lumbar and middle thoracic), it results in shortening of stature, bowing of back (kyphosis), and forward thrust of head.
   - Chronic pain from vertebral body collapse is common and disabling.
4. **Diagnostic Studies**
   - Vitamin D deficiency is very common.
   - Serum calcium, phosphate, and PTH—normal.
   - Alkaline phosphatase—usually normal, but may be slightly elevated, especially following fracture.
   - Testing for thyrotoxicosis and hypogonadism may be required.
   - Screen for celiac disease with serum IgA antitissue transglutaminase and IgA antiendomysial antibodies.
   - X-ray of spine may show demineralization or compression of vertebrae.
   - X-ray of pelvis may show demineralization.
   - Dual-energy X-ray absorptiometry (DEXA) is quite accurate and delivers negligible radiation.
   - **Osteoporosis:** bone densitometry T score ≤–2.5; osteopenia: T score ≤–1.0 to –2.5
   - Quantitative CT delivers more radiation, but is highly accurate.
5. **Management**
   - True prophylaxis begins in adolescents, at the time of bone-density formation, with adequate calcium intake, vitamin D, and exercise.
   - Calcium citrate (0.4 to 0.7 g elemental calcium) or calcium carbonate (1.0 to 1.5 g elemental calcium) is taken once daily. Vitamin D_2 800–2000 international units once daily orally.
   - Bisphosphonates—mainstay of treatment.
   - Estrogen or raloxifene for women with hypogonadism.
   - Teriparatide; subQ bone forming agent.
   - Adequate diet/smoking cessation/avoid alcohol/increase exercise.
   - Discontinue or reduce corticosteroids.
   - Fall avoidance education.
   - Periodic measurements of patient's height and bone mass to assess disease progression.

B. Osteomalacia and Rickets

1. **Etiology**
   - Most frequently caused by inadequate levels of calcium and inorganic phosphorus because of vitamin D deficiency.
   - **Vitamin D deficiency:**
     - Lack of vitamin D (poor diet, malabsorption, pollution).
     - Defective activation of vitamin D (liver and renal disease, hypoparathyroidism).

- Tissue resistance to 1,25-dihydroxy-vitamin D (phenytoin).
- Other causes include calcium malabsorption, chronic hypophosphatemia, and systemic acidosis.
- Homebound elderly patients, who are unlikely to eat dairy products (inadequate dietary vitamin D) or go out in the sun, are at increased risk for osteomalacia.

2. **Pathology**
- In contrast to osteoporosis in which the decrease in bone mineral and matrix is proportional, osteomalacia is characterized by only decreased mineralization.
- Decreased deposition of calcium and phosphorus in the bone matrix leads to changes in the epiphyses (increased width) and the bone (cortical thinning).
- When defective mineralization occurs in childhood, before the closing of epiphyseal growth plates, the disease is called rickets. Osteomalacia develops in adults.

3. **Clinical Features**
- Manifestations depend on age of onset and severity.
- **Infants and young children:**
  - Features include irritability, delayed closure of fontanelles, growth retardation, and delayed dentition.
  - Enlargement of costal cartilages (rachitic rosary), bowing of long bones.
- **Adults:**
  - Osteomalacia is typically asymptomatic at first.
  - Symptoms include diffuse skeletal pain and proximal muscular weakness; pain may be localized to hip and result in antalgic gait.
  - Hypocalcemia leads to tetany, muscle wasting, and hypotonia.
  - Fractures occur with little or no trauma.

4. **Diagnostic Studies**
- Studies aimed at possible etiologies (i.e., renal function and serum PTH).
- Serum calcium and phosphate are low; alkaline phosphatase is high.
- 1,25-Dihydroxy-vitamin D may be low.
- In adult patients, radiographic images show osteopenia, transverse radiolucent markings (pseudofractures).

5. **Management**
- Treat underlying cause.
- Vitamin D (50,000 to 100,000 U per week) and calcium; monitor urinary calcium for adjustment of doses.
- Oral calcium supplements with meals.
- Calcitriol for cases of inactive vitamin D (patients with renal failure).
- Vitamin D resistance requires treatment with large doses of calcium and phosphorus.

C. Renal Osteodystrophy
1. **Etiology**
- Group of bone disorders (osteitis fibrosa and osteomalacia) present in patients with chronic renal failure.
- Bone disorders are caused by secondary hyperparathyroidism.

2. **Pathology**
- Failing kidneys do not eliminate phosphate properly and, at the same time, poorly synthesize 1,25-dihydroxy-vitamin D; these trigger a compensatory increase in PTH.
- Mineralization disorders such as subperiosteal erosions and osteoid production are features of pathologic PTH action on bone.

3. **Clinical Features**
- Bone and proximal muscle pain in a uremic context.
- Pathologic fractures especially of vertebrae, ribs, and long bones.

4. **Diagnostic Studies**
- Increased serum phosphate and decreased serum calcium; serum vitamin D level depends on the degree of renal failure.
- Bone turnover markers are not reliable because of altered renal clearance.
- Radiographic: subperiosteal erosion, cystic (brown tumor) and fibrous anomalies of long bones.

5. **Management**
- Goal is to normalize serum phosphate and calcium levels, and, indirectly, PTH.
- Phosphate binders are used to decrease phosphate level.
- When phosphate level is controlled, calcium supplements can also include vitamin D.
- Correction of acidosis is also important.

D. Paget Disease
1. **Etiology**
- Possible consequence of a slow viral infection; genetic analyses support autosomal dominant inheritance.
- Mainly affects persons of western European descent.
- Clinical presentation before age 40 is unusual.

2. **Pathology**
- Characterized by increased formation and resorption of bone (rapid turnover).
- The lysed bone is replaced by the formation of dense trabecular bone with abnormal architecture. This process can remain localized or extend to an entire bone, or multiple bones.
- The remodeled bone has areas of weakening producing fractures and, due to its enlargement, compresses neural structures (i.e., cranial nerve VIII).

3. **Clinical Features**
- Asymptomatic patients are usually discovered as a result of an elevated alkaline phosphatase on screening, or during routine radiographic procedures.

- Symptomatic patients experience pain (predominant complaint) in the back or lower extremities, gait disturbances, increasing head size, and hearing loss.
- Common bones involved are pelvis, femur, skull, tibia, and lumbosacral spine.
- Complications—hypercalcemia, hypercalciuria, nephrolithiasis, high-output cardiac failure secondary to the increased skeletal vascularity, and osteosarcoma.

  4. **Diagnostic Studies**
     - Marked elevated serum alkaline phosphatase due to increased osteoblastic activity. Serum calcium and phosphorous typically normal.
     - Increased urinary excretion of hydroxyproline due to increased bone resorption; this test has been replaced with the detection of urinary pyridinolines or *N*-telopeptide.
     - Increased uptake on technetium bone scan, even before diagnostic changes are visible on X-ray.
     - Radiographic changes: initially—lytic lesions; later—coarser, chaotic, denser cortical bone with deformity and possible fractures.
     - X-ray abnormalities are most often seen in the pelvis, femur, and skull.

  5. **Management**
     - Asymptomatic patients, in general, require no treatment; newer guidelines require that in patients with increased bone turnover markers, therapy with bisphosphonates should be started.
     - Indications for treatment include pain, neurologic complications, fractures, hypercalcemia, and high cardiac output.
     - Aspirin and NSAIDs are used for mild-to-moderate bone pain and joint discomfort.
     - Bone resorption can be decreased with bisphosphonates and calcitonin, ensuring longer remissions.
     - Orthotic and orthopedic measures.

V. Adrenal Cortex Disorders

A. Adrenocortical Insufficiency (Addison Disease)

  1. **Etiology**
     - Primary disease (Addison disease)—insufficiency of the adrenal cortex.
     - Secondary adrenal insufficiency is due to deficient ACTH; tertiary form of disease is produced by low levels of corticotropin-releasing factor.

  2. **Pathology**
     - Progressive destruction of the adrenal gland.
     - Primary adrenocortical insufficiency is usually autoimmune process, involving all zones of the cortex, and can be associated with other autoimmune diseases. Secondary adrenocortical insufficiency appears commonly when glucocorticoid therapy is interrupted abruptly.

- Deficiency of all adrenocortical hormones: glucocorticoids, mineralocorticoids, androgens in primary adrenocortical insufficiency, and only glucocorticoids in secondary insufficiency.
- Main glucocorticoid hormone—cortisol; its deficiency affects intermediary metabolism, vascular tone, water balance, and inflammation.
- Most important mineralocorticoid—aldosterone (part of renin-angiotensin-aldosterone system); its decrease leads to changes in sodium and potassium balance. In secondary adrenocortical insufficiency, aldosterone is relatively normal.

  3. **Clinical Features**
     - Weakness, fatigue, anorexia, nausea and vomiting, abdominal pain, and weight loss.
     - Hypotension with postural drop and hypoglycemia may occur.
     - Cortisol insufficiency may cause inability to withstand surgical stress, trauma, and infection, and result in vascular collapse.
     - Aldosterone deficiency manifests by increased renal sodium loss, failure to adequately excrete potassium (neuromuscular and cardiac dysfunction), and associated volume depletion (dehydration).
     - Adrenal androgen deficiency is not significant in adults.
     - Hyperpigmentation is an important characteristic, typical to primary adrenocortical insufficiency, and present on extensor surfaces of extremities, buccal mucosa, genitalia, nipples, palmar creases, and knuckles.

  4. **Diagnostic Studies**
     - Cosyntropin stimulation is the major test for diagnosis.
     - Low morning plasma cortisol; low aldosterone levels; elevated plasma ACTH levels in Addison disease.
     - Also, in primary adrenal insufficiency—hyponatremia, hyperkalemia, metabolic acidosis.
     - Eosinophilia, normochromic normocytic anemia.
     - Secondary adrenocortical insufficiency: low level of ACTH and cortisol.

  5. **Management**
     - Acute, emergent phase with cardiovascular collapse: high-dose glucocorticoid therapy (hydrocortisone, 100 mg IV, TID).
     - Long-term management: glucocorticoid replacement therapy (prednisone and hydrocortisone) and mineralocorticoid replacement (fludrocortisone), in Addison disease.

B. Hypercortisolism (Cushing Syndrome)

  1. **Etiology**
     - Results from excessive levels of glucocorticoids.
     - Endogenous causes include ACTH-secreting pituitary tumor (Cushing disease), autonomous adrenal adenoma or hyperplasia, adrenal carcinoma, ectopic production of ACTH, and

ectopic production of corticotropin-releasing hormone.

- Exogenous cause—the most common—is the result of chronic glucocorticoid treatment.

2. **Pathology**
   - Usually, the endogenous cause is bilateral adrenal hyperplasia secondary to an ACTH pituitary secreting tumor.
   - Sustained increase in cortisol with loss of diurnal rhythm.
   - Hypercortisolism results in decreased protein synthesis, increased protein catabolism, nitrogen wasting, glucose intolerance, and changes in mineral metabolism.

3. **Clinical Features**
   - Hypertension.
   - Weight gain with central obesity, but slender extremities, "moon" facies, "buffalo hump," and fat pads in supraclavicular area.
   - Easy fatigue, muscle weakness, and wasting.
   - Easy bruising, poor wound healing, and purple abdominal striae.
   - Thinning of scalp hair, acne, and hirsutism.
   - Diminished libido, menstrual irregularities, and infertility in men.
   - Emotion disturbances (e.g., depression, psychosis, mania).
   - Osteoporosis due to inhibition of osteoblasts and stimulation of osteoclasts.

4. **Diagnostic Studies**
   - Baseline 24-hour urinary free cortisol elevation.
   - ACTH level, overnight low-dose dexamethasone suppression test, and studies for elevated late afternoon cortisol level (loss of physiologic dip) are additional screening tools.
   - Diagnostic—high-dose overnight dexamethasone suppression test.
   - Radiologic studies (MRI) for pituitary gland and adrenal enlargement and ectopic site; chest X-ray (CXR) for ectopic site, and DEXA scan for the evaluation of bone involvement.

5. **Management**
   - If exogenous—removal of agent or use of lowest dose possible.
   - If endogenous—surgical intervention on source, medication if inoperable (ketoconazole), or both.

C. Hyperaldosteronism

1. **Etiology**
   - Aldosterone-producing adrenal adenomas (65%) and bilateral adrenal hyperplasia (35%).
   - Useful to contrast Conn syndrome (primary hyperaldosteronism) with secondary hyperaldosteronism; the latter is caused by increased renin.

2. **Pathology**
   - Primary hypersecretion of aldosterone causes hypertension and hypokalemia.
   - Elevated aldosterone increases sodium reabsorption by the kidneys, resulting in the expansion of plasma volume.
   - Sodium reabsorption in exchange for potassium and hydrogen ions results in hypokalemia and metabolic alkalosis, respectively.
   - Secondary hyperaldosteronism appears in the context of high renin secretion due to renal artery stenosis and any clinical situation with decreased renal perfusion (CHF, hypovolemia), although in the latter, there is no hypertension.

3. **Clinical Features**
   - Usually, no specific symptoms.
   - Hypokalemia and hypertension.
   - Patients with primary hyperaldosteronism, despite vascular expansion, have no edema.
   - Paresthesias, proximal muscle weakness, fatigue, and decreased or absent deep tendon reflexes due to hypokalemia.

4. **Diagnostic Studies**
   - Hypokalemia with metabolic alkalosis.
   - Aldosterone/renin ratio screening in patients with hypertension.
   - Hypomagnesemia.
   - ECG changes consistent with hypokalemia (e.g., prominent U waves).
   - Low plasma renin level in primary hyperaldosteronism and high renin in the secondary form.
   - CT scan and MRI to assess adrenal or extra-adrenal mass.
   - Adrenal vein sampling is a sensitive localization technique for the measurement of aldosterone.

5. **Management**
   - Surgical intervention—treatment of choice for aldosterone-producing adenomas; angioplasty in renal artery stenosis.
   - Antihypertensive medication—spironolactone, angiotensin-converting enzyme (ACE) inhibitors, and calcium channel blockers.
   - Correct electrolyte abnormalities.

VI. Disorders of Adrenal Medulla

A. Pheochromocytoma

1. **Etiology**
   - Benign—90%; malignant—10%.
   - 0.1% to 0.5% of hypertensive patients.
   - Can be part of MEN syndromes.

2. **Pathology**
   - Tumor of chromaffin tissue from adrenal medulla that secretes catecholamines.
   - Synthesizes norepinephrine and epinephrine autonomously.
   - Paroxysmal catecholamine release may be triggered by surgery, exercise, pregnancy, and medication (tricyclic antidepressants [TCAs], opiates, metoclopramide).

3. **Clinical Features**
   - Hypertension—most consistent finding; may be sustained or acutely elevated. Hypertension due to pheochromocytoma is classically associated with paroxysmal headaches, profuse sweating, and palpitations.
   - Other symptoms—chest and abdominal pain, nausea, weakness, fatigue, weight loss (despite increased appetite).

4. **Diagnostic Studies**
   - Screening—measuring of increased 24-hour urinary excretion of catecholamines or their metabolites—metanephrines and vanillylmandelic acid.
   - Plasma catecholamines are particularly increased during a hypertensive episode.
   - MRI to visualize the tumor.

5. **Management**
   - Surgical excision, unless widespread metastases or patients with unacceptable surgical risk.
   - Before surgery, α-adrenergic blockade (phenoxybenzamine and phentolamine), *followed by* β-adrenergic blocking agents; calcium channel blockers (nifedipine) may be used to control hypertension.

VII. Diabetes Mellitus and Hypoglycemia

A. Diabetes Mellitus

1. **Etiology**
   a. **Type 1 Diabetes**
      - Pancreatic islet β-cell destruction by an autoimmune process, resulting in complete lack of insulin.
      - Type 1 diabetes is part of human leukocyte antigen associated immune-mediated diseases; not genetically predetermined, but increased susceptibility may be inherited.
      - Disease of juveniles, usual onset before age 30.
      - Environmental factors—viruses, chemicals, toxins—may act as triggers in genetically predisposed persons.
   b. **Type 2 Diabetes**
      - More than 90% of patients with diabetes in the United States have type 2 DM.
      - Epidemiologic data suggest a strong genetic influence and a familial character.

2. **Pathology**
   a. **Type 1 Diabetes**
      - Autoimmune process destroys pancreatic islet β-cells' secretion; absolute deficiency of insulin results in the accumulation of circulating glucose and fatty acids, associated with hyperosmolality and hyperketonemia.
      - Hyperglycemia induces osmotic diuresis; also, without insulin, accelerated breakdown of muscle mass and fat.

   - Dehydration and metabolic acidosis (ketoacidosis).
   b. **Type 2 Diabetes**
      - Tissue insensitivity to insulin; other contributing mechanisms: β-cell dysfunction, abnormality in postprandial glucose metabolism (impaired glucose tolerance), and excessive hepatic glucose production.
      - Obesity appears to be a cofactor in 75% to 80% of patients.
      - Maturity-onset diabetes of the young is a rare disorder, characterized by onset before age 25 years, in nonobese patients of non–insulin-dependent DM secondary to impaired glucose-induced secretion of insulin.
      - Insulin resistance—syndrome X; metabolic syndrome; chronic hypertension, atherosclerosis, central obesity, and stroke (CHAOS)—is seen in obese patients with glucose intolerance, hyperinsulinemia, and dyslipidemia. This syndrome is a precursor of diabetes; it carries a greatly increased cardiovascular risk; the major features are the central obesity and insulin resistance.

3. **Clinical Features**
   a. **Type 1 Diabetes**
      - Manifestations may have acute or subacute presentation.
      - During exacerbations: anorexia, nausea and vomiting, alteration of consciousness, diaphoresis.
   b. **Type 2 Diabetes**
      - Often asymptomatic.
      - Occasionally, with prolonged "occult" DM (blood sugars not high enough to cause symptoms), patients may already have vascular or neuropathic complications at the time of diagnosis.
      - Obesity with increased waist-to-hip ratio.
   c. **Common Features**
      - Polyuria, polydipsia, and polyphagia (3 Ps).
      - Weakness.
      - Peripheral neuropathy: paresthesia and neuropathic ulcers.
      - Autonomic neuropathy: nausea, vomiting, diarrhea, constipation, and impotence.
      - Eruptive xanthomas (when triglycerides reach high levels) on flexor surfaces of limbs and buttocks; chronic skin infections.
      - Loss of subcutaneous fat and muscle wasting, especially in poorly controlled type 1 DM.
      - Blurred vision.
      - Recurrent vulvovaginitis (candidiasis).

4. **Diagnostic Studies**
   a. **Diagnostic Criteria**
      - Fasting plasma glucose (FPG) <100 mg per dL (5.6 mmol per L) is normal; FPG 100 to 125 mg per dL indicates impaired fasting glucose;

FPG ≥126 mg per dL (7.0 mmol per dL) shows presence of diabetes.

- Random plasma glucose ≥200 mg per dL and the presence of symptoms indicate DM.
- Glycosylated hemoglobin (HbA1c) measurements reflect the state of glycemia over the preceding 8 to 12 weeks. HbA1c <5.7 is normal. HbA1c 5.7 to 6.4 indicates impaired glucose tolerance ("prediabetes"). HbA1c ≥6.5% indicates DM.
- Urinalysis may show ketonuria.

b. Criteria for Screening for Type 2 Diabetes in High-Risk Populations
- Screen all adults with cardiovascular disease, hypertension, dyslipidemia, or other risk factors for cardiovascular disease.
- Screen patients who, on previous tests, had impaired glucose tolerance or impaired fasting glucose.
- Consider screening adults with risk factors for type 2 DM (family history of DM, obesity, gestational DM, polycystic ovarian syndrome, or membership in high risk ethnic groups—African Americans, Hispanic Americans, American Indians, and Asian and Pacific Islanders).

c. Other Studies
- Microalbuminuria; albumin/creatinine ratio for glomerular evaluation. Assess electrolytes.
- Lipid profile, in insulin-resistance syndrome, shows elevated triglycerides, decreased high-density lipoprotein (HDL), and elevated LDL levels.
- Evaluate cardiac function and peripheral vessels.
- TSH (type 1 DM only)—higher incidence of autoimmune thyroid disease in these patients.
- Eye examinations—annual from the time of diagnosis for type 2 DM, and beginning 5 years after the diagnosis of type 1 DM.
- Refer to podiatrist for the treatment of calluses and deformities and for advice on footwear.

5. Management
a. Goals of Therapy
- Relieve symptoms due to hyperglycemia (3 Ps), and prevent/delay progression of complications; importance of early therapeutic intervention and aggressive follow-ups.
- To prevent morbidity and mortality, management in diabetes involves teamwork: primary provider, nutritionist, podiatrist, ophthalmologist, social worker, and psychologist.

b. Diet
- Major part of the treatment.
- Personalized according to the type of diabetes (type 2, due to obesity, usually needs low-calorie diet), age of the patient (adolescents need increased protein intake), and cultural background.

- Carbohydrates should provide 50% to 60% of total calories, proteins—15% to 20%, and the remainder should be from fat (<10% saturated fat, low cholesterol).

c. Insulin Therapy
- Absolute requirement in type 1 and sometimes used in type 2 diabetes.
- Insulin replacement using the regimen most appropriate to the patient.
- Insulin preparations include rapid acting (lispro, aspart, glulisine), short acting (regular), intermediate acting Neutral Protamine Hagedorn, or Isophane Insulin (NPH), long acting (detemir, glargine), and mixed, short/intermediate acting (70/30, 75/25, 50/50).
- Insulin is delivered subcutaneously, by injection or by infusion pumps.
- Self-monitoring of blood glucose is recommended for all patients with type 1 diabetes and should be strongly considered for patients with type 2 diabetes on insulin.
- Patient education about insulin-induced hypoglycemia.
- **Other insulin therapy complications:**
  - Somogyi phenomenon—rebound hyperglycemia following hypoglycemia; due to activation of counterregulatory systems for hypoglycemia.
  - Dawn phenomenon—early morning rise in glycemia not preceded by hypoglycemia; mediated by nocturnal secretion of GH; correct with later evening administration of slow-acting insulin.

d. Oral Antihyperglycemic Agents
- Insulin secretagogues—sulfonylureas, meglitinides, and amino acid derivatives.
- Insulin sensitizer—thiazolidinediones.
- Decreased hepatic glucose output—biguanides. (Metformin is usually considered the first-line drug for most patients.)
- Decreased glucose absorption—α-glucosidase inhibitors.

e. Incretins and Others
- GLP-1 receptor agonists (incretins): these drugs amplify glucose-induced insulin release—exenatide and liraglutide are given by subcutaneous injection.
- DPP-4 inhibitors (incretins): these drugs prolong the action of endogenous GLP-1—sitagliptin and saxagliptin are given PO.
- Others: a synthetic analogue of the human β-cell hormone, amylin—pramlintide is given subcutaneously.

f. Complementary Therapy
- As important as treating hyperglycemia is the treatment of dyslipidemia (statins) and hypertension (especially with ACE inhibitors, which are also beneficial for patients with microalbuminuria).

g. **Patient Education**
- How to administer insulin and how to do home glucose monitoring, even without insulin therapy (patient should maintain a log and bring it to each appointment).
- Signs or symptoms of hyperglycemia or hypoglycemia.
- Pathogenesis and progression of the disease and its complications.
- Lifestyle changes—exercise program, diet, weight loss (especially for patients with type 2 diabetes), and smoking cessation.

6. **Chronic Complications**
  a. **Macrovascular Complications**
  - Cardiovascular—hypertension, myocardial ischemia, and infarction.
  - Cerebrovascular—stroke and transient ischemic attacks.
  - Peripheral vascular disease (PVD).
  - In type 2 diabetes, clinical manifestations of macrovascular complications can appear even before 3 Ps.
  - Risk factors—duration of disease, increased age, hypertension, hyperinsulinemia, obesity, hypertriglyceridemia, proteinuria, increased LDL, and low HDL.
  - Pathologic mechanism—accelerated atherosclerosis and vascular thrombosis.
  - Imperative to treat early and aggressively to decrease the severity of complications.
  - Hypertension—ACE inhibitors or angiotensin receptor blockers (also, for kidney protection); all other antihypertensive classes including β-blockers (also, secondary prevention of myocardial infarction). Target blood pressure: <130/80.
  - Procoagulation state may benefit from low dose of aspirin.
  - Statins for dyslipidemia. LDL goal <100 (<70 if multiple cardiovascular risk factors).
  - Smoking cessation, treat obesity.
  b. **Microvascular Complications**
    1. **Diabetic retinopathy affects nearly all patients with type 1 diabetes and 80% with type 2, leading cause of blindness in highly developed countries.**
    - Diabetic eye disease can present as nonproliferative/proliferative retinopathy, macular edema, and premature cataracts.
    - Annual ophthalmologist appointments (dilated examination and laser therapy).
    2. **Diabetic nephropathy is the leading cause of premature death in young patients and the most common cause of end-stage renal disease in developed countries.**
    - Pathologic mechanisms—glomerular damage (sclerosis) and ischemic changes in the nephron's vasculature.

- Earliest sign—microalbuminuria (at this stage, renal function is still normal).
- The stage of persistent proteinuria can progress to nephrotic syndrome with peripheral edema, hypoalbuminemia, and decline in glomerular filtration rate.
- Frequently associated with normochromic, normocytic anemia, and hypertension.
- Importance of regular checkups; ACE inhibitors when microalbuminuria appears.
- Women with diabetes have an increased risk of developing ascending urinary tract infections (bladder stasis due to autonomic neuropathy).
    3. **Diabetic neuropathy presents in several varieties: distal symmetric, mainly sensorial polyneuropathy ("stocking-glove"); acute painful neuropathy; mononeuropathy (cranial nerves, isolated peripheral nerve); and autonomic neuropathy.**
    - Autonomic neuropathy clinically manifests as postural hypotension, gastroparesis (nausea, vomiting), diarrhea, bladder stasis, and impotence.
    - Diabetic foot—peripheral neuropathy, ischemia, and infection combine in producing tissue necrosis. Podiatrist appointments; careful feet examination at home.
    4. **Other Complications**
    - Diabetic amyotrophy: especially in older men, painful wasting of quadriceps.
    - Skin: necrobiosis diabetica, *Candida* infections; sometimes vitiligo, acanthosis.
    - Chronic infections are a marker of poor glycemic control; can affect skin, gastrointestinal tract, urinary tract, and lungs.
    - Bone and joints: signs of osteopenia; osteoporosis can develop in both genders.

7. **Acute Complications**
  a. **Diabetic Ketoacidosis**
    1. **Etiology**
    - Results from uncontrolled diabetes, and presents most commonly in patients with DM type 1; also can be seen in type 2 diabetes, during acute illness.
    - If hyperglycemia is not present, other causes of anion gap metabolic acidosis—uremia, salicylates, poisoning with alcohols (i.e., methanol), and lactic acidosis—must be considered.
    2. **Pathology**
    - Hyperglycemia associated with ketosis and high anion gap metabolic acidosis.
    3. **Clinical Features**
    - Recent onset of polyuria, polydipsia, nocturia, fatigue, weight loss, abdominal pain and tenderness, nausea, and vomiting.

- Decreased level of consciousness.
- Kussmaul breathing due to acidosis and acetone breath.
- Orthostatic hypotension with tachycardia, poor skin turgor, indicating dehydration.
- Signs and symptoms of precipitating illness.

4. **Diagnostic Studies**
   - Elevated serum glucose level (>250 mg per dL).
   - High anion gap metabolic acidosis, elevated serum acetone, elevated serum phosphate, mild-to-moderate hyperkalemia (despite total body potassium depletion), and mild-to-moderate hyponatremia (if thirst is maintained).
   - Volume depletion, associated with elevated hematocrit and azotemia.
   - Urine, blood, and throat cultures.
   - Diagnostic studies are appropriate for the precipitating illness.

5. **Management**
   - Fluid replacement—first priority; with monitoring of pH, and glucose.
   - Therapy with regular insulin—should be initiated as needed, either by infusion or intramuscular (IM); monitor and supplement potassium level.
   - Treatment of underlying cause (e.g., infection) is essential.

b. **Hyperglycemic Hyperosmolar State**
   1. **Etiology**
      - Hyperglycemic hyperosmolar state occurs almost exclusively in type 2 DM.
      - Severe hyperglycemia in the absence of ketosis/acidosis.
      - Profound dehydration due to intense osmotic diuresis from high-level hyperglycemia.
      - Often, precipitating factor, such as infection; elderly and physically impaired patients with limited access to free water.

   2. **Pathology**
      - Main mechanism—severe hyperosmolality and intense dehydration.
      - Minimal levels of insulin prevent appearance of ketosis.

   3. **Clinical Features**
      - Insidious onset (days to weeks).
      - Polyuria, polydipsia, nocturia, weight loss, and malaise.
      - Altered sensorium, progressing to coma.
      - Patients appear severely ill and dehydrated (dry mucous membranes and poor skin turgor).
      - Mortality rate >50%.

   4. **Diagnostic Studies**
      - Serum glucose levels demonstrate severe hyperglycemia (600 to 2,000 mg per dL).

- Significantly elevated serum osmolality (>320 mOsm per L).
- Absence of ketones (blood pH > 7.3).
- Low levels of potassium.
- Lactic acidosis indicates a poor prognosis.
- Complete blood count, arterial blood gases, blood and urine cultures, CXR, and other studies should be incorporated to find underlying precipitant and guide therapy.

5. **Management**
   - Fluid and electrolytes replacement—mainstay of management.
   - Insulin is required.
   - Antibiotics—if underlying infection exists.

B. **Hypoglycemia**
   1. **Etiology**
      - Hypoglycemia occurs when insulin is highly relative to the level of endogenous or exogenous supply of glucose.
      - Common cause is iatrogenic—in type 1 DM, excessive administered dose of insulin; in type 2 DM, sulfonylurea side effect.
      - Reactive (postprandial) hypoglycemia develops a few hours after eating is characterized by the presence of adrenergic symptoms, and is a rare condition.
      - Fasting hypoglycemia can be caused by hepatic failure, adrenocortical insufficiency, ethanol, insulinomas, and surreptitious administration of insulin or sulfonylureas.

   2. **Pathology**
      - Body tissues require glucose to maintain integrity and function.
      - Without adequate glucose levels, organ dysfunction develops acutely (especially CNS).

   3. **Clinical Features**
      - Symptoms begin at plasma levels of 60 mg per dL; brain function is impaired at approximately 50 mg per dL.
      - Coma and death can develop rapidly.
      - **Sympathetic response is characterized by:**
        - Hunger, diaphoresis, and anxiety.
        - Palpitations and tachycardia.
        - Tremulousness, weakness, and tingling around the mouth/fingers.
      - **Neuroglycopenic symptoms:**
        - Altered mental status and focal neurologic deficits.
        - Blurred vision and headaches.
        - Incoordination and difficulty speaking.
        - Seizure and coma.

   4. **Diagnostic Studies**
      - Low plasma glucose levels.
      - Elevated insulin level indicates insulinoma or exogenous insulin source. In endogenous source—insulinoma—C peptide is elevated.
      - Also, high levels of sulfonylureas.

5. Management
- Hypoglycemia is life-threatening.
- Emergency treatment for symptomatic hypoglycemia requires IV infusion of glucose (if patient is unable to take oral glucose), or glucagon given subcutaneously or IM.
- Glucagon stimulates endogenous glucose production.
- When patient is stable, high carbohydrate meal may be given.
- Assess for the cause of episode, including medications, diet, physical activity, and alcohol.
- Small, frequent meals (minimal amount of simple sugars) for reactive hypoglycemic patients.
- Treat underlying disorders (e.g., liver and renal disease), if present.
- Adjust oral hypoglycemic agents/insulin as required.
- Surgery for pancreatic tumor.

VIII. Obesity

A. Etiology
- One of the most common disorders in medical practice.
- Multifaceted disorder in which energy intake exceeds expenditure; lipid storage enhanced, mostly in adipose tissue.
- Obesity has a strong genetic predisposition and is influenced by sedentary lifestyle.

B. Pathology
- Increased total body fat; enlarged fat cells.
- Several mechanisms involved—enzymatic (lipoprotein lipase), hormonal (leptin), neuromediators in hypothalamus.

C. Clinical Features
- The most used indicator of obesity is the body mass index—BMI: weight/(height)^2. Values are measured in kg per m^2.
- BMI 25 to 29.9—overweight; BMI 30 to 34.9—class I obesity; BMI 35 to 39.9—class II obesity; BMI >40—class III (extreme/morbid) obesity.
- **Patients may complain of:**
  - Fatigue, shortness of breath, large joint pain, and ambulating difficulty.
  - Recurrent fungal infection under the skin folds (e.g., breast and groin).
  - Excessive accumulation of subcutaneous adipose tissue, with occasional "yellow striae.
  - Pattern of obesity—may vary from truncal distribution without limb involvement to involvement of every segment of the body.
  - Fat deposition pattern affects health risks (e.g., increased abdominal fat correlates with the risk of heart disease).
  - In severe/morbid obesity—chronic hypoventilation, left ventricular dysfunction, and arrhythmias.
- Serious psychosocial consequences.

D. Diagnostic Studies
- Laboratory abnormalities may include hyperlipidemia and glucose intolerance.
- Pertinent studies to rule out other causes may be warranted (i.e., glucocorticoid excess, tumors of hypothalamus and pituitary, hypothyroidism).

E. Management
- If assessment reveals excessive intake, nutritional factors and exercise are mainstays of therapy.
- Investigate insulin resistance and treat accordingly.
- Anorectic medications should be used cautiously.
- Underlying causes or complications should be identified and managed.
- Aggressive health care provider monitoring and support.
- For morbid obesity, bariatric surgery may be indicated.

IX. Multiple Endocrine Neoplasia

A. Etiology
- A group of familial disorders that affect multiple endocrine organs.

B. Pathology
- Autosomal dominant chromosomal abnormalities lead to hyperplasia or neoplasms.
- Types of multiple endocrine neoplasia (MEN; by organ affected):
  - 1: Wermer syndrome: Parathyroids (90% of patients with this disorder), pituitary adenoma, and pancreatic tumors—secreting insulin, gastrin, vasoactive intestinal polypeptide, and serotonin.
  - 2a: Sipple syndrome: Thyroid (medullary carcinoma producing calcitonin), parathyroids, adrenals (pheochromocytoma), and Hirschsprung disease.
  - 2b: Same tumors as type 2a, but less preponderance of parathyroid hyperplasia; also, patients with MEN 2b have a marfanoid habitus and multiple neuromas.

C. Clinical Features
- Clinical manifestations depend on the endocrine dysfunctions.

D. Diagnostic Studies
- Patients who have neoplasms in one of these glands should be evaluated for MEN syndromes (also, review family history).
  - Type 1: Measure PTH and calcium levels; image pancreas and pituitary.
  - Type 2a: Measure PTH, urinary catecholamines, and calcitonin; image adrenals.
  - Type 2b: Same as type IIa, plus mucosal neuromas and marfanoid features.

E. Management
- Treat identified neoplasia with surgery if possible—for example, parathyroidectomy.

- Cinacalcet orally is effective for hyperparathyroidism (MEN 1).
- Prevention is aimed toward screening first-degree relatives.

X. Paraneoplastic Endocrine Syndromes

A. Etiology

- Paraneoplastic endocrine syndromes are consequences of remote effects of cancer due to ectopic hormone secretion (approximately 10% of patients with advanced malignancies).

B. Pathology

- **Most common ectopic hormones:**
  - ACTH produced by small cell lung cancer and other carcinoids.
  - ADH secreted in primary lung cancers (small cell); rarely, prostate and cervical cancers.
  - PTH-related protein from squamous cell lung cancer.

C. Clinical Features

- Cushing syndrome (see V. B. 3.).
- SIADH (see I. B. 2. c.).
- Hypercalcemia of malignant disease; in cases of breast cancer and myeloma, hypercalcemia is produced by local osteolytic factors.

D. Diagnostic Studies

- Diagnosis is suggested by new endocrine symptoms in patients with known cancers.
- The most common cause of hypercalcemia, after primary hyperparathyroidism, is malignancy; therefore, if hypercalcemia is present, but serum PTH is low, malignancy must be sought.

E. Management

- Treatment of underlying cause is the main objective.
- Symptomatic relief with medications specific to each hormonal disorder.

SELECTED REFERENCES

American Diabetes Association. Standards of medical care in diabetes—2010 [position statement]. *Diabetes Care.* 2010;33:S11–S61. doi:10.2337/dc10-S011.

Barnett P, Braunstein G. Diabetes mellitus. In: Andreoli TE, ed. *Cecil Essentials of Medicine.* 5th ed. Philadelphia, PA: WB Saunders; 2001:583–598.

Bouknight AL. Thyroid physiology and thyroid function testing. *Otolaryngol Clin North Am.* 2003;36(1):9–15.

Bringhurst FR, Finkelstein JS, Seton MP. Diseases of bone and bone mineral metabolism. In: Andreoli TE, ed. *Cecil Essentials of Medicine.* 5th ed. Philadelphia, PA: WB Saunders; 2001:627–665.

Burch HB. Hyperthyroidism (thyrotoxicosis). Physicians' Information and Education Resource (pier), American College of Physicians; 2011. http://pier.acponline.org/physicians/diseases/d175/d175.html. Accessed June 6, 2011.

Bushardt RL, Turner JL, Ragucci KR, et al. Non-estrogen treatments for osteoporosis: an evidence-based review. *JAAPA.* 2006;19(12):25–30.

http://www.jaapa.com/issues/j20061201/articles/osteo1206.htm. Accessed June 19, 2007.

Cranney A, Wells GA. Hormone replacement therapy for postmenopausal osteoporosis. *Clin Geriatr Med.* 2003;19(2):361–370.

Drury PL, Howlett TA. Other endocrine diseases; diseases of many glands. In: Kumar P, Clark M, eds. *Clinical Medicine.* 5th ed. Edinburgh, Scotland: WB Saunders; 2002:1067–1068.

Evans T. Hyperthyroidism. In: Moser RL, ed. *Primary Care for Physician Assistants.* 1st ed. New York, NY: McGraw-Hill; 1998:171–173.

Fitzgerald PA. Endocrine disorders. In: Tierney LM Jr, McPhee SJ, Papadakis MA, eds. *Current Medical Diagnosis & Treatment.* 50th ed. Stamford, CT: Lange; 2011:1050–1138.

Herman-Bonert V, Friedman TC, Braunstein GD, et al. Endocrine disease. In: Andreoli TE, ed. *Cecil Essentials of Medicine.* 5th ed. Philadelphia, PA: WB Saunders; 2001:543–604.

Jochen AL, O'Shaughnessy IM. Diseases of parathyroid glands, vitamin D metabolism, and calcium homeostasis; metabolic bone disease. In: Kutty K, Shapira RM, Van Ruiswyk J, eds. *Kochar's Concise Textbook of Medicine.* 4th ed. Philadelphia, PA: Lippincott Williams & Wilkins; 2003:380–392.

Loriaux DL, Klein R, Ahmann AJ, et al. Endocrinology, metabolism, and genetics. In: Humes HD, ed. *Kelley's Essentials of Internal Medicine.* 2nd ed. Philadelphia, PA: Lippincott Williams & Wilkins; 2001:724–784.

Masharani U. Diabetes mellitus and hypoglycemia. In: Tierney LM Jr, McPhee SJ, Papadakis MA, eds. *Current Medical Diagnosis & Treatment.* 50th ed. Stamford, CT: Lange; 2011:1140–1188.

McDermott MT. Hypothyroidism. Physicians' Information and Education Resource (pier), American College of Physicians; 2011. http://pier.acponline.org/physicians/diseases/d238/d238.html. Accessed June 6, 2011.

Meunier, PJ, Kream BE, Lorenzo JA. Metabolic bone disease. In: Larsen PR, Kronenberg HM, Melmed S, et al, eds. *Williams Textbook of Endocrinology.* 10th ed. Philadelphia, PA: WB Saunders; 1993:1378–1398.

Neumann HPH. Pheochromocytoma. In: Fauci AS, Braunwald E, Kasper DL, et al, eds. *Harrison's Principles of Internal Medicine.* 17th ed. New York, NY: McGraw Hill; 2008:chap 337:2269–2275.

North American Menopause Society. Management of osteoporosis in postmenopausal women: 2006 position statement of the North American Menopause Society. *Menopause.* 2006;13(3):340–367. http://www.guideline.gov/summary/summary.aspx?doc_id=9399. Accessed June 19, 2007.

Nussbaum SR. Approach to the patient with hypercalcemia. In: Goroll AH, May LA, Mulley AG Jr, eds. *Primary Care Medicine.* 3rd ed. Philadelphia, PA: JB Lippincott; 1995:534–539.

Paauw DS, Burkholder LR, Migeon MB, eds. Thyroid disease. In: *Guide to Internal Medicine.* 1st ed. St Louis, MO: Mosby-Year Book; 1999:128–131.

Passaro MD, Ratner RE. Diabetes mellitus, type 1. Physician's Information and Education Resource (pier), American College of Physicians; 2011. http://pier.acponline.org/physicians/diseases/d257/d257-faq.html. Accessed June 6, 2011.

Potts JT Jr. Diseases of the parathyroid gland and other hyper- and hypocalcemia disorders. In: Fauci AS, Braunwald E, Kasper DL, et al, eds. *Harrison's Principles of Internal Medicine.* 17th ed. New York, NY: McGraw Hill; 2008:chap 347:2377–2396.

Powers AC. Diabetes mellitus. In: Fauci AS, Braunwald E, Kasper DL, et al, eds. *Harrison's Principles of Internal Medicine.* 17th ed. New York, NY: McGraw Hill; 2008:2275–2304.

Raisz LG. Is steroid osteoporosis preventable? N Engl J Med. 328(24):1781–1782. http://content.nejm.org/cgi/content/full/328/24/1781. Accessed June 19, 2007.

Sherwin RS. Diabetes mellitus. In: Goldman L, Ausiello D, eds. *Cecil Textbook of Medicine.* 22nd ed. Philadelphia, PA: WB Saunders; 2004:1424–1452.

Stockigt JR. Free thyroid hormone measurement—a critical appraisal. *Endocrinol Metab Clin North Am.* 2001;30(2):265–289.

Strategies for reducing morbidity and mortality from diabetes through health-care system interventions and diabetes self-management education in community settings. A report on recommendations of the Task Force on Community Preventive Services. *MMWR Morb Mortal Wkly Rep*. 2001;50(RR16):1–15.

Uwaifo GI, Ratner RE. Novel pharmacologic agents for type 2 diabetes. *Endocrinol Metab Clin North Am*. 2005;34(1):155–197.

Vijan S. Diabetes mellitus, type 2. Physician's Information and Education Resource (pier), American College of Physicians; 2011. http://pier.acponline.org/physicians/diseases/d296/d296.html. Accessed June 6, 2011.

Weissman PN. Reappraisal of the pharmacologic approach to treatment of type 2 diabetes mellitus. *Am J Cardiol*. 2001;90(5)(suppl 1):42–50.

Renal and Urinary Tract Disorders

Eric W. Cucchi • Theresa J. Riethle

I. Urethritis

A. Etiology
- Infection, reactive or posttraumatic induced inflammation of the urethra.
- Most commonly associated with sexually transmitted infections.
- Urethritis is classified as gonococcal or nongonococcal.
- Nonsexually transmitted cases are most commonly seen in diabetics, organisms vary.
- Noninfectious causes include reactive arthritis as seen in Reiter syndrome.
- Posttraumatic urethritis can occur in patients practicing intermittent catheterization.

B. Pathology
- Acute inflammation of the urethra.
- Concurrent infection with several organisms is common.

1. **Gonococcal Urethritis**
   - Incubation period is between 2 and 7 days.
   - Coinfection *Chlamydia* is present in 30% to 40% of cases.

2. **Nongonococcal Urethritis**
   - Incubation period is 7 to 14 days.
   - *Chlamydia trachomatis* is present in 50% of cases.
   - Other common etiologic agents include *C. trachomatis, Ureaplasma urealyticum*, and *Trichomonas vaginalis.*

C. Clinical Features
1. **Gonococcal Urethritis**
   - Men: Initial burning with urination with serous or milky urethral discharge, which progresses to profure, purulent discharge.
   - Women: Dysuria, urinary frequency, and urgency with copious purulent urethral discharge, possible dyspareunia. Symptoms often worse with menses.
   - Asymptomatic infection may occur in men and women.
   - Fever, rash, tenosynovitis, conjunctivitis, and arthritis can be seen with disseminated disease.
   - Local complications of gonococcal urethritis include epididymitis, penile edema, acute prostatitis, seminal vesiculitis, and periurethral abscesses.

2. **Nongonococcal Urethritis**
   - Associated with clear-to-white, scanty discharge, pruritis, and dysuria.

- Women infected with *Chlamydia* may be asymptomatic or may have symptoms of cervicitis or pelvic inflammatory disease.

D. Diagnostic Studies
1. **Gonococcal Urethritis**
   - Gram stain of discharge reveals intracellular gram-negative diplococci that may be seen in a smear or cultured from an infected site.
   - If Gram stain is inconclusive, culture on Thayer–Martin medium is recommended.

2. **Nongonococcal Urethritis**
   - Gram stain shows no organisms.
   - Culture is reliable, but difficult and expensive.
   - Nucleic acid amplification of urine or cervical/urethral samples is recommended and diagnosis confirmed whenever possible.
   - Historically, diagnosis was often made clinically and by exclusion and presumptive treatment was administered.
   - Wet prep of discharge—may show *Trichomonas.*

E. Management
1. **Gonococcal Urethritis**
   - In uncomplicated situations, ceftriaxone, 125 mg intramuscular, is the treatment of choice.
   - Also treat for concurrent chlamydial infection.
   - Effective, single-dose regimens for gonococcal urethritis also are available, such as cefpodoxime (400 mg).

2. **Nongonococcal Urethritis**
   - Chlamydial infection and infection by *Ureaplasma* respond to azithromycin 1 g orally as a single dose, and doxycycline (100 mg BID × 7 days).
   - Erythromycin, 500 mg four times a day for 7 days, is appropriate for pregnant women or patients allergic to tetracycline.
   - Infection caused by *Trichomonas* responds to Flagyl (metronidazole): 2g orally as a single dose or 250mg TID × 7 days.
   - In all cases, sexual partners also should be treated.
   - Education of patients in prevention and safe sex practices is essential.

II. Cystitis

A. Etiology
- Typically ascending infection primarily due to coliform bacteria (especially *Escherichia coli*) and, occasionally, gram-positive bacteria (enterococci).

- Female predominance and increased incidence with age.
- Owing to the longer and protected urethra in men, cystitis in men implies a pathologic process requiring further investigation.
- Risk factors include diabetes mellitus (DM), use of an indwelling catheter, obstruction, use of a diaphragm or spermicide, neurogenic bladder, pregnancy, immunocompromised state, and underlying anatomic abnormalities of the urinary tract.

B. Pathology
- In general, genitourinary (GU) tract infections occur as a result of ascension of the infecting agent up the urethra.
- Hematogenous spread is uncommon.

C. Clinical Features
- Dysuria, urinary frequency, urgency, burning, and sensation of incomplete bladder emptying are common.
- Hematuria or cloudy urine.
- Suprapubic discomfort.
- In women, symptoms may often appear after sexual intercourse.
- Physical examination is often unremarkable.
- Signs of systemic involvement (e.g., fever, nausea, or vomiting) are absent.

D. Diagnostic Studies
- Urinalysis discloses pyuria and bacteriuria with or without hematuria.
- Urine culture demonstrating bacteria >10^5 bacteria per mL confirms diagnosis.
- Additional or follow-up studies are warranted only with recurrent infections, suspicion of anatomic abnormalities, or if pyelonephritis is suspected.

E. Management
1. Acute Uncomplicated Cystitis
- Antibiotics are appropriate to the causative agent. A 3-day course of fluoroquinolones or nitrofurantoin is the recommended treatment.
- Trimethoprim/sulfamethoxazole (TMP/SMX) is becoming ineffective because of resistant organisms.
- Postcoital cystitis may require prompt voiding followed by a single dose of TMP/SMX or ciprofloxacin.
- Pregnant patients require 10- to 14-day treatment with pregnancy-safe antibiotic such as cephalexin or amoxicillin.
- Urinary analgesics (phenazopyridine, 200 mg orally three times daily), sitz baths, and fluids may provide symptomatic relief.
- Owing to the infrequent occurrence of uncomplicated cystitis in men, additional investigation is warranted and treatment is targeted to the underlying etiology.

III. Pyelonephritis
A. Etiology
- Ascending, infectious, inflammatory disease of the renal parenchyma and pelvis.
- Risk factors include underlying urinary tract abnormalities, nephrolithiasis, DM, immunocompromised conditions, elderly institutionalized women, and episode of acute pyelonephritis within the previous year.

B. Pathology
- Infection ascends from lower urinary tract most commonly.
- Most common etiologic agents are gram-negative bacteria including *E. coli*, *Proteus*, *Klebsiella*, *Enterobacter*, and *Pseudomonas*.
- Gram-positive organisms are seen less commonly and include *Streptococcus faecalis* (enterococci) and *Staphylococcus aureus* (hematogenous route).

C. Clinical Features
- Patient presents with symptoms of fever, flank pain, and shaking chills.
- Nausea, vomiting, and loose stool are also common.
- Irritative voiding symptoms are often present or were present before systemic symptoms.
- Physical examination may disclose costovertebral tenderness, fever, and tachycardia.

D. Diagnostic Studies
- Urinalysis discloses pyuria, bacteriuria with or without hematuria, and possibility of white blood cell (WBC) casts.
- Urine culture demonstrates specific offending agent.
- Complete blood count (CBC) typically shows a leukocytosis with a left shift.
- Blood cultures may be positive if sepsis suspected.
- Renal ultrasound (U/S) may reveal hydronephrosis or obstruction in complicated pyelonephritis.
- Computed tomography (CT) scanning is used if failure to respond to treatment or complicating factors are present.

E. Management
- In the outpatient setting, fluoroquinolones or TMP/SMX may be initiated for 1 to 2 weeks.
- In patients in whom complicating factors or evidence of severe infection is present, hospital admission is required.
- IV ampicillin and gentamycin or fluoroquinolones are administered until fever free for 24 hours.
- Upon discharge patients, are converted to appropriate oral antibiotic therapy to complete a 2- to 3-week course.
- Follow-up urine cultures are required after the completion of treatment.

IV. Nephrolithiasis

A. Etiology

- Calculi in the urinary tract.
- Major types of urinary stones.
- Calcium oxalate/calcium phosphate: 75% of stones.
- Magnesium ammonium phosphate (or struvite): 10% to 15% of stones.
- Uric acid: 5% to 8% of stones.
- Cystine: 1% to 3% of stones.
- Men are affected more frequently than women, in the ratio of 3:1.
- A medical history of gout, chronic urinary tract infections (UTIs), and chronic diarrhea or family history of renal calculi increases the risk of stone development.
- **Commonly used medications may increase the risk of stone formation:**
  - Antacids and carbonic anhydrase inhibitors may raise urinary pH, which facilitates calcium phosphate stone precipitation.
  - Calcium-containing antacids may increase the amount of calcium ingested and subsequently filtered by the kidney.
  - Loop diuretics may cause increased urinary calcium concentrations leading to an oversaturation state.
  - Large doses of vitamin C can result in hyperoxaluria in some patients because ascorbic acid is oxidized to oxalate.
- **Dietary factors have a significant effect on stone formation:**
  - Metabolic acidosis secondary to animal protein metabolism leads to an increased filtered load of calcium and a decrease in tubular calcium reabsorption and hypercalciuria.
  - Meats and other purine-containing foods also augment uric acid excretion, increasing both calcium-based and uric acid stones.
  - Thiazide diuretics and alcohol may increase the risk of uric acid stones.
  - Oxalate-rich foods (green leafy vegetables, such as kale, spinach, mustard greens; nuts; tea; coffee) contribute to calcium oxalate nephrolithiasis.

B. Pathology

- Stones develop as the result of growth of crystalline components in a supersaturated urine.
- Hypercalciuria is present in 40% to 60% of calcium stone formers.
- **Secondary causes include:**
  - Hyperparathyroidism, hyperthyroidism, Cushing syndrome, granulomatous diseases (sarcoidosis, tuberculosis, disseminated candidiasis), immobilization, vitamin D intoxication, rapidly progressive bone disease.

C. Clinical Features

- Often asymptomatic until obstruction.
- Patient may complain of sharp, colicky flank pain with radiation to the testicle or labia. Associated fever, chills, nausea, or vomiting may be present.
- Urinary symptoms include frequency and urgency, with or without dysuria.
- Hematuria.
- Costovertebral angle (CVA) tenderness may be present on physical examination.

D. Diagnostic Studies

1. Acute Stone Disease

- Stone analysis should be performed on recovered stones.
- Urinalysis may disclose microscopic or gross hematuria, pyuria, bacteriuria, crystals, and altered pH.
  - pH persistently <5.0 is correlated with uric acid or cystine stones.
  - pH persistently >7.2 is suggestive of struvite stones.
- CBC demonstrates an elevated WBC if infection is present.
- Electrolytes may show hypokalemia, hypercalcemia, and metabolic acidosis.
- Uric acid may be elevated.
- Creatinine may be elevated with bilateral obstruction or unilateral obstruction in a patient with one kidney.
- Radiograph: kidney, ureter, and bladder.
- Radiopaque stones are visible—calcium and struvite.
- Radiolucent stones are not visible—uric acid and cystine.
- Renal U/S can demonstrate the presence of stones and hydronephrosis secondary to obstruction. Abdominal, transvaginal, or transrectal U/S can aid in identifying calculi in the ureterovesicular junction.
- Noncontrast spiral CT is a test of choice and identifies radiopaque and radiolucent stones.

2. Chronic Stone Disease

- Analysis of stones.
- Urinalysis to determine pH.
- Parathyroid hormone (PTH) level if calcium is elevated.
- Serum calcium, phosphate, and uric acid.
- Qualitative test for urinary cystine.
- Twenty-four-hour urine collection on a random diet to ascertain volume, urinary pH and calcium, uric acid, oxalate phosphate, and citrate excretion. A second collection on a restricted calcium and sodium diet is undertaken to subcategorize patients.

E. Management

1. Acute Stone Disease

- Initial management includes fluids and analgesia. Most stones <5 mm pass spontaneously.

- Stones of 5- to 10-mm size may need to be removed in the presence of intractable pain, severe obstruction, serious bleeding, or infection.
- Extraction through lithotripsy or ureteroscopy with extraction.
- Stones >10 mm may require inpatient treatment and removal.
- Extracorporeal lithotripsy or percutaneous nephrolithotomy.

2. Chronic Stone Disease
- Asymptomatic calculi need not be treated. They should be followed with serial abdominal radiographs or renal U/S. If stones become symptomatic or grow, treatment should be instituted.
- Treatment of any underlying disorder.
- Increased fluid intake is of great importance.

V. Ureteral Stones

A. Etiology
- See IV (Nephrolithiasis).

B. Pathology
- Renal calculi may become lodged in the ureter, which interferes with the effect of peristalsis and leads to impediment of urine flow.
- Ureteral stones typically become lodged at three sites: (1) ureteropelvic junction, (2) crossing of the ureter over the iliac vessels, and (3) ureterovesical junction.
- Stones <5 mm in diameter frequently pass spontaneously.

C. Clinical Features
- See IV (Nephrolithiasis).
- Fever in association with an upper urinary tract obstruction is a medical emergency.

D. Diagnostic Studies
- Urinalysis.
- Abdominal radiographs.
- Abdominal, transvaginal, or transrectal U/S.
- Noncontrast spiral CT.

E. Management
- Conservative observation with appropriate pain medication for up to 6 weeks. Indications for intervention earlier than 6 weeks include fever, persistent nausea and vomiting, severe pain, or unresponsiveness to medications.
- Distal ureteral stones respond to in situ extracorporeal shock wave lithotripsy or ureteroscopic stone extraction.

VI. Urinary Incontinence

A. Etiology
- Multiple etiologies.
- Outflow obstruction = overflow incontinence – least common.
- Detrusor muscle hyperactivity = urge incontinence – most common.
- Urethral incompetence = stress incontinence.
- Cognitive impairment (physical or environmental barriers) = functional incontinence.
- Neurogenic bladder, loss of central nervous system (CNS) control.
- Risk factors include increasing age, female gender, multiparity, prostatic hypertrophy, dementia/spinal cord injury, multiple sclerosis, stroke, and diabetes.

B. Pathology
- Involuntary loss of urine from the bladder, which may occur while patient is asleep or awake.
- The amount of urine lost can vary greatly.
- Typically comes to medical attention when it is perceived as a social and/or health problem by the patient or patient's family.

C. Clinical Features
- Depends on the type of incontinence.
- Involuntary loss of urine, urgency, dysuria, and perineal irritation.
- Physical examination may disclose distended bladder, and digital rectal examination may show prostatic hypertrophy.
- In addition, identifying neuropsychiatric disease, impaired mobility, or pharmaceutical issues is essential.
- In women, vaginal speculum examination and bimanual pelvic examination may disclose GU pathology.

D. Diagnostic Studies
- Urinalysis is typically normal, but may show glycosuria, proteinuria, WBCs, red blood cells (RBCs), or bacteria.
- Voiding cystogram may disclose bladder or urethral pathology.
- Cystogram may disclose abnormal sphincter pressure or bladder physiology.
- Postvoiding residual measurement may show increased residual urine.
- If a postvoid residual is > 150 ml in a male, a renal ultrasound is required to rule out hydronephrosis.

E. Management
1. General Measures
- Detrusor instability—bladder training and Kegel exercises.
- Medications—oxybutynin or tolterodine (antimuscarinic agents).
- Urethral incompetence—lifestyle modifications, Kegel exercises, and biofeedback.
- Drug therapy is limited to trials with pseudoephedrine or duloxetine. Bladder suspension surgery is a last resort but most effective.

- Outflow obstruction—intermittent or indwelling catheterization.
  - Medication: bethanechol (Urecholine).
- Overflow obstruction due to prostatic enlargement—intermittent or indwelling catheterization, and surgery.
  - Medications: prazosin (Minipress), terazosin, and finasteride (Proscar).
- Cognitive impairment—direct treatment to underlying impairment.

VII. Cystic Diseases of the Kidney

A. Etiology
- **Simple cysts or solitary cysts:**
  - Account for up to 70% of all renal masses, must rule abscess, malignancy, or polycystic kidney disease.
- **Medullary sponge kidney:**
  - Autosomal dominant.
  - Common, benign disorder, present at birth, diagnosed in fourth or fifth decade.
  - Mutations in the MCKD1 or MCKD2 genes on chromosomes 1 and 16.
- **Autosomal recessive polycystic kidney disease (ARPKD):**
  - Rare. Occurs in 1 in 20,000 live births. Diagnosed in utero or in neonatal period.
- **Autosomal dominant polycystic kidney disease (ADPKD):**
  - ADPKD1—Defective gene on the short arm of chromosome 16 in 85% to 90% of cases.
  - ADPKD2—Defect on chromosome 4 in 10% to 15% of cases. Slower progression with longer life expectancy.
  - Age at onset is between 20 and 40 years.
  - Among the five leading causes of renal failure in adults, accounting for 10% of dialysis patients in the United States.

B. Pathology
- Renal cysts are epithelium-lined cavities filled with fluid or semisolid material that develop primarily from renal tubular elements.
- They are noted in isolated areas in the cortex, medulla, and interpapillary collecting ducts depending on the type of cystic kidney disease.
- One or more simple cysts are common in people >50 years of age.
- Generalized cystic diseases are associated with cysts scattered throughout the cortex and medulla of both the kidneys and can progress to end-stage renal disease (ESRD).

C. Clinical Features
- **Simple or solitary cysts:**
  - Usually asymptomatic, present on routine urographic examination.

- **Medullary cystic disease:**
  - Gross or microscopic hematuria, recurrent UTIs, or nephrolithiasis.
- **ARPKD:**
  - Presentation highly variable based on when disease is detected.
- **ADPKD:**
  - Abdominal or flank pain associated with hematuria and hypertension.
  - Extrarenal manifestations may include cerebral "berry" aneurysms, hepatic cysts, valvular heart disease, and colonic diverticula.
  - Positive family history may be obtained in the majority of patients.
  - Hypertension is present in <50% of the patients.
  - Palpable kidneys.

D. Diagnostic Studies
- **Simple or solitary cysts:**
  - Concern is to differentiate from a malignant renal mass.
  - U/S and CT are recommended procedures for evaluation.
  - Both simple and complex cysts should be reevaluated periodically.
- **Medullary sponge kidney:**
  - Intravenous pyelogram (IVP)—which shows striations in the papillary portions, which represent the accumulation of contrast in the dilated collecting ducts.
- **ARPDK:**
  - U/S reveals large echogenic kidneys.
- **Polycystic kidneys:**
  - Urinalysis may show hematuria and mild proteinuria.
  - Diagnosis is confirmed by U/S.
  - CT or MRI is recommended if sonogram is equivocal or to detect presymptomatic disease.

E. Management
- **Simple cysts:**
  - Benign cysts require observation and periodic reappraisal. If the cysts change, surgical exploration or percutaneous biopsy is recommended.
- **Medullary sponge kidney:**
  - No known treatment, provide supportive care, including, adequate fluid intake and thiazide diuretics if hypercalciuria is present.
- **ARPKD:**
  - No specific therapy. Advances in neonatal management and kidney transplant have led to survival into adulthood.
- **ADPDK:**
  - Treatment is supportive including controlling hypertension, adequate fluid intake, dialysis, and transplantation if warranted.

VIII. Renal Vascular Hypertension

A. Etiology

- Renal artery stenosis is a common cause of secondary hypertension.
- May be due to atherosclerotic narrowing of one or both renal arteries.
- In Caucasian women younger than 50 years, may be due to fibromuscular hyperplasia (or fibrous dysplasia).

B. Pathology

- Excessive renin release due to reduction of renal blood flow and perfusion pressure.

C. Clinical Features

- **May present in a manner similar to essential hypertension, but should be considered under the following circumstances:**
  - Onset below age 20 or above age 50.
  - Hypertension is resistant to three or more drugs.
  - In the presence of renal artery or epigastric bruits.
  - If concomitant atherosclerosis of the aorta or peripheral arteries is present.
  - Abrupt deterioration in renal function after the administration of angiotensin-converting enzyme (ACE) inhibitors.

D. Diagnostic Studies

- Renal arteriography is the definitive test and is suggested when suspicion is high.
- Noninvasive angiography through MRI or CT if moderate to low suspicion.
- Doppler sonography is playing an increasing role in detection and monitoring for progression.

E. Management

- Therapy is aimed at controlling the blood pressure (BP) and preserving the glomerular filtration rate (GFR).
- Medical therapy includes the use of at least three drugs: ACE inhibitors, Angiotension II Receptor Blockers (ARBs), and diuretics in most patients.
- Surgical management includes percutaneous transluminal angioplasty with or without stent placement for fibromuscular hyperplasia and discrete stenotic atherosclerotic lesions.
- Nephrectomy may be necessary in patients with severe, uncontrolled hypertension or in those with inevitable risk of losing a kidney due to ischemia.
- Close follow-up and monitoring is essential.

IX. Acute Renal Injury

A. Etiology

- **Prerenal:**
  - Forty percent to 80% of acute renal injury (ARI) cases.
  - Failure of appropriate kidney perfusion.
- **Intrinsic:**
  - Up to 50% of ARI cases.
  - Acute tubular necrosis (ATN), acute interstitial nephritis (AIN), acute glomerulonephritis (AGN).
- **Postrenal:**
  - Five percent to 10% of ARI cases.
  - Obstruction.

B. Pathology

- An abrupt decrease in GFR which results in the retention of nitrogenous wastes.

C. Clinical Features

- Typically nonspecific.
- Anorexia, asterixis, altered mental status, edema, fatigue, gastrointestinal (GI) hemorrhage, pruritis, seizures, nausea, vomiting, and weakness.
- Physical examination is variable based on the etiology of ARI.

D. Diagnostic Studies

- Serum blood chemistries for elevations of blood urea nitrogen (BUN), creatinine (although not specific for acute vs. chronic renal failure), hyperkalemia, hyperuricemia, hyperphosphatemia, and hypocalcemia.
- Urine analysis is a key initial test.
- **Prerenal**—Increased specific gravity and hyaline casts. High osmolality and urea. Decreased urine sodium.
- **Intrinsic**—AGN and vascular causes: proteinuria, hematuria, and RBC casts. In AIN: WBCs, eosinophils, and WBC casts. ATN: low urine specific gravity, high urine sodium, and "muddy brown casts."
- Pigmented casts are seen in rhabdomyolysis and hemolysis.
- **Postrenal**—values can vary based on the duration of the obstruction.
- **Special tests:**
  - U/S is helpful to evaluate postrenal causes of ARI.
  - CT, MRI, and magnetic resonance angiography are useful adjuvant testing modalities to evaluate underlying causes of ARI.
  - Renal biopsy may be diagnostic for patients where the cause of intrinsic renal failure is not clear.

E. Management

- **Prerenal:**
  - Volume repletion with appropriate fluids ± blood products.
  - Occasional use of short-term dialysis until renal function restored.
- **Intrinsic:**
  - ATN: Diuresis, correct electrolyte disorders, nutritional support with low protein diet.
  - AIN: Supportive measures with removal of inciting agent, corticosteroids, short-term dialysis.

- AGN: high-dose corticosteroids, cytotoxic agents, and/or plasmapheresis.
- **Postrenal:**
  - Identify location of obstruction and treat definitively.
- **All causes of ARI may need short-term dialysis treatment.**

X. Chronic Kidney Disease

A. Etiology

- The result of renal pathology that interferes with renal excretory and regulatory function on a chronic basis.
- The major causes of chronic kidney disease (CKD) include glomerulopathies (diabetic nephropathy), tubulointerstitial nephritis (drug hypersensitivity), hereditary diseases (polycystic kidney disease), obstructive nephropathies (prostate disease), and vascular disease (hypertension).

B. Pathology

- Progressive and irreversible deterioration of renal function caused by a variety of diseases over a period of 3 months or longer.
- The underlying primary disease is often difficult to identify when advanced renal failure is diagnosed.
- The two most common causes of CKD include DM and systemic hypertension.
- Laboratory manifestations of CKD may not occur until ≥40% of renal function is lost, and clinical manifestations may not occur until ≥80% of renal function is lost.
- The following are the five stages of CKD:
  - Stage 1—slight kidney damage with normal or increased filtration, GFR >90.
  - Stage 2— mild decrease in kidney function, GFR 60 to 89.
  - Stage 3—moderate decrease in kidney function, GFR 30 to 59.
  - Stage 4—severe decrease in kidney function, GFR 15 to 29.
  - Stage 5—kidney failure, GFR <15 or dialysis.

C. Clinical Features

- **Symptoms are nonspecific, but include:**
  - Malaise, metallic taste, pruritis, easy bruising, edema, shortness of breath, dyspnea, orthopnea, nausea, vomiting, anorexia, restless legs, altered mental status, and irritability.
  - Physical examination may reveal hypertension, pallor or jaundice, cachexia, edema, asterixis, uremic fetor, and muscle wasting.

D. Diagnostic Studies

- Laboratory evaluation is divided into two categories:
- Evaluate the etiology of CKD.
- Monitor the progression of CKD.

- Evaluation includes serial measurements of serum creatinine, urinary protein excretion, estimations of GFR, urea, calcium, phosphate, bicarbonate, alkaline phosphatase, anemia, and lipids.
- Renal U/S—evaluates the presence of the two kidneys, obstruction, and renal size and symmetry. Bilateral small kidneys (<10 cm) supports the diagnosis of CKD.
- Renal biopsy—reserved when definitive diagnosis cannot be made.

E. Management

1. **Resolution of primary cause of CKD**
   - Lifestyle modifications including low protein and potassium diet.
   - Strict diabetes and hypertension control.
   - Removal of obstructions.
   - Discontinuation or modification of medication that exacerbates CKD.
2. **Stabilization of CKD**
   - Medical therapy with ACE inhibitor or ARB.
   - Revascularization for renal artery stenosis.
   - Optimal control of comorbid conditions.
   - Minimize effects on other organ systems.
3. **Renal replacement therapy**
   - Dialysis.
   - Generally started when serum creatinine is >8 mg per dL or creatinine clearance is <10 mL per μm.
   - Hemodialysis or peritoneal dialysis.
   - Kidney transplantation.
   - Average wait for a deceased-donor transplant is 2 to 5 years depending on geographic location.
   - Requires chronic immunosuppressive therapy.
   - One- and 3-year survival for cadaveric-donor transplantation is 90% and 78%, respectively, whereas that for living-related donor transplantation is 95% and 88%, respectively.

XI. Acute Tubular Necrosis

A. Etiology

- Accounts for 85% of acute kidney injury (AKI).
- Usually induced by two etiologies. The first cause is ischemia and the second most common cause is nephrotoxins.

B. Pathology

- Ischemic damage is a result of inadequate perfusion, which may be a result of hypotension or hypoxia to the kidneys resulting in tubular injury. This destruction of the tubules results in the inability of the tubules to concentrate the urine and to reabsorb sodium.
- Nephrotoxins can be exogenous or endogenous.
- Exogenous nephrotoxins can be aminoglycosides, IV radiographic contrast, cyclosporines, and many other medications.

- Endogenous nephrotoxins include myoglobulins (seen with rhabdomyolysis), uric acid (seen with leukemias and lymphomas), Bence-Jones proteins (produced in multiple myeloma), and hemoglobin (such as seen in hemolysis).

C. Clinical Features
- There are three clinical phases of ATN: (1) injury, (2) maintenance, and (3) recovery.
- Injury is the inciting agent causing destruction of the renal tubules.
- Maintenance is described as oliguric (<500 mL of urine per day) or nonoliguric, which generally has a better prognosis. This phase generally occurs for 1 to 3 weeks, but can be longer. This is the phase that the tubules are being repaired and the damaged cells are cleared.
- The recovery phase is seen with diuresis and the improvement of the renal function.

D. Laboratory Diagnosis
- The BUN/Cr ratio is often <20:1.
- Hyperkalemia and hyperphosphatemia are often seen.
- The urine can be dark, and under microscopy, "muddy brown casts" may be seen.
- Urine sodium levels are usually elevated.

E. Management
- Mortality is 20% to 50% in inpatients, and up to 70% with underlying comorbid conditions.
- Need to avoid hypervolemia and hyperkalemia.
- Diuretics may help convert oliguric to nonoliguric AKI, but may not improve mortality/morbidity.
- Ultrafiltration may have some role if the patient also has decompensated heart failure.
- Improving nutrition may prevent catabolism.
- Correct electrolyte abnormalities.
- Remove inciting nephrotoxin or improve oxygenation/perfusion in the case of ischemic injury.

XII. Glomerulonephritis

A. Etiology
- Typically, glomerular diseases present as nephritic or nephrotic syndrome, or both.
- Accounts for 5% of all AKI.
- **Glomerular diseases presenting as nephritic syndrome:**
  - Postinfectious glomerulonephritis.
  - Immunoglobulin A (IgA) nephropathy (Buerger disease) and Henoch–Schönlein purpura.
  - Pauci-immune glomerulonephritis, which include Wegener granulomatosis, microscopic polyangiitis, and Churg-Strauss disease.
  - Idiopathic crescentic glomerulonephritis.
  - Goodpasture syndrome.
  - Essential (mixed) cryoglobulinemia.

B. Pathology
- Each underlying disease process utilizes different inflammatory pathways.
- An inflammatory process involving the glomerulus, although renal vasculature, interstitium, and tubular epithelium may be involved.
- Glomerular inflammation may result in damage to the glomerular basement membrane (GBM), mesangium, or capillary endothelium.
- The inflammatory process is often a result of formation and deposition of antigen–antibody complexes.
- Subsequently, a variety of secondary mediators of immune injury are activated (i.e., classic alternative complement pathways, neutrophils, proteolytic enzymes, superoxide radicals, monocytes, macrophages, inflammatory mediators, and vasoactive compounds).

C. Clinical Features
- Nephritic syndrome presents with edema, hypertension, and hematuria with RBC casts.
- Postinfectious glomerulonephritis—most commonly occurs 1 to 3 weeks after a group A (β-hemolytic) streptococci. It is characterized by the sudden onset of cola-colored urine (caused by RBC cast proteinemia), edema, oliguria, and varying degrees of hypertension.
- IgA nephropathy (Buerger disease) is the most common form of glomerulonephritis in the world, mostly occurring in children and young adults. It generally presents as an episode of macroscopic hematuria associated frequently with upper respiratory tract infection (50%), GI symptoms, or flu-like illness.
- Hypertension and edema are uncommon.
- Gross hematuria may occur 1 to 2 days after an infection, no latent period in contrast to postinfectious.
- Hematuria may occur in only a single episode; in some patients, recurrent episodes may occur over years.
- Approximately 50% of patients with IgA nephropathy develop progressive loss of renal function.
- Henoch–Schönlein purpura presents most commonly in male children and typically presents with palpable purpura secondary to leukocytoclastic vasculitis, arthralgias, and abdominal symptoms (e.g., nausea and colic melena). Purpuric lesions are often located on lower extremities. Patients rarely develop progressive renal disease and generally recover in several weeks.
- Pauci-immune glomerulonephritis is a small vessel antineutrophil cytoplasmic antibody (ANCA) associated vasculitides. Wegener granulomatosis, generally presents with necrotizing vasculitis that can affect the pulmonary system as well as the renal system.

- Anti-GBM glomerulonephritis is generally associated with glomerulonephritis and pulmonary hemorrhage; however, one-third of patients do not have lung involvement. More common in men than women and usually occurs in the second and third decades of life and is usually preceded by an upper respiratory infection.
- Cryoglobulin-associated glomerulonephritis occurs from the precipitation of cryoglobulins in the glomeruli and is associated with an underlying infection. Skin necrosis in the dependent areas, arthralgias, fevers, and hepatosplenomegaly. Associated with rapidly progressive glomerulonephritis.

D. Diagnostic Studies
- **Initial evaluation in a patient suspected of having glomerulonephritis includes:**
  - Urinalysis to determine hematuria, proteinuria, and cellular elements (i.e., RBCs, WBCs, and casts).
  - Twenty-four-hour urine for protein excretion and creatinine clearance to establish the presence of nephrotic syndrome and the degree of renal dysfunction.
  - Creatinine clearance.
  - Urine and serum protein electrophoresis to identify monoclonal or Bence-Jones proteins suggestive of multiple myeloma or amyloidosis.
- Additional tests: depending on history and results in initial evaluation.
  - Complement levels CH50, C3, C4, antistreptolysin titer, cryoglobulins, ANCA, anti-GBM, serum IgA, serum eosinophils, antinuclear antibody (ANA), RF, and hepatitis B and C serology.
  - Light and electron microscopy: for specific characteristics related to specific diseases.
  - Renal U/S and biopsy (pathologic diagnosis is often definitive).

E. Management
- Nephritic syndrome—treatment is directed toward correcting fluid overload, hypertension, uremia, and inflammatory injury to the kidney. Measures include sodium and water restriction, diuretic therapy and dialysis, antihypertensive medications, and imunosuppressive therapy to reduce inflammatory injury.
- Postinfectious glomerulonephritis is usually self-limiting.
  - Supportive, antibiotics for the underlying infection.
  - Most patients recover normal renal function within 2 months of onset.
  - No specific treatment other than antihypertensives, sodium restriction, and diuretics.
- IgA nephropathy.
  - ACE inhibitors or ARBs to decrease hypertension and proteinuria.
  - Corticosteroids.

- Fish oil may have some benefit to improve proteinuria.
- Patients with ESRD may need kidney transplant.
- Henoch–Schönlein purpura—most patients recover renal function completely without long-term sequelae.
- Pauci-immune glomerulonephritis treatment includes corticosteroids and cytotoxic agents (such as cyclophosphamide). Without treatment, prognosis is very poor; however, with treatment, complete remission occurs in 75% of patients. Some patients may benefit from plasmapheresis.
- Anti-GBM glomerulonephritis is treated with plasmapheresis, corticosteroids, and cytotoxic agents.
- Cryoglobulin-associated glomerulonephritis is treated with to treat the underlying infection. Some benefit may be seen with plasmapheresis, corticosteroids, cytotoxic agents, and interferon *a* (with hepatitis C infections).

XIII. Nephrotic Syndrome

A. Etiology
- May be a consequence of primary glomerulopathy or as a manifestation of one of a variety of systemic disorders.
- A majority of adult patients (50% to 70%) who present with nephrotic syndrome have an associated systemic illness.
- Most common multisystem diseases associated with this syndrome are DM, systemic lupus erythematosus (SLE), and other collagen vascular diseases and primary or secondary amyloidosis.
- Bacterial, viral, protozoan, and helminthic infections have been associated with nephrotic syndrome. Hepatitis B, hepatitis C, and HIV have also been associated with nephrotic syndrome.
- Neoplasms including solid tumors, lymphomas, and leukemias are associated with nephrotic syndrome.
- Idiopathic nephrotic syndrome, in which no identifiable cause is present, or associated systemic disease occurs in 30% to 50% of adults with nephrotic syndrome.
- Idiopathic nephrotic syndrome is secondary to one of the four forms of glomerular disease: minimal change, focal glomerular sclerosis, membranous nephropathy, or membranoproliferative glomerulonephritis.

B. Pathology
- Nephrotic syndrome is a combination of clinical and laboratory abnormalities common to a variety of disease processes, characterized by increased permeability of the glomerular capillary wall to circulating plasma proteins, primarily albumin.

- Defects in both the size-selective and charge-selective properties of the glomerular capillary membrane result in proteinuria.
- Albumin is the most abundant protein lost because it is the most abundant protein in plasma; however, urinary excretion of other proteins may also be increased.
- Minimal change disease is usually associated with allergies, Hodgkin disease, and nonsteroidal anti-inflammatory drugs (NSAIDs). Seen with fusion of foot processes on electron microscopy.
- Focal and segmental glomerulosclerosis is associated with heroin abuse, HIV, reflux nephropathy, and obesity. Seen with focal segmental sclerosis, IgM and C3 sclerotic lesions, and fusion of foot processes.
- Membranous nephropathy is associated with non-Hodgkin lymphoma, carcinoma, gold therapy, penicillamine, and SLE. Associated with thickened GBM, granular IgG and C3.
- Membranoproliferative glomerulonephropathy has two types. Type 1 is associated with upper respiratory infections (URIs). Type 1 is seen with granular C3, C1q, C4, IgG, and IgM. And type 2 is seen with C3 deposits only.

C. Clinical Features

- Most common sign of nephrotic syndrome is peripheral edema due to sodium retention as a result of renal dysfunction.
- As plasma albumin concentrations fall to <3 g per dL, ascites and anasarca develop.
- Hypercholesterolemia and hypertriglyceridemia are associated with increased hepatic production of proteins to compensate for the loss of albumin.
- Minor elevations of the platelet count and plasma concentrations of fibrinogen and factors V, VII, VIII, and X, as well as platelet hyperaggregability, occur in the patient with nephrotic syndrome.
- Exertional dyspnea suggestive of pulmonary edema is associated with severe hypoalbuminemia.
- Patients with nephrotic syndrome exhibit a predilection for arterial and venous thrombosis, especially renal vein thrombosis.
- If nephrotic syndrome is due to the presence of systemic disease, clinical manifestations pertinent to those diseases may be present.

D. Diagnostic Studies

- Quantification of urinary protein loss is necessary through 24-hour urine collection. Protein loss of >3.5 g per 24 hours is diagnostic.
- Urine dipstick analysis may be used as a screening test to determine whether increased amounts of protein, particularly albumin, are being excreted. Results, however, may be affected by urine specific gravity.
- On microscopic analysis, findings such as hematuria, cellular casts, or pyuria strongly suggest glomerular disease as the cause of nephrotic syndrome.
- Oval fat bodies, as a result of lipid deposition, are found in the urine, if there is hyperlipidemia present. They may present as "Maltese crosses" or "grape clusters" under polarized light.
- Blood chemistries associated with nephrotic syndrome include decreased serum albumin (<3 g per dL), decreased total serum protein (<6 g per dL), and elevated serum cholesterol (>200 mg per dL).
- Serum creatinine should be measured.
- Complement levels (C3, C4, CH150), fasting glucose serum and urine electrophoresis, ANA, and hepatitis B and C serology may also help determine the etiology of nephrotic syndrome.
- Renal biopsy may be used to obtain a histologic diagnosis. It should be used to differentiate glomerulopathies amenable to therapy from those diseases for which specific therapeutic interventions are of unproved benefit.

E. Management

- **Treatment issues common to all patients with nephrotic syndrome include:**
  - Protein loss—moderation of protein intake (0.6 to 0.8 g/kg/day with a GFR <25 mL per minute) may have some benefit to decrease the adverse effect of increased protein intake on renal function. Need to watch for malnutrition. Goal is generally to match protein loss with protein intake to avoid malnutrition.
  - Addition of an ACE inhibitor may reduce the amount of proteinuria.
- **Peripheral edema and ascites respond to:**
  - Dietary salt restriction.
  - Diuretics—thiazide diuretics are appropriate for mild edema; however, loop diuretics are more appropriate for fluid retention associated with pleural effusions and ascites. Addition of a metolazone or thiazide acting distal to the loop of Henle may potentiate the action of a loop diuretic if necessary.
- **Hyperlipidemia:**
  - Hypercholesterolemia and hypertriglyceridemia typically accompany nephrotic syndrome.
  - Although low-fat diet—with a weight control and exercise program—is recommended, pharmacologic intervention should be instituted, as in patients with hyperlipidemia not associated with nephrotic syndrome.
- **Nephrotic proteinuria:**
  - Increased loss of antithrombin III and other proteins involved in the clotting and fibrinolytic cascades, causing a relative hypercoagulable state increasing risk and incidence of peripheral venous thrombosis and renal vein thrombosis.
  - If thrombosis is detected, heparin therapy followed by warfarin is necessary for at least 3 to 6 months.

- **Minimal change disease:**
  - Prednisone 1 mg/kg/day, adults often require a longer course, may take up to 16 weeks and should continue several weeks after remission. Frequent recurrences may require cyclophosphamide. ESRD is rare.
- **Membranous nephropathy:**
  - Treatment depends on the risk of progression of disease. Management is based on the level of proteinuria. When <3.5 g per day, low salt diet, BP control, and ACE inhibitor. When 3.5 to 8 g per day with normal renal function, can use corticosteroids and chlorambucil or cyclophosphamide × 6 months. When the protein level is >8 g per day, should receive a corticosteroid and cytotoxic agent.
- **Focal segmental glomerular sclerosis:**
  - Treatment includes supportive care and 1 to 1.5 mg/kg/day of corticosteroids for 2 to 3 months followed by a taper.
- **Membranoproliferative glomerulonephropathy:**
  - Treated with corticosteroids and antiplatelet therapy (because of increased platelet consumption). Fifty percent progress to ESRD in 10 years. Type 2 has a worse outcome than type 1. Both types will recur after transplant; however, it is more common in type 2.

XIV. Acute Tubulointerstitial Nephritis

A. Etiology

- Drug reactions to NSAIDs (which account for 70% of all causes), antibiotics (including penicillins, cephalosporins, sulfonamides, and rifampin), diuretics, proton pump inhibitors, and miscellaneous drugs such as allopurinol, cimetidine, and phenytoin.
- **Systemic infections due to:**
  - Bacteria: *Streptococcus, Corynebacterium diphtheriae, Legionella.*
  - Viruses: Epstein–Barr virus, cytomegalovirus.
  - Others: *Mycoplasma, Rickettsia rickettsii, Toxoplasmosis, Leptospirosis, Histoplasmosis.*
- Systemic inflammatory diseases such as SLE, Sjögren, sarcoidosis, and cryoglobulinemia.
- Idiopathic such as tubulointerstitial nephritis-uveitis (TINU).

B. Pathology

- Mostly caused by T lymphocytes, with the help of plasma cells and macrophages, which appear to damage the interstitium by way of direct cytotoxicity, release of lymphokines, or both, which cause the recruitment of inflammatory cells, including eosinophils.

C. Clinical Features

- Sudden decrease in renal function in a previously asymptomatic patient; often associated with ingestion of newly prescribed drugs.
- **Signs and symptoms are associated with allergic reactions:**
  - Fever (seen in 80% of patients), transient maculopapular rash (seen in 25% to 50% of patients), bilateral or unilateral flank pain secondary to renal capsule distension, renal failure evolves over days to weeks, and arthralgias.
- TINU.
- Unknown etiology. Characterized by anterior uveitis seen usually before or after acute tubulointerstitial nephritis. Associated with bone marrow granulomas, chlamydia and mycoplasma infections. Usually seen in women and seen with weight loss and anemia and with an elevated erythrocyte sedimentation rate.

D. Diagnostic Studies

- Gross or microscopic hematuria (seen in 95% of cases).
- Peripheral eosinophilia, as well as eosinophiluria.
- Urinalysis may show pyuria, proteinuria (<1 g per 24 hours), eosinophiluria, and WBC casts.
- U/S shows normal or enlarged kidneys with increased cortical echogenicity.
- Gallium scanning may show bilaterally increased uptake of isotope; however, this is a nonspecific finding.

E. Management

- Discontinue the offending drug.
- Dialysis may be necessary in up to one-third of patients.
- Some benefit may be seen with corticosteroids at high doses, which can be administered if drug discontinuation does not lead to return to baseline renal function within a few days.
- Most patients have complete recovery of renal function, although advanced age at onset and a prolonged period of acute renal failure are poor prognostic indicators.

XV. Chronic Tubulointerstitial Nephritis

A. Etiology

- The most common cause is prolonged obstructive uropathy, vesicoureteral reflux, analgesics, and heavy metals.

B. Pathology

- Obstructive uropathy is the most common cause of chronic tubulointerstitial nephritis (CTIN). It can be caused by prostatic hypertrophy, calculi, and carcinoma of the cervix, colon, bladder, and retroperitoneal space.

- Vesicoureteral reflex is usually seen in children and is the second most common cause of CTIN. Generally associated with retrograde flow of urine from the bladder back into the ureters to the kidneys during voiding because of an incompetent ureteral sphincter. The urine then causes inflammation in the interstitium, and this inflammation can cause fibrosis.
- Increased analgesic use (cumulative intake of 3 kg or ingestion of 1 g per day for 3 years supports this diagnosis) is associated with CTIN as well as renal failure; seen with the use of acetaminophen, aspirin, and NSAIDs. Aspirin and acetaminophen are concentrated in the kidney. The process of metabolizing acetaminophen in the kidney results in oxidative tissue damage and necrosis. Aspirin and other NSAIDs are potent inhibitors of prostaglandin synthesis, and their overuse may lead to a reduction in renal medullary blood flow and result in ischemic damage.
- Environmental exposure to heavy metals, lead, and cadmium are also the causes of CTIN. Chronic exposure to lead leads to urinary concentrating defects by causing dysfunction in the proximal tubules, resulting in decreased uric acid secretion.

C. Clinical Features

- Obstructive uropathy can cause polyuria (due to insensitivity of vasopressin), which may be present and can result in dehydration and salt wasting. In contrast oliguria, due to poor glomerular filtration, can also occur. Azotemia and hypertension (HTN) may occur due to secretion of rennin-angiotensin.
- Reflux nephropathy occurs before the age of 5, but focal renal deterioration continues. Focal glomerulosclerosis and hypertension are often a sequelae, and the patient may progress to ESRD.
- Analgesic abuse can result in hematuria, mild proteinuria, polyuria, anemia (from GI bleed), and sterile pyuria, and may be present because of the necrosis caused by the analgesic medication(s). An IVP may reveal "ring shadow" sign due to the destruction of the papillae.
- Chronic exposure of heavy metals can over years results in progressive azotemia, hyperuricemia, saturnine gout, and hypertension. Hypercalciuria can occur with cadmium exposure.

D. Diagnostic Studies

1. **General Diagnostic Characteristics**
   - Small, contracted kidneys.
   - Decreased urinary concentrating and diluting ability.
   - Hyperchloremic due to type 1 and 4 renal tubular acidosis.
   - Hyperkalemia due to the distal tubules becoming aldosterone resistant.
   - Proteinuria <2 g per day because of dysfunction to the proximal tubule, so that it cannot reabsorb protein well.

2. **General Studies**
   - Urinalysis in CTIN is essentially nonspecific and may show mild proteinuria, few cells, and broad granular casts.
   - Most characteristic finding is polyuria and sodium wasting out of proportion to the degree of renal impairment, and inability to acidify urine in association with hyperchloremic metabolic acidosis (renal tubular acidosis).

3. **Obstructive Uropathy**
   - Renal U/S is useful for disclosing hydronephrosis. Antegrade or retrograde pyelography may be needed to confirm the diagnosis.
   - Urinalysis (UA) may show hematuria, pyuria, and bacteriuria.
   - May need further abdominal imaging to rule out carcinoma.

4. **Reflux Nephropathy**
   - May be diagnosed by proteinuria of >1 g per day and renal U/S or IVP demonstrating renal scarring and potentially hydronephrosis.

5. **Analgesic-Associated Disease**
   - Associated with hematuria, proteinuria, and sterile pyuria or urinalysis.
   - If gross hematuria occurs secondary to papillary necrosis, sloughed papillae may be noted in the urine.
   - IVP demonstrates a "ring shadow" sign and the papillary tip in the case of papillary necrosis.

6. **Heavy Metal Exposure**
   - May be diagnosed by performing an edetate (EDTA) test to diagnose lead nephropathy; >600 mg of lead in a 24-hour period after an IV infusion of 1 g of edetate indicates excessive lead exposure.

E. Management

- Underlying disorder responsible for renal dysfunction must be identified.
- Recovery of renal function depends on the degree of interstitial fibrosis. When evidence exists of small, shrunken kidneys, ESRD cannot be prevented, and treatment is directed toward the management of medical complications.
- In the presence of hydronephrosis, relief of the obstruction should be undertaken.
- Medical management of specific tubular dysfunction with dietary restriction of potassium, or sodium and bicarbonate supplements, may be necessary if damage is irreversible.
- Management of patients suspected of having lead nephropathy consists of chelation therapy when no evidence of marked interstitial fibrosis is present.
- Treatment of analgesic nephropathy necessitates withdrawal of all analgesics and may result in stabilization or improvement in renal function if significant interstitial fibrosis has not already resulted.

XVI. Hematuria

A. Etiology

- Can be gross hematuria or microscopic hematuria.
- Upper sources of bleeding are nephrolithiasis (40%), kidney disease (20%), renal cell carcinoma (10%), urothelial cell carcinoma (5%), trauma, medications, diabetes, and sickle cell trait disease.
- Lower sources of bleeding are infection, urothelial cell carcinoma (most common in the absences of infection), anticoagulation, trauma, and benign prostatic hypertrophy (most common form of microscopic hematuria in men).
- Hematuria associated with pyuria with or without symptoms of frequency, urgency, or dysuria suggests an infectious cause.
- Pseudohematuria may be caused by substances that impart a color to urine that may be mistaken for hematuria, such as porphyrins, myoglobin, and certain medications.

B. Pathology

- Pathology depends on underlying disease process. The clinician will need to obtain an excellent history and physical examination to help determine the underlying cause.

C. Clinical Features

- May be asymptomatic, and hematuria may be incidentally found on routine dipstick urinalysis.
- Patient may present with urethral discharge suggesting underlying infection.
- Patient may present with grossly, bloody urine with or without clots.
- The character of the hematuria may provide a clue to the site of origin (i.e., if the patient also complains of flank pain, it may suggest nephrolithiasis).
- Initial hematuria with presence of blood at the beginning of the urinary stream implies an anterior or penile urethral source.
- Terminal hematuria with presence of blood only at the end of the urinary stream is associated with bladder neck or prostatic urethral source.
- Total hematuria, presence of blood throughout the urinary stream, is associated with a bladder or upper tract source.
- Intermittent hematuria in patients younger than 40 years is less concerning for cancer. However, hematuria in patients older than 50 years should have a high concern for cancer.

D. Laboratory Diagnosis

- Hematuria is defined as >2 RBCs/high power field (HPF) on at least two occasions. However, there is no lower limit that will definitively rule out underlying disease.
- Dipstick method can detect 1 to 2 RBCs/HPF; therefore, it is as sensitive as microscopic evaluation.

However, they are not specific because they can have a high rate of false positives if there are myoglobins or oxidizing agents present. The dipstick tests can also give false positives if the patients recently ate beets or rhubarb or there was bleach or formaldehyde in the urine collection container. In men, semen can lead to a false positive.

- May see proteinuria and casts, which would suggest underlying renal disease.
- If it is unclear as to the source of hematuria, further evaluation of the underlying disease may be warranted. This workup may include the following:
  - CBC, an estimate of glomerular function (serum creatinine), sickle cell preparation, and 24-hour urine specimen to determine concentration of calcium and uric acid.
  - In patients suspected of having a bleeding disorder, a platelet count and partial prothrombin time/partial thromboplastin time should be obtained.
  - CT urography, MRI, U/S, cystoscopy, and/or IVP.
  - Biopsy is not usually needed for isolated glomerular hematuria without proteinuria or renal insufficiency.
  - In older patients or those at risk for neoplasia, cytology should be performed and a urologist should be consulted.

E. Management

- Identifiable causes should be treated.
- When neoplasm is suspected, a urologist should be consulted.
- When underlying renal disease is suspected, a nephrologist should be consulted.

XVII. Hyponatremia

A. Etiology

- Defined as a serum sodium concentration <135 mEq per L; is the most common electrolyte abnormality observed in the general hospitalized population. No age or gender prevalence exists.
- Hyponatremia is a dysfunction of water balance.
- There are three major types of hyponatremia based on serum osmolality. They are (1) isotonic hyponatremia, (2) hypertonic hyponatremia, and (3) hypotonic hyponatremia.
- Hypotonic hyponatremia is further divided based on the patient's volume status. These types are (1) euvolemic hypotonic hyponatremia, (2) hypervolemic hypotonic hyponatremia, and (3) hypovolemic hypotonic hyponatremia.
- Hypovolemic hypotonic hyponatremia is further divided into (1) extrarenal and (2) renal volume/salt losses based on the urine sodium level.

B. Pathology

- **Isotonic hyponatremia (normal serum osmolality of 280 to 295 mOsm per kg):**
  - Ninety-three percent liquids and 7% solids normally comprise plasma.
  - Any increase in plasma solids such as lipids and protein lowers the proportion of liquid in comparison with the amount of solids.
  - The increase in solids lowers the plasma sodium concentration without altering the sodium in the liquid compartment.
  - Examples: Hyperlipidemia gives a milky-appearing serum as seen in familial hyperlipidemia or nephrotic syndrome. Hyperproteinemia such as in multiple myeloma or macroglobulinemia.
- **Hypertonic hyponatremia (high serum osmolality of >295 mOsm per kg):**
  - Introduction of osmotically active solutes (such as glucose and mannitol), which do not readily penetrate the cell membrane, will increase extracellular fluid osmolality. This will create transcellular osmotic gradients and move water out of cells and into the extracellular space, which will result in increase of the extracellular water content and dilute the sodium and lower the serum sodium concentration.
  - Examples: Hyperglycemia and hypertonic therapy with mannitol.
- **Hypotonic hyponatremia (low serum osmolality of <280 mOsm per kg):**
  - Euvolemic hypotonic hyponatremia.
    - No extracellular fluid expansion or depletion relative to the amount of sodium is present.
    - Examples: syndrome of inappropriate antidiuretic hormone (SIADH), psychogenic polydipsia, beer potomania, and exercise.
- **Hypervolemic hypotonic hyponatremia:**
  - Expansion of extracellular fluid relative to the amount of sodium present.
  - These patients have edema and other signs of intravascular volume overload.
  - Examples: congestive heart failure (CHF), nephrotic syndrome, and cirrhosis.
- **Hypovolemic hypotonic hyponatremia:**
  - Depletion of extracellular fluid relative to the amount of sodium due to extrarenal or renal volume/salt loss.
  - Antidiuretic hormone (ADH) is secreted to maintain intravascular volume at the sacrifice of serum osmolality resulting in water and salt loss.
  - Extrarenal volume/salt loss (low urine sodium of <10 mEq per L in the setting of a low serum osmolality of <280 mOsm per kg).
  - Examples: dehydration, diarrhea, and vomiting.
- **Renal volume/salt loss (high urine sodium of >20 mEq per L in the setting of a low serum osmolality of <280 mOsm per kg):**
  - Examples: diuretics, ACE inhibitors, nephropathies, mineralocorticoid deficiency, and cerebral salt wasting.

C. Clinical Features

- Patients may be asymptomatic with a serum Na^+ in the range of 130 to 135 mEq per L.
- Symptoms are common with a serum Na^+ of <125 mEq per L.
- Uncommon for a serum Na^+ of <120 mEq per L to be acute.
- Symptoms include nausea, weakness, muscle cramps, and orthostatic hypotension.
- Neurologic symptoms and can be a change in mental status, lethargy, disorientation, obtundation, coma, and seizure (Na^+ of 115 to 118 mEq per L).
- Slow progression of hyponatremia may be asymptomatic because the brain has time to shift idiogenic osmoles and change intracellular tonicity to match the extracellular tonicity so that the brain does not become edematous. This can occur over weeks to months, and patients can then tolerate very low sodium levels.
- If hyponatremia occurs rapidly, over hours to days, the brain does not have time to shift the idiogenic osmoles and can result in varying levels of severity based on the rapidity and degree of hyponatremia.
- Neurologic symptoms are common because the brain is confined in the skull, and therefore more damage occurs when the brain is edematous.

D. Diagnostic Studies

- Sodium level.
- BUN, creatinine to evaluate for renal dysfunction.
- Serum osmolality and urine sodium levels.
- **Additional studies to help determine underlying cause:**
  - Serum glucose, each 100 mg per dL rise in plasma glucose decreases serum sodium by approximately 1.5 mEq per L.
  - Urine dipstick for glucose and protein.
  - Serum albumin.
  - Serum cholesterol.
  - Serum electrophoresis when multiple myeloma is suspected.
  - Thyroid-stimulating hormone level to rule out hypothyroidism.
  - CT scan of the head if pituitary or CNS disorder is considered.
  - Chest X-ray to rule out pulmonary pathology if SIADH.

E. Management

- Inpatient management is needed if hyponatremia is symptomatic or acute, and/or the patient is asymptomatic with a serum sodium <125 mEq per dL.
- Treatment should be thought of to correct the water imbalance rather than replete sodium.

- Isotonic hyponatremia will require fluid restriction to 1,000 mL per day, and treatment of the underlying condition.
- Treatment of hypertonic hyponatremia is to correct the underlying cause (i.e., correct hyperglycemia).
- A loop diuretic may be added to enhance free water excretion if the patient has hypervolemic hypotonic hyponatremia.
- Euvolemic and hypervolemic hypotonic hyponatremia can sometimes be treated with vasopressin antagonists in the inpatient setting.
- Hypovolemic hypotonic hyponatremia treatment consists of volume replacement with isotonic crystalloid.
- Severe symptomatic hyponatremia may need to be repleted with hypertonic crystalloid (such as 3% saline), in the rate of 1 to 1.5 mL/kg/hour, and not to correct the serum sodium more than 10 to 12 mEq/L/day.
- Avoid too rapid a correction, as the osmotic imbalance may cause water to preferentially enter brain cells leading to cerebral edema and potentially severe neurologic impairment (central pontine myelinolysis).
- Monitor electrolytes frequently, every 1 to 2 hours in the early treatment phase.
- Treat underlying and/or precipitating events (stop thiazide diuretics, thyroid hormone replacement therapy when indicated).

XVIII. Hypernatremia

A. Etiology
- Defined as a serum sodium >145 mEq per L.
- Hypernatremia is always hyperosmolar and is usually hypovolemic because of excess water loss.
- Often accompanied by an impaired thirst mechanism.
- Occurs most commonly in hospitalized, elderly patients.
- Lactulose, mannitol osmotic therapy, and diabetes insipidus (DI), both central and nephrogenic, can cause hypernatremia (see Chapter 9).
- May occur with diarrhea in infants.
- Occurs after the administration of hypertonic fluids.

B. Pathology
- Intact thirst mechanism usually prevents hypernatremia, and its presence is associated with conditions in which access to water is limited.
- One must determine whether the hypernatremia is accompanied by a normal, decreased, or increased extracellular fluid volume because total body sodium content is the major determinant of extracellular volume.
- Hypertonicity results from increased solutes in the extracellular fluid that do not cross the cell membrane (i.e., sodium, mannitol, or glucose).

- Hyperosmolality results from increased solutes (i.e., urea or alcohol) that freely cross all membranes and may be present without hypertonicity.
- The brain attempts to shift idiogenic osmoles and change intracellular tonicity to match the extracellular tonicity so that the brain does not shrink.

C. Clinical Features
- Severity correlates with the extent of hyperosmolality.
- Thirst may initially be present, but as the sodium levels continue to rise the thirst mechanism may become dysfunctional.
- Dry mouth and mucous membranes, decreased tears, decreased salivation, oliguria, and orthostatic hypotension.
- Fever, hyperventilation, hyperthermia, delirium, and coma.
- Polydipsia, polyuria, and nocturia.
- Brain shrinkage may result in intracranial hemorrhages, permanent neurologic damage, or death.
- Osmotic demyelination syndrome is uncommon.

D. Diagnostic Studies
- Serum osmolality is always >290 mOsm per kg, which represents a hyperosmolar state.
- Urine osmolality >400 mOsm per kg indicates renal water-conserving ability is functioning, and therefore the free water loss is from extrarenal causes such as sweating, loss from the respiratory tract, and GI losses. Renal losses of free water are seen in severe hyperglycemia and osmotic diuresis.
- Urine osmolality <250 mOsm per kg with hypernatremia is characteristic of DI.
- Salt ingestion typically shows increased urine sodium, increased urine osmolality.
- Dehydration has decreased urine sodium and increased urine osmolality.

E. Management
- General measures include correcting the cause of the fluid loss, replacing water, and repletion of electrolytes as needed.
- Removal of salt from diet in the case of hypervolemic hypernatremia.
- Acute hypernatremia has a free water deficit similar to the amount of weight loss.
- Calculate free water deficit for chronic hypernatremia:

$$\text{Volume (L) to be replaced} = \text{Current body weight (kg)} \times ([\text{Serum sodium}] - 140)/140$$

- Fluid therapy should be administered over 48 hours with a goal of decreasing serum sodium to 1 mEq/L/hour. In response to increased plasma osmolality, brain cells synthesize solutes that increase osmotic flow of water back into the brain cells to regulate their volume. This process is initiated 4 to 6 hours after dehydration and takes several days to reach a steady state. A too-rapid correction of hypernatremia may cause water to preferentially enter brain cells, causing cerebral edema and severe neurologic impairment.

- Hypernatremia with hypovolemia that is causing hemodynamic instability should be treated with isotonic (0.9%) saline, otherwise, 0.45% saline is adequate.
- In patients with hypernatremia with euvolemia, water drinking or 5% dextrose and IV water results in the excretion of excess sodium in the urine.
- In patients with hypervolemic hypernatremia, provide water as 5% dextrose in water to reduce hyperosmolality and loop diuretics (in severe renal insufficiency, hemodialysis may be required).

XIX. Hypokalemia

A. Etiology

- Serum potassium <3.5 mEq per L is considered hypokalemia.
- Always associated with a total body potassium deficit.
- Deficits arise from poor intake or from excessive loss of body fluids.
- **Nonrenal causes of hypokalemia:**
  - Vomiting and nasogastric suctioning.
  - Metabolic alkalosis increases the magnitude of potassium loss by increasing renal potassium secretion.
  - Malabsorption of nutrients in patients with small bowel disorders or decreased intake.
  - Colon losses during episodes of diarrhea or induced losses from laxatives, enemas, or colon preparation before lower endoscopy.
  - Villous adenoma and Zollinger–Ellison syndrome.
- **Renal losses:**
  - Diuretic treatment (most common cause in outpatients), digoxin intoxication.
  - Renal tubular acidosis I and II or parenchymal disease.
  - Adrenal hormones.
  - Primary hyperaldosteronism (second most common, generally occurs due to underlying heart or liver disease).
  - Secondary hyperaldosteronism (CHF, cirrhosis, nephrotic syndrome, rennin-producing tumors, and Bartter syndrome).
  - Excessive glucocorticoid excess (Cushing disease and exogenous glucocorticoid administration).
  - Genetic disorders.
  - Hypomagnesemia.

B. Pathology

- Hypokalemia can occur as a result of shift of potassium from outside to inside the cell, GI loss (vomiting or diarrhea), insufficient intake, or renal potassium loss.

- "Redistribution hypokalemia" is seen when potassium taken up by the cell which is stimulated by insulin in the presence of glucose. It is also facilitated by β-adrenergic stimulation of the Na-K-ATPase pump, whereas α-adrenergic stimulation blocks it.
- Aldosterone regulates potassium uptake in the distal tubules.
- Magnesium is a cofactor for potassium uptake and for maintaining adequate intracellular potassium levels.

C. Clinical Features

- Any level of hypokalemia may potentially be dangerous.
- Neuromuscular—skeletal muscle weakness and cramps.
- Smooth muscle involvement may result in constipation and ileus.
- Hypokalemia causes vasoconstriction and ischemia.
- When potassium level is <2.5 mEq per L, flaccid paralysis, hypercapnia, tetany, and rhabdomyolysis may be present.
- Cardiac involvement leads to ventricular dysrhythmias, hypotension, cardiac arrest.
- Hypokalemia causes "proarrhythmic" effects of patients taking digoxin.
- Hypokalemia causes acid secretion by the kidney causing metabolic alkalosis.
- Renal involvement causes polyuria and nocturia due to impaired concentration ability.
- Hypertension may suggest aldosterone or mineralocorticoid excess.

D. Diagnostic Studies

- Serum potassium <3.5 mEq per L is diagnostic of hypokalemia.
- Urine potassium of <20 suggests extrarenal losses, and a urine potassium of >40 suggests renal losses.
- Electrocardiogram (ECG).
- Findings include frequent premature ventricular contractions, decreased amplitude and broadening of T waves, prominent U waves, depressed ST segments, and, in severe deficits, atrioventricular block.
- ECG findings occur more frequently with worsening hypokalemia.
- **Special tests:**
  - Plasma renin and aldosterone levels to differentiate adrenal from nonadrenal causes.
  - If patient is acidotic and hypertension is not present, renal tubular acidosis should be considered.
  - A high urine chloride level in the absence of hypertension and acidosis suggests hypokalemia secondary to diuretics or Bartter syndrome; a low urine chloride suggests vomiting as the probable cause.

E. Management

- General measures include treatment of underlying cause.
- Mild-to-moderate deficiency may be treated with oral potassium phosphate in doses of 40 to 120 mEq/L/day.
- Potassium chloride (KCl) is suitable for all forms of hypokalemia, especially ones associated with hypochloremia.
- IV potassium replacement is indicated in patients with severe hypokalemia and those who cannot take oral supplements.
- If the serum potassium level is >2.5 mEq per L without ECG abnormalities, potassium can be given in the rate of 10 mEq/L/hour IV in concentrations not exceeding 40 mEq per L.
- In emergent situations (serum potassium <2.5 mEq per L), the rate of administration should not exceed 20 mEq/L/hour and maximum recommended concentration is 60 mEq per L. To replace potassium safely using higher concentrations, it should be administered through central venous access. These patients should have potassium levels checked every 4 to 6 hours.
- Continue to monitor ECGs and watch for signs of hyperkalemia.
- If hypomagnesaemia is present, it must be repleted.

XX. Hyperkalemia

A. Etiology

- Most commonly associated with AKI.
- A common electrolyte disorder with plasma potassium concentration >5.0 mEq per L.
- Severe hyperkalemia (>6.5 mEq per L) can be life-threatening, causing ventricular fibrillation and death.
- Total body potassium concentration is approximately 4,000 mEq per L, and mostly concentrated intracellularly.
- May be due to increased potassium load, translocation of potassium between cellular compartments, or factitious.

B. Pathology

- Spurious causes of hyperkalemia can be associated with hemolysis, thrombocytosis/leukocytosis, repeated fist clenching during blood draw, and blood drawn from a line with potassium infusion.
- Decreased excretion can result in hyperkalemia from acute kidney disease or CKD, renal secretory defects, decreased rennin/aldosterone, and medications that inhibit potassium secretion.
- Potassium can also shift from the intracellular to extracellular spaces causing hyperkalemia. This can occur from burns, rhabdomyolysis, hemolysis, severe infections, internal bleeding and extreme exercise,

metabolic acidosis, hypertonicity, decreased levels of insulin, and medications.
- Excess intake of potassium can also result in hyperkalemia.

C. Clinical Features

- Half of all patients with serum potassium >6.5 mEq per L have no ECG findings.
- Effects of hyperkalemia constitute a medical emergency.
- Hyperkalemia can cause bradycardia, PR prolongation, and peaked T waves progressing to widened QRS complexes and then sine waves.
- Patients are initially hyperreflexic, but then progress to flaccid paralysis, because of decreased neuromuscular transmission.
- Hyperkalemia also causes vasodilation.

D. Diagnostic Studies

- Mild hyperkalemia is 5.5 to 5.9 mEq per L, moderate is 6 to 6.9 mEq per L, and severe is ≥7 mEq per L. A serum potassium >7.5 mEq per L will require immediate intervention.
- **Special tests:**
  - Cortisol and aldosterone levels to confirm suspected mineralocorticoid deficiency.

E. Management

- Confirm laboratory value is real.
- Discontinue potassium-sparing drugs or dietary potassium.
- Determine underlying cause; if hyperkalemia is severe (>6.5 to 7 mEq per L), treat it first then determine underlying cause.
- Emergent treatment is indicated if cardiac toxicity or muscular paralysis is present.
- IV β-agonists, sodium bicarbonate, and insulin will temporarily shift potassium into the cell within a few minutes of administration.
- A source of dextrose should be given with insulin boluses to prevent hypoglycemia.
- Intravenous calcium gluconate will stabilize the cardiac membrane.
- Cation exchange resins, given orally or rectally, help with excretion of potassium in the GI tract within 1 to 2 hours after administration.
- Loop diuretics, or other nonpotassium sparing diuretics, can aid in the excretion of potassium from the kidneys if the kidneys are not in overt failure.
- In severe cases, dialysis can be used to excrete potassium and works immediately upon initiation of treatment.

XXI. Disorders of Calcium

A. Calcium

- Ninety-nine percent of calcium is stored in bone.
- 0.01% of calcium is stored in solution in body fluid.

- Fifty percent of calcium is bound to protein (mostly albumin), 10% is bound to other complexes, and the remaining 40% is "free" or ionized calcium.
- Ionized calcium is the physiologically active form.
- Normal serum total calcium level is 9 to 10 mg per dL.
- Normal serum ionized calcium level is 4.6 to 5.4 mg per dL.
- Serum ionized calcium is the most accurate measurement of serum calcium concentration.
- Functions of ionized calcium include neuromuscular function, smooth muscle contraction, plasma membrane stability, and permeability.
- Vitamin D is required for adequate absorption of calcium within intestines.

B. Hypocalcemia

1. Etiology
- Hypoalbuminemia is the most common cause of low calcium levels in the serum. When the albumin level is <4 g per dL, the serum calcium level decreases by 0.8 to 1 mg per dL for every drop in albumin of 1 g per dL.
- CKD is the most common cause of hypocalcemia because of decreased Vitamin D_3 production and increased hyperphosphatemia.
- Sepsis, acute pancreatitis, and postthyroid surgery.
- Hypoparathyroidism.
- Vitamin D deficiency.
- Alkalosis, blood transfusions, drugs (cimetidine, phenytoin), hyperphosphatemia, and calcitonin secretion with medullary carcinoma of the thyroid.

2. Pathology
- Hypocalcemia is a result of decreased intestinal absorption (vitamin D deficiency due to renal failure or nutritional deficiencies), decreased calcium intake, decrease in PTH levels, and deposition of ionized calcium into soft tissues or bone.
- Hypocalcemia causes a lowering of the excitation threshold of the neuromuscular and cardiovascular systems, thereby making these nerves more sensitive to stimulation and impulses.
- Hypocalcemia causes a reduced contractile force in both vascular smooth muscle and cardiac muscle.

3. Clinical Features
- **General**
  - Generally, patients with hypocalcemia are asymptomatic.
  - Weakness/fatigue.
- **Neurologic**
  - Skeletal muscle cramps and tetany, hyperactive deep tendon reflexes, paresthesias of lips and fingertips, and laryngospasm with stridor that may lead to fatal asphyxia, seizures, and confusion.
  - Chvostek sign is defined as a contraction of the facial muscle in response to tapping facial nerve anterior to the ear.
  - Trousseau sign is defined as carpal spasm occurring after 3 minutes following inflation of BP cuff to proximal arm, just above systolic pressure.
- **GI**
  - Abdominal pain.
- **Cardiac**
  - Arrhythmias, QT segment prolongation, heart block, ventricular fibrillation, hypotension, and heart failure.
- **Skeletal**
  - Abnormal dentition, rickets, osteomalacia, and osteodystrophy.
- **Hypocalcemia from chronic hyperparathyroid**
  - Cataracts and calcification of basal ganglia.

4. Diagnostic Studies
- Total serum Ca^{2+}: low to <9.0 mg per dL.
- Ionized Ca^{2+}: low to <4.0 mg per dL or <2.0 mEq per L.
- Commonly, hyperphosphatemia and hypomagnesemia are noted.
- ECG demonstrates prolongation of QT interval.

5. Management of Hypocalcemia
- **If the patient is asymptomatic:**
  - Oral calcium carbonate.
  - Vitamin D preparations such as ergocalciferol or calcifediol.
  - Magnesium replacement therapy, if low.
  - If total serum calcium is low, and the ionized Ca^{2+} level is normal, then no calcium replacement is needed.
- **If the patient is symptomatic:**
  - IV calcium gluconate 10% solution (92 mg of calcium per 10 mL).
  - IV calcium gluconate has a short duration and therefore continuous infusions is generally required.
  - IV calcium chloride 10% solution (272 mg of calcium per 10 mL) is more caustic to venous than the gluconate preparation.
  - Maintenance of serum Ca^{2+} level at 7 to 8 mg per dL.
  - Treat hypomagnesemia, if present.
  - Monitor serum calcium, other electrolytes—as appropriate, frequently (every 4 to 6 hours).

C. Hypercalcemia

1. Etiology
- Increased calcium intake, milk-alkali syndrome, hyperparathyroid (most common), multiple myeloma, Paget disease, adrenal insufficiency, acromegaly, neoplasm, Zollinger–Ellison, excessive vitamin D or A intake, medications, and sarcoidosis.

2. Pathology
- Hypercalcemia causes an increase of the excitation threshold of the neuromuscular and cardiovascular systems, thereby requiring an increased level of stimulus or impulse to trigger a response.

3. **Clinical Features**
   - **General**
     - Malaise, weakness, polydipsia, and dehydration.
   - **Neurologic**
     - Muscle weakness with hyporeflexia, hypotonia, tremor, lethargy, confusion, stupor, and coma.
   - **Cardiovascular**
     - Arrhythmias.
   - **Renal**
     - Polyuria, nocturia, rénal calculi, and nephrogenic DI, which is caused by increased calcium in the collecting ducts resulting in decreased response to ADH.
   - **GI**
     - Nausea, vomiting, abdominal pain, constipation, ileus, peptic ulcer disease, and pancreatitis.
   - **Musculoskeletal**
     - Muscle weakness, bone pain, fractures, and deformities.

4. **Diagnostic Studies**
   - Total serum calcium is >11 to 12 mg per dL.
   - Ionized serum calcium is >6 mg per dL or <2.7 mEq per L.
   - ECG demonstrates shortened QT interval.

5. **Management**
   - Primary disease or cause identified and controlled.
   - Correct dehydration caused by increased Ca^{2+} levels interfering with ADH and ability of the kidney to concentrate urine.
   - Hydration with IV fluids forces urinary excretion of calcium.
   - Patients with cardiac or renal disease may require adjustment of fluid replacement and/or peritoneal dialysis or hemodialysis.
   - IV furosemide can also be used to enhance Ca^{2+} excretion and prevent volume overload.
   - Thiazides may worsen hypercalcemia.
   - Replacement of K^+ and Mg^{2+} is usually necessary.
   - **Additional treatment options for specific disease:**
     - *Metastatic bone disease:*
       - Calcitonin (rapid, mild inhibition of bone resorption) and pamidronate (delayed onset, most potent inhibition of bone resorption).
     - *Sarcoidosis, vitamin A or D intoxication, multiple myeloma, leukemia, or breast cancer:*
       - Glucocorticoids (increases calcium urinary excretion, decreases GI absorption of calcium, and interfere with lymphoid neoplastic tissue growth).
   - Neoplasms producing PTH-like activity, consider irradiation or resection.
   - Surgical resection of the parathyroid glands in the setting of medically refractory hyperparathyroidism.

XXII. Disorders of Phosphorus

PHOSPHORUS
- Mainly inorganic phosphates in the plasma.
- Intracellular phosphorus is 70% and intraskeletal phosphorus is 29%.
- Serum phosphorus is approximately <1% of total body phosphorus.
- Phosphorus levels are based on renal excretion and release from bone caused by PTH (major factor), intestinal absorption caused by 1,25-dihydroxy-vitamin D_3, and intercellular and extracellular shifts.
- Since PTH and vitamin D are involved in the metabolism of phosphorus and calcium, often if there is a disorder of phosphorus, there will be a disorder of calcium present as well.

HYPOPHOSPHATEMIA

A. **Etiology**
- Diminished supply or decreased intestinal absorption such as starvation, refeeding syndrome, decreased intake, and vitamin D deficiency.
- Increased loss from medications, hyperparathyroid, and hyperthyroid.
- Intracellular shift caused by increased glucose, anabolic steroids, hungry bone syndrome, respiratory alkalosis, diabetic ketoacidosis, postoperative phase, trauma, sepsis, and salicylate toxicity.
- Electrolyte abnormalities such as hypercalcemia and hypomagnesemia.
- Common in patients who abuse alcohol.

B. **Pathology**
- Pathology is based on the underlying disease process.
- Severe hypophosphatemia results in decreased affinity of hemoglobin for oxygen.

C. **Clinical Features**
- Severe hypophosphatemia (<1 mg per dL) can result in rhabdomyolysis, paresthesias, encephalopathy, irritability, confusion, dysarthria, seizures, and coma.
- Since serum phosphorus levels do not reflect the total amount of phosphorus, low levels of serum phosphorus may be asymptomatic.
- May see respiratory failure or failure to wean in ventilated patients because of diaphragmatic weakness:
  - Arrhythmias are uncommon.
  - Hemolysis and petechial hemorrhages.
  - Anorexia, muscle and bone pain, and fractures.
- Severe hypophosphatemia is a high prognostic indicator of mortality in sepsis.

D. **Diagnostic Studies**
- Serum phosphate levels <2.5 mg per dL.
- Urine phosphate >20 mg per dL suggests renal loss.
- PTH levels may be elevated.
- Bone biopsy may show osteomalacia.
- If creatinine kinase (CK) levels are elevated, it may suggest rhabdomyolysis.

E. Management
- Phosphate repletion with oral replacement of sodium or potassium phosphate.
- IV phosphate repletion can result in hypocalcemia.
- Moderate or chronic hypophosphatemia (1 to 2.5 mg per dL) is generally asymptomatic and does not require repletion.
- Severe hypophosphatemia (<1 mg per dL) may require IV replacement and when able should be switched to an oral regimen.
- Monitor phosphate levels when repleting, as well as calcium, potassium, and magnesium levels, and correct any other electrolyte abnormality.
- Phosphate repletion in hypoparathyroidism, hypercalcemia, and CKD should be done with caution.

HYPERPHOSPHATEMIA

A. Etiology
- Most commonly seen in CKD, but may also be seen in AKI, hypoparathyroidism, and acromegaly because of decreased excretion.
- Phosphate shifts into the extracellular space from increased intake, increased levels of vitamin D, rhabdomyolysis, cellular lysis, and metabolic or respiratory acidosis.
- Multiple myeloma, hyperbilirubinemia, hypertriglycemia, and hemolysis are all causes of pseudohyperphosphatemia.

B. Pathology
- Pathology is determined by the underlying cause.
- Hypercalcemia seen with hyperphosphatemia suggests underlying malignancy.

C. Clinical Features
- Signs and symptoms are based on the underlying disease.

D. Diagnostic Studies
- Phosphate level is elevated.
- Tests ordered will be based on the underlying disease.

E. Management
- Treat the underlying disease.
- Oral phosphate binders such as calcium carbonate, calcium acetate, sevelamer carbonate, lanthanum carbonate, and aluminum hydroxide.
- Sevelamer, lanthanum, and aluminum hydroxide are used if there is hypercalcemia in addition to the hyperphosphatemia.
- Aluminum hydroxide can cause neurotoxicity if used for a prolonged period of time.
- Dialysis can be used in AKI and CKD.

XXIII. Disorders of Magnesium

MAGNESIUM
- Normal magnesium levels are 1.5 to 2.5 mEq per L.
- One percent of total body magnesium is within the extracellular fluid.
- One-third of serum magnesium is bound to protein.
- Two-thirds of serum magnesium is in the cation form.
- Excretion of magnesium is primarily from the kidneys.
- Hypomagnesemia and hypermagnesemia both can decrease PTH production.
- Magnesium concentration disorders are usually associated with changes in calcium levels and can be associated with changes in potassium levels.

HYPOMAGNESEMIA

A. Etiology
- Hypomagnesemia caused by decrease absorption from chronic diarrhea, small bowel bypass, increased gastric suction, alcoholism, and malnutrition.
- Increased renal loss from diuretics, hyperaldosteronism, hyperparathyroid, hyperthyroid, hypercalcemia, hypervolemia, tubulointerstitial disease, medications, and kidney transplantation can all cause hypomagnesemia.
- Diabetes, hungry bone syndrome, respiratory alkalosis, and pregnancy are all other potential causes of hypomagnesemia.

B. Pathology
- Pathology is determined by the underlying cause.
- Severe hypomagnesemia can cause decreased resistance to PTH in end organs and result in hypocalcemia that is resistant to repletion until the magnesium level is normalized.
- Increased renal excretion of potassium can be secondary to hypomagnesemia, and therefore the hypokalemia may be resistant to repletion until the magnesium level is normalized.

C. Clinical Features
- Signs and symptoms are similar to those of hypokalemia and hypocalcemia.
- Weakness, hyperreflexia, cramps, hyperirritability, tremors, athetoid movements, jerking, nystagmus, a Babinski reflex, confusion, disorientation, hypertension, tachycardia, and ventricular arrhythmias.

D. Diagnostic Studies
- Magnesium level is <1.5 mEq per L.
- Urinary magnesium level of greater than 10 to 30 mg per day or a fractional excretion of >2% suggests a renal loss of magnesium.
- Calcium and potassium levels may also be low.
- ECG may see a prolonged QT and prolonged ST.
- PTH levels may be low.

E. Management
- For chronic, mild, or asymptomatic hypomagnesemia, may treat with magnesium oxide orally.
- For severe or symptomatic hypomagnesemia, may treat with IV magnesium sulfate.
- Replete potassium and calcium levels.
- Monitor electrolyte levels and watch for hypermagnesemia.

HYPERMAGNESEMIA

A. Etiology
- Hypermagnesemia is usually associated with CKD or increased intake of magnesium.

B. Pathology
- Pathology is determined by the underlying cause.
- Severe hypermagnesemia (>5 mEq per L) can depress PTH and cause hypocalcemia. This can be seen in patients with preeclampsia receiving magnesium therapy.

C. Clinical Features
- Signs and symptoms can be muscle weakness, hyperreflexia, mental obtundation, flaccid paralysis, ileus, urinary retention, confusion, hypotension, cardiac arrest, or respiratory muscular paralysis.

D. Diagnostic Studies
- Magnesium level >2.5 mEq per L.
- If CKD is present, may also see a rise in BUN/Cr and other electrolyte abnormalities.
- ECG may show a prolonged PR, widened QRS, and peaked T waves.

E. Management
- Decrease the magnesium intake.
- Calcium will antagonize magnesium and should be given IV.
- Dialysis can be performed for patients with CKD.

XXIV. Acid–Base Disturbances

A. Normal Physiology
1. Etiology
- Acid–base balance is dependent on the maintenance of the hydrogen (H^+) ion concentration in body fluids, especially in the extracellular space, where it is more easily measured.
- H^+ ions at cellular levels have a low concentration compared with that of other ions.
- Normal pH is 7.35 to 7.45, even minor deviations can affect physiologic responses.
- Acidosis is when pH is <7.35, resulting from exposure to an acid load. *Acidemia* is the term when the arterial pH has been measured and reflects this change.
- Alkalosis is when pH is >7.45, resulting from an alkaline load; alkalemia is when this is reflected by the measured pH.
- Total venous CO_2 is a better measurement of bicarbonate because it is almost in all the bicarbonate form within the serum. Therefore, the CO_2 level is ±3 mEq per L of the actual serum bicarbonate level.

2. Pathology
- Normal physiologic processes cause increased amounts of carbonic acid and noncarbonic acids. The body has processes that correct these under normal circumstances.

- **Acid–Base homeostasis is maintained by:**
  - Buffer: internal, rapid changes that work within a fraction of a second to change strong acids and bases (alkalines) into weak ones.
  - Respirations: because CO_2 and H^+ are closely connected, altering rate and depth of respiration can compensate for pH shifts. Takes approximately 1 to 3 minutes for an adjustment to occur.
  - CO_2 and $H_2O = H_2CO_3$ (carbonic acid) $= H^+$ and HCO_3^- (bicarbonate).
  - H^+ can then be secreted into the tubules and HCO_3^- into blood at the level of the proximal tubules. These changes in secretion can also be reversed. Can take hours or days to see changes.

B. Metabolic Acidosis
1. Etiology
- Characterized by decreased bicarbonate and decreased pH.
- Separated into two categories: with increased anion gap or without increased anion gap.
- Caused by one of two things: increased acid other than carbonic acid or loss of bicarbonate.
- Anion gap is a measurement of the difference between anions, which are negatively charged, and cations, which are positively charged [$(Na^+) - (HCO_3^- + Cl^-)$], normally equals 8 to 16 mEq per L.
- Cations are usually slightly greater in concentration.
- **Metabolic acidosis with an increased or widened anion gap includes:**
  - Lactic acidosis.
  - Ketoacidosis—DM, alcohol (ETOH) abuse, and starvation.
  - Intoxication overdose (salicylates, methanol, and ethylene glycol).
  - Uremia.
- **Metabolic acidosis with normal anion gap includes:**
  - Diarrhea.
  - Mild renal insufficiency.
  - Diuretic treatment.
  - Renal tubular acidosis types I (classic distal), II (proximal), and IV (hyporeninemic-hypoaldosteronemic).

2. Pathology
- Pathology of metabolic acidosis is due to underlying causes.
- Patients may hyperventilate to cause a respiratory alkalosis as a compensation mechanism.

3. Clinical Features
- If pH is >7.2, usually will be well tolerated.
- Symptoms depend on underlying cause.

4. Diagnostic Studies
- Arterial blood gases (ABGs) show $\downarrow HCO_3^-$ and $\downarrow$pH.
- May see a $\downarrow PCO_2$ if there is a compensatory respiratory response.
- Calculation of anion gap.

- Other studies as needed for underlying cause.
5. **Management**
   - Treat underlying cause.
   - Varying practices on administration of bicarbonate to correct acidemia. If patient is given too much, it can lead to overcompensation, resulting in respiratory acidosis, and hypokalemia. Usually, correction of initial cause is enough to resolve the acidemia.
   - Alkali administration for type I and II RTA. Type IV renal tubular acidosis (RTA) may need potassium restriction.

C. Metabolic Alkalosis
1. **Etiology**
   - Characterized by increased bicarbonate and increased pH.
   - Happens in two ways: by adding bicarbonate or by the loss of H^+ ions.
   - If lost H^+ through stomach, will always be associated with the accompanying loss of chloride.
   - Mechanisms causing a primary metabolic alkalosis:
     - Vomiting/too aggressive suctioning of gastric contents.
     - Diuretics (depletion of K^+ leads to the stimulation of proximal tube secretion and H^+, causing the so-called contraction alkalosis).
     - Overcorrection of bicarbonate in cardiac arrest or respiratory acidosis.
     - Volume depletion (especially as the kidney tries to compensate for other problems, i.e., diuretics, chloride depletion).
     - Adrenal cortical overactivity.
2. **Pathology**
   - Pathology of the metabolic alkalosis is due to the underlying cause.
   - Patients hypoventilate to increase PCO_2, as a compensation mechanism.
3. **Clinical Features**
   - Weakness, irritability, hyporeflexia, and tetany.
   - Hypoventilation.
   - Orthostatic hypotension.
   - Rarely symptoms other than those of underlying illness.
4. **Diagnostic Studies**
   - ABGs show $\uparrow HCO_3^-$ and $\uparrow$pH.
   - May see a $\uparrow CO_2$ if there is a compensatory respiratory response.
   - Check for urine chloride levels.
   - Other studies as needed for underlying cause.
5. **Management**
   - Mild alkalosis is well tolerated.
   - Severe alkalosis (pH > 7.6) needs immediate treatment.
   - Treat underlying cause.
   - Acetazolamide will increase renal bicarbonate excretion.
   - Fluids with sodium chloride (NaCl) as determined by underlying causes.

- Administration of KCl as determined by underlying causes.

D. Respiratory Acidosis
1. **Etiology**
   - Hypoventilation leading to increased PCO_2.
   - Disorders that result in hypoventilation may cause respiratory acidosis.
   - Chronic obstructive pulmonary disease (COPD).
   - Paralysis of chest/respiratory muscles (i.e., trauma and neuromuscular disorders).
   - Narcotic or sedative-hypnotic overdose.
2. **Pathology**
   - May have an acute or chronic respiratory acidosis.
   - Renal compensation occurs with increased H^+ excretion and increased reabsorption of HCO_3^- at proximal renal tubules.
3. **Clinical Features**
   - Symptoms depend on underlying cause.
   - CNS depression: as PCO_2 regulates blood flow to brain and increases cerebrospinal fluid pressure, leads to generalized CNS depression.
   - Cardiac output decreases, leading to decreased blood flow to organs.
   - Asterixis and myoclonus.
4. **Diagnostic Studies**
   - ABGs show $\uparrow PCO_2$ and $\downarrow$pH.
   - May see a $\uparrow HCO_3^-$ if there is a compensatory metabolic response.
   - Studies determined by underlying cause.
5. **Management**
   - Treat underlying cause.
   - Hyperventilate to "blow off" excess CO_2 if an acute respiratory acidosis.

E. Respiratory Alkalosis
1. **Etiology**
   - Hyperventilation leading to decreased PCO_2.
   - Disorders that result in hyperventilation may cause respiratory alkalosis.
   - Psychiatric disorders, anxiety—most common.
   - Fever.
   - Head injury.
   - CVA.
   - Pulmonary disorders—asthma, pneumonia, and fibrosis.
   - Acetylsalicylic acid—in extremely high doses, it increases respirations by directly affecting the respiratory center.
2. **Pathology**
   - Renal compensation occurs with decreased H^+ excretion and decreased HCO_3^- reabsorption in the proximal renal tubules.
3. **Clinical Features**
   - Carpal/pedal spasm.
   - Tetany, paresthesias, and perioral numbness.
   - Light-headedness.
   - Anxiety.

- Cardiac output increases due to alkalemia, but can then decrease if the pH is >7.7.
- Symptoms also depend on underlying cause.

4. **Diagnostic Studies**
   - ABGs show ↓PCO_2 and ↑pH.
   - May see a ↓HCO_3^- if there is a compensatory metabolic response.
   - Studies determined by need, depending on underlying cause.

5. **Management**
   - Treat underlying cause.
   - Evaluate underlying cause, then may need to control ventilation to increase CO_2, although usually only in severe cases.

F. **Mixed Acid–Base Disturbances**
   1. **Etiology/Pathology**
      - Many patients present with two to three concomitant acid–base disturbances.
      - Most common combination is respiratory acidosis with a compensatory metabolic alkalosis; COPD with new onset CHF (sodium restriction and diuresis leading to metabolic alkalosis).
      - pH from any combination can be high, normal, or low, depending on which is more acute or severe, whether they add to each other or cancel each other out.
      - The only combination that cannot coexist is respiratory alkalosis and respiratory acidosis because one is secondary to hypoventilation and the other to hyperventilation.

G. **Steps to Determine Acid–Base Disturbance**
   1. **Look at the pH is high, low, or normal?**
      - High means alkalosis.
      - Low means acidosis.
      - Normal does not mean there are no abnormalities.
   2. **Look at the CO_2 and the HCO_3 for the primary acid–base disorder (or the reason the pH is high or low).**
      - High $PaCO_2$ (nmL 35 to 45) means respiratory acidosis.
      - Low $PaCO_2$ (nmL 35 to 45) means respiratory alkalosis.
      - High HCO_3 (nmL 24 to 32) means metabolic alkalosis.
      - Low HCO_3 (nmL 24 to 32) means metabolic acidosis.
   3. **Is there an appropriate compensation?**
      - Need to calculate the compensation (see Table 10-1).
      - The purpose of the compensation equations are to determine a second, if any, acid-base disorder or whether there is an appropriate compensation by the opposite molecule (HCO_3 or CO_2).

TABLE 10-1.   Compensatory Changes in Simple Acid–Base Disorders

Metabolic Acidosis

Primary change: HCO_3^- decreased
Predicted compensation[a]: $PaCO_2 = (10.5 \times HCO_3^-) + 8 \pm 2$

Metabolic Alkalosis

Primary change: HCO_3^- increased
Predicted compensation[b]: $PaCO_2 = (0.9 \times HCO_3^-) + 9$

Respiratory Acidosis

Primary change: $PaCO_2$ increased
Predicted compensation
Acute acidosis: HCO_3^- increases 1 mEq/L for every 10 mm Hg increase in $PaCO_2$
Chronic acidosis: HCO_3^- increases 3.5 mEq/L for every 10 mm Hg increase in $PaCO_2$

Respiratory Alkalosis

Primary change: $PaCO_2$ decreased
Predicted compensation
Acute alkalosis: HCO_3^- decreases 2 mEq/L for every 10 mm Hg decrease in $PaCO_2$
Chronic alkalosis: HCO_3^- decreases 5 mEq/L for every 10 mm Hg decrease in $PaCO_2$

[a]Full compensation may require 12 hours.
[b]Actual compensation is erratic and only approximated by this formula.
From Fishman M, Hoffman A, Klausner R, et al. Fluids, electrolytes, and pH homeostasis. In: Fishman M, Hoffman A, Klausner R, et al, eds. *Medicine*. 3rd ed. Philadelphia, PA: JB Lippincott; 1991:chap 21:159–172, with permission.

4. **Is there an anion gap?**
   - Only needed to perform if you find a metabolic acidosis.
   - Sodium level—(HCO_3^+ chloride).
   - Greater than 16 means there is an anion gap.
5. **Is there a third disorder?**
   - If there is an anion gap acidosis, check a Delta–Delta gap.
   - Delta–Delta is calculated by the equation change in the anion gap divided by the change in the bicarbonate level ($\Delta AG / \Delta HCO_3$).
   - If there is another acid causing the anion gap that is *not the HCO₃*, then you need to see what the HCO_3 is doing: if it is higher than it should be, it is an alkalosis, or if it is lower than it should be, it is an acidosis.
   - In other words, a separate acid is causing the pH to change. You still need to know what the bicarbonate is doing. The Delta–Delta is how you determine this.
   - If the Delta–Delta gap is <1, then that means there is a nonanion gap acidosis superimposed on the top of an anion gap metabolic acidosis.
   - If the Delta–Delta gap is >1.5, then that means there is a metabolic alkalosis superimposed on the top of an anion gap metabolic acidosis.

SELECTED REFERENCES

Adrogue HJ, Gennari FJ, Galla JH, et al. Assessing acid-base disorders. *Kidney Int.* 2009;76:1239–1247.

Adrogue HJ, Madias NE. Hypernatremia. *N Engl J Med.* 2000;342(20):1493–1499.

Badr KF, Brenner BM. Vascular injury to the kidney. In: Fauci AS, Braunwald E, Kasper DL, et al, eds. *Harrison's Principles of Internal Medicine.* 17th ed. New York, NY: McGraw-Hill; 2008:1811–1812.

Cho KC. Electrolyte and acid base disorders. In: McPhee SJ, Papadakis MA, eds. *Current Medical Diagnosis and Treatment.* 50th ed. New York, NY: McGraw Hill; 2011:841–868.

Cooper MS, Gittoes NJL. Diagnosis and management of hypocalcemia. *BMJ.* 2008;336:1298–1302.

Geerse DA, Bindels AJ, Kuiper MA, et al. Treatment of hypophosphatemia in the intensive care unit: a review. *Crit Care.* 2010;14:R147.

Hruska KA, Mathew S, Lund R, et al. Hyperphosphatemia of chronic kidney disease. *Kidney Int.* 2008;74:148–157.

Kumar J, Walker PD. Major nonglomerular disorders. In: Andreoli TE, Carpenter C, Griggs RC, eds. *Cecil Essentials of Medicine.* 7th ed. Philadelphia, PA: Saunders Elsevier; 2007:319–321.

Meng MV, Stoller ML, Walsh TJ. Urologic disorders. In: McPhee SJ, Papadakis MA, eds. *Current Medical Diagnosis and Treatment.* 50th ed. New York, NY: McGraw Hill; 2011:904–905.

Morris CG, Low J. Metabolic acidosis in the critically ill: part 2. Causes and treatment. *Anaesthesia.* 2008;63:396–411.

Parham WA, Mehdirad AA, Biermann KM, et al. Hyperkalemia revisited. *Tex Heart Inst J.* 2006;33:40–47.

Rose BD, Fletcher RH. Evaluation of hematuria in adults. http://www.uptodate.com/contents/evaluation-of-hematuria-in-adults. Updated December 24, 2009. Accessed May 21, 2011.

Rosen S, Stillman IE. Acute tubular necrosis is a syndrome of physiologic and pathologic dissociation. *J Am Soc Nephrol.* 2008;19:871–875.

Smellie WSA, Shaw N, Bowlees R, et al. Best practice in primary care pathology: review 9. *J Clin Pathol.* 2006;60:966–974.

Stoller ML, Kane CJ, Meng MV. Urologic disorders. In: Tierney LM, McPhee SJ, Papadakis MA, eds. *Current Medical Diagnosis and Treatment.* 48th ed. New York, NY: McGraw-Hill; 2009:827–847.

Sutton LE, Atkinson HH. The aging patient. In: Andreoli TE, Carpenter C, Griggs RC, et al, eds. *Cecil Essentials of Medicine.* 7th ed. Philadelphia, PA: Saunders Elsevier; 2007:1173–1174.

Watnick S, Morrison G. Kidney disease. In: McPhee SJ, Papadakis MA, eds. *Current Medical Diagnosis and Treatment.* 50th ed. New York, NY: McGraw Hill; 2011:869–903.

Male Reproductive Disorders

Jose "Pepe" E. Barcega • Patrick C. Auth

I. Disorders of the Testes

A. Testicular Torsion

1. **Definition**
   - Rotation of the testicle and spermatic cord with its blood vessels causes obstruction of blood flow.

2. **Etiology**
   - Unknown.
   - Most common in teenage boys (average age 16 to 17.5 years); also occurs in neonates (extravaginal); however, it may occur at any age.
   - Incidence decreases with age.
   - Often difficult to differentiate from epididymitis.
   - The differential diagnosis of acute scrotal pain includes testicular torsion, torsion of the appendix testis, appendix epididymis, and epididymitis.

3. **Pathology**
   - Incomplete fixation of the tunica vaginalis and posterior scrotal wall exists.
   - Unilateral cremaster muscle contraction can result in torsion.

4. **Clinical Features**
   - Acute onset of severe testicular, scrotal, inguinal, or lower abdominal pain. Possibly nausea and vomiting.
   - Recent history of trauma, an athletic event, strenuous physical activity; however, it may occur during sleep.
   - There is an increased number of young boys presenting to the emergency department with nonspecific abdominal pain, initially diagnosed with viral syndrome or gastroenteritis, only to return in 1 to 2 days with a testicular torsion.
   - On examination, reveals a swollen, tender, retracted testicle that often lies in the horizontal plane (bell clapper deformity).
   - Cremasteric reflex absent on the affected side.
   - "Blue dot sign" at the upper pole of the testicle—sign of testicular appendix torsion.

5. **Diagnostic Studies**
   - Gold standard—radionucleotide study used to detect blood flow to the testes.
   - Ultrasound (U/S) demonstrates diminished blood flow to the affected testicle with up to 98% accuracy in children.
   - Emergency exploration is necessary for diagnosis.
   - Urine is usually clear with a normal urinalysis, one-third of cases there is a peripheral leukocytosis.

6. **Management**
   - A surgical emergency.
   - While awaiting surgical intervention, manual detorsion of the affected testis should be attempted.
   - Ancillary studies should not delay operative intervention, because testicular infarction will occur within 6 to 12 hours after torsion.
   - Acute torsion must be differentiated from hernia, orchitis, epididymitis, urolithiasis.
   - Urgent urologic consultation and urgent surgery—detorsion, orchidectomy may be warranted, if gonad infracted.
   - Ischemia of the testicle may result in irreversible damage.

B. Acute Epididymitis

1. **Definition**
   - Acute inflammation, infection of epididymis.
   - Must rule out testicular torsion.

2. **Etiology/Pathology**
   - **Bacterial**
     - In younger age group (men younger than 40 years), it is usually sexually transmitted and associate with urethritis. The causative organisms are *Chlamydia trachomatis, Neisseria gonorrhoeae*, and *Ureaplasma*.
     - In older men (men 40 years of age and older), underlying structural urologic abnormalities, bacterial prostatitis, or a history of recent genitourinary tract manipulation is present. Gram-negative urinary pathogens (e.g., *Escherichia coli, Klebsiella*) are typically causative agents. Amiodarone has been associated with self-limited epididymitis, which is a dose-dependent phenomenon.
   - **Traumatic or chemical**
     - Seen in young men, due to sterile urine reflux.

3. **Clinical Features**
   - Gradual onset of pain in the testicle, scrotum, inguinal canal, lower abdomen.
   - Symptoms may follow acute physical strain (heavy lifting), trauma, or sexual activity.
   - The onset of pain in epididymitis is most often more gradual (1 to 2 days) than that of testicular torsion.
   - Younger patients may have concurrent symptoms of dysuria and penile discharge consistent with urethritis.

- Older patients may have symptoms consistent with prostatitis.
- On examination, a firm, tender mass along the testicle may be palpable and can progress to more diffuse mass with swelling of the scrotum.
- A urethral discharge should be sought because asymptomatic urethritis may be present, especially in patients younger than 40 years.

4. Diagnostic Studies
- Urinalysis often shows pus, bacteria; however, absence of both does not rule out diagnosis.
- In the sexually transmitted variety, Gram staining the urethral discharge may be diagnostic of gram-negative intracellular diplococcic (*N. gonorrhoeae*). White cells without visible organisms on urethral smear represent nongonococcal urethritis, and *C. trachomatis* is the most likely pathogen.
- Culture of epididymal aspirates in patients for whom medical therapy fails, or in those who develop recurrences without a diagnosis of cause.
- U/S often helpful in differentiating epididymitis from testicular torsion or other causes of scrotal masses.

5. Management
- Bed rest, scrotal elevation, ice to the affected area.
- Nonsteroidal anti-inflammatory drugs (NSAIDs), analgesics for pain and swelling.
- Antibiotics based on suspected etiology (i.e., chemical: tetracycline, NSAID; gonococcal: ceftriaxone, tetracycline, NSAID; *Chlamydia*: ceftriaxone, tetracycline, NSAID; *E. coli*: trimethoprim/sulfamethoxazole, NSAID; *Klebsiella*: trimethoprim/sulfamethoxazole, NSAID).

C. Orchitis

1. Definition
- Rare condition consisting of infection of the testicle.

2. Pathology
- Most common presentation as a sequelae to mumps in postpubertal males (seen in 25% of adult males with mumps); presents within 1 to 2 weeks after primary infection.
- Syphilis and other viral infections also have been implicated.
- Untreated epididymitis can progress to the testicle, resulting in epididymo-orchitis.
- Bacteria typical cause in this setting.

3. Clinical Features
- Unilateral or, rarely, bilateral swelling of testicle.
- Fever.
- Malaise.
- History of recent mumps, preceding or concurrent parotid swelling supports mumps orchitis.

4. Diagnostic Studies
- U/S is helpful in differentiating orchitis from other testicular and scrotal pathology.

5. Management
- Symptomatic; bed rest, anti-inflammatory agents, scrotal elevation.
- Treat underlying illness and consider urology referral.

D. Hydrocele, Spermatocele, and Varicocele

1. Definition
- Hydrocele—cystic fluid-containing testicular mass.
- Spermatocele—cystic fluid- and sperm-containing testicular mass.
- Varicoceles—cystic veracious vein-containing mass of testicle.

2. Pathology
- Idiopathic fluid accumulation between layers of the tunica vaginalis.
- May be due to trauma, tumor, fluid overload, infection.
- Inadequate venous return due to obstruction of pampiniform plexus. Left spermatic vein drains into left renal vein, whereas the right drains directly into the inferior vena cava, explaining the preponderance of left varicoceles.

3. Clinical Features
- Slow-growing, painless masses.
- On examination, swelling with standing and transillumination typically present.
- Swelling can make palpation of testicle and epididymis difficult.
- Varicoceles often have "bag of worms" appearance, which represents twisting and dilation of pampiniform plexus.
- Rule out testicular tumor because swelling may obscure mass.

4. Diagnostic Studies
- U/S useful in differentiating cystic from solid masses, testicular from extratesticular masses.
- Complete blood cell count may be helpful to rule out infections such as epididymitis.

5. Management
- Most often, no treatment is necessary unless for infertility (decreased sperm count secondary to increased temperature).
- Then, surgical treatment may be of benefit.

E. Undescended Testicle

1. Etiology
- Cryptorchidism—one of the most common congenital disorders.
- Incidence approximately 1% to 3% at birth.
- Reason unclear, but may result from chromosomal disorders.
- Incidence greater in premature and low-birth-weight infants.

2. Pathology
- Testes located outside scrotum, typically in inguinal canal, but also in abdominal cavity or other ectopic places.

3. Clinical Features

- On examination, one or both testes are absent from external scrotal sac.
- May be palpated in inguinal canals.
- Must assess for testes descended, but retracted due to a strong cremasteric reflex.

4. Diagnostic Studies

- U/S may assist in locating testes.

5. Management

- Most cryptorchid testes will descend spontaneously during first year of life.
- Orchiopexy is the treatment of choice after age 2.
- If discovered after puberty, orchiectomy typically performed because the undescended testicle is a cancer risk.
- Human chorionic gonadotropin (hCG) injections may stimulate descent in some instances.

F. Male Infertility

1. Etiology/Pathology

- Males contribute to couple's infertility in >25% of instances.

2. Clinical Features

- Inability to conceive after 1 year of trying under a physician's guidance/fertility consultation.

3. Diagnostic Studies

- Evaluate external sexual organs, especially testes for varicocele and cryptorchidism.
- Semen analysis after 3 to 5 days abstinence, evaluated for number, shape, motility of sperm.
- Hormone studies: luteinizing hormone (LH), follicle-stimulating hormone (FSH), testosterone levels are checked (Table 11-1).
- Testicular biopsy, vasography may be used in some patients with azoospermatism.

TABLE 11–1.   Evaluation of the Infertile Male

Abnormality	Etiology
↑FSH, ↑LH LH, ↓, testosterone	Primary testicular failure
↓FSH, ↓LH, ↓testosterone	Hypothalamic pituitary disease
NI to ↓FSH, ↑LH, ↑testosterone	Azoospermia/severe oligospermia? Partial androgen resistance
NI FSH, LH, testosterone	? Obstruction of epididymis or vas deferens
↑FSH, nl LH, nl testosterone	

From Hume HD, ed. *Kelley's Essentials of Internal Medicine.* 2nd ed. Philadelphia, PA: Lippincott Williams & Wilkins; 2001:733, with permission.

4. Management

- The treatment of male infertility is outlined in Table 11-2.

G. Primary Tumors of the Testes

1. Etiology/Pathology

- Most common neoplasm in men of age 20 to 35.
- More often involves the right testicle.
- Approximately 5% of testicular cancer develops in patients with a history of cryptorchidism.
- These diseases can be divided into two categories: seminoma and nonseminomatous.
- Seminoma is defined by its general lack of marker production and excellent therapeutic response to radiation therapy.
- Nonseminomatous germ cell tumors may be pure histologic type or composed of a mixture of two or more types—that is, embryonal carcinoma,

TABLE 11–2.   Treatment of Male Infertility

Category	Cause	Treatment
No treatment	Primary testicular failure	AID or adoption; androgen replacement if necessary
Specific treatment	Hypogonadotropic hypogonadism	Gonadotropins/GnRH
	Hyperprolactinemia	Bromocriptine
Potentially helpful treatment	Sexual dysfunction	Counseling
	Obstructive azoospermia	AIH
		Vasovasostomy or epididymovasostomy, microsurgical retrieval of spermatozoa followed by IVF
Value of treatment controversial	Varicocele	Varicocele ligation
	Sperm autoimmunity	High-dose glucocorticoids, IVF
	Genital tract infection	Antibiotics
	Idiopathic oligospermia, asthenospermia, or teratozoospermia	IVF, tubal embryo or zygote transfer; micromanipulation

AID, artificial insemination with donor sperm; GnRH, gonadotropin-releasing hormone; AIH, artificial insemination with husband sperm; IVF, *in vitro* fertilization.
From Hume HD, ed. *Kelley's Essentials of Internal Medicine.* 2nd ed. Philadelphia, PA: Lippincott Williams & Wilkins; 2001:733, with permission.

teratocarcinoma, endodermal sinus (yolk sac) tumors, and choriocarcinoma.

2. Clinical Features
- Painless enlargement of the testis.
- Testicular mass.
- Rarely: secondary hydroceles, gynecomastia.
- Stage I, confined to testis; stage II, retroperitoneal nodal involvement; and stage III, involvement elsewhere (usually lung).

3. Diagnostic Studies
- Evaluate hCG, α-fetoprotein, and LDH.

4. Management
- Orchiectomy and retroperitoneal irradiation.

II. Disorders of the Penis

A. Impotence

1. Definition
- Consistent inability to generate or maintain an erection.

2. Etiology/Pathology
- Neurologic, vascular, endocrine disorders, as well as trauma/surgery, drugs, and psychogenic causes contribute.
- Based on underlying cause.
- Lack of neurologic intervention, blood supply, and circulating hormones are some predisposing factors.

3. Clinical Features
- Thorough sexual history taking should disclose duration, nature of onset of impotence.
- Abrupt onset more likely suggests psychogenic causes, especially if morning erections persist.
- Gradual worsening of symptoms indicates systemic cause.

4. Diagnostic Studies
- Thorough medical history and physical examination to assess signs and symptoms of systemic diseases.
- Examination of genitals, auscultation for bruits; perineal pinprick sensation; rectal tone; prostate examination; penis for plaques or deformities; and testes for size, shape, position.
- Evaluation of impotence not standardized.
- Initial history and physical and basic laboratory work including testosterone level.
- Additional hormonal testing should be done if testosterone level is low.
- Clinical suspicion should be used to evaluate other possible etiologies.
- Nocturnal penile tumescence used to evaluate sleep erections (differentiates organic from psychogenic causes).
- Duplex U/S scanning used most frequently to determine penile blood flow.
- Angiography used for patients who may be surgical candidates.

5. Management
- Testosterone injections used if levels are low.
- Drugs such as yohimbine and trazodone have been tried.
- Intracorporeal injection therapy with prostaglandin (PGE_1), combination of papaverine and phentolamine, Caverject also used.
- Vacuum pumps, penile revascularization, penile prosthesis provide relief.
- Psychotherapy also may be of benefit in treating psychogenic impotence.
- Sildenafil (Viagra) has been approved for use in select patients. Its use is contraindicated in patients using other forms of nitrates; potential hypotensive effects of nitrates with its use.

B. Priapism

1. Definition
- Disorder consisting of prolonged erections without sexual excitation.
- Pathologic erection in which both corpora cavernosa are engorged with stagnant blood.
- Infection and impotence are common complications.

2. Etiology/Pathology
- Idiopathic—40% to 50%.
- Sickle cell disease—11%.
- Drugs and alcohol—20%.
- Injection of erectile-aiding agent—30%.
- Trauma—<10%.
- Divided into high-flow (arterial) or low-flow (venous) status (latter most common).
- Main causes of infertility—varicocele, 30% to 40% of patients.
- Others—hormonal, chromosomal, idiopathic, duct obstruction, cryptorchidism, torsion, infections.

3. Clinical Features
- Erection, with glans penis and corpus spongiosum typically not engorged.
- Low flow—very painful.
- High flow—little or no pain usually secondary to trauma.
- End result—ischemia with necrosis, infarction, infection, urinary retention, impotence.

4. Diagnostic Studies
- Magnetic resonance imaging used to detect thrombosis associated with priapism.

5. Management
- Goal of treatment—detumescence and preserving potency.
- Terbutaline given orally or subcutaneously occasionally reverses priapism.
- In low-flow cases, injections directly into the corpora with α-adrenergic agents, phenylephrine unless contraindicated (patients with cardiac or cerebrovascular history).
- Needle aspiration of corpora.

- Recurrent or prolonged episodes require surgical treatment.
- Attempt to treat underlying disease process; sickle cell patients often benefit from hydration, ± transfusions.
- Ice packs, pressure dressings, cold and hot enemas, nitrates, hypotensive agents have been tried.

C. Paraphimosis

1. Definition
- Entrapment of a retracted foreskin that cannot be reduced behind the coronal sulcus.
- If the paraphimosis is not promptly reduced, arterial blood supply becomes compromised, and the glans may necrose.

2. Clinical Features
- Pain, swelling, and erythema of the foreskin.
- If severe, the constriction causes edema and venous engorgement of the glans, which can lead to arterial compromise with subsequent tissue necrosis.

3. Management
- Squeezing the glans firmly for 5 minutes to reduce the swelling can lead to successful reduction of the foreskin.
- Using the index fingers to pull the prepuce distally while pushing the glans into the prepuce.
- Local infiltration of anesthesia with vertical incision of the constricting band can be performed by the urologist if manual reduction fails.

III. Disorders of the Prostate

A. Prostatitis

1. Definition
- Acute or chronic bacterial infection.
- Inflammation of the prostate gland.
- Nearly half of all men experience symptoms of prostatitis in their lives.

2. Etiology/Pathology
- Causative agents for acute bacterial prostatitis include gram-negative bacilli (most often *E. coli*) and *Pseudomonas* species and less commonly by gram-positive organisms (e.g., enterococci); however, *Chlamydia* and *Trichomonas* are noted in the younger age groups. Chronic bacterial prostatitis may evolve from acute bacterial prostatitis; many men have no history of acute infection. Gram-negative rods are the most common etiologic agents, but only one gram-positive organism (*Enterococcus*) is associated with chronic infection.
- Some patients have complaints consistent with prostatitis, but no organism can be identified.

3. Clinical Features

ACUTE
- Symptoms include dysuria, fever, chills, perineal discomfort/pain, irritative and obstructive voiding symptoms associated with low back and perineal discomfort.
- Perineal or suprapubic pain; exquisite tenderness is common on rectal examination.
- Prostatic massage should not be performed because of the risk of bacteremia.
- Rectal examination shows tender, "boggy" prostate.

CHRONIC
- Symptoms typically milder than those in acute form.
- Chronic prostatitis is a cause of relapsing urinary tract infection in men.
- Perineal or suprapubic discomfort, often dull and poorly localized.
- Fever uncommon.
- Rectal examination can be normal.

4. Diagnostic Studies
- Urinalysis, expressed prostatic massage secretions, postmassage urine should be analyzed for leukocytes and bacteria.
- Vigorous prostatic massage should be avoided in acute setting to avoid bacteremia.

5. Management
- Antibiotics should be chosen on likely etiology.
- Some patients with acute prostatitis require intravenous antibiotics, hospitalization.
- Supportive therapy with sitz baths, analgesics, and stool softeners.
- Helpful, but nonspecific, is a 4- to 6-week course of antibiotic, regardless of etiology.
- Treatment for chronic prostatitis is usually unsatisfactory due to the inability of antimicrobial agents to diffuse into prostatic fluid.
- Trimethoprim-sulfamethoxazole has resulted in moderately high cure rates, treatment must be prolonged (8 to 12 weeks), and relapse is frequent.

B. Benign Prostatic Hyperplasia (BPH)

1. Definition
- Benign enlargement of prostatic gland.

2. Etiology/Pathology
- Etiology unclear, but androgens (testosterone) are a factor, as demonstrated by lack of this condition in castrated men.
- Hyperplasia of stromal and glandular elements of prostate.
- Gland enlargement creates urethral narrowing that affects bladder emptying, which can lead to bladder wall hypertrophy distention.
- In severe hypertrophy, ureters dilate, hydronephrosis and renal impairment ensue.
- Prevalence almost universal in aging men.
- Twenty percent in men aged 41 to 50, 50% in men aged 51 to 60, and >90% in men aged 80 and older.
- Symptoms are also age related.
- At age 55, approximately 25% of men report obstructive voiding symptoms, at age 75, 50% of men report a decrease in the force and caliber of the urinary stream.

3. **Clinical Features**
   - Obstructive symptoms; hesitance, decreased force and caliber of stream, sensation of incomplete bladder emptying, double voiding (urinating a second time within 2 hours), straining to urinate, and postvoid dribbling.
   - Irritative symptoms; urgency, frequency, and nocturia.
   - Rectal examination discloses enlarged uniform prostate, nontender and free of nodules.
   - Size does not always correlate with degree of symptoms.

4. **Diagnostic Studies**
   - Careful history with attention to medication use, particularly anticholinergic agents that can cause difficulty urinating.
   - Abdominal examination may disclose distended bladder.
   - Rectal examination should be performed, gently palpating contour of prostate, note size and consistency of the prostate.
   - Urinalysis, blood urea nitrogen, and creatinine levels should be ordered.

5. **Management**
   - Patient education regarding the condition is essential.
   - Avoidance of drugs that can worsen symptoms.
   - Observation versus medical versus surgical treatments should be based on the degree of symptoms and whether renal impairment is present.
   - Selective α_1-blockers such as prazosin (Minipress), terazosin (Hytrin), and doxazosin (Cardura) often provide improvement of symptoms.
   - Hormonal therapy with finasteride (Proscar), a 5α-reductase inhibitor, reduces prostate size and symptoms.
   - Combination therapy: α-blockers and 5α-reductase inhibitor (e.g., long-term combination therapy with doxazosin and finasteride) is safe and overall clinical progression of BPH significantly more than either drug alone.
   - Transurethral resection of prostate removes the zone of the prostate around the urethra leaving the peripheral portion of the prostate and prostate capsule, useful in eliminating symptoms, but carries a slight risk of anesthesia, postoperative sexual dysfunction.
   - Consider open simple prostatectomy when the prostate is too large to remove endoscopically.
   - Transurethral laser-induced prostatectomy under transrectal U/S guidance is a minimally invasive procedure; advantages of laser surgery include outpatient surgery, minimal blood loss, and rare occurrence of transurethral resection syndrome; disadvantages of laser surgery include lack of tissue for pathologic examination, longer postoperative catheterization time, and more frequent irritative voiding complaints.

IV. Disorders of Testosterone Secretion

A. Male Hypogonadism

1. **Etiology/Pathology**
   - Caused by insufficient testosterone secretion by the testes themselves (more common), or due to decreased gonadotropin secretion of the pituitary gland.
   - Other causes: alcohol, chronic illness, Cushing syndrome, hemochromatosis.
   - The deficiency of testosterone contributes to erectile dysfunction (ED) and can produce osteoporosis.

2. **Clinical Features**
   - Decreased libido, ED, fatigue, depression.
   - Physical signs: diminished sexual hair growth, decrease of testicular mass, loss of muscle mass with increase in weight.

3. **Diagnostic Studies**
   - Decreased morning serum testosterone level.
   - LH and FSH should be measured; they are elevated in patients with testicular dysfunction and low in patients with pituitary (secondary hypogonadism) disorders.

4. **Management**
   - Testosterone replacement therapy should be started only after evaluation for prostate cancer.
   - Forms of replacement: oral preparations, intramuscular, and transdermal (skin patches).

SELECTED REFERENCES

Bates B, ed. *A Guide to Physical Examination and History Taking*. 10th ed. Philadelphia, PA: JB Lippincott; 2008.

Bennett JC, Plum F, eds. *Cecil Textbook of Medicine*. 22nd ed. Philadelphia, PA: WB Saunders; 2004.

Bondesson JD. Urologic conditions. In: Knoop KJ, Stack LB, Storrow AB, et al, eds. *The Atlas of Emergency Medicine*. 3rd ed. New York, NY: McGraw-Hill; 2010:chap 8. http://www.accessmedicine.com/content.aspx?aID=6002004. Accessed January 7, 2012.

David AK, Johnson TA Jr, Phillips DM, et al, eds. *Family Medicine: Principles and Practice*. 6th ed. New York, NY: Springer-Verlag; 2003.

DeCherney AH, Nathan L, eds. *Current Obstetric and Gynecologic Diagnosis and Treatment*. 11th ed. New York, NY: McGraw-Hill; 2011.

DeGowin RL, ed. *Degowin and Degowin's Diagnostic Examination*. 9th ed. New York, NY: McGraw-Hill; 2009.

Doherty GM, ed. *Current Surgical Diagnosis and Treatment*. 13th ed. Norwalk, CT: McGraw-Hill Companies; 2010.

Geisler WM, Krieger JN. Epididymitis and the acute scrotum syndrome. In: Klausner JD, Hook EW III, eds. *CURRENT Diagnosis and Treatment of Sexually Transmitted Diseases*. New York, NY: McGraw-Hill; 2007:chap 6. http://www.accessmedicine.com/content.aspx?aID=3027157. Accessed January 7, 2012.

Gillenwater JY, Grayhack JT, Howards SS, et al, eds. *Adult and Pediatric Urology*. 4th ed. St Louis, MO: Mosby; 2002.

Goroll AH, May LA, Mulley AG, eds. *Primary Care Medicine, Office Evaluation and Management of the Adult Patient*. 6th ed. Philadelphia, PA: Lippincott-Raven; 2009.

Greenfield LJ, Mullholland MW, Oldham KT, et al, eds. *Essentials of Surgery, Scientific Principles in Practice*. Philadelphia, PA: Lippincott-Raven; 2010.

Hatcher RA, Trussell J, Stewart F, et al, eds. *Contraceptive Technology*. 17th ed. New York, NY: Ardent Medica; 1998.

Isselbacher KJ, ed. *Harrison's Principles of Internal Medicine*. 18th ed. New York, NY: McGraw-Hill; 2011.

Kavoussir LR, ed. *Campbell-Walsh Urology*. 7th ed. Philadelphia, PA: WB Saunders; 2007.

La Rochelle J, Shuch B, Belldegrun A. Urology. In: Brunicardi FC, Andersen DK, Billiar TR, et al, eds. *Schwartz's Principles of Surgery*. 9th ed. New York, NY: McGraw-Hill; 2010:chap 40. http://www.accessmedicine.com/content.aspx?aID=5025145. Accessed January 7, 2012.

Mackett CW III, Nusbaum MR. Adult sexual dysfunction. In: South-Paul JE, Matheny SC, Lewis EL, eds. *CURRENT Diagnosis and Treatment in Family Medicine*. 3rd ed. New York, NY: McGraw-Hill; 2011:chap 18. http://www.accessmedicine.com/content.aspx?aID=8151380. Accessed January 7, 2012.

Meng MV, Stoller ML, Walsh TJ. Urologic disorders. In: McPhee SJ, Papadakis MA, Rabow MW, eds. *CURRENT Medical Diagnosis and Treatment 2012*. New York, NY: McGraw-Hill; 2012:chap 23. http://www.accessmedicine.com/content.aspx?aID=11857. Accessed January 7, 2012.

Mengel MB, Schwiebert LP, eds. *Ambulatory Medicine the Primary Care of Families*. 3rd ed. Norwalk, CT: Appleton & Lange; 2001.

Nicks BA, Manthey DE. Male genital problems. In: Tintinalli JE, Stapczynski JS, Cline DM, et al, eds. *Tintinalli's Emergency Medicine: A Comprehensive Study Guide*. 7th ed. New York, NY: McGraw-Hill; 2011:chap 96. http://www.accessmedicine.com/content.aspx?aID=6362635. Accessed January 7, 2012.

Noble J, Greene HL II, Levinson W, et al, eds. *Textbook of Primary Care Medicine*. 3rd ed. St. Louis, MO: Mosby; 2001.

Reirden DH, Sigel EJ, Nyquist A. Sexually transmitted infections. In: Hay WW, Levin MJ, Sondheimer JM, et al, eds. *CURRENT Diagnosis and Treatment: Pediatrics*. 20th ed. New York, NY: McGraw-Hill; 2011:chap 42. http://www.accessmedicine.com/content.aspx?aID=6592312. Accessed January 7, 2012.

Schwartz SI, ed. *Principles of Surgery*. 8th ed. New York, NY: McGraw-Hill; 2005.

Tierney LM Jr, McPhee SJ, Papadakis MA, eds. *Current Medical Diagnosis and Treatment*. 50th ed. New York, NY: McGraw-Hill/Appleton & Lange; 2011.

Tintinalli JE, Krome RL, Ruiz E, eds. *Emergency Medicine: A Comprehensive Study Guide*. 7th ed. New York, NY: McGraw-Hill; 2011.

Female Reproductive Disorders

Grace P. Landel • Robin Wempe • Margaret Schwedler

FEMALE REPRODUCTIVE DISORDERS

- Carcinomas are addressed in Chapter 16 "Surgery Disorders."

I. Infections (Table 11–3)

A. Diseases Characterized by Vaginal Discharge

1. **Bacterial Vaginosis (BV)**
   a. **Etiology/Pathology**
   - Most common cause of vaginitis.
   - Overgrowth of normal vaginal flora (*Gardnerella vaginalis, Mobiluncus* species, anaerobic gram-negative rods, and *Peptostreptococcus* species).
   - Marked decrease in the lactobacilli acidophilus that maintains vaginal pH.
   - Overall prevalence of 29.2%; 45.2% among women who reported having sex with another women

   b. **Clinical Features**
   - Copious watery, foul-smelling (fishy, rotten smell), gray-white discharge.
   - May be associated with pruritus.
   - No associated lesions.
   - May be asymptomatic (>50%).

   c. **Diagnostic Studies**
   - Saline wet mount: clue cells and marked decrease of lactobacilli, few white blood cells (WBCs).
   - Positive "whiff test" (fishy odor) with 10% potassium hydroxide (KOH).
   - pH > 4.5.
   - Can do Gram stain of discharge if unsure of diagnosis (large number of small gram-negative bacilli and a relative absence of lactobacilli).

   d. **Complications**
   - Associated with preterm labor, premature rupture of membranes, chorioamnionitis, postpartum endometritis, posthysterectomy vaginal cuff cellulitis, postabortion infection, and pelvic inflammatory disease (PID).
   - May experience recurrence despite treatment.

   e. **Management**
   - **Metronidazole**
     - 500 mg orally twice a day for 7 days; or
     - 0.75% gel, one full applicator (5 g) intravaginally, once a day for 5 days; or
     - 750 mg extended release tablets PO once daily for 7 days.
   - **Clindamycin**
     - Two percent cream, one full applicator (5 g) intravaginally at bedtime for 7 days; or
     - Three hundred milligram PO BID for 7 days; or
     - One hundred milligram ovules intravaginally once at bedtime for 3 days; or
     - Clindesse vaginal cream: one full applicator (5 g) intravaginally one time dose.
   - Chronic or recurrent infection: 0.75% metronidazole gel, one full applicator (5 g) intravaginally two times a week for 4 to 6 months.
   - Avoid douching—promotes loss of vaginal lactobacilli.
   - Unclear if sexually transmitted; treating partners is not necessary.
     - Use of condoms by male partners associated with a reduced risk of recurrence.
     - Consider screening female partners because BV is frequently found in both members of monogamous lesbian couples.

2. **Trichomoniasis**
   a. **Etiology/Pathology**
   - Caused by infestation of *Trichomonas vaginalis*, a unicellular flagellate protozoan.
   - Sexually transmitted.

   b. **Clinical Features**
   - Copious, frothy, yellow-green vaginal discharge, usually worse after menses or during pregnancy.
   - May have foul odor, and secondary vulvitis.
   - May have pruritus or pain.
   - Generalized vaginal erythema and cervical petechiae "strawberry cervix."
   - Often, simultaneous infection of urinary tract.
   - Male sex partners may develop urethritis or balanitis, but usually are asymptomatic.

   c. **Diagnostic Studies**
   - Saline wet mount shows motile trichomonads, increased WBCs: sensitivity approximately 60% to 70%.
   - pH >5.0.
   - May be seen on Pap smear.
   - OSOM Trichomonas Rapid Test (immunochromatographic capillary flow dipstick technology): sensitivity >83%, specificity >97%.
   - Affirm VP III (nucleic acid probe test): sensitivity >83%, specificity >97%.

TABLE 11–3. Comparisons of Infections

Diseases Characterized by Vaginal Discharge

	Etiology/ Pathology	Clinical Features	Diagnostic Studies	Complications	Management
Bacterial vaginosis	Overgrowth of normal vaginal flora Marked decrease in the lactobacilli acidophilus that maintains vaginal pH Most common cause of vaginitis	Copious watery, foul-smelling, gray-white discharge May be associated with pruritus; no associated lesions May be asymptomatic (>50%)	Wet mount: clue cells, few WBCs, decrease of lactobacilli Positive "whiff test" pH >4.5	Recurrence common; unclear if sexually transmitted; treating partners is not necessary, but consider screening female partners May be associated with preterm labor, PROM, chorioamnionitis, postpartum endometritis, posthysterectomy, vaginal cuff cellulitis, postabortion infection, and PID	Metronidazole orally or intravaginally Clindamycin orally or intravaginally Avoid douching—promotes loss of vaginal lactobacilli Use condoms with male partners
Trichomoniasis	*T. vaginalis*, sexually transmitted	Malodorous, frothy, yellow-green vaginal discharge Pruritus or pain Vaginal erythema Cervical petechiae Male partners may develop urethritis or balanitis, but usually asymptomatic atic	Wet mount: WBCs, motile trichomonads, pH >4.5 Rapid tests available	Associated with perinatal complications Increased incidence in the transmission of HIV	Metronidazole Tinidazole Treat partner Spermicidal agents decrease transmission Evaluate for other STIs
Vulvovaginal Candidiasis	Overgrowth of *C. albicans*	Vaginal discharge, pruritus, dysuria, ± dyspareunia Erythematous, edematous vulva, ± excoriations Thick, cottage cheese-like discharge	KOH: budding hyphae and spores. pH ≤4.5	May be unrefractory in pregnancy, HIV infection, and diabetes mellitus	Intravaginal options: Butoconazole Clotrimazole Miconazole Nystatin Terconazol Oral: Fluconazole Prevention
Cytolytic vaginitis	Overgrowth of lactobacilli	Nonodorous white to opaque vaginal discharge, vaginal and/or vulvar itching, vaginal or vulvar burning	Saline wet preparation: copious amounts of lactobacilli and a large number of epithelial cells pH between 3.5 and 4.5	None documented	Discontinue tampon use; sitz bath with sodium bicarbonate or sodium bicarbonate douche

(Continued)

TABLE 11–3.   Comparisons of Infections *(Continued)*

	Etiology/ Pathology	Clinical Features	Diagnostic Studies	Complications	Management
Gonorrhea	*N. gonorrhoeae* Coinfection with *Chlamydia* common	Incubation period—3 to 5 days Asymptomatic or purulent vaginal discharge, urinary frequency, dysuria, chronic cervicitis	Culture Nucleic acid hybridization tests NAAT	May cause PID, infertility, increased risk of ectopic pregnancy, disseminated infection, arthritis Neonatal gonococcal conjunctivitis/ pharyngitis/ respiratory/ systemic infection	Ceftriaxone Cefixime Treat for *Chlamydia* Notify and treat partners Avoid sexual activity for 7 days following treatment
Chlamydia	*C. trachomatis* Most common cause of cervicitis Cause of LGV in tropical countries Coinfection with gonorrhea common	May be asymptomatic May cause mucopurulent cervicitis, urinary frequency, dysuria, abdominal pain, PID, and/ or postcoital bleeding	LCR test: most sensitive/ specific Others: culture, direct fluorescent antibody, DNA probe test, enzyme immunoassay	PID, infertility, ectopic pregnancy, premature labor and delivery Postpartum infection Atypical cytologic findings on Pap smear	*Recommended*: Azithromycin Doxycycline *Alternatives:* Erythromycin Ofloxacin Levofloxacin Test for gonorrhea Treat partners LGV: doxycycline Avoid sexual activity for 7 days following treatment
		Diseases Characterized by Genital Ulcers			
Genital HSV infections	Herpes simplex virus Transferred during symptomatic and asymptomatic viral shedding Sexually transmitted	Primary outbreak: 2–7 days from exposure, resolves in 2–6 weeks Prodromal symptoms Multiple vesicles erode into painful ulcers Fever, malaise, inguinal lymphadenopathy, dysuria or other urinary symptoms With cervical infection: profuse watery discharge Virus remains in the sacral ganglia— recurrence in the same location Some outbreaks are asymptomatic	Viral culture for HSV Serum antibody titers Tzanck smear: multinucleated giant cells	HSV infection during pregnancy associated with congenital malformations C-section if active herpetic lesions or prodromal symptoms at time of delivery Prophylactic oral acyclovir after 36 weeks	Self-limiting infection, lesions heal spontaneously Dosing varies depending on first episode, suppression therapy or episodic treatment for recurrence Acyclovir Famciclovir Valacyclovir
Syphilis	*T. pallidum*	*Primary*: Painless ulcer, 10–90 days after exposure	Darkfield examination for spirochete	Neurosyphilis	Benzathine penicillin G 2.4 million units IM

Diseases Characterized by Genital Ulcers

	Etiology/ Pathology	Clinical Features	Diagnostic Studies	Complications	Management
	Contracted by direct contact with an infectious moist lesion May be congenital	Lesions heal in 1–5 weeks ± painless lymphadenopathy *Secondary:* Generalized, maculopapular rash, condyloma lata, fever, sore throat, diffuse adenopathy, patchy alopecia Develops average ~6 weeks (0.5–6 months) after initial infection, resolves in 2–6 weeks Serology positive in this stage *Latent:* Infectious in the first 1—2 years of latency *Tertiary:* Occurs 4–20+ years after initial infection in one-third of untreated patients	Serologic tests: become positive 1–4 weeks after the 1° lesion appears VDRL, RPR, FTA-ABS For neurosyphilis, CSF finding useful for monitoring resolution following treatment	Jarisch–Herxheimer reaction Congenital syphilis	*For primary, secondary syphilis and latent (of <1 year): one dose* *For late latent:* weekly dose for 3 weeks (7.2 million units total) Treat partners Offer HIV testing
Chancroid	*H. ducreyi* Uncommon in the US sexually transmitted, lesions on the hands have occurred. Incubation period is 3–5 days	Soft, painful, shallow, genital ulcer Multiple, small papules or vesicles may develop Lesion produces heavy, foul, contagious discharge Painful inguinal adenitis common, with abscess formation	Clinical diagnosis Culture is diagnostic, but positive in less than one-third of cases PCR available (not FDA-cleared)	Secondary infections, scarring	Azithromycin Ceftriaxone Erythromycin Ciprofloxacin

Others

	Etiology/ Pathology	Clinical Features	Diagnostic Studies	Complications	Management
HPV	Virus with double-stranded DNA Five types with oncogenic potential Two types linked to genital warts	Most asymptomatic Flat, papular, or pedunculated growths May have vaginal discharge, pruritus. postcoital bleeding	Pap smear—characteristic changes when high risk oncogenic types present Nucleic acid tests Acetowhite staining of epithelium Colposcopy and biopsy	Associated with cervical dysplasia Condylomas may proliferate during pregnancy and resolve after delivery	*Office treatment:* Podophyllin Cryotherapy TCA BCA Surgical removal *Outpatient treatment:* Podofilox Aldara (imiquimod)

(Continued)

TABLE 11–3. Comparisons of Infections (Continued)

Others

	Etiology/ Pathology	Clinical Features	Diagnostic Studies	Complications	Management
	Sexually transmitted				*Prevention:* Quadrivalent HPV vaccine (Gardasil)
PID	*N. gonorrhoeae* *C. trachomatis* Other microbes Risks: multiple partners, not using condoms	*Acute:* Appears ill May have fever, abdominal tenderness, purulent vaginal discharge, cervicitis, cervical motion tenderness, adnexal tenderness or mass, uterine tenderness *Chronic:* Less-severe symptoms, with a history of PID in the past	Wet mount. CBC, ESR, C-reactive protein (β-hCG. Gram stain Culture for gonorrhea and chlamydia Pelvic U/S Culdocentesis	Infertility Ectopic pregnancy Chronic pelvic pain	*Acute:* Antibiotics to cover gonorrhea, chlamydia, anaerobes NSAIDs *Chronic:* Antibiotics for 2–3 weeks and NSAIDs Surgery Screen partners for STIs and treat, if necessary
TSS	Toxins produced by *S.aureus*	Sudden onset of high fever, watery diarrhea, nausea, vomiting, sore throat, headache, diffuse macular rash, myalgias Appear acutely ill, fever ≥39° C (102.2° F) Tachycardia, dehydration, hypotension, erythematous rash, erythematous conjunctiva and pharynx, muscle and abdominal tenderness Pelvic examination should be done, remove tampon if present Multisystem involvement	CBC with differential, electrolytes, UA, BUN, creatinine, LFTs Culture suspected sources of the staphylococcal toxins	May progress to hypotensive shock in <48 hours Death	Admission to hospital Supportive measures Search for source and treat Antistaphylococcal antibiotics
Bartholin gland cyst/ abscess	Retained secretions from duct obstruction leads to gland enlargement May be infected by gonococcus, *E. coli*, *Staphylococcus*	*Not infected:* Nontender unilateral vulvar mass in the area of the Bartholin gland *Infected:* painful, unilateral vulvar mass, with associated inflammation and edema	Culture exudates	Recurrence	Simple asymptomatic cyst: no treatment I&D, may require marsupialization

- Culture: most sensitive specific but not commonly done.
  - **d. Complications**
    - Associated with perinatal complications.
    - Increased incidence in the transmission of HIV.
  - **e. Management**
    - Metronidazole 2 g PO in a single dose, or 500 mg BID + 7 days.
    - Tinidazole 2 g PO in a single dose.
    - Must treat partner also, who is usually asymptomatic.
    - Spermicidal agents (nonoxynol-9 etc.) decrease the transmission of *Trichomonas*.
    - Evaluate for other sexually transmitted infections (STIs).
3. **Vulvovaginal Candidiasis**
   - **a. Etiology/Pathology**
     - Caused from overgrowth of *Candida albicans* (present in normal vaginal flora), due to a change in normal vaginal environment.
     - Consider *Candida glabrata*, if KOH is negative, but yeast is suspected clinically.
   - **b. Clinical Features**
     - Vaginal discharge, pruritus of vulva and vaginal introitus, burning when urine touches the skin (secondary to inflammation and excoriation), vulva feels swollen, sore, ± dyspareunia.
     - Erythematous, edematous vulva, possibly with excoriations from scratching.
     - Vagina may have thick, cottage cheese-like discharge.
   - **c. Diagnostic Studies**
     - Budding hyphae and spores visible with 10% KOH solution.
     - Normal vaginal pH (<4.5).
     - Gram stain if suspect C. *glabrata*.
     - Yeast culture rarely indicated.
   - **d. Complications**
     - Yeast infections may be unrefractory in pregnancy, HIV infection, and diabetes mellitus.
   - **e. Management**
     - **Intravaginal options**
       - Butoconazole:
         - Two percent cream 5 g intravaginally for 3 days.
         - Butoconazole 1-sustained release, single intravaginal application.
       - Clotrimazole:
         - One percent cream 5 g intravaginally for 7 to 14 days.
         - One hundred milligram vaginal tablet for 7 days.
         - One hundred milligram vaginal tablet, two tablets for 3 days.
       - Miconazole:
         - Two percent cream 5 g intravaginally for 7 days.

- One hundred milligram vaginal suppository, one suppository for 7 days.
- Two hundred milligram vaginal suppository, one suppository for 3 days.
- One thousand and two hundred milligram vaginal suppository, one suppository for 1 day.
- Nystatin 100,000-unit vaginal tablet, one tablet for 14 days.
- Tioconazole 6.5% ointment 5 g intravaginally in a single application.
- Terconazole:
  - About 0.4% cream 5 g intravaginally for 7 days.
  - About 0.8% cream 5 g intravaginally for 3 days.
  - About 80 mg vaginal suppository, one suppository for 3 days.
- **Oral:** Fluconazole 150 mg PO, one tablet in single dose.
- Discuss vulvovaginal hygiene: keep vulva dry; wear 100% cotton underwear; avoid tight-fitting clothing, feminine deodorant products, bubble baths.
4. **Cytolytic Vaginitis**
   - **a. Etiology/Pathology**
     - Caused by an overgrowth of lactobacilli.
     - Etiology remains unknown.
     - Often misdiagnosed as BV or candidiasis.
   - **b. Clinical Features**
     - Variable symptoms: may include white vaginal discharge, vaginal and/or vulvar pruritus, vulvar burning or vulvar dysuria, and/or dyspareunia.
     - Minimal exam findings: may include white or opaque discharge, tenderness with speculum insertion and/or slightly erythematous vulvar and vaginal tissue.
   - **c. Diagnostic Studies**
     - Saline wet preparation: copious amounts of lactobacilli and a large number of epithelial cells.
     - pH 3.5 to 4.5.
   - **d. Management**
     - Discontinue tampon use to decrease vaginal acidity.
     - Sitz bath with 2 to 4 tbsp of sodium bicarbonate.
     - Sodium bicarbonate douche with 1 tbsp of sodium bicarbonate to 1 pint of water.
     - Treatment may have to be repeated before relief is achieved.
5. **Gonorrhea**
   - **a. Etiology/Pathology**
     - *Neisseria gonorrhoeae* contracted by sexual contact with an infected person.
     - Coinfection with *Chlamydia* common.
   - **b. Clinical Features**
     - Incubation period: 3 to 5 days.
     - Usually asymptomatic.

- If symptomatic: vaginal discharge, urinary frequency, dysuria, rectal discomfort from perineal spread.
- Can progress to PID, disseminated infection, arthritis.

c. **Diagnostic Studies**
- **Nucleic acid amplification tests (NAAT)**—most sensitive and specific:
  - Endocervical specimen.
  - Vaginal specimen.
  - Urine.
- **Culture:**
  - Endocervical specimen.
- **Nucleic acid hybridization tests:**
  - Endocervical specimen.
- **Gram stain:**
  - Not specific for endocervical specimens, therefore not recommended.

d. **Complications**
- May cause PID, infertility, increased risk of ectopic pregnancy secondary to tubal scarring, neonatal conjunctivitis.

e. **Management**
- **Recommended regimens—one time dose:**
  - Ceftriaxone 250 mg IM; or
  - Cefixime 400 mg: 1 tablet or 10 cc (200 mg per 5 mL) PO.
- **Alternative regimens—one time dose:**
  - Ceftizoxime 500 mg IM; or
  - Cefoxitin 2 g IM, administered with probenecid 1 g PO; or
  - Cefotaxime 500 mg IM.
- Also treat with Azithromycin 1 g PO × one for presumptive coinfection with chlamydia.
- Partners within the last 60 days, or last partner if >60 days, should be notified and treated.
- Avoid sexual activity for 7 days following treatment.

f. **Screening—U.S. Preventive Services Task Force (USPSTF) Recommendations**
- All sexually active women and men under the age of 26.
- Any woman or man at increased risk for infection: positive for other STIs, new or multiple sexual partners, erratic condom use, having sex for drugs or money.

6. *Chlamydia*
a. **Etiology/Pathology**
- *Chlamydia trachomatis* contracted by sexual contact with an infected person.
- Most common cause of cervicitis.
- Cause of lymphogranuloma venereum (LGV) in tropical countries.
- Coinfection with gonorrhea common.

b. **Clinical Features**
- May be asymptomatic.
- May cause mucopurulent cervicitis, urinary frequency, dysuria, abdominal pain, PID, and/or postcoital bleeding.
- Discharge tends to be less purulent and painful, and more watery than discharge of gonorrhea.

c. **Diagnostic Studies**
- Culture, direct fluorescent antibody, enzyme immunoassay, DNA probe test.
- Ligase chain reaction (LCR) test is the most sensitive and specific. Can be run on a urine specimen.

d. **Complications**
- PID, infertility, ectopic pregnancy.
- Premature labor and delivery.
- Postpartum infection.
- Atypical cytologic findings on Pap smear.

e. **Management**
- **Recommended regimens:**
  - Azithromycin: 1 g once; or
  - Doxycycline: 100 mg PO BID × 7 days.
- **Alternative regimens:**
  - Erythromycin base 500 mg PO QID × 7 days; or
  - Erythromycin ethylsuccinate 800 mg PO QID × 7 days; or
  - Ofloxacin 300 mg PO BID × 7 days; or
  - Levofloxacin 500 mg PO once daily for 7 days.
- Also test for gonorrhea.
- Partners within the last 60 days, or last partner if >60 days, should be notified and treated.
- Avoid sexual contact for 7 days after treatment.
- For LGV: doxycycline 100 mg BID × 21 days.

f. **Screening—USPSTF Recommendations**
- All sexually active women and men under the age of 26.
- Any woman or man at increased risk for infection: positive for other STIs, new or multiple sexual partners, erratic condom use, having sex for drugs or money.

B. **Diseases Characterized by Genital Ulcers**
1. **Genital HSV Infections**
a. **Etiology/Pathology**
- Herpes simplex virus (HSV).
- Transferred during both symptomatic and asymptomatic viral shedding.
- Sexually transmitted (oral, anal, or vaginal intercourse) through direct contact with contaminated secretions or mucosal surfaces.

b. **Clinical Features**
- Primary outbreak occurs 2 to 7 days from the time of exposure.
- Prodromal symptoms (itch/tingle) may be experienced prior to the development of multiple vesicles that erode into painful ulcers on labia and around introitus.

- May have fever, malaise, and inguinal lymph-adenopathy in severe infections.
- Dysuria or other urinary symptoms, including urinary retention, may develop.
- Herpes outbreaks on the cervix cause a profuse watery discharge and no other symptoms.
- Lesions are self-limited, resolving in 2 to 6 weeks.
- The virus remains in the sacral ganglia and can recur any time with lesions.
- Some outbreaks are asymptomatic.

c. **Diagnostic Studies**
- Viral culture for HSV.
- Serum antibody titers.
- Tzanck smear reveals multinucleated giant cells.

d. **Complications**
- If pregnant woman has active herpetic lesions or prodromal symptoms at the time of delivery, C-section is indicated to prevent neonatal transmission (60% fetal mortality rate, with vaginal delivery; 40% to 50% chance of transmission during active primary infection, 5% during recurrent infection). Consider prophylactic oral acyclovir after 36 weeks.
- HSV infection during pregnancy also associated with congenital malformations.

e. **Management**
- Self-limiting infection, lesions heal spontaneously.
- **First episode:**
  - Acyclovir 400 mg PO TID × 7 to 10 days or 200 mg PO 5 times a day × 7 to 10 days.
  - Famciclovir 250 mg PO TID a day for 7 to 10 days; or
  - Valacyclovir 1 g PO BID for 7 to 10 days.
- **Suppression therapy for ≥6 recurrences per year:**
  - Acyclovir 400 mg PO BID.
  - Valacyclovir 1.0 g PO BID.
- **Episodic therapy for recurrent herpes:**
  - Acyclovir 400 mg PO TID for 5 days.
  - Acyclovir 800 mg PO BID for 5 days.
  - Acyclovir 800 mg PO TID for 2 days.
  - Famciclovir 125 mg PO BID for 5 days.
  - Famciclovir 1,000 mg PO BID for 1 day.
  - Valacyclovir 500 mg PO BID for 3 days.
  - Valacyclovir 1.0 g PO once a day for 5 days.

f. **Screening—USPSTF Recommendations**
- Screening not recommended.

2. **Syphilis**
a. **Etiology/Pathology**
- *Treponema pallidum* (a spirochete).
- Contracted by direct contact with an infectious moist lesion.
- Site of infection may be the hand as a consequence of touching a lesion.
- May be congenital.

b. **Clinical Features**
- **Primary:** chancre (indurated, firm, painless papule, or ulcer with raised borders); develops 10 to 90 days after exposure to infection. It can occur anywhere on skin or mucous membrane. The lesions heal in 1 to 5 weeks. May be associated with painless lymphadenopathy.
- **Secondary:** caused by the spirochetes entering the bloodstream. Self-limited, generalized, maculopapular rash develops 2 weeks to 6 months (average ~6 weeks) after initial infection, resolves in 2 to 6 weeks. Skin lesions common in 80% of patients, classically affecting the palms and soles. Condyloma lata, fever, sore throat, diffuse adenopathy, and patchy alopecia may be present. Serology positive in this stage.
- **Latent:** period after resolution of the lesions of primary and secondary infection, or the finding of a reactive serologic test without a history of therapy. Infectious in the first 1 to 2 years of latency.
  - Early latent stage: infection of <1 year.
  - Late latent stage: infection of >1 year.
- **Tertiary:** occurs 4 to 20+ years after initial infection in one-third of untreated patients. Commonly causes skin, cardiac, and neurologic problems, can affect any organ system.

c. **Diagnostic Studies**
- Identification of the organism: darkfield examination of specimens from cutaneous lesions. Requires experience.
- Serologic tests: become positive 1 to 4 weeks after the primary lesion appears.
  (1) **Nontreponemal tests:** Venereal Disease Research Laboratory (VDRL) test, rapid reagin (RPR) test, and automated reagin test for screening procedures in the field.
  (2) **Treponemal antibody tests:** the fluorescent treponemal antibody absorption (FTA-ABS) test and microhemagglutination assay for *T. pallidum* detect antibody against *Treponema* spirochetes.
- For neurosyphilis, cerebrospinal fluid (CSF) findings are unreliable for excluding the diagnosis, but are useful for monitoring resolution following treatment.

d. **Complications**
- Neurosyphilis may develop.
- **Jarisch–Herxheimer reaction:**
  - Febrile reaction occurring in 50% to 75% of patients with early syphilis treated with penicillin.
  - Occurs 4 to 12 hours after injection; lasts 24 hours.
  - Uncertain cause.
  - Generally benign.
- With pregnancy in an infected woman, the baby will have congenital syphilis.

e. **Management**
- For primary, secondary, and latent syphilis (of <1 year): benzathine penicillin G 2.4 million units intramuscular (IM) once.
- For late latent: benzathine penicillin G 2.4 million units IM once weekly for 3 weeks (7.2 million units total).
- Partners should be notified and treated.
- Offer HIV testing to all patients diagnosed with syphilis due to high rates of coinfection.

f. **Screening—USPSTF Recommendations**
- Persons at increased risk for syphilis infection.
- All pregnant women.

3. **Chancroid**
a. **Etiology/Pathology**
- *Haemophilus ducreyi* (gram-negative bacillus).
- Uncommon in the United States.
- Sexually transmitted, lesions on the hands have occurred.
- Incubation period is 3 to 5 days.

b. **Clinical Features**
- Soft, painful, shallow, genital ulcer, circumscribed by a bright red zone of congestion.
- Multiple, small papules or vesicles may develop.
- Lesion produces heavy, foul, contagious discharge.
- Painful inguinal adenitis common, often with abscess formation.

c. **Diagnostic Studies**
- Culturing is diagnostic, but positive in less than one-third of cases.
- PCR testing available, although not FDA-cleared.
- Rely on clinical diagnosis; probable diagnosis made if:
  - One + painful genital ulcers.
  - No evidence of syphilis by darkfield examination or serology.
  - Negative HSV test.
  - Clinical presentation is typical for chancroid.

d. **Complications**
- Secondary infections, scarring.

e. **Management**
- Azithromycin 1 g once; or
- Ceftriaxone 250 mg IM once; or
- Erythromycin 500 mg PO TID × 7 days; or
- Ciprofloxacin 500 mg PO BID × 3 days.

4. **Lymphogranuloma Venereum**
- Uncommon in the United States and in women.

5. **Granuloma Inguinale**
- Uncommon in the United States.

C. **Others**
1. **Human Papilloma Virus (HPV)**
a. **Etiology/Pathology**
- Virus with double-stranded DNA.
- More than 20 types of HPV identified: Types 16, 18, 31, 33, and 35 appear to have the most oncogenic potential and are considered "high risk."
- Types 6 and 11 are associated with genital condyloma and considered "low risk."
- When vulvar lesions are present, the entire lower tract is usually involved.
- Sexually transmitted, both partners infected.
- Condyloma lesions, aka warts, are benign and not related to the development of cervical cancer.

b. **Clinical Features**
- Most types cause an asymptomatic infection.
- Flat, papular, or pedunculated growths.
- Warts are either external or internal.
- With florid condylomas, may have vaginal discharge and pruritus.
- Postcoital bleeding may occur.
- Massive proliferation seen in immunosuppression (pregnancy, HIV infection, diabetes, renal transplant) and treatment often is difficult.

c. **Diagnostic Studies**
- Characteristic changes may be present on Pap smear when high-risk types of HPV are present.
- Nucleic acid tests.
- Acetowhite staining of epithelium with dilute acetic acid solution.
- Colposcopy and biopsy.

d. **Complications**
- Associated with cervical dysplasia, regular Pap smears recommended.
- Condyloma may proliferate during pregnancy and spontaneously resolve following delivery.

e. **Management**
- Most lesions respond within 3 months of treatment.
- **Office treatment:**
  - Podophyllin resin 10% to 25% in a compound tincture of benzoin applied to each wart (not in pregnancy) repeated weekly. Wash off after 1 to 4 hours to reduce local irritation.
  - Cryotherapy internally.
  - Trichloroacetic acid or bichloroacetic acid (BCA) 80% to 90% applied to each wart, repeated weekly if needed.
  - Surgical removal, tangential shave excision, curettage, or electrosurgery.
- Most lesions respond within 3 months of treatment.
- **Outpatient treatment:**
  - Not in pregnancy.
  - Podofilox (0.5% solution of gel), apply BID × 3 days, repeat weekly for up to 4 weeks.
  - Imiquimod (Aldara), applied externally overnight three times a week for up to 16 weeks.
- **Prevention:**
  - Quadrivalent HPV vaccine (Gardasil).
    - Three-dose schedule, second and third doses—2 and 6 months after the first dose.

- Routine vaccination of females aged 11 to 12 years; can be started as young as age 9 years. Recommended up to 26 years of age.
- Screenings for cervical cancer and HPV DNA or HPV antibody prior to vaccination are not needed.
- No therapeutic effect on current infection.
- May be used in immunocompromised and lactating women, not given in pregnancy.

2. **Pelvic Inflammatory Disease**
   a. **Etiology/Pathology**
      - Infectious inflammation of upper genital tract (uterus, fallopian tubes, ovaries, pelvic peritoneum).
      - Polymicrobial infection, caused most commonly by *N. gonorrhoeae* and *C. trachomatis.*
      - Other microbes may be present.
      - Having multiple partners, not using condoms puts patients at high risk.
   b. **Clinical Features**
      - Patient is usually in reproductive years with a history of unprotected sex.
      - Onset often associated with menses or dilation and curettage (D&C).

      ACUTE
      - Appears ill.
      - May have fever, abdominal tenderness, purulent vaginal discharge, cervicitis, cervical motion tenderness, adnexal tenderness or mass, uterine tenderness.

      CHRONIC
      - Less-severe symptoms, with a history of PID diagnosis in the past.
   c. **Diagnostic Studies**
      - Wet mount—BV, *Trichomonas* and/or WBCs may be present.
      - Blood work: complete blood count (CBC) (increased WBCs); ESR (increased); β-human chorionic gonadotropin (β-hCG) (rule out ectopic); C-reactive protein (elevated).
      - Gram stain: gram-negative kidney-shaped diplococci in polymorphonuclear leukocytes.
      - Cervical cultures for gonorrhea and chlamydia.
      - Pelvic ultrasound (U/S): most valuable for following abscess progression or regression.
      - Culdocentesis, if appropriate.
   d. **Complications**
      - Increases risk of infertility.
      - Ectopic pregnancy.
      - Chronic pelvic pain.
      - Occasionally patient ends up with diagnostic laparoscopy because symptoms may mimic acute appendicitis.
   e. **Management**
      - Screen partners for STIs and treat, if necessary.

- Inpatient or outpatient treatment, depending on the severity of symptoms.
  - All pregnant or immunocompromised women with PID should be hospitalized.
- Antibiotic therapy needs to cover gonorrhea, chlamydia, anaerobes.
- Pain management with nonsteroidal anti-inflammatory drugs (NSAIDs).

CHRONIC
- Antibiotics for 2 to 3 weeks and NSAIDs.
- Surgery (TAH-BSO) if associated with intractable pelvic pain and/or tubo-ovarian abscess.

3. **Toxic Shock Syndrome (TSS)**
   a. **Etiology/Pathology**
      - Toxins produced by *Staphylococcus aureus.*
   b. **Clinical Features**
      - Sudden onset of high fever, watery diarrhea, nausea, vomiting, headache, myalgias, diffuse macular rash, sore throat.
      - Tachycardia, dehydration, possibly hypotension.
      - Appear acutely ill, fever $\geq39°$ C ($102.2°$ F); erythematous, sunburn-like rash is seen over the face, proximal extremities; erythematous conjunctiva and pharynx; muscle and abdominal tenderness.
      - Pelvic examination should be done, remove tampon if present.
      - Mucosal lesions should be sought, and a culture for *S. aureus* performed.
      - Multisystem involvement is the rule (three or more of the following involved: muscular, mucous membranes, renal, hepatic, hematologic, CNS).
   c. **Diagnostic Studies**
      - Assess for effects on various organ systems: CBC with differential, electrolytes, urine analysis (UA), blood urea nitrogen (BUN), creatinine, liver function tests (LFTs), blood and throat cultures, CSF culture, if indicated.
      - Culture suspected sources of the staphylococcal toxins.
   d. **Complications**
      - May progress to hypotensive shock in <48 hours.
      - Thirty percent of women who suffer from TSS have recurrences (greatest risk is in the first three menstrual cycles after the original episode).
      - Mortality rate 3% to 6%.
      - Major causes of death from TSS are adult respiratory distress syndrome, disseminated intravascular coagulation, and hypotension.
   e. **Management**
      - Admission to hospital.
      - Supportive measures (e.g., intravenous fluids, blood pressure support, analgesics).

- Search for source and treat (e.g., removal of vaginal products, exploration of recent surgical wounds).
- Antistaphylococcal antibiotics.

4. **Bartholin Gland Cyst/Abscess**
   a. **Etiology/Pathology**
      - Duct obstruction leads to enlargement of the gland from retained secretions, often complicated with infection by gonococcus, *E. coli*, *Staphylococcus*, for example.
   b. **Clinical Features**
      - Nontender unilateral vulvar mass in the area of the Bartholin gland if not infected.
      - Painful, unilateral vulvar mass, with associated inflammation and edema if infected.
   c. **Diagnostic Studies**
      - Culture exudate.
   d. **Complications**
      - Recurrence.
   e. **Management**
      - Simple asymptomatic cyst requires no treatment.
      - Incision and drainage (I&D).
      - May require marsupialization.
      - Recurrent infections may require excision or marsupialization of the gland for permanent drainage.

II. Disorders of the Cervix

A. Cervical Polyps
1. **Etiology/Pathology**
   - Result of focal endocervical hyperplasia of unknown etiology. May be related to hyperestrogenism.
   - May be covered with squamous, columnar, or squamocolumnar epithelium. Often attached by a long stalk.
   - Common; occur at any age, but more common in multigravidas over 20.
   - Most are benign; although low risk for cancer (0.5%—dysplasia; 0.5%—malignant), all should be removed and sent for pathologic diagnosis.
2. **Clinical Features**
   - May be asymptomatic, found on examination.
   - Symptoms:
     - Bleeding: intermenstrual, postcoital, heavy and/or prolonged.
     - Vaginal discharge—leukorrhea.
   - Soft, smooth, red approximately 0.5 to 1 cm × 1 to 2 cm growth protruding from cervical opening, or seen in the endocervical canal with the use of an endocervical speculum.
   - Fragile, may bleed on contact.
3. **Diagnostic Studies**
   - Remove polyp and send for pathologic diagnosis.
   - Polyps may be seen on transvaginal pelvic U/S, hysterosalpingogram, or saline infusion sonohysterography.

- Culture for concomitant infections if abnormal discharge is present.
4. **Complications**
   - Cause of previously unexplained infertility.
   - Cervicitis, endometritis, and parametritis.
   - Salpingitis.
5. **Management**
   - Removal, usually done in office by twisting at the pedicle with hemostat (usually curative).

B. Nabothian Cysts
1. **Etiology/Pathology**
   - Mucus-secreting columnar endocervical epithelium become covered by squamous cells.
   - Secretions accumulate.
2. **Clinical Features**
   - Smooth, clear, or yellow nodule visible on examination; may be palpable.
   - Several millimeters to 3 cm in diameter.
3. **Diagnostic Studies**
   - None.
4. **Complications**
   - None.
5. **Management**
   - No treatment necessary.

III. Disorders of the Uterus

A. Fibroid Tumors (Leiomyoma)
1. **Definition**
   - Benign tumors of the uterus.
2. **Etiology**
   - True etiology unknown.
   - Most common pelvic tumor in females.
   - More common in African American than Caucasian females.
   - Responsive to hormones; grow during reproductive years.
3. **Pathology**
   - Benign growths, primarily of smooth muscle, originating in the myometrium.
   - Usually multiple.
   - Classification based on anatomic location.
4. **Clinical Features**
   - About 50% to 65% are asymptomatic.
   - Symptoms may include abnormal uterine bleeding (most common), pelvic pain or heaviness, dysmenorrhea, anemia, back pain, premature labor.
   - Uncommon symptoms due to the pressure of a large fibroid: increased urinary frequency, hydronephrosis, stress incontinence, dyspareunia, constipation, lower extremity edema.
   - Enlarged, irregularly contoured uterus on bimanual examination.
   - May be palpable during abdominal examination.
5. **Diagnostic Studies**
   - β-hCG: rule out pregnancy.
   - CBC count: anemia common, leukocytosis with acute degeneration or infection.

- Sedimentation rate: may be elevated with acute degeneration or infection.
- Pelvic U/S: document size and position of fibroids.
- Intravenous pyelogram: rule out hydronephrosis.
- Consider endometrial biopsy to rule out endometrial cancer as a cause of bleeding.

6. **Complications**
   - Anemia secondary to menorrhagia.
   - Degeneration: caused by ischemia when a fibroid outgrows its blood supply; a painful condition that may present as an acute abdomen; sarcomatous (malignant) degeneration is rare.
   - Pregnancy (rapid growth can occur due to hormones): degeneration leading to pain; premature labor; obstruction requiring C-section; postpartum hemorrhage.
   - Possible link to fertility: myomectomy for endocavitary fibroids.
   - Spontaneous abortion.

7. **Management**
   a. **Nonpregnant, Asymptomatic Patient**
      - Follow with bimanual examination every 6 months or serial pelvic U/S to follow growth. Fibroids may shrink after menopause; consequently, postmenopausal fibroid growth considered malignancy until proven otherwise.
   b. **Symptomatic**
      - **Conservative treatment:**
        - Progestin therapy for abnormal bleeding. GnRH agonists create temporary menopause and are used frequently preoperatively (fibroid tumors shrink in the absence of estrogen stimulation).
        - Mirena (levonorgestrel-releasing intrauterine device [IUD]) to treat menorrhagia.
      - **Surgical treatment:**
        - *Myomectomy*—removes fibroids and preserves the uterus (and fertility). Depending on the location of tumors may be able to be done by laparoscope or hysteroscope.
        - *Hysterectomy*—performed when fertility is not an issue. Curative.
        - *Embolization*—embolizing agent infused into the uterine artery supplying the fibroid.

IV. Disorders of the Ovaries

A. Ovarian Cysts

1. **Definition**
   - Cystic enlargement of any of the normal ovarian structures.
   - Fluid-filled sacs often related to ovulation.
   - Common in reproductive years, usually unilateral.

2. **Etiology/Pathology**
   - Follicular cysts represent a mature follicle that fails to rupture.
   - Corpus luteum cysts develop as a result of bleeding into center of corpus luteum.

- Theca lutein cysts are associated with elevated levels of chorionic gonadotropin. They can be associated with hydatidiform mole, choriocarcinoma, and chorionic gonadotropin or clomiphene therapy and, rarely, with normal pregnancy.

3. **Clinical Features**
   - May be asymptomatic and an incidental finding on pelvic examination.
   - May cause a change in menstrual cycle, aching pelvic pain, dyspareunia, abnormal uterine bleeding.
   - Palpable adnexal mass on bimanual examination.
   - Ruptured cyst can present as an acute abdomen.

4. **Diagnostic Studies**
   - β-hCG to rule out pregnancy.
   - Pelvic U/S to confirm diagnosis.

5. **Complications**
   - Bleeding, torsion (surgical emergency), rupture causing symptoms of an acute abdomen.

6. **Management**
   - Cysts usually resolve spontaneously over the next few menstrual cycles.
   - Oral contraceptives have been used in the past to aid in resolution. Data do not support increased rate of resolution.
   - If no resolution occurs, or if demonstrated continued growth is present, laparoscopic cystectomy to rule out malignancy.

B. Polycystic Ovarian Syndrome

1. **Definition**
   - Endocrine syndrome characterized by anovulation, obesity, hirsutism, bilaterally enlarged polycystic ovaries, menstrual irregularity, insulin resistance, and infertility.

2. **Etiology/Pathology**
   - Etiology unknown.
   - Abnormal gonadotropin secretion with excessive androgen production with pituitary suppression.

3. **Clinical and Associated Features**
   - Anovulatory cycles.
   - Menstrual abnormalities, including amenorrhea.
   - Hirsutism (50%), obesity (80%), amenorrhea (50%), abnormal uterine bleeding (30%), enlarged ovaries on bimanual examination.
   - Metabolic syndrome.

4. **Diagnostic Studies**
   - Luteinizing hormone (LH) and follicle-stimulating hormone (FSH): rule out premature ovarian failure.
   - Thyroid-stimulating hormone (TSH): rule out thyroid disorder.
   - Prolactin level: rule out pituitary adenoma.
   - Lipid panel to evaluate for dyslipidemia.
   - Glucose tolerance test to evaluate for insulin resistance.
   - Testosterone (elevated), DHEA-S (elevated in 50% of patients), and 17-hydroxyprogesterone.

5. **Complications**
   - Infertility, hirsutism, and endometrial hyperplasia.
   - Increased risk of early-onset type 2 diabetes mellitus, cardiovascular disease, endometrial and breast cancer.
6. **Management**
   - Treat patient symptoms.
   - Oral contraceptives regulate menstrual cycle and prevent endometrial hyperplasia; cyclic progestin can also be used.
   - Hirsutism: Spironolactone (decreases androgenic action in target organs); antiandrogens (flutamide or finasteride); low-dose OCP (results after 6 to 12 months); depilation, and electrolysis.
   - Dexamethasone for high DHEA-S levels.
   - Obesity: weight reduction may help to restore ovulation.
   - Infertility: induce ovulation with drugs: clomiphene (stimulates ovaries); oral hypoglycemics (reduce hyperandrogenemia and hyperinsulinemia). Refer if needed.
   - Monitor lipids, glucose; consider screening carotids starting at 30 and coronary calcium starting at 45.

V. Disorders of the Breasts
   - **See also Chapter 16: "Surgery Disorders," "III. Disorders of the Breast"**
A. Mastitis
   1. **Etiology/Pathology**
      - *Congestive*: bilateral breast engorgement occurring 2 to 3 days postpartum.
      - *Infectious*: Uncommon complication of breast feeding; due to nipple trauma; infection with *S. aureus* or *Candida*.
      - More common in first-time nursing mothers.
   2. **Clinical Features**
      - *Congestive*: bilateral breast pain and swelling, low-grade fever, may have axillary lymphadenopathy.
      - *Infectious*: presents 1 week postpartum; usually unilateral breast pain; fever, chills; findings confined to one quadrant of the breast with tenderness, swelling, erythema and warmth; ± nipple discharge; ± abscess formation (edema and fluctuation).
   3. **Diagnostic Studies**
      - Culture of abscess if draining.
      - CBC, although not necessary.
   4. **Complications**
      - Abscess.
   5. **Management**
      - *Congestive*: if woman does not want to breastfeed—tight-fitting bra, ice packs, avoiding breast stimulation, analgesics. If she does want to breastfeed, supportive therapy only—manually emptying breasts completely after baby is done breastfeeding, analgesics, local heat, and continuing to nurse.

   - *Infectious*: supportive measures as above, with antibiotic therapy (antistaphylococcal) or fluconazole 200 mg PO daily.
   - Abscess: surgical I&D, discontinue breastfeeding, and suppress lactation.

VI. Other Disorders
A. Pelvic Organ Prolapse
   1. **Definition**
      - Herniation of one of the pelvic organs, classified by their location.
        - Anterior vaginal wall: cystocele.
        - Apical: uterine prolapse.
        - Posterior vaginal wall: rectocele.
   2. **Etiology/Pathology**
      - Relaxation, injury, congenital or developmental weakness of pelvic support structures.
      - Risk factors: age, obesity, activities that increase pressure on the pelvic floor—multiparity, chronic coughing, repetitive heavy lifting.
      - Staging is based on position of the prolapse to the hymen, graded 0 (no prolapse) to IV (complete prolapse).
   3. **Clinical Features**
      - Condition may affect quality of life.
      - Symptoms include pressure or discomfort in the vagina or pelvis; low back pain; urinary symptoms including stress incontinence and urinary tract infection (UTI) symptoms without dysuria; sensation of something protruding from the vagina (somewhat relieved by lying down); dyspareunia; difficulty with defecation; sexual dysfunction due to a feeling of laxity.
      - Examination: bulging mass, more prominent with increased intraabdominal pressure.
      - Also evaluate for urinary incontinence.
   4. **Diagnostic Studies**
      - Usually not needed.
      - Pelvic U/S if questionable pelvic mass is present.
      - Voiding cystourethrography (VCUG): for evaluation of bladder and bladder support.
   5. **Complications**
      - Not common.
      - Ulceration of the protruding vaginal tissue, which can lead to cellulitis.
      - UTI or urinary obstruction.
      - Urinary or fecal incontinence.
   6. **Management**
      - Kegel exercises: strengthen pelvic floor.
      - Pessary: provides symptomatic relief.
      - Hormone replacement therapy: to improve symptoms due to atrophy.
      - Surgery: only curative treatment; procedure dependent on the type of prolapse.

B. Endometriosis

1. **Etiology/Pathology**
   - Cause is unknown, may be due to retrograde menstruation.
   - Endometrial tissue is found outside of the uterus.
   - Occurs in women of reproductive age.
2. **Clinical Features**
   - Asymptomatic or infertility.
   - Dysmenorrhea and dyspareunia, premenstrual low back, pelvic, or rectal pain.
   - Pelvic examination: usually normal; may find a tender mass or nodules in the adnexa, posterior fornix or rectovaginal septum; fixed uterus and cervical motion tenderness.
3. **Diagnostic Studies**
   - None of value. Diagnosed with direct visualization at laparotomy or laparoscopy.
4. **Complications**
   - Infertility.
   - Otherwise rare: symptoms due to adhesions; obstruction of ureters or bowel; ovarian torsion.
5. **Management**
   - **Conservative treatment:**
     - Premenstrual/menstrual pain: NSAIDs; analgesics with or without narcotics.
     - Prevention of ovulation with decrease in hormone levels: continuous use of oral contraceptive pills, patch or ring for 6 to 12 months; danazol for 4 to 6 months; GnRH analogs for 6 months; progestins.
   - **Surgical treatment:**
     - Laparoscopic ablation of lesions.
     - Hysterectomy with bilateral oophorectomy for women no longer interested in childbearing.

C. Stress Incontinence

- *(Urinary incontinence is addressed in Chapter 10 "Renal and Urinary Tract Disorders").*

1. **Etiology/Pathology**
   - Involuntary urinary leakage that occurs with increased intraabdominal pressure (coughing, sneezing, laughing, exertion).
   - Due to pelvic floor muscle laxity and insufficiency of the urethral sphincter.
   - Risk factors include vaginal delivery, obesity, chronic cough, heavy lifting, straining, strenuous exercise.
2. **Clinical Features**
   - Patient leaks urine with coughing, sneezing, laughing, exercising, straining.
   - Examination: evaluate pelvic support structures; evaluate for estrogen effect (atrophy); anal wink reflex for neurologic defects.
   - Observe for urine leakage with Valsalva.
   - Cotton-tipped applicator test: checks for bladder neck hypermobility—positive if >30° rotation is present.
3. **Diagnostic Studies**
   - UA with culture and sensitivity to rule out UTI.
   - Cystoscopy and urodynamic testing to evaluate function and rule out abnormal pathology.
4. **Complications**
   - Social and psychological effects.
   - Side effects of various treatment modalities.
   - Chafing.
5. **Management**
   - Establish bladder capacity through voiding diary. Prevent bladder filling to this capacity through fluid restriction, avoiding/decreasing alcohol, and caffeine consumption.
   - Strengthen pelvic floor muscles: Kegel exercises or electrical stimulation.
   - Biofeedback.
   - Prescription: α-adrenergic agonists (oxybutynin and ephedrine), estrogen replacement therapy (systemic or local), pessary use if cystocele or urethrocele is present.
   - Collagen injection.
   - Surgery to restore bladder neck position.

D. Osteoporosis

- *(Addressed in Chapter 9 "Endocrine Disorders").*

VII. Menstrual Disorders

A. Disorders of Menstruation

1. **Definition**
   - *Normal menstrual cycle*: 24 to 38 days, lasting 4.5 to 8 days; average blood loss of 30 mL (range: spotting to 80 mL).
   - *Amenorrhea*: absence of menstrual periods.
   - *Cryptomenorrhea (hypomenorrhea)*: unusually light flow, may be only spotting.
   - *Menopause*: cessation of menses for 6 months, not due to pregnancy.
   - *Menorrhagia*: normal intervals of heavy or prolonged flow.
   - *Metrorrhagia*: bleeding between menstrual cycles.
   - *Menometrorrhagia*: irregular intervals, varying amounts and duration of flow.
   - *Oligomenorrhea*: interval >36 days.
   - *Polymenorrhea*: interval <21 days.
2. **General Approach**
   - History including family history, a menstrual and reproductive history, and a general medical history including medications used, and nutritional, exercise, and emotional assessments.
   - Physical examination looking for abnormal genital anatomy (including imperforate hymen, enlarged fibroid uterus), signs of androgen excess, estrogen deficiency, or an endocrinopathy.
3. **Diagnostic Studies**
   - Blood: β-hCG; CBC with differential (thrombocytopenia, anemia); thyroid studies.
   - Pap smear: screen for cervical cancer.

- Wet mount: cervical or vaginal infection, for example, *Trichomonas*.
- Endometrial biopsy: rule out endometrial hyperplasia.
- Pelvic U/S: confirm fibroids, detect polyps, masses.
- Hysteroscopy: allows for direct visualization of the uterine cavity with removal or biopsy of lesions.

4. **Management**
   - Treat according to cause.

B. Amenorrhea

1. **Definition**
   - *Primary*: no menarche by age 13 (girls without development of secondary sexual characteristics) or by age 15 (those with secondary sexual characteristics).
   - *Secondary*: cessation of menses after the onset of menarche, lasting 3 or more months.

2. **Pathology**
   - Amenorrhea is a symptom not a disease. Most common cause is pregnancy.
   - Primary amenorrhea: causes include developmental anomalies or absence of reproductive organs, ovarian failure, hypogonadotropic hypogonadism, androgen insensitivity, chronic anovulation.
   - Secondary amenorrhea: causes include CNS, pituitary gland, thyroid gland, adrenal gland, ovarian, or uterine dysfunction; prolonged, continuous, strenuous exercise.

3. **Diagnostic Studies**
   - Document abnormal growth and development, secondary sex characteristics, evidence of endocrine disorders, normal reproductive tract.
   - Genetic karyotyping may be indicated in primary amenorrhea.
   - Depends on history and physical exam findings: β-hCG, TSH, serum prolactin, testosterone, DHEA-S, FSH, LH, estradiol level.

4. **Complications**
   - Abnormal development, infertility, endometrial hyperplasia, osteoporosis.

5. **Management**
   - Depends on etiology and patient's wishes regarding fertility.
   - Underlying medical problems should be corrected, often menses then resumes.

C. Menopause

1. **Definition**
   - Cessation of menses due to loss of ovarian function.
   - Premature menopause: ovarian failure before age 40.

2. **Etiology/Pathology**
   - Average age of onset in the United States, 51.3 years (range 45 to 55).
   - May occur naturally, surgically, or secondary to medical therapy (chemotherapy, radiation).
   - Occurs sooner in smokers than in nonsmokers, type-1 diabetics, women who live at high altitudes, vegetarians, women who are undernourished.
   - Climacteric (perimenopausal period) is a result of oocyte depletion.
   - FSH raises and estrogen levels decline, causing characteristic signs and symptoms.

3. **Clinical Features**
   - Menstrual cycle irregularities until menstruation has ceased for 1 year.
   - Hot flushes and night sweats.
   - Mood swings, trouble sleeping.
   - Atrophic changes of vulva and vagina, causing vaginal dryness, which leads to dyspareunia.
   - Pelvic relaxation and bladder problems.
   - Hair and skin thinning, with growth of facial and body hair.

4. **Diagnostic Studies**
   - Serum FSH and LH levels are elevated and plasma estradiol.

5. **Complications**
   - Osteoporosis and fractures.
   - Increased risk of cardiovascular disease.
   - Psychosexual changes.
   - Increased risk of endometrial cancer.

6. **Management**
   - Vaginal atrophy: transdermal, intravaginal estrogen.
   - Hot flushes: estrogens, progestins, clonidine, selective serotonin-reuptake inhibitors (SSRIs), gabapentin.
   - Osteoporosis prevention/treatment: calcium, vitamin D, regular exercise, bisphosphonates, calcitonin, estrogens (with or without progestins), selective estrogen receptor modulators (raloxifene).
   - Risk/benefit of hormone replacement therapy (HRT) must be carefully considered.

D. Postmenopausal Bleeding

1. **Definition**
   - Vaginal bleeding after menopause.

2. **Etiology/Pathology**
   - *Uterine causes*: fibroids, endometrial problems (hyperplasia, polyp, carcinoma).
   - *Cervical causes*: cancer, polyp, erosion.
   - Also atrophic vaginitis and HRT.
   - *Any* report of vaginal bleeding from a postmenopausal woman not on HRT, or from a woman on HRT with abnormal bleeding, is suspicious for cancer.

3. **Clinical Features**
   - Examine for friability of vaginal mucosa and cervix, evidence of cervical polyp, uterine or ovarian masses.

4. **Diagnostic Studies**
   - Pelvic examination.
   - Pap smear.
   - Pelvic U/S.
   - Endometrial biopsy.
   - Hysteroscopy with D&C (often diagnostic and therapeutic).

5. **Complications**
  - Anemia.
  - Surgery often necessary.
6. **Management**
  - Depends on etiology.

E. Dysmenorrhea

1. **Etiology/Pathology**
   - **Primary dysmenorrhea:**
     - Painful menstruation associated with uterine contractions mediated by prostaglandins.
     - No associated pelvic pathology.
     - Pain usually begins 1 to 2 years after the onset of menarche; may become more severe with time.
   - **Secondary dysmenorrhea:**
     - Pain caused by pelvic pathology (e.g., endometriosis, PID, IUD).
     - Onset generally after the age of 25.
2. **Clinical Features**
   - Pelvic pain with the onset of menses that may radiate to the back of the legs, low back.
   - May be accompanied by nausea, vomiting, diarrhea, headache.
   - Usually lasts 1 to 3 days.
   - Exam normal or may have uterine tenderness in primary dysmenorrhea. In secondary dysmenorrhea, may have findings related to the cause.
3. **Diagnostic Studies**
   - Cervical cultures (rule out cervicitis).
   - Secondary dysmenorrhea: depends on suspected cause (e.g., laparoscopy, MRI).
4. **Complications**
   - May be so severe, woman is unable to function adequately at home or work.
5. **Management**
   - Symptomatic treatment: heat, rest, vitamin E.
   - Antiprostaglandin (NSAID): works best when started before the onset of severe symptoms.
   - Oral contraceptives/Depo-Provera/contraceptive vaginal ring: suppress ovulation and significantly reduce symptoms.
   - If above treatment fails: laparoscopy to rule out causes of secondary dysmenorrhea.

F. Premenstrual Syndrome (PMS)

1. **Etiology/Pathology**
   - Multifactorial, poorly understood; disease versus constellation of symptoms.
   - Occurs during reproductive years.
   - True etiology unknown: may include serotonin dysfunction or be related to ovarian function.
   - Premenstrual dysphoric disorder (PMDD): more severe form of PMS.
2. **Clinical Features**
   - Symptoms include a feeling of weight gain, aggressiveness, lower extremity edema, bloating, breast pain, depression, food cravings, headache, inability

to concentrate, irritability, lethargy, libido change, skin disorders.
   - Symptoms occur during the luteal phase (7 to 14 days before the onset of menses), are relieved within 2 to 3 days of the onset of menses, and there are at least 7 symptom-free days in the follicular phase of the cycle.
   - Symptoms must be documented in at least three consecutive cycles.
   - Psychiatric history important.
   - Essentially normal physical examination.
3. **Diagnostic Studies**
   - Rule out thyroid disorder and anemia.
4. **Complications**
   - Underlying psychiatric illness may be present.
5. **Management**
   - Treat patient's symptoms, for example:
     - Breast pain: bromocriptine, danazol.
     - Bloating: spironolactone, calcium carbonate.
     - Mood disorders, especially for PMDD: SSRIs either daily or on symptomatic days; monophasic OCP (20 μg ethinyl estradiol and 3 mg drospirenone).
     - Water retention: spironolactone.
   - Aerobic exercise; decrease or eliminate caffeine and alcohol; low salt complex carbohydrates diet; calcium supplementation.
   - Psychiatric referral may be necessary for underlying psychiatric disease.

VIII. Infertility

A. Definition

- One year of unprotected intercourse without resulting pregnancy.

B. Etiology/Pathology

- Male partner contributes to approximately 40% of cases of infertility; a combination of factors is common.
- Female: anovulatory cycles; congenital or acquired problems in fallopian tubes, cervix, or uterus.
- Sixty percent of couples will achieve a pregnancy within 3 years, in the absence of identifiable causes of infertility.

C. Clinical Features

- May have a history of menstrual irregularity, hirsutism, galactorrhea, dyspareunia, pelvic pain, IUD use, PID, diethylstilbestrol (DES) exposure.
- Sexual history is important: frequency of penis in vagina intercourse, ejaculation, use of lubricants, prior contraceptive use.
- Speculum and bimanual examination, breast examination (galactorrhea), skin examination (hirsutism).

D. Diagnostic Studies
- Postcoital microscopy on ovulatory day looking at number of motile sperm in the cervical mucus and their survival rate.
- Verification of ovulation:
  - Measure the serum progesterone level at the midpoint of the secretory phase (21st day) to evaluate for adequate luteal function.
  - Basal body temperature elevation during the luteal phase.
  - Endometrial biopsy.
  - Change in cervical mucus.
- Hysterosalpingogram for tubal patency and uterine cavity structure.
- Laparoscopy with instillation of dye: diagnostic for tubal dysfunction; able to identify and treat endometriosis, other pelvic pathology, PID; lysis of adhesions.

E. Complications
- Risks associated with surgical procedures.
- Emotional and physical stress.

F. Management
- Best handled by an infertility specialist.
- Treatment based on etiology:
  - *Nonpatent tubes*: repair surgically.
  - *Anovulation or oligoovulation (treatment depends on cause)*:
    - Rule out underlying endocrine disorders. Women start ovulating after endocrine problems have been corrected.
    - Polycystic ovary: induce ovulation with clomiphene citrate.
    - Exercise-induced anovulation: reduce exercise level and weight gain; -hCG therapy.
    - Hyperprolactinemia: bromocriptine therapy.
  - *Antisperm antibodies:* condom usage for 6 months.

IX. Contraceptive Counseling (Table 11-4)
- Women should be advised of their contraceptive options and choose the method appropriate for themselves based on personal preference, health risks, and cost. Predicted pregnancy rate of 85% in a year without use of contraception.

A. Natural Family Planning (Fertility Awareness Methods)
- Involves abstaining from intercourse during fertile period.
- Requires a regular menstrual cycle and specific determination of ovulation, using basal body temperature charting, cervical mucus evaluation, and/or urine tests and patient motivation.
- Can be used with a barrier method during most fertile phase of cycle, increasing effectiveness.
- Abstaining from intercourse during fertile days, leaves few days of the month for intercourse.
- Failure rate dependent on the method used and the patient.
- No protection from STIs.

B. Coitus Interruptus
- Male withdraws penis from vagina before ejaculation.
- Failure rate due to sperm in the preejaculatory fluid, premature ejaculation, and/or the deposition of semen on the vulva.
- No protection from STIs.

C. Spermicide: Nonoxynol-9
- Mechanical barrier and toxic to sperm.
- Comes in vaginal jelly, cream, gel, suppository, film, and foam.
- Available without a prescription.
- Most effective when used with other forms of birth control.
- Nonoxynol-9 can cause microabrasians to the vaginal mucosa, therefore increasing the risk of HIV transmission; sex workers and women with multiple partners should be discouraged from using methods that contain nonoxynol-9.

D. Barrier Methods
- Physical barrier between ejaculate and vagina.
1. Condoms
- Male (latex, polyurethane, lambskin) and female (polyurethane), both of which offer protection from STIs.
- Available without a prescription.
- Highly effective in preventing pregnancy, especially when used in combination with a spermicidal jelly, foam, or insert.
- May decrease sensitivity for partners.
- Female condom is awkward to use for some women; external ring may cause irritation.
- Female condom: only female-controlled birth control with STI and pregnancy protection.
- Latex allergy may deter use of male condoms; lambskin condoms do not prevent STIs.
2. Diaphragm
- Requires pelvic examination and fitting by a trained health care professional.
- Should be used with spermicidal jelly in the cup for maximum effectiveness.
- Can be inserted several hours before intercourse, and must remain in place for 6 to 24 hours after intercourse.
- Small risk of TSS if left in place too long.
- Additional spermicidal jelly must be inserted into vagina with an applicator between each act of intercourse.
- Device requires a prescription.
- Can be messy and difficult to insert and remove.
- Effective when used properly.

TABLE 11–4.   Comparisons of Birth Control Methods (Predicted Pregnancy Rate of 85% in a Year without Use of Contraception)

Barrier Methods: Physical Barrier between Ejaculate and Vagina

	Description	OTC/RX	Typical Failure Rate during First Year of Use	STI Protection	Others
Condoms: male	Latex, polyurethane, lambskin sheath	OTC	18%	Yes	Some contain nonoxynol-9 More effective if used with spermicide
Condoms: female	Polyurethane sheath with two rings to stabilize it in the vagina	OTC	21%	Yes	Only female-controlled birth control with STI and pregnancy protection More effective if used with spermicide
Diaphragm	Rubber cuplike device that holds spermicide against the cervix	RX	12%	±	
Fem-cap	Smaller rubber cuplike device that fits over the cervix, holding spermicide	RX	14%	±	
Contraceptive sponge	One-time use sponge with nonoxynol-9	OTC	Nulliparous: 12% Parous: 24%	±	

Hormonal Methods

	Description	OTC/RX	Typical Failure Rate	STI Protection	Others
Combination oral contraceptive pills	Contain estrogen and progestin—type varies	RX	9%	No	Contraindications for use Many noncontraceptive benefits Not for smokers >35
Progestin-only pills "Mini-pill"	Oral contraceptive pill without estrogen	RX	9%	No	May be used by women who cannot use estrogens, including lactating women Menstrual irregularities Must take at consistent time
Plan B	Two tablets of 0.75 mg levonorgestrel ingested 12 hours apart, or both tablets at once; initiated within 5 days of unprotected intercourse	OTC ≥18 RX <18	1% when taken within 72 hours	No	
Implanon	Single rod implant, releases 68 pg of etonogestrel daily	RX	0.05%	No	Office visit for insertion Lasts for 3 years
Depo-Provera	Depo medroxyprogesterone acetate IM	RX	6%	No	Office visit every 3 months for injection

(Continued)

TABLE 11–4. **Comparisons of Birth Control Methods (Predicted Pregnancy Rate of 85% in a Year without Use of Contraception) (*Continued*)**

Hormonal Methods

	Description	OTC/RX	Typical Failure Rate	STI Protection	Others
Ortho Evra	Transdermal patch that delivers 150 pg norelgestromin and 20 pg ethinyl estradiol daily	RX	9%	No	Applied once a week for 3 consecutive weeks followed by 1 week off May be less effective in women ≥198 lb
NuvaRing	Flexible plastic ring that releases 120 pg of the etonogestrel and 15 pg of ethinyl estradiol	RX	9%	No	Inserted intravaginally for a 3-week period, then removed for 1 week, during which withdrawal bleeding is expected

Others

	Description	OTC/RX	Typical Failure Rate	STI Protection	Others
Natural family planning Cervical mucus Symptothermal Calendar (rhythm) Standard days	Avoid intercourse or use contraception during fertile times	N/A	Up to 24%	No	Classes available
Coitus interruptus	Withdrawal of penis from vagina before ejaculation	N/A	22%	No	
Spermicide Nonoxynol-9	Mechanical barrier and toxic to sperm	OTC	28%	Slight, not HIV	Vaginal jelly, cream, gel, suppository, film, foam
IUD Mirena (levonorgestrel) ParaGard (Copper T 380A)	Intravaginal device	RX	Mirena 0.2% ParaGard 0.8	No	Mirena: 5 years ParaGard: 10 years History of PID—absolute contraindication
Sterilization	Permanent blocking of the fallopian tubes by either mechanical, or chemical means		0.5%	No	Surgical procedure Considered permanent; reversal difficult

3. **FemCap**
   - Silicone rubber cap with brim and strap for removal; acts as a barrier by completely covering the cervix.
   - Used with spermicidal jelly.
   - Can be inserted several hours prior to intercourse and must remain in place for at least 8 hours; however, can remain in place for up to 48 hours.
   - Risk of toxic shock if left in place too long.
   - No additional jelly needed between acts of intercourse.
   - Requires a prescription, but no fitting required; size is determined by obstetrical history.
   - Can be messy and difficult to insert and remove.
   - Effective when used properly.
4. **Contraceptive Sponge**
   - Polyurethane sponge containing nonoxynol-9 for single use only.
   - Moistened with tap water prior to insertion.
   - May be inserted a few hours prior to intercourse, but must be left in place for at least 6 hours after the last act of intercourse; should not be left in place for more than 24 hours.
   - Risk of toxic shock if left in place too long.
   - No prescription needed.
   - Check for current availability; method available as of fall 2011.

E. **Hormonal Methods**
   - Prevent pregnancy by inhibiting ovulation, thickening cervical mucus, and altering the quality of the endometrium.
   - Women who smoke have a higher risk of death from cardiovascular disease, and should stop combined

hormonal methods at age 35 if they continue to smoke.
- Use cautiously in women with diabetes, HTN, hyperlipidemia, and history of biliary tract disease.

1. **Oral Contraceptives**
   a. **Combination (Containing an Estrogen and a Progestin)**
      - Requires an office visit and prescription.
      - Woman must remember to take a pill every day, consistently.
      - Many side effects and contraindications; however, when used correctly, are more than 99% effective against preventing pregnancy.
      - Most side effects are tolerable.
      - Offers no protection against STIs.
      - Noncontraceptive benefits include improving dysmenorrhea, controlling menstrual cycle and flow, protection against ovarian cysts, ovarian and endometrial cancer; improvement of acne; positive effect on bone mass.
      - Women who smoke have a higher risk of death from cardiovascular disease, and should stop the pill at age 35 if they continue to smoke.
      - Use cautiously in women with diabetes, HTN, hyperlipidemia, and history of biliary tract disease.
   b. **Combination Oral Contraceptives Containing Progestin Drospirenone**
      - Diuretic effect may be beneficial for women who experience water retention and bloating during menses.
      - Only combined oral contraceptive approved by the FDA for treatment of PMDD.
      - Should not be used by women with kidney, liver, or adrenal disease.
      - May increase potassium levels.
   c. **Progestin Only Pills (No Estrogen)**
      - Requires office visit and prescription.
      - Fewer contraindications.
      - May be used by breastfeeding women.
      - Slightly less effective in preventing pregnancy than combination pills.
      - No protection from STIs.
      - Menstrual irregularity from amenorrhea to menometrorrhagia.
      - Woman must remember to take a pill every day, consistently.
   d. **Emergency Contraception: Multiple Formulas, Plan B Is Most Commonly Used**
      - Consists of two tablets of 0.75 mg levonorgestrel ingested 12 hours apart, initiated within 72 hours of unprotected intercourse.
      - Evidence-based medicine: taking both 0.75 mg tablets at once has shown to have greater efficacy at preventing pregnancy.
      - In addition, studies have shown that Plan B may be effective for up to 5 days following unprotected intercourse.
      - Over-the-counter for women over 18, by prescription for 17 and under.
      - Patients are advised to seek medical attention if menses have not begun within 21 days after treatment.
      - Paraguard (Copper IUD or IUC) can also be used as emergency contraception if inserted within 5 days of unprotected intercourse.

2. **Implantable/Injectable/Long-Acting Progestins**
   a. **Implanon**
      - Single-rod implant, releases 68 μg of etonogestrel daily.
      - Prevents ovulation in most women for 3 years.
      - Similar side effects as with other progesterone only methods.
      - Menstrual irregularity from amenorrhea to menometrorrhagia.
      - Requires prescription and office visit for placement.
      - No protection from STIs.
      - Highly effective.
   b. **Norplant Implants**
      - Wyeth Pharmaceuticals voluntarily removed Norplant from the US market on July 26, 2002, due to limitations in product component supplies. Wyeth does not plan to reintroduce it.
      - Patients need to switch to other forms of birth control after the removal at the 5-year expiration date.
   c. **Depo-Provera (Depo Medroxyprogesterone Acetate)**
      - Injectable progesterone; prevents pregnancy for 3 months at a time.
      - Similar menstrual disturbances as with other progesterone only methods.
      - Requires prescription.
      - No protection from STIs.
      - Highly effective.
      - Weight gain and irregular bleeding are common complaints.

3. **Other Hormonal Options**
   a. **Ortho Evra**
      - Transdermal patch that delivers 150 μg norelgestromin and 20 μg ethinyl estradiol daily into the circulation.
      - Applied once a week for 3 consecutive weeks followed by 1 week off.
      - Efficacy similar to that of oral contraceptives, but compliance may be better.
      - May be less effective in women ≥198 lb.
      - Requires prescription and office visit.
      - No protection from STIs.
   b. **NuvaRing**
      - Flexible plastic ring that releases 120 μg of the etonogestrel and 15 μg of ethinyl estradiol daily into the circulation.

- Inserted intravaginally for a 3-week period, then removed for 1 week, during which withdrawal bleeding is expected.
- Efficacy is comparable with that of combination oral contraceptives.
- Requires prescription and office visit.
- May be removed for intercourse, but must be replaced within 3 hours to maintain continued efficacy.
- No protection from STIs.

F. Intrauterine Device (IUD or IUC)
- Exact mechanism of action is not currently known, may inhibit sperm transport or disrupt the uterine lining.
- Progesterone IUC has additional mechanism of cervical mucus thickening.
- Device placement (and removal) in the uterus must be done by a trained health care professional.
- Two types available:
  - Mirena (releases levonorgestrel): 5 years.
    - Similar menstrual disturbances as with other progesterone only methods.
  - ParaGard (Copper T 380A): 12 years.
    - May cause menorrhagia in some women.
- No protection against STIs.
- Highly effective.

G. Continuous Cycling
- All combined contraceptive methods may be prescribed for continuous use by skipping the placebo or off week.
- Good option for women with menstrual migraines, dysmenorrhea, menorrhagia, endometriosis, recurrent ovarian cysts, anemia, or PMS.
- Will require additional prescriptions to cover year's supply, which may not be covered under insurance or funding.

H. Irreversible Methods: Voluntary Female Sterilization
- Women should choose this method only if they are absolutely sure that they are finished with childbearing.
  1. **Tubal Ligation**
     - A permanent mechanical blocking of the fallopian tubes achieved through a surgical procedure in which the lumen of the tube is interrupted.
     - Requires surgery.
  2. **Transcervical Approach: Essure**
     - Chemical or coils are used to scar the proximal portion of the tubes or cornua.
     - Can be done in office or clinic and requires local anesthesia only.
  3. **For All Forms of Sterilization**
     - Reversal is difficult and rarely successful.
     - If failure occurs, it is often an ectopic pregnancy.
     - No protection from STIs.
     - No alteration of menstrual pattern.

- Highly effective.
- No long-term side effects.

X. General Guidelines for Women's Health Maintenance

A. Health Maintenance
- Women should have gynecologic examinations annually from age 18, or when sexually active. Risk factors such as smoking, alcohol intake, drug use, sexual promiscuity, obesity, sedentary lifestyle, and abuse should be discussed.
- **Cervical cancer screening:**
  - Pap smear screening should be initiated at the age of 21.
  - Screening is recommended every 2 years between the ages of 21 and 29 as long as cytology results are negative.
  - Screening may be decreased to every 2 to 3 years in women aged 30 and older who have had three or more negative cytology results in a row and no history of cervical intraepithelial neoplasia (CIN 2) or CIN 3.
  - For women over the age of 30, screening should be done no more than every 3 years if combined with HPV DNA testing.
  - Screening may be discontinued in women between the ages of 65 and 70 years who have had three or more negative cytology test results in a row and no history of abnormal results in the past 10 years.
  - Women who have a history of DES exposure in utero require annual Pap smears.
  - HIV+ women with should have annual screening regardless of the cytology results.
  - Discontinue routine screening in any woman who has had a total hysterectomy for benign reasons and negative history for high-grade CIN.
- **Breast cancer screening—Breast self-examination (BSE):**
  - Value of BSE debated; for women who choose to do BSE, review proper technique; must be done monthly by woman age ≥20, immediately after menstruation or on Days 5 to 7 of cycle.
  - Clinical breast examination should be performed at least every 3 years in women between the ages of 20 and 39, then annually after the age of 40.
  - Mammogram guidelines currently are conflicting.
    - USPSTF recommends baseline mammogram at age 50, then every other year until the age of 74. Mammogram screening should be performed every other year beginning at age 40 only in women with risk factors.
    - ACS continues to recommend baseline screening beginning at age 40 and continuing annually.
- The decision to continue with screening mammograms after the age of 65 should be based on the

patient's comorbidities, expected life span, and patient's preference. It is generally not recommended to continue routine screening after the age of 65 to 75.
- If there is a family history of breast cancer in a first-degree relative, baseline mammogram should be done 10 years before the age at which the family member was diagnosed.
- **Colon cancer screening—done starting at age 50:**
  - Annual fecal occult blood test.
  - Sigmoidoscopy every 5 years or colonoscopy every 10 years.
- **Cholesterol screening**—every 5 years.

B. Wellness Promotion
- Smoking cessation; smoking specifically increases the risk of developing cervical cancer.
- Cease substance use/abuse.
- Regular exercise.
- Proper nutrition/weight management.
- Stress reduction/management.
- Immunization updates.

XI. Management of Pap Smear Results
- (See also Chapter 16 "Surgical Disorders.")

A. Normal Pap Smear Result
- Repeat in 2 years for women between the ages of 21 and 29; repeat every 2 to 3 years in women over the age of 30, but no more than every 3 years if HPV DNA testing is also done.
- Women with HIV, and those with a history of DES exposure in utero, should be screened annually.

B. Abnormal Pap Smear Result
1. **Infection**
   - Treat the specified infection.
   - If normal cytology, follow-up in 2 to 3 years.
2. **Reactive and Reparative Changes**
   - Rule out infection.
   - If cytology is negative, follow-up in 2 to 3 years.
3. **Squamous Cell Abnormalities**
   - Atypical squamous cells of undetermined significance.
     - If HPV negative, repeat in 1 year.
     - If HPV positive, colposcopy needed.
   - Low-grade squamous intraepithelial lesion (SIL): colposcopy, biopsy, and treatment. Repeat Pap smear at 6 and 12 months, or have HPV testing in 1 year.
   - High-grade SIL: colposcopy, biopsy, and treat. Close follow-up for 2 years.
   - Squamous cell cancer: refer to gynecologist for colposcopy and treatment.

SELECTED REFERENCES

Center for Disease Control and Prevention. Sexually transmitted diseases treatment guidelines, 2010. *MMWR Recomm Rep.* 2010;59(RR-12):1–110.

DeCherney AH, Nathan L, Goodwing TM, eds. *Current Obstetric and Gynecologic Diagnosis and Treatment.* 10th ed. New York, NY: McGraw-Hill; 2006.

Gibbs R, Karlan B, Haney A, et al. *Danforth's Obstetrics and Gynecology.* 10th ed. Philadelphia, PA: Lippincott Williams & Wilkins; 2008.

Hatcher RA, Trussell J, Nelson AL, et al, eds. *Contraceptive Technology.* 20th revised ed. New York, NY: Ardent Media; 2011.

McPhee SJ, Papadakis MA, Rabow MW, eds. *Current Medical Diagnosis and Treatment 2012.* New York, NY: McGraw-Hill; 2012.

Zieman M, Hatcher R, Cwiak C, et al. *Managing Contraception for Your Pocket. 2010–2012 Edition.* Atlanta, GA: Bridging the Gap Foundation; 2010.

Complicated Pregnancies

Melissa M. Kagarise • Jill M. Cavalet

I. Rh Alloimmunization

A. Definition
- Material antibodies that can bind to fetal red blood cells (RBCs) resulting in hemolytic disease in the newborn.

B. Etiology
- Rhesus factor (Rh) alloimmunization (also isoimmunization or erythroblastosis fetalis) is caused by incompatibility between fetal and maternal blood. Mother Rh-negative and fetus Rh-positive (mother Rh-negative, father Rh-positive).

C. Pathology
- Rh antigens are lipoproteins located on the red cell membrane. Patients who lack a specific red cell antigen produce an antibody if exposed to the antigen.
- This antibody may be harmful following an incompatible blood transfusion or a second hemorrhage between a mother and an incompatible fetus. This condition is potentially dangerous in subsequent pregnancies.
- Rh-negative women who delivered or will deliver an Rh-positive fetus will become immunized and must be treated to prevent subsequent erythroblastosis.
- Infection, hemorrhage at delivery, threatened abortion, placenta previa, abruption, and C-section can transfer fetal blood to mother.
- Maternal antibody is transferred to fetus. The fetus' red cells get damaged. Hemolysis responds with erythropoiesis. Further hemolysis.

D. Clinical Features
- Hemolytic disease in the newborn.
  - Hemolysis, bilirubin release, anemia.
- Fetal hepatosplenomegaly.
- Fetal icterus (kernicterus).
- Fetal heart failure.
- Fetal hydrops—fluid accumulation in at least two of the following extravascular areas.
  - Pericardial effusion, pleural effusion, ascites, subcutaneous edema.
- Fetal death.

E. Diagnostic Studies
- **Pregnant woman**
  - ABO blood group.
  - Rh-D type.
  - Indirect erythrocyte antibody screen (Titers of 1:8 to 1:32 are associated with fetal hemolysis).
  - Kleihauer–Betke test used to detect the presence of fetal RBCs in maternal circulation.
  - Indirect Coombs test to determine sufficient antibody.
- **Fetus-monitor for fetal anemia in second trimester**
  - Amniotic fluid assessment—increasing bilirubin levels positive sign.
  - Ultrasound (U/S) of middle cerebral artery for peak velocity—increase in flow secondary to decrease viscosity of blood in fetal anemia.
  - Percutaneous umbilical blood sampling (PUBS) for direct measurement of fetal hematocrit.
  - Paternal blood type and Rh status is helpful.

F. Management
- **Prevention, mother**
  - About 300 μg Rh immune globulin (RhIG) intramuscularly (IM) for Rh-negative mother and Rh-positive or Rh-unknown father:
    - At 28 weeks gestation.
    - With procedures or conditions with possibility of fetal-to-maternal bleeding.
    - After ectopic pregnancy.
    - After spontaneous, threatened, or induced abortions or vaginal bleeding.
    - Within 72 hours of delivery of an Rh-D positive infant.
- **Baby**
  - Moderate–severe anemia requires transfusion of antigen-negative RBCs through U/S-guided transfusion into umbilical vein.

II. Genitourinary Infections

A. Definition
- Infection of the genitourinary tract caused by various organisms.

B. Etiology
- Bladder and ureters under pressure from uterus with decreased voiding patterns and smooth muscle relaxation from elevated progesterone levels may contribute to increased risk for genitourinary infections.

1. **Lower Urinary Tract Infections (UTIs) and Asymptomatic Bacteriuria**
   a. **Pathology:** *Escherichia coli.*
   b. **Clinical features**
      - Asymptomatic.
      - Dysuria, frequency, urgency.
   c. **Diagnostic studies**
      - Urine analysis (U/A) and culture and sensitivity at onset of prenatal care or symptomatology.
   d. **Management**
      - Seven to ten days treatment with cephalosporin, nitrofurantoin, or sulfonamide.
      - Repeat cultures following treatment.
2. **Upper UTIs (Pyelonephritis)**
   a. **Pathology:** *E. coli* **and gram-negative aerobes.**
   b. **Clinical features**
      - Fever, malaise, dehydration.
      - Costovertebral tenderness/back pain.
      - Premature labor.
      - Maternal sepsis with high morbidity.
   c. **Diagnostic studies**
      - U/A with culture and sensitivity.
   d. **Management**
      - Admit for inpatient treatment.
      - IV hydration, antipyretics.
      - IV antibiotics with cephalosporin or penicillin and aminoglycosides.
      - Tocolytic therapy to halt contractions if preterm labor (PTL) develops.
      - Repeat cultures following treatment.
3. **Vaginitis**
   a. **Pathology**
      - Bacterial vaginosis (previously termed *Gardnerella* vaginitis or *Haemophilus vaginalis* vaginitis).
      - Candidiasis: *Candida albicans.*
      - Trichomoniasis: protozoan parasite *Trichomonas vaginalis.*
   b. **Clinical features**
      - Bacterial vaginosis: abnormal, odorous discharge.
      - Candidiasis: white, curd-like discharge, pruritus, dysuria.
      - Trichomoniasis: vaginal itching and discharge with or without odor, occasionally foamy with cervical erosion.
   c. **Diagnostic studies**
      - Bacterial vaginosis: wet mount for clue cells.
      - Candidiasis: potassium hydroxide smear for budding yeast.
      - Trichomoniasis: wet mount for *T. vaginalis* and white cells.
   d. **Management**
      - Bacterial vaginosis: 7-day course of metronidazole or clindamycin.
      - Candidiasis: 7-day course of vaginal azoles.
      - Trichomoniasis: one-time dose of metronidazole 2 g.

4. **Sexually transmitted disease**
   Sexually transmitted infection (STI) is the more current term and is replacing sexually transmitted disease (STD). Also, STI will include someone who is infected but does not have any symptoms-therefore covering a broader area.
   a. **Pathology**
      - *Chlamydia: Chlamydia trachomatis,* most common STD.
      - Herpes simplex infection: Herpes simples virus types 1 and 2.
      - *Neisseria gonorrhoeae.*
   b. **Clinical features**
      - *Chlamydia.*
        - Asymptomatic, urethritis, mucopurulent cervicitis.
      - Herpes simplex infection.
        - Ulcerated tender vesicles with crusting.
      - *Neisseria gonorrhoeae.*
        - Asymptomatic or nonspecific symptoms.
        - Purulent discharge from urethra, cervix or vagina, may be greenish or yellow.
   c. **Diagnostic studies**
      - *Chlamydia.*
        - Culture.
        - Direct fluorescent antibody staining, enzyme immunoassay.
        - Nucleic acid hybridization and amplification tests (NAATs).
      - Herpes simplex.
        - Culture of vesicles for the identification of HSV.
        - Polymerase chain reaction (PCR) testing.
        - Serologic testing for HSV-1 and HSV-2 immunoglobulin.
      - *Neisseria gonorrhoeae.*
        - Culture, NAAT.
        - PCR for at-risk women.
   d. **Management**
      - *Chlamydia.*
        - Azithromycin 1 g dose once **or** 7-day course of amoxicillin.
        - Retest 3 months after treatment.
      - Herpes simplex.
        - Acyclovir if symptoms are severe or for suppression starting at 36 weeks to reduce viral shedding.
        - Cesarean delivery only if active lesions on vulva, in vagina, or on cervix at the time of labor or rupture of membranes.
      - *Neisseria gonorrhoeae.*
        - Ceftriaxone 125 mg IM or ciprofloxacin 500 mg orally in a single dose.
        - All neonates receive routine prophylactic ophthalmic ointment (erythromycin or tetracycline) for the prevention of gonococcal ophthalmia.

5. **Group Streptococcus**
   a. **Pathology:** *Streptococcus agalactiae*.
   b. **Clinical features**
      - Asymptomatic in pregnant woman.
      - Manifestations in newborn can include septicemia, pneumonia, or meningitis.
   c. **Diagnostic studies**
      - Rectovaginal culture for group B streptococci (GBS) in all women between 35 and 37 weeks gestation.
   d. **Management**
      - Penicillin, ampicillin, cefazolin, clindamycin, or vancomycin prophylaxis for positive culture, and with PTL, premature rupture of membranes, maternal fever in women with unknown status, ideally within 4 hours of labor.

6. **Syphilis**
   a. **Pathology:** *Treponema pallidum*.
   b. **Clinical features**
      - Painless ulcer at site initially.
      - Skin rash in 1 to 3 months.
      - Condyloma lata lesions in woman.
      - Newborn symptoms develop up to 14 days after delivery and include maculopapular rash, hepatosplenomegaly, jaundice.
   c. **Diagnostic studies**
      - Serologic screening of all women with Venereal Disease Research Laboratory.
      - Rapid plasma reagin (RPR).
      - Sometimes treponemal-specific tests (FTA-ABS & TP-PA).
   d. **Management**
      - Benzathine penicillin G 2.4 million units IM as a single dose.
      - Patient should receive a follow-up RPR test for syphilis 1 month after treatment to document decreasing titer.
      - If patients are sensitive to penicillin, they usually require desensitization.

7. **HIV/AIDS**
   a. **Pathology**
      - Human immunodeficiency virus (HIV) that becomes incorporated into CD4+ cells (lymphocytes, monocytes, and some neural cells).
   b. **Clinical features**
      - Wide range of presentations common with HIV/AIDS diagnosis.
      - Candidiais, bacterial vaginosis, genital herpes, syphilis may be common in pregnancy.
      - Decline in absolute CD4+ counts.
   c. **Diagnostic studies**
      - Enzyme-linked immunosorbent assay (ELISA).
      - Western blot if positive ELISA.
      - Rapid HIV testing is an alternative for at-risk women of unknown infection status presenting in labor.
      - Viral load and CD4+ counts monthly in HIV positive pregnant women.
   d. **Management**
      - Antiretroviral therapy.
         - Zidovudine (AZT) 100 mg orally five times daily has been shown to reduce viral transmission to the fetus.
      - Vaccinations.
      - Should be followed at a high-risk clinic, internist specializing in treating HIV-positive persons, or a maternal fetal medicine specialist.
      - Planned cesarean at 38 weeks for women with viral load >1,000 copies per mL.

8. **Chorioamnionitis, Inflammation of Fetal Membrane**
   a. **Pathology**
      - Ascending genital tract infection most commonly caused by *Bacteroides* and *Prevotella* species, *E. coli*, anaerobic streptococci, and GBS.
   b. **Clinical features**
      - Maternal fever.
      - Maternal tachycardia.
      - Uterine or abdominal tenderness.
      - Fetal tachycardia, distress.
   c. **Diagnostic studies**
      - Transabdominal amniocentesis for culture.
   d. **Management**
      - Parenteral antibiotic.
         - Ampicillin (2 g every 6 hours) or penicillin (5 million units every 6 hours) plus gentamicin (1.5 mg per kg every 8 hours).
      - C-section for fetal distress and poor biophysical profile (BPP).

III. Genetic/Chromosomal Disorders

A. Definition
   - Congenital abnormality in fetus.

B. Etiology
   - Chromosomal abnormalities.
   - Single gene (Mendelian) disorders.
   - Polygenic or multifactorial disorders.
   - Teratogenic disorders.
   - Risk factors.
   - Advanced maternal age (>35 years).
   - Previous pregnancy affected by abnormality.
   - History of early pregnancy loss.
   - Advanced paternal age (>50 years).
   - Ethnicity.

C. Pathology
   - Chromosomal and gene replication errors within the cell's DNA.

D. Clinical Features
   - Estimated that 50% of early spontaneous abortions and 5% of stillborns are due to an abnormal chromosomal number.
   - Clinical traits or features of newborn will vary depending on specific genetic disorder.

- Chromosomal: trisomy 21 (Down syndrome).
  - Mental retardation.
  - Cardiac abnormalities.
  - Respiratory infections.
  - Leukemia.
  - Polygenic disorders.
  - Hydrocephaly.
  - Neural tube defects.
  - Cleft lip and palate.
  - Pyloric stenosis.
- In instances where the patient has not begun prenatal care until later in her pregnancy, a pelvic U/S may detect physical deformities such as neck webbing, neural tube disorders, anencephaly, cardiac malformations, growth restrictions, or dwarfism.

E. Diagnostic Studies
- Serum triple screen at 15 to 18 weeks to assess risk for Down syndrome, trisomy 18 and 13.
  - α-Fetoprotein (AFP).
  - Human chorionic gonadotropin (hCG).
  - Pregnancy-associated plasma protein A.
- U/S for nuchal transparency.
- Amniocentesis for karyotyping (Down syndrome) between 15 and 20 weeks gestation.
- Chorionic villus sampling for DNA evaluation.
- PUBS or cordocentesis after 20 weeks gestation for fetal blood analysis and DNA analysis.
- Fetal blood sampling and fetal biopsy for DNA sampling.

F. Management
- Genetic counseling for couples at increased risk for genetic abnormalities.
- Introduction to maternal fetal medicine specialist.
- Pregnancy should be treated as high risk.
- Depends on genetic abnormality and severity.
- Option for termination of pregnancy.
- Postpartum support groups in instances of fetal demise or termination.
- Postpartum genetic counseling.
- Folic acid supplementation may prevent occurrence and recurrence of neural tube defects.

IV. Abortions

A. Definition
- Expulsion of all or part of the products of conception before the completed 20th week of conception. Incidence estimated to be 50% of all pregnancies, most occurring during the first 7 weeks.

B. Etiology
- Fetal chromosomal abnormalities (50% of all cases).
- Maternal infections.
- Uterine defects.
- Endocrine abnormalities.
- Malnutrition.
- Immunologic factors.
- Physical trauma.

C. Pathology
- Death of embryo.
- Hemorrhage, inflammation, and necrosis at the site of implantation.
- Detachment of gestational sac with uterine contractions for expulsion of the products of conception.

1. **Spontaneous Abortion**
   a. **Definition**
   - Expulsion of all or part of products of conception before the completed 20th week of conception; miscarriage. Incidence estimated to be 50% of all pregnancies.
   b. **Clinical features**
   - Passage of products of conception.
   - Maybe associated bleeding, cramping, contractions, and cervical changes.
   c. **Management**
   - Emotional support to family.
   - Administer Rh immunoglobulin, if needed.
   - Submit any product of conception (POC) to pathology, if present.

2. **Complete Abortion**
   a. **Definition**
   - Expulsion of all the products of conception before the 20th completed week of gestation.
   b. **Clinical features**
   - Passing of entire conceptus.
   - Pain and bleeding cease after passage of tissue.
   - Cervical os closed.
   - Uterus small and nontender.
   c. **Management**
   - Emotional support to family.
   - Administer Rh immunoglobulin, if needed.
   - Submit any POC to pathology, if present.

3. **Incomplete Abortion**
   a. **Definition**
   - Expulsion of part of products of conception before the 20th completed week of gestation. Typically no viable conceptus.
   b. **Clinical features**
   - Passage of part of POC.
   - Retained tissue.
   - Continuous bleeding that can be profuse.
   - Boggy uterus with dilated os.
   - Cramps.
   c. **Management**
   - Dilation and evacuation (D&E).
   - Pitocin.
   - Rh immunoglobulin, if needed.
   - Submit any POC to pathology.
   - Emotional support.

4. **Inevitable Abortion**
   a. **Definition**
   - Bleeding or cramping before the 20th completed week with continuous and progressive dilation of the cervix and rupture

of membranes, no expulsion of the products of conception.

b. Clinical features
- Moderate effacement of the cervix.
- Cervical dilation >3 cm.
- Rupture of the membranes.
- Bleeding for >7 days.
- Persistence of cramps.

c. Management
- D&E for retained tissue.
- Emotional support to family.
- Administer Rh immunoglobulin.
- Submit POC to pathology.

5. Threatened Abortion
a. Definition
- Bloody vaginal discharge before the 20th completed week with or without uterine contraction.

b. Clinical features
- Vaginal bleeding ranges from spotting to profuse, brown to bright red, precedes uterine contraction or back pain.
- Blood in vaginal vault.
- Bleeding from cervical opening.
- Cervix is closed and uneffaced.
- No evidence of passage of tissue.

c. Diagnostic studies
- Serial β-hCG levels.
  - Decreasing β-hCG levels suggests probable loss of pregnancy.
- Pelvic U/S to determine gestational age and viability.
  - Abnormal gestational sac, small embryo with slow heart rate suggests probable loss of pregnancy.

d. Management
- No treatment modalities are available other than time.
- Rest at home, instruct patient to call if symptoms persist or increase.
- Reassure patient that it is not her fault.
- Symptoms remain mild or cease. Follow β-hCG every 3 days until the pattern of increasing levels and uterine growth are proven.

6. Missed Abortion
a. Definition
- Death of fetus before the 20th complete week of gestation; products of conception remain in utero.

b. Clinical features
- Loss of symptoms of pregnancy.
- Decrease in uterine size.
- Embryo has succumbed, no passage of tissue.
- Maybe brownish vaginal discharge.
- Cervix is firm and closed.

c. Diagnostic studies
- β-hCG decreased.
- U/S to evaluate suspected missed abortion.
- Pregnancy test may be negative.

d. Management
- First trimester—suction curettage.
- Second trimester—D&E or induction of labor with prostaglandin E_2 (PGE_2) suppositories 20 mg vaginally every 4 hours or misoprostol 200 mg tablets vaginally every 4 hours.
- Emotional support to family.

7. Septic Abortion
a. Definition
- Retained products of conception have become infected, including uterine and adjacent organ infection.

b. Clinical features
- Severe abdominal pain.
- Fever/chills.
- Uterine tenderness.
- Normal to decreased bowel sounds.
- Brown to bloody, foul-smelling vaginal discharge.
- Cervix may be nondilated with motion tenderness.
- Shock.
- Hemorrhage.
- Possible renal failure.

c. Diagnostic studies
- Complete blood count (CBC) count (leukocytosis), urinalysis, electrolytes, blood urea nitrogen (BUN) and creatine, type and screen, coagulation studies.
- Anaerobic and aerobic cultures from blood, cervix, POC.
- Cervical cultures for gonorrhea and *Chlamydia*.
- Abdominal radiographs to evaluate for free air or foreign bodies, rule out perforation.
- Chest X-ray.

d. Management
- Admission to hospital.
- Broad-spectrum antibiotics.
- Removal of POC, D&E.
- Hysterectomy may be needed if treatment does not resolve infection.

8. Recurrent Miscarriage
a. Definition
- Three or more consecutive spontaneous pregnancy losses.

b. Clinical features
- Clinical features reflective of type of spontaneous miscarriage.

c. Diagnostic studies for etiologic evaluation
- Radiographic or direct visualization of uterus for structural defects.
- Endometrial biopsy or luteal-phase serum progesterone levels to investigate possible luteal phase defect (LPD).

- Evaluation for polycystic ovarian syndrome (PCOS).
- Genetic testing.
- Antiphospholipid autoantibodies for evaluation of antiphospholipid syndrome (APS).
  d. Management
- LPD—25 mg progesterone vaginal suppository twice daily.
- PCOS—metformin.
- APS—anticoagulation therapies.
  9. Induced Abortion
  a. Definition
- Voluntary termination of pregnancy surgically or pharmaceutically.
  b. Clinical features
- Surgical abortion.
  - Dilation and curettage (D&C) procedure for 5 to 13 weeks gestation.
  - D&E procedure for >12 weeks gestation.
- Pharmaceutical (medication) abortion for gestations up to 49 days.
  - Mifepristone 200 to 600 mg PO on Day 1.
  - Misoprostol 400 to 800 μg PO or p.v. on Day 3 if abortion has not occurred after mifepristone.
  - Methotrexate 50 mg per m^2 IM or 25 to 50 mg PO—has not been FDA approved for early medication abortion.
  c. Diagnostic studies
- Screening for cervical gonorrhea and *Chlamydia*.
- U/S for accurate estimation of gestational age.
- Rh(D) typing.
  d. Management
- Preprocedure counseling.
- Administration of RhIG if indicated.

V. Ectopic Pregnancy

A. Definition
- Implantation of a fertilized ovum outside the uterine cavity. Leading cause of maternal death in first trimester due to hemorrhagic complications.

B. Etiology
- High risk.
  - History of ectopic pregnancy.
  - Tubal damage secondary to ligation, surgery, pathology, or infection.
  - Intrauterine contraceptive devices.
  - Assisted reproductive technology is associated with 5% increased risk for ectopic pregnancies.
- Moderate risk.
  - Infertility.
  - History of genital infections.
  - Multiple sexual partners.
- Low risk.
  - History of pelvic infections.
  - Cigarette smoking.
  - Previous abdominal or pelvic surgery.

C. Pathology
- Implantation of a fertilized ovum outside the uterine cavity, incidence by location:
  - Fallopian tube 98.3%.
  - Abdominal 1.4%.
  - Ovarian and cervical 0.15% each.

D. Clinical Features
- *Classic*: pelvic or abdominal pain, bleeding, cervical motion tenderness, adnexal mass in a pregnant woman.
- *Others*: amenorrhea or irregular periods with abdominal pain.
- **Rupturing or ruptured ectopic pregnancy:**
  - Severe abdominal pain, dizziness, nausea, vomiting, weakness, shock.
  - Syncope or dizziness may be present.
  - Adnexal or cervical motion tenderness.
  - Constitutes a true medical emergency.

E. Diagnostic Studies
- Serial serum β-hCG—can indicate ectopic pregnancy if levels rise <66% over 2 days, plateau or decrease.
- Transvaginal U/S—98.9% sensitivity and 84.4% specificity.
  - Absence of intrauterine products of conception.
- Presence of noncystic, extraovarian adnexal mass.
- Uterine evacuation with histologic evaluation when β-hCG and U/S are indeterminate.
- Laparoscopy—infrequently necessary for diagnosis when serial β-hCG, U/S, and uterine sampling utilized.
  - Allows direct visualization and possible removal of ectopic pregnancy before rupture.
- Exploratory laparotomy—when ruptured ectopic is suspected or proven.

F. Management
- Expectant management for falling β-hCG levels under 1,000 mIU per mL.
  - Spontaneous resolution in 67% of ectopic pregnancies.
- Medical management for unruptured ectopic pregnancies ≤4 cm.
  - Mulitple-dose methotrexate.
    - Methotrexate 1 mg per kg and leucovorin 0.1 mg per kg alternating day dosing for maximum of four doses each.
    - β-hCG monitoring on Day 0 and then odd-numbered days, successful when 15% drop between two successive blood draws.
  - Single-dose methotrexate.
    - Methotrexate 50 mg per m^2 single dose.
    - β-hCG monitoring on Days 0, 4, and 7, successful when 15% drop in levels from Day 4 to 7.
  - Two-dose methotrexate.
    - Methotrexate 50 mg per m^2 on Days 0 and 4.

- β-hCG monitoring on Days 0, 4, and 7, successful when 15% drop in levels from Days 4 to 7.
- Surgical management for ruptured ectopic pregnancy or contraindicated methotrexate therapy.
  - Laparoscopic salpingostomy—first choice "Gold standard" for unruptured tubal pregnancies <2.0 cm.
  - Explorative laparotomy and salpingectomy—alternatives.
- Administer Rh immunoglobulin if indicated.

VI. Cervical Insufficiency (Formerly Cervical Incompetence)

A. Definition
- Premature cervical dilation in the second trimester with higher risk of preterm birth.

B. Etiology
- Often no identifiable risk factors present.
- Previous procedures or trauma to cervix.
- Structure defects in uterus or cervical connective tissue.
- Diethylstilbestrol exposure in utero.
- Prior spontaneous or induced abortions.
- Multiple gestation.

C. Clinical Features
- Patient may be asymptomatic.
- Gradual and painless dilatation and effacement of cervix.
- History of painless cervical dilation with preterm delivery.

D. Diagnostic Studies
- Serial digital examination for shortening and effacement of cervix.
- U/S may detect cervical funneling or shortened cervix.
- Evaluate for PTL, rupture of membranes, chorioamnionitis, and fetal anomalies in women who have a short cervix.

E. Management
- Patients with a history of recurrent loss of pregnancy due to incompetent cervix should be followed early with frequent, gentle pelvic examinations and U/S.
- Weekly injections of 17α-hydroxyprogesterone caproate have shown effectiveness for nonsurgical therapy.
- Utilization of pessaries has demonstrated success in studies.
- Prophylactic, therapeutic, or emergent cerclage (surgical suture technique of the cervical os) may be necessary.
- Corticosteroids administered to woman at 24 to 34 weeks gestation to reduce complication risks of preterm delivery.

VII. Preterm Labor

A. Definition
- Regular uterine contractions with progressing cervical changes (dilation, effacement) occurring before 37 weeks gestation.
- Accounts for 75% of all neonatal morbidity and mortality.

B. Etiology
- Prior history of preterm delivery.
- Multiple gestations.
- African American race.
- Preterm, premature rupture of the fetal membranes (PPROM).
- Infections (e.g., chorioamnionitis) caused by prostaglandin endotoxin-producing bacteria (*Streptococcus, Fusobacterium, Gardnerella vaginalis*).
- Dehydration.
- Incompetent cervix.
- Uterine trauma.
- Placental abnormalities (e.g., abruptio placentae, placenta previa).

C. Clinical Features
- Low, dull backache.
- Pelvic or abdominal pressure.
- Cramps with or without diarrhea.
- Vaginal discharge increase or change (e.g., "bloody show").
- Contractions, often without pain.
- Contractions may be visible on a fetal monitor.

D. Diagnostic Studies
- Pelvic examination (sterile speculum examination), if PPROM is ruled out a bimanual examination may be done.
  - Cervical dilation and effacement with possible premature rupture of membranes.
    - Cervical dilation ≥3 cm and 80% effacement = PTL.
    - Cervical dilation 2 to 3 cm and <80% effacement = PTL likely, unconfirmed.
    - Cervical dilation <2 cm and <80% effacement = PTL unlikely.
  - Mucus bloody vaginal discharge or "bloody show" may be present. If more significant bleeding, evaluate for placenta previa or abruption placentae.
  - Nitrazine and fern test.
- Transvaginal U/S, cervical length.
  - Cervical length <20 mm with contractions = PTL.
  - Cervical length 20 to 30 mm with contractions = PTL likely.
  - Cervical length >30 mm without/without contractions = PTL likely.
- Fetal fibronectin test of cervicovaginal fluid for the presence of protein that is strongly associated with PTL if present between 20 and 34 weeks gestation.
  - Transabdominal U/S to assess fetus (weight, position) and amniotic fluid.

- Anovaginal GBS culture.
- Cervical cultures for *Chlamydia* and gonorrhea.
- Wet mount for bacterial vaginosis, *Trichomonas*, or yeast.

E. Management
- Continuous fetal monitoring.
- Tocolytic therapy—suppress uterine activity—contraindicated with intrauterine infection, severe preeclampsia, severe fetal anomaly.
  - β-Adrenergic agonists (ritodrine and terbutaline) titrate till halt of uterine contractions or development of side effects.
  - Magnesium sulfate ($MgSo_4$).
  - Calcium channel blockers (nifedipine).
  - Prostaglandin synthetase inhibitor (indomethacin).
- Antenatal corticosteroids—accelerate fetal lung maturity.
  - Single course given if between 24 and 32 weeks gestation, maximum benefit when administered within 7 days of delivery.
  - Betamethasone 12 mg IM every 24 hours for total of two doses.
  - Dexamethasone 6 mg IM every 12 hours for a total of four doses.
- Antibiotics, GBS prophylaxis, hydration therapy and bed rest may be beneficial.
- Delivery should occur in a hospital equipped with neonatal intensive care.
- C-section is usually done for premature breech infants who weigh under 2,000 g.

VIII. Hyperemesis Gravidarum

A. Definition
- An abnormal condition of pregnancy associated with severe nausea and vomiting, weight loss, electrolyte imbalance, and ketonuria most often occurring in the first or second trimester.

B. Etiology/Pathology
- Unclear, thought to be multifactorial.
- May be related to rapidly rising serum levels of hormones.
- Social and psychological factors may contribute.
- Risk factors include primigravida, multiple gestations, molar pregnancy, previous hyperemesis gravidarum.

C. Clinical Features
- Morning sickness—mild nausea and vomiting, usually resolved by 16th week of gestation.
- Hyperemesis gravidarum—severe nausea and vomiting.
- Weight loss of up to 5% of pregravid weight.
- Dehydration.
- Acidosis from starvation.
- Alkalosis from loss of hydrochloric acid in vomitus.
- Hypokalemia.

D. Diagnostic Studies
- Follow weight.
- Urinalysis for ketones.
- Electrolytes, liver function tests (LFTs), CBC and peripheral blood smear, thyroid function tests.
- Sonogram.

E. Management
- Depends on symptom severity.
- Morning sickness—usually no treatment necessary.
- Vitamin supplementation may be needed, vitamin B_6 10 to 25 mg, three times daily.
- Alternative therapies having shown benefit in research include ginger (250 mg four times daily) and acupuncture.
- Medications for antiemetic therapy doxylamine, 12.5 mg, three or four times daily and may add promethazine, 12.5 to 25 mg taken orally or rectally every 4 hours or dimenhydrinate, 50 to 100 mg taken orally or rectally every 4 to 6 hours.
- Severe hyperemesis gravidarum—admission.
- IV hydration, multivitamin and thiamin supplementation, electrolyte correction, IV antiemetic medications.
- Total parenteral nutrition for lack of response to other therapies.
- If the pregnant woman does not respond to medical treatment, a psychiatric consult is advised.

IX. Gestational Diabetes Mellitus (GDM)

A. Definition
- Glucose intolerance during pregnancy resulting in maternal hyperglycemia.

B. Etiology
- Risk factors:
  - History of diabetes type 1, type 2 or gestational diabetes.
  - Family history of diabetes.
  - Prior macrosomic, malformed, or stillborn infant.
  - In current pregnancy, presence of fetal macrosomia, polyhydramnios, multiple gestations.
  - Older maternal age.
  - Obesity.

C. Pathology
- Increases in serum insulin levels, sensitivity, estrogen, progestin, and cortisol for maternal fat accumulation resulting in increased insulin resistance.

D. Clinical Features
- GDM affects most body systems, and the woman may present with:
  - Hypoglycemia.
  - Hyperglycemia.
  - Recurrent urinary infections.
  - Vaginal infections.

- Hypertension.
- Hydramnios.
- Retinopathy.
- Stocking/glove neuropathy.
- Infant presentation:
  - Macrosomia.
  - Polyhydramnios.
  - Neonatal hypoglycemia.
  - Hypocalcemia.
  - Hyperbilirubinemia.
  - Congenital anomalies.
  - Respiratory distress.

E. Diagnostic Studies

- All pregnant women are screened at 24 to 28 weeks gestation for gestational diabetes.
- About 50-g oral glucose challenge without regard to time of day or last meal; plasma sample taken at 1 hour.
  - Level of 140 mg per dL or less is considered normal.
  - Level >140 mg per dL, patient should receive a 3-hour oral glucose tolerance test (OGTT).
- OGTT overnight fasting with a fasting blood sugar draw followed by 100-g glucose load; plasma glucose drawn at 1, 2, and 3 hours.
  - Two of the four plasma glucose levels above normal is diagnostic of GDM.
  - See Table 12-1, criterion values for diagnosis of GDM.
- Pelvic U/S to evaluate fetus for growth and abnormalities, and amniotic fluid for amount.

F. Management

- Glucose control to obtain and maintain euglycemia, monitor with frequent home blood glucose checks four times daily (fasting and 1 to 2 hours following meals).
- Optimal glucose levels for fasting is <95 mg per dL and <120 mg per dL after meals.
- Glycosylated hemoglobin (HbA$_1$c) drawn monthly to evaluate control.
- Nutritionist for diabetic diet counseling.
  - Calorie intake should be 24 (for overweight women), 30 (normal weight), and 40 (underweight) kcal per kg daily.
  - Diet should be 20% protein, 40% fat, and no more than 40% carbohydrate.
- Exercise.
- Pharmacologic therapy initiated when diet is ineffective.
  - Insulin, therapy of choice.
  - Does not cross the placenta and will not affect the fetus directly.
  - Maternal weight and gestational age dictate insulin dosing.
    - Total daily dosing during first trimester: 0.8 U per kg actual body weight; second trimester 1.0 U per kg actual body weight; third trimester 1.2 U per kg actual body weight.
    - Total daily dose is split between morning and evening. Often, NPH and regular insulin combinations are used.
    - Two-thirds of total daily dose given before breakfast (two-thirds of NPH and one-third regular).
    - Remaining one-third of total daily dose divided into 1/2 of that given as regular before dinner and remaining given as NPH at bed.
  - Glyburide may be an acceptable alternative to insulin in GDM. Research has shown similar glucose control as insulin but higher rate of preeclampsia and need for infant photo therapy.
    - Start at 2.5 mg in morning and titrate up to max 10 mg every 12 hours.
- Fetal monitoring.
  - Biweekly starting at about 32 weeks of gestational age.
  - Daily fetal "kick counts" monitored.
  - Fetal heart rate monitoring.
  - Nonstress test (NST).
  - BPP (U/S tests fetal respiration, tone, flexion/extension, amniotic fluid levels) or contraction stress test if NST nonreactive.
  - U/S monitoring of fetus for macrosomia and shoulder dystocia.
  - Early delivery—at 38 weeks, the fetus should be evaluated by pelvic U/S for weight. If macrosomic, >4,500 to 5,000 g, an elective C-section should be performed.
  - Before delivery, U/S-guided amniocentesis should be performed, and amniotic fluid analyzed for the

TABLE 12–1. Criterion Values for Diagnosis of GDM from Results of OGTT		
Time Since 100-g Glucose Load (h)	**Modified O'Sullivan Scale**	**Carpenter & Coustan Scale**
Fasting	105	95
1	190	180
2	165	155
3	145	140

Values are plasma glucose levels in mg per dL.
From *The Johns Hopkins Manual of Gynecology and Obstetrics*. 3rd ed. Baltimore, MD: Lippincott Williams & Wilkins; 2006:164, with permission.

level of phospholipid, phosphatidylglycerol, an indicator of fetal lung maturity.
- Fetal intrauterine demise common with noncompliant patients.
- If PTL develops in the patients with diabetes, magnesium sulfate is the tocolytic agent of choice, as many of the others exacerbate diabetes-related problems.
- If there is a risk of preterm delivery, corticosteroids should be given for fetal lung maturity, but remember to be careful as corticosteroids have a hyperglycemic effect.

X. Hypertensive Disorders in Pregnancy

A. Chronic Hypertension
1. Definition
- Hypertension before pregnancy or before the 20th week of gestation, or persistence past 12 weeks postpartum.
- Mild: systolic blood pressure (BP) 140 mm Hg or higher, diastolic 90 mm Hg or higher, on two separate occasions at least 6 hours apart and not more than 1 week apart.
- Severe: systolic BP ≥180 mm Hg, diastolic ≥110 mm Hg.
- High risk of developing superimposed preeclampsia or eclampsia.

2. Diagnostic Studies
- CBC, glucose screen, electrolyte panel, BUN/creatinine levels, serum urea nitrogen, uric acid, calcium.
- U/A, note proteinuria; also obtain urine culture.
- Coagulation studies such as PT, PTT, fibrin split products.
- Twenty-four hour urine calcium measurement.
- ECG.
- Pelvic U/S to monitor fetus.

DIFFERENTIAL DIAGNOSIS
- Gestational hypertension, preeclampsia.

3. Management
MILD CHRONIC HYPERTENSION
- Prenatal visits every 2 to 4 weeks, weekly beginning at 34 to 36 weeks.
- Monitor BP and urine for protein frequently.
- Check fundal height.
- Ask about symptoms/signs of preeclampsia.
- Fetal monitoring begins at 32 to 34 weeks.
- Delivery by week 39 to 40.

SEVERE CHRONIC HYPERTENSION
- Most clinicians begin pharmacologic treatment at 150/100 mm Hg.
- May need more frequent prenatal visits to monitor.
- Monitor BP, proteinuria, and fetal growth.
- Assess for preeclampsia.
- If end-organ involvement, monitor for exacerbation.

- U/S for fetal growth every 2 to 4 weeks beginning at 32 to 34 weeks.
- Delivery after week 38 or when fetal lungs are mature.
- Methyldopa is first-line therapy in pregnancy.
- Labetalol or calcium channel blockers may be used.

B. Gestational Hypertension
1. Definition
- Hypertension detected after the 20th week of pregnancy without proteinuria. Resolves by 12 weeks postpartum. May also occur within 48 to 72 hours after delivery.

2. Management
- Outpatient treatment; some recommend withholding antihypertensives so as not to mask severe preeclampsia.
- If antihypertensives are used, hydralazine or labetalol are recommended.
- Continue to follow BP measurements and proteinuria closely (as noted above), as the majority of these patients progress to preeclampsia later in pregnancy.
- Draw baseline CBC, BUN, creatinine. Some practitioners recommend following a uric acid level. A rise indicates progression to preeclampsia.

XI. Preeclampsia

A. Definition
- Hypertension and proteinuria after the 20th week of gestation.
- Edema is no longer part of the diagnostic criteria because it occurs too frequently in normal pregnancies.
- Can occur prior to 20th week in trophoblastic disease or multiple gestation.
- Categorized as mild and severe.

B. Etiology
- Largely unknown. Incidence is 2% to 7% in nulliparous women.

C. Risk Factors
- Nulliparity.
- Previous preeclampsia/eclampsia; family history of preeclampsia.
- Multiple gestation (i.e., twins).
- Thyroid disease.
- Extremes of age.
- Preexisting hypertensive, vascular, autoimmune, or renal disease.
- Pregestational diabetes.
- Obesity.
- Fetal hydrops.
- Trisomy 13.
- Hydatidiform mole.

D. Clinical Features
1. Mild Preeclampsia
- Systolic BP ≥140 mm Hg and/or diastolic BP ≥90 mm Hg on two separate occasions at least 6 hours apart (but no >1 week apart).

- Proteinuria >300 mg in 24-hour period (or >+1 on urine dipstick).

2. **Severe Preeclampsia**
   - Systolic BP ≥160 mm Hg and/or diastolic BP ≥110 mm Hg on two occasions as noted above.
   - Or any of the following:
     - Proteinuria: >5 g in a 24-hour period (or +3 to +4 on urine dipstick).
   - Oliguria <500 mL in 24 hours.
   - Thrombocytopenia.
   - Pulmonary edema.
   - HELLP syndrome (special entity, **H**emolysis, **E**levated **L**iver enzymes, **L**ow **P**latelets).
   - Restriction of fetal growth.
   - Other symptoms include:
   - Epigastric/upper right quadrant pain.
   - Nausea, vomiting.
   - Dyspnea.
   - Lack of fetal movement.
   - PTL.
   - Elevated LFTs.
   - Headache.
   - Visual disturbances/scotomata.
   - Altered mental status.

E. **Diagnostic Studies**
   - Recognize preeclampsia early.
   - Obtain BP measurements on two occasions with patient in left lateral position.
   - U/A for protein.
   - CBC, coagulation factors (PT, PTT, fibrin split products), BUN and creatinine levels, LFTs, if severe form.
   - Pelvic U/S to monitor fetus.

F. **Management**
   - **Mild:**
     - Only cure for preeclampsia is delivery.
       - Deliver if at 34 to 36 weeks gestation or more.
       - Restrict activity; bed rest for mild preeclampsia is controversial.
       - Daily weights and urine dipstick; weekly 24 hour urine.
       - Twice weekly NSTs and/or BPPs weekly.
       - BP control.
       - Seizure prevention.
   - **Severe:**
     - Continue to monitor mother and fetus, control BP, and prevent seizures.
     - Patient should be hospitalized for moderate to severe preeclampsia.
     - MgSO₄ IV reduces patient's BP and helps prevent seizures, but not used until diagnosis of severe preeclampsia or start of labor.
     - Other BP lowering agents may be necessary (e.g., hydralazine, labetalol, nifedipine).
     - Monitor fetal well being, continuous heart rate, U/S, BPP.

- Consider amniocentesis to evaluate fetal lung development if fetus is 30 to 37 weeks. If lungs are immature, give corticosteroids. If fetus is between 26 and 30 weeks, give corticosteroids.
- Depending on the patient's condition, delivery of a preterm infant may be delayed for steroid treatment to facilitate lung maturity. If the patient is at term, she should be delivered by induced vaginal delivery or by C-section.

G. **Complications**
   - Abruptio placentae.
   - Liver failure/rupture/HELLP.
     - Congestive heart failure.
   - Renal failure.
   - Cerebrovascular accident (CVA).
   - Adult respiratory distress syndrome.
   - Fetal distress/demise.

XII. Eclampsia

A. **Definition**
   - Occurrence of convulsions, coma, or both in a woman with preeclampsia.
   - Life threatening for mother and fetus.
     - Can occur antepartum (most commonly), intra- or postpartum.

B. **Etiology**
   - Unknown.
   - Incidence is 0.05% to 0.10% in the United States, but higher in developing countries.

C. **Clinical Features**
   - Abrupt tonic–clonic seizure of 1 to 2 minutes duration, followed by postictal state.
   - May include headache, visual changes, epigastric pain.
   - Cardiorespiratory arrest may follow.
   - Pulmonary aspiration.
   - Other neurologic symptoms may be present.

D. **Diagnostic Studies**
   - Studies as for preeclampsia (see XI.).

   DIFFERENTIAL DIAGNOSIS
   - Until proven otherwise, a seizure during pregnancy should be considered eclampsia.
   - Others include epilepsy, encephalitis, meningitis, cerebral tumor, and CVA.

E. **Management**
   - Airway, breathing, circulation.
   - Protect the patient from injury.
   - Treat hypertension as in preeclampsia.
   - Drugs—MgSO₄ to prevent recurrence of seizure.
   - Deliver fetus after patient is stabilized—be prepared for emergency C-section.
   - Monitor for pulmonary edema; careful attention to fluid status.
   - Monitor urine output with use of indwelling Foley catheter.

XIII. Placenta Previa

A. Definition

- The presence of placental tissue in the lower uterine segment over, or adjacent to, the cervical os.
- Results in complete or partial coverage of the cervix, ahead of presenting fetal part.
- Average presentation of first bleeding episode is 29 to 30 weeks.
- Bleeding is a result of separation of placenta from lower uterine segment and cervix.

TOTAL (COMPLETE) PLACENTA PREVIA

- Internal cervical opening covered completely.

PARTIAL/MARGINAL PLACENTA PREVIA (PREVIOUSLY CATEGORIZED SEPARATELY)

- Placenta lies within 2 to 3 cm of the cervical os, but not covering it.

B. Etiology

- Unknown. Incidence is 0.5% to 1.0% in all pregnancies.

C. Risk Factors

- Previous uterine surgery, C-section.
- Advanced age.
  - Prior endometrial trauma, D&C, D&E.
- Minority patient.
  - Abnormality of endometrial vascularity.
- Delayed ovulation.
- Multiparity.
- Cigarette smoking.

D. Clinical Features

- Spotting during first and second trimesters.
- Sudden painless vaginal bleeding in third trimester.
- Usually soft, nontender uterus.
- Patients with no prenatal care may present with severe vaginal bleeding.
- Prenatal patients usually receive a U/S between the 12th and 20th weeks of gestation, which allows for diagnosis prior to the onset of bleeding.

E. Diagnostic Studies

- Transvaginal U/S—to localize the placenta.
- Additional U/S are necessary to establish the degree of previa, because the placenta may migrate.
- Abdominal examination, uterine tone.
- Fetal heart rate.
- Monitor mother's vital signs.
- CBC, platelet count, coagulation studies—in patients with significant bleeding.
- Amniocentesis—to determine lung maturity.
- Digital examination is contraindicated if placenta previa is present.

F. Management

- Treatment depends on the extent of bleeding, gestational age, and status of the cervix.
- Hospitalization with hemodynamic stabilization.
- Maternal and fetal monitoring.
- Steroids between 24 and 34 weeks for fetal lung development.
- Rh0(D) immunoglobulin to Rh-negative mothers.
- Pelvic rest.
- Preterm patients with one to two episodes of mild bleeding are treated with bed rest and tocolysis, if needed.
- Follow closely and monitor CBC.
- May progress to term and deliver vaginally (marginal placenta), or by C-section (total previa).
- Patients with severe hemorrhage or third bleeding episode should be resuscitated and delivered by urgent C-section.
- Usually, if a mother is hospitalized on three separate occasions, she will remain in the hospital until delivery.
- If a patient is not bleeding during third trimester, confirm previa through U/S, pelvic rest, patient education of warning signs, avoid strenuous activity, and check fetal U/S every 3 or 4 weeks.

G. Complications

- Longer hospital stay.
- C-section.
- Abruptio placentae.
- Postpartum hemorrhage (PPH).
- Malpresentation.

XIV. Abruptio Placentae

A. Definition

- Premature partial or complete separation of the placenta from its normal implantation.
  - One of the leading causes of fetal mortality.
- Classified according to clinical findings:
- Grade 1, mild abruption. Slight bleeding.
- Grade 2, moderate or partial abruption.
- Grade 3, large or complete abruption (least common).
  - Grade 3 and complete separation should be considered life threatening to mother and fetus.
  - Figure 12-1 shows common features of different types of abruption.

B. Etiology

- Primary etiology is unknown.
- Occurs in approximately 1 of 120 births.
- Abruption accounts for 10% to 15% of perinatal mortality.

C. Risk Factors

- Maternal hypertension (strongly associated with grade 3).
- Blunt abdominal trauma (initially often grade 1, can progress rapidly to grade 3).
- Previous abruptio placentae.
- Chorioamnionitis.
- Multiple gestation.
- Poor nutrition (folic acid deficiency).
- Cigarette smoking; drug abuse (alcohol, cocaine).
- Advanced maternal age.
- Uterine anomalies or myomas.
- Thrombophilia defects.

D. Pathology
- Separation is initiated by bleeding into decidua basalis.
- Decidua splits and placenta is sheared off.
- Blood may extravasate into and through myometrium.

E. Clinical Features
- Abruption may be life-threatening or, depending on grade, may be asymptomatic and only be discovered on delivery of placenta.
- Vaginal bleeding in third trimester (80%).
- Uterine tenderness.
- Abdominal pain or back pain.
- Premature labor.
- May be fetal distress.
- Severe cases can lead to hypovolemic shock, disseminated intravascular coagulopathy (DIC), fetal distress, demise, uterine tetany.

F. Diagnostic Studies
- Pelvic U/S of fetus, placenta, and uterus.
- Fetal heart rate monitor and tocometry may show hypertonic contractions with elevated baseline and various degrees of abnormal heart rate patterns.
- Coagulation studies—PT, PTT, fibrin, fibrin split products.

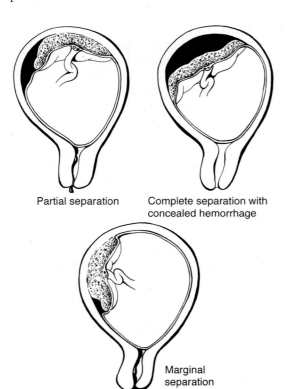

Partial separation

Complete separation with concealed hemorrhage

Marginal separation

FIGURE 12–1. **Various degrees of separation of a normally implanted placenta.** (From Scott JR. Placenta previa and placental abruption. In: Scott JR, DiSaia PS, Hammond GB, Spellacy WN, eds. *Danforth's Obstetrics and Gynecology*. 8th ed. Philadelphia, PA: Lippincott Williams & Wilkins; 1999:412, with permission.)

- CBC with platelet count, hematocrit, blood type and screen depending on the severity of bleeding, BUN, and creatinine.
- U/A.

DIFFERENTIAL DIAGNOSIS
- Placenta previa (abruptio placentae has abdominal discomfort and painful contractions, placenta previa does not).

G. Management
- **Mild abruption**—no treatment may be necessary.
- Follow closely in labor unit until fetal maturity; may be confused with premature or early labor; expect vaginal delivery.
- After abdominal trauma, patients should be observed closely for at least 24 hours.
- May place Foley catheter to measure urine output which should be >0.5 to 1.0 mL per kg per hour.
- Administer Rh0(D) immunoglobulin to Rh-negative individuals.
- **Moderate-to-severe abruption with signs of fetal distress**, loss of fetal heart tones, or maternal signs of shock require immediate resuscitation and delivery by C-section.
- Patients should be cross-matched for 4 to 6 units of blood.
- Repeat coagulation studies and CBC to evaluate for DIC.
- **Moderate-to-severe abruption with no signs of fetal distress or maternal hypotension**: vaginal delivery may be attempted with gentle induction of labor with Pitocin, as long as no evidence of fetal distress or maternal complications is present.
- Postdelivery of infant and placenta, patient may still develop complications and should be treated symptomatically.

XV. Multiple Gestations

A. Definition
- Gestation and delivery of two or more fetuses.
  - One of the most common high-risk conditions.
  - Twin gestation is the most common form.

B. Etiology
- Ethnic background—more common in African Americans than Caucasians or Asians.
- Maternal age—more common in women between 30 and 40 years of age.
- Infertility therapy.
- Hereditary—increased incidence in families.

C. Pathology
- Dizygotic twins (fraternal)—more common type (1 in 90 pregnancies); two separate ova are fertilized. The placentation is always diamniotic and dichorionic.
- Monozygotic twins (identical)—single ovum is fertilized and splits into distinct persons (1 in 250 pregnancies). May have diamniotic and dichorionic

placenta; however, much more common is monoam-niotic, monochorionic placenta (Figure 12-2).

D. Clinical Features
- Fundal height above normal for EGA.
- The patient may have earlier and more severe pressure in pelvis.
- Excessive maternal weight gain.
- Nausea.
- Backache.
- Varicosities.
- Constipation, hemorrhoids.
- Abdominal distentions.
- Difficulty breathing.
- Multiplicity of small parts.
- Two fetal hearts detected.
- Two fetuses palpated.

E. Complications
- Higher incidence of complications compared with singletons:
  - PTL.
  - Preeclampsia.
  - Abruption.
  - Anemia.
  - Hydramnios.
  - UTI.
  - PPH.
  - C-section.
- For the fetus, most common problems are:
  - Low birth weight.
  - Prematurity.
  - Congenital abnormalities.
  - Incidence higher in monozygotic twins.
  - Discordance.
  - Vanishing twin.
  - Monoamniotic cord entanglement.
  - Twin-to-twin transfusion syndrome.

- Molar pregnancy and fetus.
- Delayed delivery.

F. Diagnostic Studies
- More than one heartbeat on auscultation.
- External examination—multiple heads and small parts.
- Higher levels of β-hCG, AFP, human placental lactogen, or estriol.
- Majority of multiple pregnancies are diagnosed by U/S scanning.

G. Management
- After diagnosis of multiple gestation, patient must be treated as high risk.
- Patient must be seen more frequently, as well as receive regular vaginal examination and U/S to evaluate for premature contractions, and for fetal growth and well-being.
- The role of bed rest is still being studied. Starting at approximately 24 weeks may be helpful for reducing complications and increasing fetal weight; 81% of perinatal mortality occurs before gestational week 29.
- Depending on fetal positions and gestational age, placental type, and mother's parity, vaginal delivery may be possible.
- In instances of monoamniotic monochorionic placentas or presenting twin breech, C-section is the best course.

XVI. Abnormalities of Labor
A. Definition
- Dystocia is defined as an abnormal progression of labor that may result in modes of delivery other than spontaneous vaginal.

B. Etiology
- **Protraction or arrest of active labor may be caused by:**
  - Abnormalities of power (uterine contractions, cervical resistance).

Zygote	Dizygotic	Monozygotic		
Day of division		0–3	3–8	8–13
Placenta				
Central membrane	2 Amnion 2 Chorion	2 Amnion 2 Chorion	2 Amnion	None

FIGURE 12–2. Types of placentation in monozygotic and dizygotic twinning. (From Spellacy WN. Multiple pregnancies. In: Scott JR, DiSaia PS, Hammond GB, Spellacy WN, eds. *Danforth's Obstetrics and Gynecology*. 8th ed. Philadelphia, PA: Lippincott Williams & Wilkins; 1999:294, with permission.)

- Abnormalities of the passenger (fetal size, presentation, position).
- Abnormalities of passage (maternal pelvimetry).

C. Clinical Features
- At first prenatal visit, especially in the case of primigravida, pelvic sizing is important.
- If noted early that the outlet may not be appropriate, patient must be watched more closely during labor.
- In instances of fetal size or presentation causing cephalopelvic disproportion, careful evaluation should be done to determine the mode of delivery.

D. Diagnostic Studies
- No laboratory studies are available that allow for prediction of abnormal labors.
- Pelvic U/S helps evaluate fetal position, presentation.
- MRI may help with some estimation of pelvimetry.
- X-ray, the original method of pelvimetry, is not commonly used today.

E. Management
- Identify the specific abnormality and determine if the problem is correctable.
- Management options vary considerably from observation to C-section.
- Augmentation with oxytocin is recommended in certain conditions.
  - Malposition—attempt at version; if unsuccessful, C-section is usually performed.
- Attempts can be made to change fetal head's position to more favorable one.
- C-section delivery is usually performed in cases of cephalopelvic disproportion, fetal abnormalities such as hydrocephalus and abnormal head positions.
- Use of forceps or vacuum can sometimes accomplish a change of position or help guide and deliver the fetal head.

XVII. Malpresentations

A. Definition
- Any presentation of presenting part other than vertex—breech, transverse position, face presentation, brow presentations, compound presentation.
- Breech presentation is the most common malpresentation.

B. Etiology
- Associated with both fetal and maternal abnormalities.
- Small fetus (increased motility).
- Decreased fetal muscle strength and tone (myotonic dystrophies, chromosomal abnormalities).
- Hydrocephalus or anencephaly.
- Multiple gestations.
- Abnormally implanted placenta (obstructive normal descent).
- Multiparity (laxity of maternal abdominal and uterine musculature).
- Uterine tumor or anomalies.

C. Clinical Features
- In most instances, presenting part of the fetus can be determined before the 36th week by pelvic examination ± U/S.
- Chances of spontaneous conversion of malpresentation decreases with EGA.
- Mode of delivery depends on position.
- Risk of cord prolapse is greatest with incomplete and compound presentations.
- Risk of injury to baby increased with vaginal delivery in nonexpert hands.

D. Diagnostic Studies
- U/S—primary tool for determining fetal position.
- Vaginal/pelvic examination.
- Leopold maneuvers.

E. Management
- In cases of breech or transverse lie, external cephalic version may be attempted after 36 weeks (40% revert to original lie).
- C-section is recommended for most malpresentations.

XVIII. Shoulder Dystocia

A. Definition
- An acute obstetrical emergency, when one (usually the anterior) or both shoulders of the fetus become lodged at the pubic symphysis after delivery of the head.
- Brachial plexus injury (Erb palsy) may result.

B. Etiology
RISK FACTORS
- Macrosomia (mother diabetic); history of macrosomic newborn.
  - Maternal obesity.
  - Multiparity.
  - Post-term gestation.
- Bony pelvic abnormality.
- Uterine abnormalities.
- Abnormal contractions.

C. Clinical Features
- Rapid or precipitous descent should warn the clinician of possible shoulder dystocia.
- Condition must be recognized quickly because it could be fatal for the fetus if too much time is taken to deliver the shoulder.

D. Management
- The first-line treatment is McRoberts maneuver: maternal hyperflexion of the hips and abduction of knees and legs to increase pelvic opening. Suprapubic pressure is applied.
- A second-line choice is to perform the Wood corkscrew maneuver by rotating the posterior shoulder toward the fetal back. Rubin maneuver may be performed (hand inserted into the vagina and digital pressure applied to posterior aspect of anterior shoulder toward the fetal chest).

- It may be necessary to fracture one or both of the clavicles if none of the above are successful. Clavicles should be broken using the thumb and fracturing the bones away from the lungs.
- As a last resort, the Zavanelli maneuver involves cephalic replacement and C-section delivery.
- The longer it takes to deliver the fetus, the greater the chance for neuropsychiatric disorders and trauma to the fetus.
- After delivery, the mother may be left with the equivalent of a fourth-degree tear. The wound must be closed properly, or the mother may suffer from rectovaginal fistulae or rectal incontinence.
- The patient is given stool softeners, and wound is checked daily for evidence of hematoma or infection.

XIX. Postpartum Fever and Sepsis

A. Definition
- Infections that occur in the immediate postpartum period causing fever, sepsis, or both.
- Fever >38°C on at least two occasions (measured at least 4 hours apart) after the first 24 hours postpartum.

B. Etiology
RISK FACTORS
- C-section.
- Breech presentation.
- Prolonged labor.
- Lengthy duration of ruptured membranes.
- Low socioeconomic status.
- Obesity.
- Immunosuppression/diabetes.
- Vaginal infections, especially bacterial vaginosis.
- Multiple vaginal examinations.

C. Clinical Features
ENDOMETRITIS
- Rare after vaginal delivery.
- Usually presents second to seventh postpartum day.
- Infection is usually polymicrobial in nature.
- Patient presents with complaints of abdominal pain, high fever, chills, purulent/foul lochia.

UTIs
- UTIs, especially pyelonephritis in postpartum period.
- Usual presentation—fever, chills, frequency, and back pain.
- Check for CVA tenderness.
- If fever persists more than 48 to 72 hours after antibiotic treatment, consider other problems such as wound infection, ovarian vein thrombosis, pelvic abscess, septic pelvic thrombophlebitis, mastitis.

WOUND INFECTION
- Pain, redness, and swelling in the area of incision.

SEPTIC PELVIC VEIN THROMBOPHLEBITIS
- Persistent fever, elevated WBC, no evidence of UTI, endometritis, or abscess.

D. Diagnostic Studies
- CBC plus peripheral blood smear.
- Urinalysis.
- Blood and urine cultures; genital cultures.
- In instances of suspected phlebitis or abscesses, pelvic U/S, computed tomography scan, or MRI may identify possible sources.

E. Management
- Patient should be admitted and started on IV antibiotics after culture and sensitivity; appropriate antibiotics may be ampicillin/sulbactam, gentamicin, clindamycin, ampicillin, or combinations thereof.
- In most instances, patients respond in 24 to 48 hours.
- If patient does not respond in 3 to 4 days, other conditions should be considered and appropriate subspecialist may be consulted.
- Prophylactic antibiotics after C-section are recommended.

XX. Postpartum Hemorrhage

A. Definition
- Emergent condition traditionally defined as bleeding in excess of 500 mL with vaginal delivery or >1,000 mL with C-section.
- Current criteria include bleeding that produces signs and symptoms, and requires a blood transfusion; 10% drop in hematocrit from admission to postpartum period.
- Early PPH occurs ≤24 hours postpartum; late PPH occurs ≥24 hours, up to 6 to 12 weeks postpartum.

B. Etiology/Pathology
- Most common cause: uterine atony (unable to contract and control bleeding).
- Severe vaginal or perineal tears, retained placenta, uterine rupture, or uterine inversion.
- Congenital bleeding disorders or other coagulation defects.
- DIC (caused by preeclampsia, sepsis, abruptio placentae, or amniotic fluid embolus).
- Accounts for a minimum of 25% maternal deaths worldwide.
- Incidence difficult to estimate due to lack of uniform definition of PPH.

C. Clinical Features
- Hypovolemic shock—pale, clammy skin; hypotension; tachycardia; delayed capillary refill; narrowed pulse pressure.

D. Diagnostic Studies
- Vital signs.
- CBC, peripheral blood smear, PT, PTT, fibrinogen, fibrin split products.
- Type and cross-match for possible transfusion.

E. Management
- Evaluate excessive bleeding and identify/treat probable cause.

TABLE 12–2.	Three Categories of Postpartum Mood Disorders		
	Postpartum Psychosis	**Postpartum Depression**	**Maternity Blues**
Incidence (%)	0.1–0.2	=10	50–80
Average time	2–3 days PP	2 weeks to 12 months PP	1–5 days PP
Average duration	Variable	3–14 months	2–3 days, resolution within 10 days
Symptoms	Similar to organic brain syndrome: confusion, attention deficit, distractibility, clouded sensorium	Irritability, labile mood, difficulty falling asleep, phobias, anxiety; symptoms worsen in the evening	Mild insomnia, tearfulness, fatigue, irritability, poor concentration, depressed affect
Treatment	A psychotic pharmacotherapy, antidepressant, 50% of patients also meet depression criteria	Antidepressant, pharmacotherapy, psychotherapy	Time, reassurance, watchful waiting; leads to PPD in 20% of patients

From Beckmann CR. *Obstetrics and Gynecology*. 5th ed. Baltimore, MD: Lippincott Williams & Wilkins; 2005:130, with permission.

- For uterine atony—bimanual massage and give oxytocin IV. If unsuccessful, other agents include methylergonovine or misoprostol. Balloon catheter or packing are next line options, whereas operative measures are a last resort.
- For retained placenta—manual removal and manage atony as above.
- If present, repair lacerations and correct coagulation defects.

XXI. Postpartum Depression (Table 12-2)

A. Definition
- Criteria for major depressive disorder are met; see clinical features below.
- Usually occurs 2 weeks to 12 months postpartum.
- Differential diagnosis includes the following:
  - Postpartum "baby" blues—common condition possibly caused by decreasing progesterone. Self-limiting and resolved within 2 weeks.
  - Postpartum psychosis—a rare, but serious, condition which may require hospitalization due to impairment and risk of harm to mother or baby.

B. Etiology/Pathology
- Psychosocial and/or biochemical factors such as prior history of depression, family history/genetic factors, poor social support, stressful life events, trauma during birth.
- Incidence is between 10% and 15% of all pregnancies.

C. Clinical Features
- The onset of postpartum depression can vary from the immediate postpartum period to several weeks following delivery.
- Symptoms may include depressed mood, anhedonia, difficulty concentrating, guilt, suicidal ideation, anxiety, and sleep or appetite changes.
- Patients may feel lonely, isolated, unable to care for self or baby.

- In early stages, clinicians should be attuned to patient complaints and changes in mood, affect, and appearance.

D. Diagnostic Studies
- Thyroid function should be assessed, as depression may be due to hypothyroidism.
- Order additional diagnostic studies as needed, to rule out other organic causes of depression.
- Postpartum depression must be taken seriously. Patients should be screened during pregnancy and postpartum period. Evaluate mood, affect, appearance, and risks for harm to mother or baby.

E. Management
- Evaluate the severity of the condition and the potential for harm. Evaluate the need for a psychiatric evaluation.
- Antidepressant medications and/or psychotherapy are recommended for treatment.

SELECTED REFERENCES

Beckman CRB, Ling FW, Barazansky BM, Herbert WN, Laube DW, Smith RP, eds. *Obstetrics and Gynecology*. 6th ed. Baltimore, MD: Lippincott Williams & Wilkins; 2010.

DeCherney AH, Nathan L, Goodwin TM, Lauger N, eds. *Current Diagnosis and Treatment Obstetrics and Gynecology*. 10th ed. New York, NY: McGraw Hill; 2007.

Gabbe SG, Niebyl JR, Simpson JL, eds. *Obstetrics: Normal and Problem Pregnancies*. 5th ed. Philadelphia, PA: Churchill Livingstone; 2007.

Gibbs RS, Karlan BY, Haney AF, Nygaard I, eds. *Danforth's Obstetrics and Gynecology*. 10th ed. Philadelphia, PA: Lippincott Williams & Wilkins; 2008.

Goodwin TM. Hyperemesis gravidarum. *Obstet Gynecol Clin N Am*. 2008;35:401–417.

Hacker NF, Gambone JC, Hobel CJ, eds. *Hacker and Morre's Essentials of Obstetrics and Gynecology*. 5th ed. Philadelphia, PA: Saunders Elsevier; 2010.

Houry DE, Salhi BA. Acute complications of pregnancy. In: Marx JA, ed. *Rosen's Emergency Medicine Concepts and Clinical Practice*. 7th ed. Philadelphia, PA: Mosby Elsevier; 2010.

Pridjian G, Benjamin TD. Update on gestational diabetes. *Obstet Gynecol Clin N Am*. 2010;37:255–267.

Hematologic Disorders

Elizabeth Quinlan-Bohn

I. Anemia

A. General Definition, Red Cell Morphology

- Anemia occurs when hemoglobin (Hgb) in blood is too low to fulfill oxygen (O_2) demands of the body.
- Can be measured by a decrease in the red blood cell (RBC) volume (hematocrit [HCT]) or decrease in the amount of Hgb.

ADULT NORMALS

- Males: 4.4 to 5.9×10^6 per mm^3.
- Females: 3.8 to 5.2×10^6 per mm^3.
- Hgb consists of protein called globin composed of four polypeptide chains and four nonprotein pigments (heme) that contain iron to carry O_2—Hgb A ($\alpha_2\beta_2$), Hgb A_2 ($\alpha_2\delta_2$), and Hgb F ($\alpha_2\gamma_2$).

HGB—ADULT NORMALS

- Males: 13.3 to 17.7 g per dL.
- Females: 11.7 to 15.7 g per dL.
- Normal adult blood contains Hgb A (95% to 98%), Hgb A_2 (1.5% to 3.5%), and Hgb F (<2%).
- HCT—percentage of blood volume that is RBCs, usually approximately three times the Hgb concentration.
- Example: A patient with an Hgb of 12 g per dL would have an approximate HCT of 36%.

HCT—ADULT NORMALS

- Males: 40% to 52%.
- Females: 35% to 47%.
- Factors that may account for variations in normal values: increased HCT due to secondary erythrocytosis among tobacco smokers and people living at high altitudes; decreased HCT due to dilutional effect from plasma volume expansion of pregnancy.
- HCT values may be artificially high or low in hypovolemia/hypervolemia.
- Gold standard—RBC mass, a nuclear medicine test that measures milliliter RBCs per kilogram of body weight, generally obtained only in the evaluation of abnormally elevated values (polycythemia).

ERYTHROCYTE INDICES

- Erythrocyte indices classify RBCs by size and Hgb content:

1. **Mean Cell Volume or Mean Corpuscular Volume (MCV)**
   - Measure of average RBC size.

NORMOCYTIC CELLS

- Have an MCV of 80 to 100 fL.

MICROCYTIC CELLS

- Have an MCV of <80 fL.

MACROCYTIC CELLS

- Have an MCV of >100 fL.

2. **Mean Corpuscular Hgb Concentration (MCHC)**
   - Measure of average Hgb concentration per RBC.
   - Percentage of Hgb in RBC.
   - Measure of *color*.

NORMOCHROMIC CELLS

- Have an MCHC of 32 to 36 g per dL.

HYPOCHROMIC CELLS

- Have an MCHC of <32 g per dL.

HYPERCHROMIC CELLS

- The MCHC cannot exceed 37 g per dL, as this is the maximum amount of Hgb that RBC can contain. No real hyperchromic cells exist except the spherocyte secondary to decreased surface–volume ratio.

3. **Mean Corpuscular Hgb (MCH)**
   - Measure of the average amount of Hgb per RBC.
   - Measure of *weight*.
   - **NOTE:** MCH does not take into account cell size—should be correlated with MCV.

NORMOCHROMIC CELLS

- Have an MCH of 26 to 34 pg.

HYPOCHROMIC CELLS

- Have an MCH of <26 pg.

HYPERCHROMIC CELLS

- Have an MCH of >34 pg.

4. **Reticulocyte**
   - Immature RBC with no nucleus and residual ribonucleic acid and mitochondria that lives in bone marrow 2 to 3 days; is then extruded into peripheral blood where it lives in this form for another day or 2.
   - Laboratory normals—0.5% to 1.5% of all RBCs.
   - Values higher than these indicate increased production of RBCs.
   - Elevated reticulocyte count indicates increased production of RBCs. Must take into account that an increased reticulocyte count does not always indicate a hyperproliferative bone marrow and also

must determine the corrected reticulocyte count (CR):

- CR = (% reticulocytes) × (patient's HCT/normal HCT).

B. Blood Loss (Acute and Chronic)

ACUTE BLOOD LOSS

1. Etiology

- Acute blood loss caused by hemorrhage from such disorder as trauma.
- Massive gastrointestinal (GI) bleed.
- Ruptured aneurysm.

2. Pathology

- Blood loss of >1,500 mL causes cardiovascular collapse.

3. Clinical Features

- Patient may complain of dizziness, lightheadedness, or both, or be stuporous or comatose.
- Physical examination may show tachycardia, hypotension, orthostatic change in pulse and blood pressure, melena, hematemesis, trauma.

4. Diagnostic Studies

- Laboratory values may be normal initially; then increased white blood cells (WBCs) with neutrophil predominance, decreased platelets, increased reticulocytes, occasionally nucleated RBCs in peripheral blood, heme-positive stool (if GI source of blood loss).

5. Management

- Maintain volume by placing two large-bore intravenous (IV) lines and transfuse with fluids, blood, albumin as clinically indicated.
- When site of blood loss is identified, treat underlying condition.

CHRONIC BLOOD LOSS

- May be due to occult bleeding.
- Patients usually present with signs/symptoms of iron deficiency anemia.
- Perform appropriate diagnostic studies—for example, upper GI test, upper endoscopy, colonoscopy, flexible sigmoidoscopy, arteriogram, pelvic examination, ultrasound (U/S).
- Then correct underlying disorder.

C. Microcytic Anemia
Iron Deficiency Anemia

1. Etiology

- Caused by blood loss (e.g., menstruation, chronic GI blood loss, and genitourinary blood loss), inadequate dietary intake, states of increased utilization (e.g., pregnancy), malabsorption (e.g., postgastrectomy, celiac sprue, chronic achlorhydria, and atrophic gastritis).

EPIDEMIOLOGY

- Most common anemia worldwide.
- Can occur at any age.
- Common cause of iron deficiency in developing countries is hookworm infestation in areas where this parasite is endemic.

2. Pathology

- Iron is absorbed most efficiently in the duodenum.
- Occurs gradually; initially, iron stores depleted and RBC count normal (iron deficiency without anemia).
- No stored iron remains.
- Total iron-binding capacity (TIBC) increases.
- After all stores depleted, RBC formation continues with low serum iron values (<30 μg per dL), transferrin saturation falls to <15%.
- MCV then decreases, with anisocytosis, poikilocytosis, hypochromia.

3. Clinical Features

- History—may be of multiple pregnancies, excess menstrual bleeding, alcoholism, poor diet, gastric surgery, celiac sprue, peptic ulcer disease.
- Symptoms—depending on the degree of anemia, the patient may be asymptomatic or may have symptoms including fatigue, weakness, palpitations, dyspnea on exertion, dizziness, syncope, bleeding, bruising, melena, bright red blood per rectum, headache, confusion, depression, pica, muscle weakness, angina, dysphagia due to pharyngeal web (Plummer–Vinson syndrome).
- Physical examination—may show hypotension, tachycardia, pallor, ecchymoses, pale palpebral conjunctiva, glossitis, cheilosis, heme-positive stool, hemorrhoids, pelvic masses, koilonychia.

4. Diagnostic Studies

- Decrease in RBCs, Hgb, HCT.
- Serum iron <30 μg per dL.
- Serum ferritin (SF) <20 μg per L. (Because SF is an *acute-phase reactant*, in the presence of microcytic MCV and anemia, SF may be higher than 20 μg per L and may still support a diagnosis of iron deficiency anemia, depending on underlying medical conditions.)
- Increased TIBC.
- Transferrin saturation of <15%.
- Microcytosis (MCV <80 fL).
- Hypochromia (MCHC <30 g per dL and MCH <26 pg).
- Anisocytosis, poikilocytosis on peripheral blood smear.
- Platelet count may be increased.
- "Gold standard"—bone marrow biopsy with iron stain to assess bone marrow iron stores. However, bone marrow is not routinely required to diagnose iron deficiency and would generally only be indicated if etiology of anemia was uncertain.

5. Management

- Treat underlying disorder, if any.
- Administer oral iron (e.g., FeSO$_4$ 325 mg PO TID, taken between meals) until iron levels normal. If patient experiences GI side effects while taking oral iron, it may be beneficial to start patient on FeSO$_4$ 325 mg PO once daily, and

gradually increase dose as tolerated, until therapeutic dose of $FeSO_4$ 325 mg PO TID is achieved. **NOTE:** Enteric-coated forms of oral iron are not well absorbed and should generally be avoided.

- Monitor response to treatment by checking to determine whether reticulocyte count increases. Period of maximum reticulocytosis generally occurs approximately 1 week after starting oral iron therapy.
- Hgb should normalize in 6 to 10 weeks, but oral iron should be continued until iron stores replete (generally requires continuation of oral iron therapy for approximately 6 months following normalization of Hgb). It is important to follow the SF level during iron replacement therapy to document repletion of iron stores.
- Occasionally, due to inability to take oral iron supplement or intestinal malabsorption, patients cannot receive oral iron therapy and must be given parenteral iron. Parenteral iron therapy in the form of iron dextran may be administered by intramuscular (IM) injection (using Z-track technique in the buttock) or IV fusion; dosage is calculated based on the patient's body weight and Hgb. Parenteral iron therapy has significant potential systemic side effects including, but not limited to, fever, rash, arthralgias, lymphadenopathy, splenomegaly, and anaphylaxis. Patients must receive a test dose to assess for hypersensitivity, before a course of iron dextran treatment is started, because of the risk of anaphylaxis.

Thalassemia
1. Etiology
- Hereditary disorder resulting from inherited defect in the synthesis of globin chains, resulting in decreased or absent α- or β-globin chain production.
- Most common among Southeast Asian, Mediterranean, and African American populations.

2. Pathology
- Chromosomes 11 and 16 are responsible for globin chain synthesis. One gene on chromosome 11 is responsible for the synthesis of β chains, and two genes on chromosome 16 are responsible for the synthesis of α chains.
  - Due to gene deletion or point mutations that cause decrease in synthesis or production of globin chains, either α or β chains, of Hgb.
  - Deficiency or total absence of α-globin chains results in the α-thalassemia disorders, and deficiency or total absence of β-globin chains results in the β-thalassemia disorders.

3. Clinical Features
- Presentation varies widely depending on whether person has α- or β thalassemia and whether they are homozygous or heterozygous.

- α-Thalassemia severity depends on the number of α-globin genes present (normally 4).
- Three α-globin genes present—silent carrier state, involves deletion of one of four alleles on chromosome 16; the patient is clinically normal.
- Two α-globin genes present—α-thalassemia minor (also known as α-thalassemia trait) with microcytic anemia; the patient is clinically normal.
- One α-globin gene present—known as Hgb-H disease. Only a small amount of Hgb A is formed, and the excess β-globin chains form tetramers of Hgb H (β_4). Clinical findings include microcytic chronic hemolytic anemia; pallor and splenomegaly may be present.
- Total absence of α-globin genes (hydrops fetalis), resulting in no fetal or adult Hgb synthesis, and is inconsistent with life.
- β Thalassemia minor found in heterozygotes with mild microcytic anemia, clinically normal.
- β Thalassemia intermedia—mild homozygous form with microcytic hemolytic anemia, hepatosplenomegaly, bony deformities.
- β Thalassemia major—severe homozygous form with severe anemia and hepatosplenomegaly, bony deformities, osteopenia, fractures.

4. Diagnostic Studies
- Microcytic anemia that varies according to severity of disease.
- On peripheral blood smear target cells, basophilic stippling, nucleated RBCs may be seen.
- Hgb electrophoresis testing is indicated for the diagnosis of β-thalassemia and more severe forms of α-thalassemia.

NOTE: In patients with α-thalassemia silent carrier state or α-thalassemia trait, Hgb electrophoresis will generally be normal; DNA mutation analysis is required to make the definitive diagnosis.

- Thalassemia should be suspected in patients with microcytosis, normal iron levels.

COMPLICATIONS
- Frequent transfusion requirements may result in iron overload causing cardiomyopathy, congestive heart failure, hepatomegaly, death.
- Misdiagnosis as iron deficiency anemia results in inappropriate iron therapy.

5. Management
- Mild disease generally requires no treatment.
- Genetic counseling should be given.
- Severe forms of thalassemia may require splenectomy, RBC transfusion with chelation therapy, folic acid, vitamin C.

Acquired Sideroblastic Anemia of Lead Poisoning
1. Etiology
- Lead poisoning among children may be caused by ingestion of lead paint chips, soil or water contaminated with lead.

- Factory workers exposed to lead may inhale it.
- Also known as *plumbism*, lead poisoning may affect 2 million preschool children annually.

2. **Pathology**
   - Lead poisons enzymes, causing cell death.
   - Shortens life span of RBCs.
   - Lead poisoning inhibits multiple enzyme steps required in heme synthesis, causing abnormal heme synthesis and resulting in an acquired sideroblastic anemia.

3. **Clinical Features**
   - Children with lead toxicity may complain of abdominal pain, fatigue. Chronic lead toxicity may cause learning disability or other neurologic or behavioral problems.
   - On examination, they may be pale, ataxic, with slurred speech, or may be seizing or comatose.
   - Adults may have symptoms of abdominal pain, headache, peripheral neuropathies, and be pale, ataxic, with loss of memory, and foot or wrist drop. A *lead line* may be present along the gum line (dark blue-gray line along gingival border).

4. **Diagnostic Studies**
   - Peripheral blood smear: microcytic, hypochromic anemia with basophilic stippling of RBCs.
   - Bone marrow examination: ringed sideroblasts may be present.
   - Increased serum iron level, normal or decreased TIBC, increased transferrin saturation and SF levels.
   - X-rays of long bones may show lead lines (increased density of metaphyseal plates).
   - Children should be screened for lead levels according to currently accepted pediatric guidelines.
   - Acceptable lead level in children: <10 μg per dL.

5. **Management**
   - Remove source of lead.
   - Specific treatment recommendations for lead poisoning are dependent on multiple factors (e.g., blood lead level and clinical presentation of patient). The decision regarding whether chelation therapy is indicated should, therefore, be made in consultation with a medical toxicologist.

D. Macrocytic Anemia
Megaloblastic Anemia: Vitamin B$_{12}$ (Cobalamin) Deficiency

1. **Etiology**
   - Most common cause of vitamin B$_{12}$ deficiency is not inadequate intake, but inability to absorb; most adults have enough vitamin B$_{12}$ stores to last 3 years.
   - Those at risk for vitamin B$_{12}$ deficiency due to inadequate intake are strict vegetarians (e.g., veganism).

2. **Pathology**
   - Following ingestion of B$_{12}$-containing food, vitamin B$_{12}$ is bound to intrinsic factor (IF), and the vitamin B$_{12}$–IF complex is transported through the intestine and then absorbed in the terminal ileum.
   - Vitamin B$_{12}$ is required for the synthesis of homocysteine to methionine, a main reaction in DNA synthesis.
   - It is theorized that a low vitamin B$_{12}$ level causes folate to be "trapped" and, therefore, to be unavailable for DNA synthesis.
   - Vitamin B$_{12}$ is present in all animal products (e.g., milk, eggs, and meat).
   - Vitamin B$_{12}$ deficiency may lead to defective myelin synthesis in the central nervous system (CNS) and subsequent neurologic dysfunction.
   - Vitamin B$_{12}$ deficiency may be caused by pernicious anemia, poor diet, malabsorption (e.g., due to partial or total gastrectomy, ileal resection, tropical sprue, small bowel lymphoma, inflammatory bowel disease, and pancreatic insufficiency), nitrous oxide (N$_2$O) inhalation, small intestine parasite infestation (fish tapeworm), bacterial overgrowth of small intestine, drugs (e.g., metformin, cholestyramine, neomycin, and colchicine), congenital disorders (e.g., transcobalamin II deficiency).

3. **Clinical Features**
   - Patient may complain of symptoms of anemia or neurologic dysfunction (e.g., paresthesias, ataxia, weakness, and change in mental status), anorexia, diarrhea.
   - Gastric atrophy and achlorhydria are present in pernicious anemia.
   - On examination, assess for pallor, decrease in position and vibratory sense, Romberg sign, Babinski sign, neuropathy, glossitis.

4. **Diagnostic Studies**
   - Anemia may not be present in 25% of patients with vitamin B$_{12}$ deficiency.
   - Neuropsychiatric symptoms due to vitamin B$_{12}$ (cobalamin) deficiency may occur when anemia or macrocytosis is not yet present.
   - If present, anemia is typically macrocytic with MCV of 110 to 140. **NOTE:** In the setting of combined deficiencies (e.g., concurrent iron deficiency and vitamin B$_{12}$ deficiency), MCV may be normal.
   - Hypersegmented neutrophils (≥5 lobes), serum B$_{12}$ <100 μg per mL, anisocytosis, poikilocytosis, macroovalocytes, decreased WBCs, decreased platelets.
   - Bone marrow may show megaloblasts, erythroid hyperplasia.
   - Increased serum lactate dehydrogenase (LDH) and increased indirect bilirubin may be present because of underlying hemolysis and increased cell turnover.
   - Serum IF antibodies are present in majority of patients with pernicious anemia, and are highly specific for this diagnosis in patients with megaloblastic anemia and elevated levels of IF antibodies.

- Parietal cell antibodies are present in 90% of patients with pernicious anemia, and support a diagnosis of pernicious anemia, but are not specific for this condition.
- Elevated serum gastrin levels in pernicious anemia.
- Schilling test is a two-step test utilizing radiolabeled B_{12} to determine whether underlying cause of B_{12} deficiency is pernicious anemia. This test is rarely used and has been largely replaced by parietal cell and IF antibody testing.
- If vitamin B_{12} levels low-normal and vitamin B_{12} deficiency is suspected, check serum levels of methylmalonic acid (MMA) and homocysteine.
- Elevated serum levels of both MMA and homocysteine confirm the diagnosis of B_{12} deficiency.

5. **Management**
  - Management of megaloblastic anemia due to vitamin B_{12} deficiency generally involves parenteral administration of vitamin B_{12}. However, the specific dosage regimen and duration of vitamin B_{12} supplementation depend on the underlying cause of vitamin B_{12} deficiency.
  - Vitamin B_{12} is available for administration in oral, nasal, or parenteral forms of delivery. When treating megaloblastic anemia due to vitamin B_{12} deficiency, initial vitamin B_{12} supplementation is generally given by parenteral route of administration. When hematologic parameters have normalized, nasal and oral forms of vitamin B_{12} are available as alternatives to continued parenteral treatment, for maintaining normal vitamin B_{12} levels. Patients receiving oral or nasal forms of vitamin B_{12} must be followed closely to ensure that normal vitamin B_{12} levels are being maintained.
  - Parenteral vitamin B_{12} is typically administered by IM injection and also may be administered by subcutaneous injection.
  - **NOTE:** Upon instituting vitamin B_{12} (cobalamin) replacement therapy, the patient must be monitored closely. *Patients may develop severe life-threatening hypokalemia requiring potassium supplementation.* Therefore, serum potassium levels must be followed closely during treatment.
  - **NOTE:** Folate administration in sufficient doses may treat the underlying anemia of vitamin B_{12} deficiency while allowing the vitamin B_{12} deficiency-related neurologic dysfunction to progress. Therefore, patients with megaloblastic anemia should be evaluated for vitamin B_{12} deficiency and folate deficiency, and empiric treatment with a trial of folate is not recommended.

Pernicious Anemia
1. **Etiology**
  - Hereditary autoimmune disorder is commonly present among Northern European and African American populations.

- Occurrence is rare before age 35.
- Most common cause of cobalamin deficiency.
- If family history exists of pernicious anemia, risk increases 20-fold.
- Patients also may have other autoimmune diseases—for example, autoimmune immunoglobulin A (IgA) deficiency, polyglandular endocrine insufficiency (e.g., Graves disease, thyroiditis, vitiligo, and hypoparathyroidism), and type I diabetes mellitus.

2. **Pathology**
  - Pernicious anemia is an autoimmune disorder characterized by immune-mediated atrophy of the gastric parietal cells, resulting in absent gastric acid and IF secretion. Lack of IF made by gastric parietal cells causes inability to absorb vitamin B_{12} in gut; therefore, it manifests itself as vitamin B_{12} deficiency anemia.
  - Atrophic gastritis leads to increased risk of gastric cancer among persons with pernicious anemia.

3. **Clinical Features/Diagnostic Studies**
  - See Vitamin B_{12} deficiency section, discussed earlier.

4. **Management of Pernicious Anemia**
  - A typical replacement schedule for the treatment of pernicious anemia is as follows: initially, 1,000 μg vitamin B_{12} IM daily for the first week, followed by 1,000 μg vitamin B_{12} IM once weekly for 1 month, followed by 1,000 μg vitamin B_{12} IM once monthly thereafter. Patients with pernicious anemia require lifelong vitamin B_{12} treatment.

  COMPLICATIONS
  - Spinal cord damage due to vitamin B_{12} deficiency is generally irreversible.
  - Other CNS abnormalities (e.g., dementia) also may be irreversible if present >6 months.

Megaloblastic Anemia: Folate Deficiency
1. **Etiology**
  - Folate—abundant in citrus fruits, green leafy vegetables (also in meat, eggs, liver).
  - Total body stores generally last 3 to 6 months.
  - Deficiency may be caused by inadequate dietary intake (e.g., hemodialysis patients and elderly persons). Folate deficiency associated with alcoholism is likely multifactorial (e.g., dietary malabsorption, decreased intracellular folate metabolism, and decreased hepatic storage of folate).
  - Other causes of folate deficiency include folate-antagonist drugs that interfere with DNA synthesis (e.g., methotrexate, trimethoprim, and pyrimethamine), increased folate utilization (e.g., pregnancy, exfoliative skin disorders, hemolytic anemia, and malignancy), malabsorption (e.g., tropical sprue, celiac disease, inflammatory bowel disease, small bowel lymphoma, and significant small bowel resection), congenital disorders (e.g.,

5-methyltetrahydrofolate transferase deficiency), and anticonvulsant medications.

2. **Pathology**
   - Folate absorption occurs primarily in the jejunum.
   - Folate is required for important steps in DNA synthesis.
   - Folate deficiency results in slow nuclear development with large cytoplasm, decreased RBC life.

3. **Clinical Features**
   - Similar to vitamin B_{12} deficiency, but without neurologic abnormalities.

4. **Diagnostic Studies**
   - Macrocytic anemia.
   - Hypersegmented neutrophils ($\geq$5 lobes).
   - Decreased serum folate level.
   - Decreased RBC folate level.
   - Normal serum B_{12} level.
   - **NOTE:** The serum folate level is sensitive to recent dietary intake of folate-containing foods. Therefore, a serum RBC folate level also should generally be checked.

   COMPLICATIONS
   - Deficiency in pregnancy may lead to neural tube defects.

5. **Management**
   - Folic acid—1 mg per day orally.

E. **Normocytic Anemia**

   Hemolytic Anemia: Glucose-6-Phosphate Dehydrogenase Deficiency

   1. **Etiology**
      - Glucose-6-phosphate dehydrogenase (G6PD) deficiency is an X-linked recessive disorder.
      - Occurs in 10% to 15% of African American males in the United States (G6PD A-variant).
      - Also present among Mediterranean population (G6PD Mediterranean variant).
      - Clinical G6PD deficiency occurs almost exclusively in males. Female carriers are variably clinically affected.

   2. **Pathology**
      - G6PD deficiency results in oxidation of Hgb to methemoglobin that then forms precipitants known as Heinz bodies, which cause membrane damage, osmotic fragility, rigid cells.
      - Damaged cells are removed by spleen.
      - Infection or exposure to drugs causes hemolysis.
      - Some drugs known to cause this condition—dapsone, quinine, quinidine, nitrofurantoin, primaquine, sulfonamides, aspirin.
      - Fava beans may also be implicated, causing a severe hemolytic episode among affected persons.

   3. **Clinical Features**
      - Patients may complain of jaundice, dark urine, abdominal and low back pain.
      - Physical examination may be normal until crisis occurs.

4. **Diagnostic Studies**
   - Laboratory studies may be normal in the time between acute hemolytic episodes.
   - During acute hemolytic episode, characteristic laboratory test results include an elevated reticulocyte count and an elevated unconjugated (indirect) bilirubin level.
   - Peripheral blood smear may show bite cells. Heinz bodies (seen with special stain preparation known as *Heinz body preparation*) may be present.
   - Perform enzyme assay for G6PD.
   - **NOTE:** Patients with the G6PD A-variant will have *normal* G6PD levels immediately following the hemolytic episode because the new cells are not yet G6PD deficient. Therefore, it is advisable to wait several weeks after the hemolytic episode before checking the G6PD level in these patients.

   COMPLICATIONS
   - Renal failure (rare).

5. **Management**
   - Avoid offending drugs, food, or both.
   - Usually self-limiting.

Hemolytic Anemia: Sickle Cell Anemia

1. **Etiology**
   - Hgb S occurs when valine substitutes for glutamic acid on the β-chain.
   - Decreased solubility of Hgb S in hypoxic tissues leads to sickle-shaped cells.

2. **Pathology**
   - Sickled cells have difficulty passing through small capillaries, leading to blockage and tissue necrosis.
   - Sickled cells are destroyed, resulting in hemolytic anemia.
   - Sickle cell trait does not result in clinical problems unless patients are subjected to severe hypoxia.

   EPIDEMIOLOGY
   - Autosomal recessive disorder.
   - Eight percent of African American persons are heterozygous for Hgb S (known as sickle cell trait).
   - 0.15% of African American children in the United States are homozygous for Hgb S (sickle cell anemia).
   - Frequency is highest in Africa, particularly where *Plasmodium falciparum* is common, and is thought to be so because the Hgb S carrier state offers a protective advantage by conferring increased resistance to *P. falciparum* malaria infection.

3. **Clinical Features**
   - Usually appears about 6 months of age when fetal Hgb is replaced with Hgb S.
   - Early signs are delayed growth and development, fevers, and infection.
   - Infarctions may result in skin ulceration, painful crises, retinopathy, ischemic necrosis of bones, renal dysfunction, hyposplenism, hepatic dysfunction, priapism.

- Hemolytic anemia may result in jaundice, gallstones.
- Decreased O_2 affinity of Hgb S results in pulmonary hypertension, congestive heart failure, and symptoms of fatigue and shortness of breath.

4. **Diagnostic Studies**
   - Hgb electrophoresis shows Hgb S ($\alpha_2\beta^s_2$) of 85% to 98%, Hgb F ($\alpha_2\gamma_2$) of 2% to 20%, and Hgb A2 ($\alpha_2\delta_2$) of 2% to 4% in sickle cell anemia.
   - Sickle cell trait has Hgb S ($\alpha_2\beta^s_2$) of 40% and Hgb A ($\alpha_2\beta_2$) of 60%.
   - Normocytic normochromic anemia.
   - Reticulocytosis.
   - Sickled cells, Howell-Jolly bodies, and target cells on peripheral smear.
   - Increased WBC count and thrombocytosis may be seen.

COMPLICATIONS
   - Chronic multisystem failure from end-organ damage.
   - Heart failure, stroke.
   - Acute chest syndrome.
   - Skin ulcers.
   - Recurrent infections.
   - Bilirubin gallstones.
   - Osteonecrosis (femoral or humeral head).
   - Aplastic crisis (from infection with parvovirus B19 or folate deficiency).
   - Median age of death is 35 years old if >3 crises per year and 50 years old if <3 crises per year.

5. **Management**
   - Genetic counseling for heterozygous carriers.
   - Avoid dehydration, treat infections aggressively.
   - Analgesics and O_2 administration during painful crises.
   - Hydroxyurea is a cytotoxic drug that has been shown to be beneficial in reducing the frequency of acute pain crises; generally considered in the treatment of patients who are more severely affected with manifestations of sickle cell disease (e.g., frequent severe acute pain crises, increased risk of stroke, and history of acute chest syndrome).
   - Folic acid supplementation.
   - Children should be immunized for *Haemophilus influenzae* type B, pneumococcus, and meningococcus, and should receive prophylactic penicillin up to age 6.
   - Allogeneic stem cell transplantation is the only potentially curative treatment available for sickle cell disease; has significant associated risks, and therefore patients must be carefully selected and have a human leukocyte antigen matched donor.
   - RBC transfusion therapy is clinically indicated in the management of sickle cell disease, in situations requiring increased O_2-carrying capacity of the blood, decreased amount of sickle Hgb present in the blood, and increased Hgb concentration (e.g., acute chest syndrome, splenic sequestration, and preoperative transfusion).

F. **Anemia of Chronic Disease**
   1. **Etiology**
      - Caused by underlying chronic inflammatory conditions such as chronic infection, inflammatory bowel disease, rheumatoid arthritis, and malignancy.
      - Most common anemia of hospitalized patients.
   2. **Pathology**
      - Unclear, but may be attributed to decreased RBC life span, block in the release of iron from macrophages, cytokine inhibition of erythropoietin (EPO).
   3. **Clinical Features**
      - Consistent with underlying disease.
      - Usually asymptomatic.
   4. **Diagnostic Studies**
      - Mild normochromic normocytic anemia most common, although also may present with hypochromic microcytic anemia; Hgb is usually not <9 to 10 mg per dL.
      - Normal or elevated SF; decreased serum iron; decreased TIBC.
      - Bone marrow iron stores are normal or increased, with decreased or absent sideroblasts.
      - Clinically, anemia of chronic disease is a diagnosis of exclusion.
   5. **Management**
      - Treat the underlying disease. The anemia often improves when the underlying inflammatory condition is treated successfully.
      - No role exists for iron therapy in the treatment of anemia of chronic disease.
      - The anemia is generally mild and typically does not require blood transfusion.

II. Malignant Diseases

A. **Lymphoma**
   Hodgkin Disease/Hodgkin Lymphoma
   1. **Etiology/Pathology**
      - No consistent chromosomal abnormalities are identified.
      - Malignant disorder of lymphoreticular system characterized by Reed–Sternberg cells (large cells with multiloculated or bilobed nucleus with halo around prominent inclusion-like nucleoli) in the background of benign lymphocytes, plasma cells, histiocytes.
      - Role of Epstein–Barr virus (EBV) in etiology is suggested by increased risk of Hodgkin disease (HD) in young adults with the history of infectious mononucleosis; frequent coinfection with EBV among patients with human immunodeficiency virus (HIV) related Hodgkin lymphoma.

- In contrast to non-Hodgkin lymphoma (NHL), Hodgkin lymphoma tends to spread in an orderly, predictable fashion to adjacent sites of lymph tissue.

EPIDEMIOLOGY

- Bimodal age distribution with increased incidence after 10 years of age, and first peak occurring approximately in the 20s, and second peak occurring after 50 years of age.
- Approximately 85% of children who have HD are boys.
- Wide geographic range of incidence; higher social class or education, small family size, and early birth order are more at risk.

2. **Clinical Features**

- Patients may complain of painless lump in the neck, fever, drenching night sweats, weight loss, malaise, generalized pruritus.
- Alcohol ingestion may cause pain in lymph nodes.
- Physical examination may disclose lymphadenopathy often starting initially in the cervical and supraclavicular regions, spreading contiguously to adjacent lymph node groups. Common extranodal sites of involvement include spleen, liver, lung, and bone marrow.
- *Pel-Ebstein fever pattern* may be present (period of days or weeks during which fever is present, alternates with periods during which patient is afebrile).

3. **Diagnostic Studies**

- Chest X-ray (CXR) may show mediastinal adenopathy.
- Laboratory tests may show anemia, elevated sedimentation rate, elevated serum LDH, decreased lymphocytes, eosinophilia, increased platelets with mild leukocytosis.
- Workup should include HIV serology.
- Positron emission tomography (PET)/computed tomography (CT) scan of the chest, abdomen, and pelvis.
- Bilateral bone marrow biopsy is also often required for staging.
- Excisional lymph node biopsy is needed for diagnosis.
- The World Health Organization (WHO) has adopted a classification system including *classic HD* (nodular sclerosis, mixed cellularity, lymphocyte rich, and lymphocyte depleted) and *nodular lymphocyte-predominant Hodgkin disease* (LPHD) (Table 13-1).
- Routine staging laparotomy is no longer recommended for all patients with a diagnosis of HD. The indications for staging laparotomy vary depending on clinical stage of patient at the time of diagnosis and anticipated treatment plan.

COMPLICATIONS

- Spinal cord compression.
- Late treatment-related complications include cardiac and pulmonary disease (related to prior

TABLE 13–1.	WHO Classification: Morphologic Subtypes of HD
Classic HD	
• Nodular sclerosis • Mixed cellularity • Lymphocyte rich • Lymphocyte depleted	
Nodular LPHD	
• Immunohistochemical studies distinguish nodular LPHD from classic HD—classic HD ($CD15^+$, $CD30^+$) and nodular LPHD ($CD20^+$, $CH45^+$, $CD15^-$, variably reactive for CD30)	

Adapted from Govindan R, Arquette MA, eds. *The Washington Manual of Oncology*. New York, NY: Lippincott Williams & Wilkins; 2002, with permission.

irradiation and/or chemotherapy side effects) and second malignancy (e.g., secondary acute leukemia, NHL, and solid tumors).
- Hypothyroidism occurs in approximately 50% of patients who received neck irradiation and occurs within 1 to 20 years after radiation treatment.
- Infertility (related to pelvic irradiation and certain chemotherapy regimens).
- Diminished cell-mediated immunity.

4. **Management**

- Treatment of HD depends on the stage of disease according to the Ann Arbor Staging System, which classifies disease stage based on anatomic location as well as the presence or absence of "B" symptoms.
  - **Ann Arbor Staging System:**
  - Stage I: Involvement of single lymph node region or single extralymphatic organ or site (Stage IE).
  - Stage II: Involvement of two or more lymph node regions on the same side of the diaphragm; also can include localized involvement of an extralymphatic organ or site (Stage IIE).
  - Stage III: Involvement of lymph node regions on both sides of the diaphragm; also can include localized involvement of an extralymphatic organ or site (Stage IIIE), or involvement of the spleen (Stage IIIS), or both (Stage IIISE).
  - Stage IV: Diffuse or disseminated involvement of one or more extralymphatic organs, with or without associated lymph node involvement.
    - "A": B symptoms not present.
    - "B": Patient with history of fever (>38°C), drenching night sweats, weight loss >10% of body weight in previous 6 months.
    - "X": Bulky disease; mediastinal widening greater than one-third of the diameter of the chest or lymph node mass >10 cm in any dimension.

- "E": Involvement of a single extranodal site contiguous or proximal to a known site.
- Treatment of classic HD:
  - **Early-stage classic HD without B symptoms or bulky disease:** Early-stage HD (Stages IA and IIA) in the absence of B symptoms or bulky disease has previously been treated with extended field radiation therapy alone. Recent clinical trials are studying the potential benefits of treating these patients with both limited chemotherapy and involved field radiation therapy (IFRT) or chemotherapy alone, in an effort to diminish the long-term, treatment-related toxicities (e.g., cardiac toxicity and second malignancies).
  - Patients with early-stage disease and without B symptoms or bulky disease have a favorable prognosis, with reported long-term, disease-free survival rates of approximately 80% to 90%.
  - **Early-stage classic HD with B symptoms or bulky disease:** Less favorable due to the presence of B symptoms or bulky disease. Therefore, these patients generally receive combined modality treatment, with chemotherapy followed by IFRT; More than 75% of patients can be cured with this treatment approach.
  - **Advanced-stage classic HD:** Treatment approach for advanced stage (Stages III and IV) HD includes combination chemotherapy with or without radiation therapy. Approximately 60% to 70% of patients with advanced HD can be cured with combination chemotherapy.
  - **Nodular lymphocyte predominant HD:** This subtype of HD follows a more indolent course and is associated with a favorable prognosis. Most patients are first seen with early-stage disease (Stages I and II), and the treatment approach typically includes IFRT only. For the infrequent patient with nodular LPHD who has advanced disease (Stages III and IV), treatment involves combination chemotherapy. Approximately, 10-year overall survival rate is 80%, and among the 20% of patients with nodular LPHD relapse, the 10-year overall survival rate is approximately 70%.

Non-Hodgkin Lymphoma
1. **Etiology/Pathology**
   - Malignancy of lymphoreticular system.
   - Classified functionally as B cell or T cell.
   - Morphologically defined as small, intermediate, large cell.
   - Several classification systems currently exist for non-Hodgkin lymphoma (NHL):
     - Working Formulation (developed in 1982) classifies NHL as low- intermediate-, or high-grade. NHL may be further classified based on clinical behavior and Working Formulation categories (Table 13-2).

TABLE 13–2. Classification of NHL Based on Clinical Behavior and Working Formulation

Indolent NHL

- Small lymphocytic (low grade)
- Follicular, small-cleaved cell (low grade)
- Follicular, mixed small-cleaved and large cell (low grade)
- Diffuse, small-cleaved cell (intermediate grade)

Aggressive NHL

- Follicular, large cell (intermediate grade)
- Diffuse, mixed small and large cell (intermediate grade)
- Diffuse, large cell (intermediate grade)
- Diffuse, large cell immunoblastic (high grade)
- Small, noncleaved cell (high grade)
- Lymphoblastic (high grade)
- Burkitt lymphoma (high grade)

Adapted from Mazza JJ, ed. *Manual of Clinical Hematology.* 3rd ed. New York, NY: Lippincott Williams & Wilkins; 2002; and Pillot G, Chantler M, Magiera H, et al, eds. *The Washington Manual Subspecialty Consult Series: Hematology and Oncology Subspecialty Consult.* New York, NY: Lippincott Williams & Wilkins; 2004, with permission.

- In 1993, the Revised European American Lymphoma (REAL) classification was developed. The WHO accepted the REAL classification with some modifications (2001), and this was further updated in 2008 (Table 13-3).
- Cytogenic abnormalities are common.

EPIDEMIOLOGY
- Median age—50 years.
- Incidence increases with age.
- Approximately 60,000 new cases of NHL are diagnosed annually in the United States.
- Increased incidence of NHL has been noted among persons with HIV disease.
- Over the last several decades, there has been an increased incidence of NHL associated with pesticides and organic solvents.

2. **Clinical Features**
   - Two-thirds of patients have persistent painless lymphadenopathy including retroperitoneum, mesentery, pelvis.
   - One-third of sites are extranodal; symptoms vary according to the site.
   - Fever, night sweats, weight loss are much less common than in HD.
   - Pruritus is rare.
   - Laboratory tests may show only anemia, elevated serum LDH, and elevated erythrocyte sedimentation rate (ESR).
   - Workup should include HIV serology.

TABLE 13–3. World Health Organization Classification of Lymphoid Neoplasms 2008

Precursor B- and T-Cell Neoplasms	Mature T-Cell and NK Cell Neoplasms
Precursor B-lymphoblastic leukemia/lymphoma	T-cell prolymphocytic leukemia
Precursor T-lymphoblastic leukemia/lymphoma	T-cell large granular lymphocytic leukemia
	Chronic lymphoproliferative disorder of NK cells
Mature B-Cell Neoplasms [a]	
	Aggressive NK cell leukemia
Chronic lymphocytic leukemia/small lymphocytic lymphoma	EBV-positive T-cell lymphoproliferative diseases of childhood
B-cell prolymphocytic leukemia	Systemic EBV-positive T-cell lymphoproliferative disease of childhood
Lymphoplasmacytic lymphoma/Waldenström macroglobulinemia	Hydroa vacciniforme-like lymphoma
Splenic marginal zone B-cell lymphoma	Adult T-cell leukemia/lymphoma
Hairy cell leukemia	Extranodal NK/T-cell lymphoma, nasal type
Splenic B-cell lymphoma/leukemia, unclassifiable	Enteropathy-type T-cell lymphoma
Splenic diffuse red pulp small B-cell lymphoma	Hepatosplenic T-cell lymphoma
Hairy cell leukemia-variant	Subcutaneous panniculitis-like T-cell lymphoma
Plasma cell neoplasms	Mycosis fungoides
MGUS	Sézary syndrome
Plasma cell myeloma	Primary cutaneous CD30+ T-cell lymphoproliferative disorders
Solitary plasmacytoma of bone	Primary cutaneous anaplastic large cell lymphoma
Extraosseous plasmacytoma	Lymphomatoid papulosis
Monoclonal immunoglobulin deposition diseases	Primary cutaneous peripheral T-cell lymphomas, rare subtypes
Extranodal marginal zone B-cell lymphoma (MALT lymphoma)	Primary cutaneous gamma-delta T-cell lymphoma
Nodal marginal zone B-cell lymphoma	Primary cutaneous CD8+ aggressive epidermotropic cytotoxic T-cell lymphoma
Follicular lymphoma	Primary cutaneous CD4+ small/medium T-cell lymphoma
Primary cutaneous follicle center lymphoma	Peripheral T-cell lymphoma, not otherwise specified
Mantle cell lymphoma	Angioimmunoblastic T-cell lymphoma
DLBCL	Anaplastic large cell lymphoma, ALK-positive
T-cell/histiocyte-rich large B-cell lymphoma	Anaplastic large cell lymphoma, ALK-negative
Primary DLBCL of the CNS	
Primary cutaneous DLBCL, leg type	**Immunodeficiency-associated Lymphoproliferative Disorders**
EBV-positive DLBCL of the elderly	Lymphoproliferative diseases associated with primary immune disorders
DLBCL associated with chronic inflammation	Lymphomas associated with HIV infection
Lymphomatoid granulomatosis	PTLD
Primary mediastinal (thymic) large B-cell lymphoma	Plasmacytic hyperplasia and infectious mononucleosis-like PTLD
Intravascular large B-cell lymphoma	Polymorphic PTLD
ALK-positive large B-cell lymphoma	Monomorphic PTLD
Plasmablastic lymphoma	Classic Hodgkin lymphoma type PTLD
Large B-cell lymphoma arising in HHV8-associated multicentric Castleman disease	Other iatrogenic immunodeficiency-associated lymphoproliferative disorders
Burkitt lymphoma/leukemia	
B-cell lymphoma, unclassifiable, with features intermediate between DLBCL and Burkitt lymphoma	
B-cell lymphoma, unclassifiable, with features intermediate between DLBCL and classic Hodgkin lymphoma	

[a]B- and T/NK-cell neoplasms are grouped according to major clinical presentations (predominantly disseminated/leukemic, primary extranodal, predominantly nodal). NK, natural killer; MGUS, monoclonal gammopathy of undetermined significance; MALT, mucosa-associated lymphoid tissue; DLBCL, diffuse large B-cell lymphoma; ALK, anaplastic lymphoma kinase; PTLD, posttransplant lymphoproliferative disorders; HHV8, human herpesvirus-8. From Friedberg JW, Mauch PM, Rimsza L, et al. Non-Hodgkin lymphomas. In: DeVita JT Jr, Lawrence TS, Rosenberg SA, et al, eds. *DeVita, Hellman, and Rosenberg's Cancer: Principles and Practice of Oncology.* 9th ed. Philadelphia, PA: Lippincott Williams & Wilkins; 2011, with permission.

3. **Diagnostic Studies**
   - Lymph node biopsy is needed for diagnosis, and an excisional lymph node biopsy is preferable.
   - Staging uses Ann Arbor classification (see HD, above).
   - CXR, CT scan of chest, abdomen, pelvis.
   - Bilateral bone marrow biopsies are often indicated for staging.
   - Lumbar puncture if CNS involvement.

- Treatment, prognosis depend on staging and histologic subtype.
4. **Management**
    - The Ann Arbor Staging System is used in the staging of NHL (see HD section, above).
    - Indolent lymphomas are generally not curable with standard treatments. The disease may respond well to chemotherapy or radiation therapy and may achieve a partial or complete remission. However, recurrence of disease is common.
    - For patients with limited disease (Stages I and II) indolent NHL, involved IFRT or IFRT with combination chemotherapy is a standard treatment approach. For patients with advanced-stage (Stages III and IV) indolent NHL who are asymptomatic, treatment is not always indicated; close observation without initial therapy may be appropriate in certain situations. For patients with advanced-stage (Stages III and IV) indolent NHL who are symptomatic, single agent or combination chemotherapy regimens may be effective in inducing a remission.
    - Stages I and II aggressive NHL generally require treatment with combination chemotherapy for several cycles, followed by involved IFRT. For Stages III and IV aggressive NHL, combination chemotherapy is generally the treatment of choice. Depending on the pathologic subtype and extent of disease, prophylactic CNS treatment using intrathecal chemotherapy also may be indicated.
    - There may be a role for consideration of autologous or allogeneic stem cell transplant (SCT) in cases of relapsed intermediate- or high-grade NHL.

Multiple Myeloma (Plasma Cell Myeloma)
1. **Etiology/Pathology**
    - Malignant proliferation of plasma cells.
    - In multiple myeloma, all five classes of immunoglobulin are produced, with a single immunoglobulin produced in excess; therefore, monoclonal gammopathy.

    EPIDEMIOLOGY
    - Usually presents in older adults; only 2% of patients are younger than 40 years at the time of diagnosis.
    - Incidence increases with age; average age of diagnosis is 60 years.
    - More men than women are affected, with increased incidence among African American population.
    - Exposure to radiation, benzene, herbicides, and insecticides may play a role.
2. **Clinical Features**
    - Patients may complain of bone pain, often in the spine and ribs (70%), at the time of diagnosis, resulting from osteolytic bone lesions or pathologic fractures.

- Bone marrow infiltration results in a normocytic, normochromic anemia; thrombocytopenia; and leucopenia.
- Bone resorption causes osteopenia and hypercalcemia.
    - Primary amyloidosis may coexist with a diagnosis of multiple myeloma.
    - Clinical findings may include macroglossia, carpal tunnel syndrome, skin involvement (e.g., periorbital ecchymosis), congestive heart failure, and nephrotic syndrome, among others.
- Fatigue, weakness, nausea, vomiting, bleeding, bruising (secondary to platelet dysfunction), or infection also may be presenting symptoms depending on the extent of disease.

3. **Diagnostic Studies**
    - Diagnosis is made by serum protein electrophoresis and urine protein electrophoresis, demonstrating a monoclonal protein (M-protein) spike, followed by immunofixation electrophoresis to further identify the specific heavy-chain class and light-chain type in the M-protein. Diagnosis is confirmed by bone marrow biopsy.
    - Bence Jones protein (monoclonal immunoglobulin light chains) in urine.
    - Normochromic, normocytic anemia is present in approximately two-thirds of patients at the time of diagnosis. *Rouleaux formation* of RBCs may be present on peripheral blood smear.
    - ESR elevation is commonly present.
    - Obtain complete baseline serum chemistry panel to evaluate calcium, total protein, albumin, LDH, blood urea nitrogen (BUN), creatinine, electrolytes, uric acid, and liver function tests (LFTs).
    - Serum C-reactive protein (marker for interleukin 6 activity, which stimulates myeloma cell growth) and serum β_2 microglobulin (reflects tumor burden in multiple myeloma) level should also be checked (Table 13-4).
    - Hypercalcemia may be present. Need to calculate corrected serum calcium level if serum albumin is low: (Corrected Ca^2) = (serum Ca^2) + [0.8 × (4.0 − patient's serum albumin)].
        - **Example:** Albumin = 2.0 mg per dL; Calcium = 12.0 mg per dL; Corrected Ca^2 = 12.0 + 1.6 = **13.6**.
    - Renal function tests may show renal insufficiency in approximately 50% of patients at the time of diagnosis.
    - Plain films show lytic bone lesions.
    NOTE: Because the bone lesions of multiple myeloma are generally purely lytic, a bone scan is not a useful diagnostic test. It is preferable to obtain a skeletal survey (plain film radiographs of skull, vertebrae, ribs, pelvis, and long bones) to assess for the extent of bony involvement.

TABLE 13–4. **International Staging System for Multiple Myeloma**

Stage	Serum β_2-microglobulin (mg/L)	Serum Albumin (g/dL)	Median Survival (Months)
I	<3.5	≥3.5	62
II	<3.5	<3.5	44
	OR		
	3.5–5.5	—	
III	>5.5	—	29

Note: — indicates that stage is determined based on serum β_2-microglobulin level, regardless of serum albumin level.
Adapted from Cashen AF, Wildes TM, Henderson KE, et al, eds. *The Washington Manual Subspecialty Consult Series: Hematology and Oncology Subspecialty Consult.* 2nd ed. Philadelphia, PA: Lippincott Williams & Wilkins; 2008:143; and Greipp PR, Miguel JS, Durie BGM, et al. International staging system for multiple myeloma. *J Clin Oncol.* 2005;23(15):3412–3420. http://jco.ascopubs.org/content/23/15/3412.full. Accessed February 22, 2012, with permission.

- Serum β_2 microglobulin level can be a useful prognostic indicator; elevated level tends to be associated with a less favorable prognosis.
- Bone marrow with mature and immature plasma cells, diffuse or in sheets, >30%.
- In asymptomatic patients, multiple myeloma may be suspected if routine laboratory tests show hypercalcemia, increased serum protein, anemia; diagnosis should then be confirmed by further testing.

COMPLICATIONS
- Renal failure.
- Recurrent infections with *Streptococcus pneumonia*, *Staphylococcus aureus*, *H. influenzae*, *Pseudomonas aeruginosa*, *Escherichia coli*, or *Klebsiella*.
- Spinal cord compression.
- Carpal tunnel syndrome.
- Visual disturbances.
- Pathologic bone fractures.

4. **Management**
- Asymptomatic patients with Stage I disease may be monitored closely for signs or symptoms of disease progression, although initiation of treatment is not generally warranted in the absence of symptoms.
- For patients with Stages II or III disease, early consideration should be given to evaluation for future autologous SCT. In patients who will be undergoing SCT, use of alkylating agents should be avoided, and induction chemotherapy typically includes treatment with regimens including thalidomide, lenalidomide, or bortezomib (e.g., bortezomib/dexamethasone), followed by SCT. In

patients who are not felt to be good candidates for SCT, standard induction chemotherapy regimens may include use of an alkylating agent such as melphalan and prednisone (MP) or melphalan/prednisone/thalidomide (MPT).
- Combination chemotherapy followed by autologous SCT has been shown to be an effective treatment option in selected patients, resulting in higher complete response rates and overall survival, when compared with standard systemic chemotherapy.
- Radiation therapy is generally reserved for palliative treatment of localized lesions, lesions causing spinal cord compression, or prophylactic treatment of large lytic lesions in long bones at risk for pathologic fracture.
- Supportive measures, aggressive hydration to delay renal insufficiency, bisphosphonates, such as pamidronate (Aredia) or zoledronic acid (Zometa), have been shown to delay skeletal disease in patients with multiple myeloma, decrease bone pain, and improve quality of life.

B. **Acute Lymphoblastic Leukemia**
1. **Etiology/Pathology**
- Malignant proliferation of lymphoid stem cells in bone marrow that invade lymph nodes, spleen, liver, other organs.
- May be classified as B-cell or T-cell origin.
- FAB (French-American-British) classification has three subtypes of acute lymphoblastic leukemia (ALL) (L1–L3) based on morphology, heterogeneity of lymphocytes.
- Has propensity for CNS, gonads.

EPIDEMIOLOGY OF ALL
- The incidence of ALL peaks between age 2 and 4 years, then decreases to fairly steady levels, with increasing incidence again after age 50 years. Approximately, 75% of ALL cases occur among patients who are <15 years of age.
- Most common childhood malignancy.
- Cause is generally unknown; however, several genetic syndromes are associated with an increased risk of developing ALL (e.g., Down syndrome and ataxia-telangiectasia syndrome).

2. **Clinical Features**
- Patients may complain of fever, fatigue, weight loss, irritability, anorexia, bone pain, arthralgias, bleeding.
- If CNS involvement is present at the time of diagnosis, patient also may complain of headache, stiff neck, visual disturbances, vomiting.
- On physical examination, there may be pallor, fever, petechiae, bruises, hepatosplenomegaly, lymphadenopathy, stiff neck, papilledema, cranial nerve palsies, seizures, change in mental status.
- Hepatosplenomegaly and lymphadenopathy can be seen.

3. Diagnostic Studies

- WBC typically varies from 5,000 to 100,000 per mm^3; however, it may be <5,000 or >100,000 per mm^3 at the time of diagnosis.
- Anemia, neutropenia, thrombocytopenia are commonly present at the time of diagnosis.
- Hypercellular bone marrow with >30% lymphoblasts.
- WBC differential often shows blast cells in peripheral blood at the time of diagnosis.
- Elevated serum uric acid may be present.
- Elevated serum LDH level often may be present.
- CXR: Anterior mediastinal mass may be present and is suggestive of T-cell ALL.
- Cerebrospinal fluid may show blast cells, with increased protein, decreased glucose.
- Presence of Philadelphia chromosome (t[9;22] [q34;q11]) in ALL is a poor prognostic sign.

COMPLICATIONS

- Chemotherapy causes immunosuppression and results in increased risk of infections.
- *Pneumocystis jiroveci* pneumonia: Trimethoprim/sulfamethoxazole (Bactrim) for prophylaxis during chemotherapy treatment.
- Sterility (related to chemotherapy).
- Metabolic complications arising during chemotherapy treatment, including *tumor lysis syndrome* (hyperuricemia, hyperkalemia, hypocalcemia, hyperphosphatemia) with associated increased risk of cardiac arrhythmias, and acute renal failure.

4. Management

APPROACH TO TREATMENT OF CHILDREN WITH ALL

- Approximately, 98% of children with ALL achieve a complete remission within 4 weeks of starting induction chemotherapy, and current clinical trial results suggest approximately 70% of children diagnosed currently with ALL can expect to be cured; children with favorable prognostic indicators may have an even better prognosis.
- Initial treatment is known as *induction chemotherapy*, and the goal of treatment is to induce a complete remission. Typical regimens include vincristine, glucocorticoid, L-asparaginase. CNS prophylaxis must be included in the initial treatment, and typically involves intrathecal chemotherapy. Cranial irradiation may be indicated for certain high-risk patients. Due to potential toxicities associated with irradiating the developing brain of a child, more recent clinical trials are studying the potential effectiveness of replacing cranial irradiation with intrathecal chemotherapy and high-dose systemic chemotherapy, while restricting use of cranial irradiation to high-risk patients.
- Following induction of remission, the patient receives *consolidation/intensification* chemotherapy.

- After completion of the consolidation/intensification treatment phase, the patient must receive *maintenance chemotherapy* for approximately 2 to 3 years.
- Allogeneic stem cell transplantation is generally reserved for the treatment of relapsed disease and typically is not recommended for children with standard-risk ALL during the first complete remission.

APPROACH TO TREATMENT OF ADULTS WITH ALL

- ALL in adulthood is associated with decreased long-term survival when compared with that of children with ALL. Approximately, 60% to 90% of adults with ALL can expect to achieve a complete remission with induction chemotherapy treatment, although many of these patients suffer a relapse of their disease. The overall cure rate for adults with ALL is approximately 30% to 40%. Presence of poor prognostic factors (e.g., age > 60 years, Philadelphia chromosome-positive, long time to achieve first remission, and high WBC at the time of diagnosis) generally is associated with reduced survival.
- As with treatment of childhood ALL, the goal of initial treatment is to induce a complete remission using *induction chemotherapy* using multiple chemotherapy drugs. Typical regimens include vincristine, glucocorticoid, and an anthracycline drug. L-Asparaginase may also be included in some treatment regimens. Following the remission induction, the patient receives *consolidation therapy* with additional chemotherapy. Consolidation treatment also generally includes CNS prophylaxis using intrathecal chemotherapy and/or cranial irradiation. For adults with ALL, the (induction + consolidation) treatment typically takes approximately 6 months following diagnosis; then followed by the *maintenance chemotherapy* phase. The optimal duration of maintenance treatment is under investigation, although it generally continues until approximately 2 to 3 years from the time of diagnosis.
- Clinical trials are ongoing regarding the role of tyrosine kinase inhibitors (e.g., imatinib) in the treatment of patients with ALL who are Philadelphia chromosome-positive.
- Allogeneic SCT for selected adult patients with ALL has been associated with improved long-term, disease-free survival rates.
- Relapse is common in adult ALL; patients may be considered for further reinduction chemotherapy, followed by autologous or allogeneic SCT.

C. Chronic Lymphocytic Leukemia

1. Etiology/Epidemiology

- Usually occurs in adults older than 50 years.
- Men outnumber women 2:1.

- The disease is rare among Asian persons.
- Cause of chronic lymphocytic leukemia (CLL) is unknown; however, evidence exists to suggest that hereditary and cytogenetic factors may have a role. CLL is associated with some common cytogenetic abnormalities (e.g., trisomy 12 and 13q deletion). There also have been familial clusters of patients identified, with relatives having 2- to 3-fold increased risk of CLL compared with that of the general population.
- CLL is the most common form of adult leukemia in Western countries.
- There have not yet been any proven environmental factors leading to increased CLL risk.

2. **Pathology**
   - Caused by proliferation of mature-appearing lymphocytes in peripheral blood that invade bone marrow, spleen, lymph nodes.
   - Usually of B-lymphocyte origin (>90%), with monoclonal surface immunoglobulin expressed by >90% of patients.
   - WHO classification of lymphoid neoplasms recognizes CLL and small lymphocytic lymphoma (SLL) (a type of NHL) as being on the same clinical spectrum. CLL manifests as a "leukemic" lymphoid process, with more prominent involvement of the peripheral blood than is present in SLL.

3. **Clinical Features**
   - May have no signs or symptoms.
   - In 25% of patients, CLL is noted initially on routine complete blood count.
   - Patients may complain of weakness, fatigue, dyspnea on exertion, infections.
   - On physical examination, lymphadenopathy, hepatosplenomegaly often seen. Advanced disease also may be associated with weight loss, fever, or bruising.

4. **Diagnostic Studies**
   - Elevated WBC count of 15,000 to 100,000 per mm^3 in 70% to 95% of cases.
   - Absolute lymphocyte count >5,000 per mm^3 (required criteria to distinguish between CLL and SLL).
   - Peripheral blood smear: mature-appearing lymphocytes with characteristic *smudge cells* present.
   - Anemia may be present and may be multifactorial (e.g., splenic sequestration, autoimmune hemolytic anemia, and bone marrow infiltration).
   - Thrombocytopenia may be present and may be multifactorial (e.g., splenic sequestration, autoimmune thrombocytopenia, and bone marrow infiltration).
   - Bone marrow: >30% well-differentiated lymphocytes.
   - Hypogammaglobulinemia is often present.
   - CXR: To evaluate for pleural effusion, infiltrates, and adenopathy associated with the disease.

- Direct Coombs test (direct antiglobulin test) will be positive in the presence of autoimmune hemolytic anemia associated with CLL.

COMPLICATIONS
- Approximately, 10% of patients may develop Coombs-positive warm antibody hemolytic anemia, and approximately, 5% of patients may develop autoimmune thrombocytopenia during the course of their disease.
- Hypogammaglobulinemia leads to impaired immunity and subsequent infection.
- Approximately, 5% of patients with CLL undergo transformation into a more aggressive lymphoma (*Richter syndrome*).
- Pancytopenia often is associated with advanced disease and may result in life-threatening infections.

5. **Management**
   - As CLL is often an indolent disease, no indication for treatment of an asymptomatic patient with stable disease generally exists. Decision whether to initiate treatment is based on several clinical indicators including disease stage, as well as presence or absence of systemic symptoms (fever, sweats, weight loss), evidence of advanced disease, whether lymphadenopathy is causing mechanical obstruction or significant physical discomfort, and if rapid doubling time for peripheral blood lymphocyte count exists.
   - Two staging systems are available for the staging of CLL: (1) the Binet staging system and (2) the modified Rai classification system.
   - **Binet Staging System:**
     - Lymph node groups—cervical, axillary, inguinal, liver, spleen.
     - Stage A: Lymphocytosis with <3 lymph node groups involved; no anemia or thrombocytopenia.
     - Stage B: Lymphocytosis with >3 lymph node groups involved.
     - Stage C: Anemia and/or thrombocytopenia regardless of number of lymph node groups.
   - **Modified RAI Classification System:**
     - Stage 0: Lymphocytosis of peripheral blood and bone marrow (>40% lymphocytes in bone marrow; >5,000 per μL blood lymphocytes).
     - Stage I: Stage 0 + lymphadenopathy.
     - Stage II: Stage 0 or I + splenomegaly and/or hepatomegaly.
     - Stage III: Stage 0, I, or II + anemia (Hgb <11 μ per dL).*
     - Stage IV: Stage 0, I, or II + thrombocytopenia (platelet count <100,000 per μL).†

---

* Anemia or thrombocytopenia is not due to autoimmune destruction.
† See note above.

- Chemotherapy options include single-agent chemotherapy—purine analogs (e.g., fludarabine and cladribine); combination chemotherapy utilizing alkylating agents (e.g., cyclophosphamide), monoclonal antibodies (e.g., Rituximab), and/or purine analogs.
- For treatment of autoimmune hemolytic anemia or autoimmune thrombocytopenia associated with CLL, glucocorticoid treatment is indicated (e.g., prednisone 1 mg/kg/day orally as starting dose, to be gradually tapered once blood counts have stabilized).
- Splenectomy may be indicated for patients with CLL and autoimmune hemolytic anemia or autoimmune thrombocytopenia who do not respond adequately to glucocorticoid therapy.
- Local radiation therapy may be indicated to relieve symptoms caused by lymphadenopathy or splenomegaly.

D. Acute Myelogenous Leukemia

1. Etiology/Epidemiology

- Acute myelogenous leukemia (AML) accounts for approximately 80% of all new cases of adult acute leukemias. Primarily occurs in adults older than 50 years, but also may occur in young adults, children.
- In most cases, the cause of AML is unknown. However, some risk factors have been identified including prior treatment with certain chemotherapy agents, exposure to ionizing radiation, benzene exposure, congenital disorders (e.g., Down syndrome).
- Can be preceded by chronic myelogenous leukemia, polycythemia vera, idiopathic myelofibrosis, or myelodysplastic syndromes (MDSs).

2. Pathology

- Caused by proliferation of abnormal myeloid cells (precursors of erythrocytes, granulocytes, monocytes, platelets) that do not mature.
- Classified by FAB classification into eight subtypes (M_0 to M_7) based on the degree of differentiation, maturation of predominant cells.

3. Clinical Features

- Patient may complain of fever, fatigue, weakness, bleeding, bruising, recurrent infection.
- Bone pain, CNS occurrence rare.
- Hepatosplenomegaly and lymphadenopathy are less common than in acute lymphocytic leukemia.
- Gingival hypertrophy, skin infiltration by leukemia (*leukemia cutis*) may be present in patients with acute monocytic leukemia (M_5 variant).
- Retinal hemorrhages may be present (due to thrombocytopenia).
- Bleeding symptoms due to disseminated intravascular coagulation (DIC) may be present, particularly with acute promyelocytic leukemia (M_3 variant).
- Leukostasis may occur, especially if WBC >100,000 per mm^3, and may cause CNS manifestations (e.g., confusion, headache, and cranial nerve deficits) or severe respiratory distress (due to leukostasis in the pulmonary vasculature). Emergent leukapheresis is indicated.

4. Diagnostic Studies

- Normocytic normochromic anemia is often present.
- Peripheral blood smear: The presence of Auer rods in the blast cytoplasm is pathognomonic for AML.
- Decreased neutrophils; absolute neutrophil count (ANC) is often low, and approximately 50% of patients have ANC <1,500 at the time of diagnosis.
- WBCs may be low, normal, high.
- Bone marrow hypercellular with >30% blasts.
- Serum uric acid and serum LDH may be elevated (related to increased cell turnover).
- Thrombocytopenia is often present.
- If the WBC >100,000, additional laboratory findings may be present, including *pseudohypoxemia* (as a result of O_2 consumption by blast cells in vitro), *pseudohyperkalemia* (as a result of elevated WBC), and *pseudohypoglycemia* (as a result of glucose consumption by blast cells in vitro).

COMPLICATIONS

- Chemotherapy causes immunosuppression, with resultant increased risk of infections.
- Leukostasis may occur; typically associated with WBC >100,000 per mm^3.
- Bleeding complications may occur because of thrombocytopenia, DIC.
- *Tumor lysis syndrome* may occur during chemotherapy treatment (see above, **Acute Lymphocytic Leukemia Complications**).

5. Management

- The prognosis for AML varies significantly and is dependent on multiple factors including age at diagnosis, whether AML occurred de novo or is secondary to toxin exposure, or preceding MDS. In addition, the cytogenetic profile is also a useful prognostic factor. Poor prognostic factors include advanced age at the time of diagnosis, unfavorable cytogenetic profile, secondary AML due to toxin exposure (e.g., benzene, alkylating agent chemotherapy, and ionizing radiation), poor performance status at the time of diagnosis, and AML preceded by myelodysplasia.
- As with ALL, initial phase of treatment is known as *induction chemotherapy*. Multiple effective induction chemotherapy regimens are available and generally include an anthracycline (e.g., daunorubicin and idarubicin) in combination with cytosine arabinoside (Ara-C). Complete remission may be obtained in 70% to 80% of patients 60 years and younger and in 50% of older patients.

- Induction chemotherapy is then followed by postinduction treatment, and options generally include additional chemotherapy with high-dose Ara-C, autologous SCT, allogeneic SCT. The decision regarding which treatment to offer depends largely on the prognostic category of the patient. Patients with poor prognostic factors are at significant risk for relapse and generally should be considered for allogeneic SCT after induction. Patients with good prognostic factors would typically be offered additional chemotherapy as the postinduction treatment, with a significant chance for cure with this approach. For patients who have intermediate prognostic factors, management must be considered on an individual basis.
- In case of relapse, consider stem cell transplantation.

E. Chronic Myelogenous Leukemia

1. Etiology/Epidemiology
- Median age at presentation is 45 to 55 years.
- Chronic myelogenous leukemia (CML) accounts for approximately 15% of all cases of leukemia in adults.
- Cause is unclear; however, increased incidence of CML has been noted among persons with a history of organic solvent exposure (such as benzene) and among persons with a history of exposure to high levels of ionizing radiation (e.g., Hiroshima and Nagasaki).

2. Pathology
- CML is a myeloproliferative disorder caused by proliferation of myeloid cells that retain their capacity to differentiate.
- Chronic phase is characterized by elevated WBCs >100,000 per mm^3 with <5% blasts in blood or bone marrow.
- Accelerated phase (>5%, <30% blasts in blood or bone marrow) is often heralded by worsening anemia and refractory response to treatment.
- Acute blast crisis phase (>30% blasts in blood or bone marrow) is an aggressive phase of the disease, as CML evolves into a secondary acute leukemia.
- Most patients who transform into an acute blast phase have disease poorly responsive to therapy and will die in this phase.
- Philadelphia chromosome-negative CML is associated with a poor prognosis.

3. Clinical Features
- May be asymptomatic.
- Patient may complain of left upper quadrant (LUQ) pain secondary to enlarged spleen, or weight loss, fever, arthralgias, bleeding.
- Physical examination may disclose marked splenomegaly, hepatomegaly, lymphadenopathy (rare), ecchymoses, bone tenderness.

4. Diagnostic Studies
- WBCs elevated >100,000 per mm^3 with increased numbers of granulocytes, especially neutrophils.
- WBC differential also may show an increase in basophils and eosinophils.
- Normocytic normochromic anemia may be present.
- Chromosomal abnormality—presence of Philadelphia chromosome t(9;22). Approximately 90% of patients with CML are Philadelphia chromosome-positive.
- Low leukocyte alkaline phosphatase (LAP) score.
- Elevated serum B$_{12}$ level.
- Thrombocytosis may be present at the time of diagnosis.
- Peripheral blood smear: WBCs present at all stages of maturation.

5. Management
- The majority of patients with CML are in *chronic phase* at the time of diagnosis. Treatment options for newly diagnosed patients with CML diagnosed in chronic phase include tyrosine kinase inhibitors (e.g., imatinib), chemotherapy followed by allogeneic SCT, α interferon (interferon α[IFN-α]), or hydroxyurea (Droxia and Hydrea).
- Allogeneic SCT is a potentially curative option and should be considered early in disease for selected patients; best chance for success if done in chronic phase.
- Treatment options for acute blast phase of CML are limited.
- **For patients who develop a secondary AML:**
  - Imatinib may be helpful in inducing a remission. If remission is achieved, consideration should be given to allogeneic SCT, if patient is eligible and a donor is available.
- **For patients who develop a secondary ALL:**
  - Imatinib may be helpful in inducing a remission. If remission is achieved, consideration should be given to allogeneic SCT, if patient is eligible and a donor is available. If patient has a relapse following treatment with imatinib, consideration may be given to treatment with an ALL chemotherapy regimen (e.g., vincristine/prednisone), which can occasionally be helpful in allowing patients to return to chronic phase for a period of time.
- Average survival time for patients with CML is approximately 5 to 7 years in chronic phase; 3 months in acute blast crisis phase.

III. Platelet Disorders
A. Acquired Coagulopathy

Disseminated Intravascular Coagulation
1. Etiology/Pathology
- Disseminated intravascular coagulation (DIC)—consumption of coagulation factors resulting from intravascular activation of coagulation process with secondary activation of fibrinolysis, which may lead to either hemorrhage or thrombosis.

- Most common causes—infection (usually gram-negative endotoxins), complications of pregnancy, massive tissue injury, malignancy, hypoxia, acidosis, snakebite, cancer, acute promyelocytic leukemia (M_3 variant of AML).

EPIDEMIOLOGY
- DIC occurs in 1/1,000 hospitalized patients.
- Twenty percent are asymptomatic.
- Most often occurs in young or elderly patients.

2. **Clinical Features**
- Acute—may present as sudden onset of bleeding, hemorrhage (80% to 90%).
- Chronic—bleeding symptoms may be mild or patient may be asymptomatic.
- Thrombosis may occur and generally involves small or midsize vessels.
- May see hematuria, GI bleed, epistaxis, petechiae, bleeding from surgical or venipuncture sites or uterus.
- Thrombi may infarct the heart, kidney, brain, liver, pancreas, causing shock secondary to increased vascular permeability and hypotension.

3. **Diagnostic Studies**
- Decreased platelets, decreased fibrinogen level, increased prothrombin time (PT)/partial thromboplastin time (PTT), elevated fibrin-split products (FSPs), elevated D-dimer level, elevated thrombin time.
- Peripheral blood smear: schistocytes and low platelet count are generally present.
- Low levels of clotting factors V, VIII.

COMPLICATIONS
- Renal failure.
- Exsanguination.
- Mortality rates—50% to 60%.

4. **Management**
- Timely and appropriate treatment of the underlying disorder is of paramount importance when managing a patient with DIC.
- Although there is a theoretical concern that giving a patient in DIC transfusion support may worsen the condition, current clinical recommendations seem to support the use of blood products for patients in DIC with documented factor deficiencies who are actively bleeding, or who require surgery or other invasive procedures, and are at high risk for bleeding. In this situation, transfusion support with appropriate blood products would generally be given (e.g., platelets, fresh frozen plasma [FFP], and cryoprecipitate).
- If thrombosis is occurring, it may be appropriate to consider initiating anticoagulation with heparin. However, the decision regarding whether to use heparin anticoagulation for a patient with DIC must always be determined on an individual basis, and the associated potential risks and benefits must be considered carefully. In the absence of thrombosis, heparin anticoagulation as a treatment for acute DIC is rarely indicated.

B. **Thrombotic Thrombocytopenic Purpura**
1. **Etiology/Pathology**
- Although the underlying mechanism for the development of thrombotic thrombocytopenic purpura (TTP) is not entirely understood, the etiology of TTP is thought to be due, in part, to a deficiency of a von Willebrand factor (vWF) cleaving proteolytic enzyme responsible for cleaving high molecular weight vWF molecules into their usual length. Elevated levels of high molecular weight vWF molecules are believed to be associated with abnormal platelet aggregation. This enzyme deficiency may either be inherited or caused by the inhibition of the enzyme by an antibody.
- TTP may be idiopathic or related to other underlying causes—for example, drug-induced (e.g., mitomycin C), pregnancy, HIV infection, connective tissue disease.
- Thrombi form in capillaries and arterioles.
- May be acute, chronic, relapsing.

EPIDEMIOLOGY
- Affects young adults 20 to 50 years of age.
- Rare disorder.
- Affects women more than men.

2. **Clinical Features**
- Patients may complain of headache, confusion, seizures, jaundice, visual defects, abdominal pain, bleeding, fever.
- A *pentad of clinical findings* characterizes this condition: microangiopathic hemolytic anemia, thrombocytopenia, CNS abnormalities, fever, renal dysfunction.
- Patients may appear pale with purpura, petechiae, jaundice, abdominal tenderness, and neurologic examination may show abnormal findings (e.g., confusion and seizures).

3. **Diagnostic Studies**
- Thrombocytopenia.
- Anemia.
- Peripheral blood smear: evidence of microangiopathic hemolysis including schistocytes, helmet cells, nucleated RBCs, polychromasia.
- Increased reticulocytes.
- Elevated BUN and creatinine.
- Elevated serum LDH.
- Elevated serum indirect bilirubin.
- Leukocytosis with a neutrophil predominance may be present.
- Coagulation tests—PT/international normalized ratio (INR), PTT—are normal, which differentiates it from DIC.
- Direct Coombs test is negative.
- Hemoglobinuria may be present.

COMPLICATIONS

- Without treatment, mortality rate is >90% because of multiorgan failure. With treatment, the mortality rate is <30%.
- Chronic renal failure (CRF).
- In some patients, the disease follows a chronic, relapsing course.

4. **Management**
   - Prompt initiation of plasma exchange (plasmapheresis) is the mainstay of therapy and is generally done on a daily basis, until the platelet count normalizes, the neurologic abnormalities resolve, and serum LDH level returns to near normal. The frequency of plasmapheresis is then generally tapered gradually over the following 1 to 2 weeks; however, it may take longer for some patients to achieve a disease remission.
   - Splenectomy may have a role in the treatment of patients who have a suboptimal response to plasmapheresis or continue to require plasmapheresis after 4 to 6 weeks.
   - Corticosteroids also have a role in the treatment of patients with TTP and are sometimes given in addition to plasmapheresis.
   - It is unclear whether the use of antiplatelet agents (e.g., aspirin and dipyridamole) confers any additional benefit in the treatment of TTP.
   - Renal dialysis if CRF occurs.

C. **Idiopathic (Autoimmune) Thrombocytopenic Purpura**
   1. **Etiology/Pathology**
      - Idiopathic thrombocytopenic purpura (ITP) is an acquired autoimmune disorder characterized by isolated thrombocytopenia, without other apparent causes or underlying conditions contributing to the thrombocytopenia. An autoantibody is produced that binds to platelets. The antibody-coated platelets are then bound to splenic macrophages and destroyed in the spleen. The thrombocytopenia occurs as a result of splenic sequestration and accelerated platelet destruction.
      - In children, ITP usually occurs acutely, 1 to 3 weeks after viral illness, and is often self-limited.
      - Viral antigen–antibody immune complexes thought to bind to platelet receptors.
      - Adults usually have more chronic form with no predisposing cause.
      - In adult ITP, an autoantibody forms against platelet membrane antigen, thereby destroying platelets.

   EPIDEMIOLOGY
      - Most common form of thrombocytopenia.
      - Occurs predominantly in young children and young women (usually younger than 40 years).
      - Peak incidence for childhood ITP is from 2 to 4 years of age.
      - May be associated with HIV infection.

2. **Clinical Features**
   - Bruising, petechiae, purpura are seen commonly at the time of diagnosis.
   - Mucocutaneous bleeding is commonly present (e.g., epistaxis and gingival bleeding).
   - Adult women may have menorrhagia.
   - Hemorrhagic bullae in the mouth of children.
   - No fever or hepatosplenomegaly. **NOTE:** If splenomegaly is present, need to question the diagnosis of ITP, as presence of enlarged spleen suggests other underlying diagnosis.
   - Intracranial hemorrhage is an infrequent occurrence; however, it is the most common cause of death among adult patients with ITP.

3. **Diagnostic Studies**
   - Hallmark—thrombocytopenia (<20,000 per mm^3 in acute form, 30,000 to 80,000 per mm^3 in chronic form).
   - Peripheral blood smear: Platelets may be normal in size or may appear enlarged. **NOTE:** It is important to evaluate the peripheral smear to rule out platelet clumping that can cause *pseudothrombocytopenia*.
   - WBC and Hgb are generally normal.
   - Coagulation studies (PT/INR, PTT) are normal.
   - Bone marrow may show increased number of megakaryocytes.
   - Serum platelet autoantibodies may be present in chronic cases.
   - HIV test may be indicated in patient with risk factors.

4. **Management**
   - Avoidance of trauma and medications that can cause bleeding (e.g., aspirin and other nonsteroidal anti-inflammatory drugs [NSAIDs]) should be advised.
   - **Treatment of childhood ITP:**
     - Childhood ITP is often a self-limited disease, and specific treatment is not always recommended, particularly if the symptoms are mild. However, children do generally receive treatment.
     - Common treatment approach for childhood ITP is the use of intravenous immunoglobulin (IVIG).
     - Because of the considerable risks of serious infection following splenectomy, consideration of splenectomy for the treatment of childhood ITP is generally reserved for selected patients with demonstrated severe thrombocytopenia and associated bleeding concerns.
   - **Treatment of adult ITP:**
     - For patients who are clinically stable, treatment is generally initiated with prednisone (1 mg/kg/day); the platelet count typically begins to increase within 1 week. After the platelet count has normalized, the prednisone dose can be tapered down

gradually to the lowest effective dose that will allow the platelet count to remain in an acceptable range. Other treatment options include IVIG, anti-Rh(D) immune globulin (can only be used in Rh+ patients who have not undergone removal of spleen).

- Given the more chronic course typical of adult ITP, patients may need further treatment. For a patient who has not responded to a trial of steroid treatment, or who continues to require high steroid doses to maintain an acceptable platelet count, splenectomy may be beneficial to consider. If a patient does not respond to steroid trial or splenectomy, some favorable responses have been observed using other agents (e.g., danazol, azathioprine, and cyclophosphamide). Thrombopoietin analogs are also available for the treatment of chronic refractory adult ITP (e.g., romiplostim and eltrombopag).
- In the case of life-threatening bleeding when a more rapid increase in the platelet count is needed, the patient is typically treated with IVIG and parenteral glucocorticoid therapy (e.g., methylprednisolone). Although there is generally no role for platelet transfusion in the treatment of ITP (because the transfused platelets will have limited survival given the presence of antiplatelet antibody), in the setting of life-threatening hemorrhage, consideration may be given to the administration of platelet transfusion in an attempt to achieve hemostasis.

IV. Factor Deficiencies
A. Hemophilia A and B

Hemophilia A (Classic Hemophilia)
1. Etiology/Pathology
- X-linked recessive disorder affecting only males (with rare exceptions); results in deficiency of coagulation factor VIII.
- Mild form if level of coagulation factor VIII activity is 6% to 30%; severe form if level of coagulation factor VIII activity is <1%.
- First episode of bleeding usually occurs when patient is <18 months old.

EPIDEMIOLOGY
- After von Willebrand disease (vWD), the most common congenital bleeding disorder.
- Occurs in 1/10,000 males births.
- Eighty percent of all patients with hemophilia have hemophilia A.

2. Clinical Features
- Patients may complain of pain in weight-bearing joints.
- Bleeding into joints occurs (hemarthroses). Commonly affected joints include knees, ankles, elbows.
- Patients also can bleed into muscles, the GI tract, or base of the tongue.
- Severe disease is associated with spontaneous bleeding; mild disease typically is associated with bleeding due to trauma or surgery, and spontaneous bleeding is rare.

3. Diagnostic Studies
- Decreased levels of factor VIII. Specific assay for factor VIII activity is necessary for diagnosis.
- Increased PTT, normal PT, normal bleeding time, normal fibrinogen.
- Mixing study: Mixing plasma of normal patients with that of plasma from a patient with hemophilia A will result in normal PTT.

COMPLICATIONS
- Hemarthroses may lead to joint deformities.
- Some patients transfused with factor VIII develop inhibitors to it and need to be identified and managed differently.
- Lack of normalization of the PTT mixing study is diagnostic of factor VIII anticoagulant activity (inhibitor).

4. Management
- Infusion of factor VIII concentrate to levels of 25% to 100%. Optimal level for factor VIII replacement is dependent on the underlying situation (e.g., patient with only mild bleeding may require only 25% factor VIII level for control of bleeding).
- Desmopressin acetate (DDAVP) may cause transient rise in factor VIII levels for several hours. **NOTE:** With repeated doses of DDAVP, tachyphylaxis occurs.
- Avoid trauma.
- Avoid medications that may cause bleeding (e.g., aspirin and other NSAIDs).
- Avoid IM injections.
- Genetic counseling for carriers.

Hemophilia B (Christmas Disease)
1. Etiology
- Occurs in 1/30,000 male births.
2. Etiology/Pathology
- X-linked recessive disorder affecting only males (with rare exceptions); results in deficiency of coagulation factor IX.
3. Clinical Features
- See **Hemophilia A**.
4. Diagnostic Studies
- Decreased levels of factor IX. Specific assay for factor IX activity is necessary for diagnosis.
- Increased PTT, normal PT, normal bleeding time, normal fibrinogen.
- Mixing study: Mixing plasma of normal patients with that of plasma from a patient with hemophilia B will result in normal PTT.

COMPLICATIONS

- Risk of thrombosis secondary to proteins (activated coagulation factors) is related to the use of some preparations of factor IX concentrate; risk has been significantly diminished with the availability of higher purity factor IX concentrates.
- Lack of normalization of the PTT mixing study is diagnostic of factor IX anticoagulant activity (inhibitor).

5. Management
- Infusion of factor IX concentrate.
- Avoid medications that may cause bleeding (e.g., aspirin and other NSAIDs).
- Avoid IM injections.
- Genetic counseling for carriers.

B. von Willebrand Disease

1. Etiology/Pathology
- Autosomal dominant disorder that results from deficient or defective vWF and causes *ineffective platelet adhesion*.
- Platelet aggregation is normal.
- vWF is produced in megakaryocytes and endothelial cells; it also functions to bind factor VIII and protects it from breaking down; therefore, decreased vWF also may cause reduced levels of factor VIII.

EPIDEMIOLOGY

- Most common inherited bleeding disorder; affects approximately 1% of population.
- Affects both men and women.

2. Clinical Features
- Patients may commonly have mucosal bleeding (e.g., epistaxis and gingival bleeding) or increased menstrual bleeding.
- Spontaneous hemarthroses do not generally occur.
- GI bleeding is less common.
- Bleeding is worsened by aspirin.

3. Diagnostic Studies
- Prolonged bleeding time (usually, but wide fluctuations can occur); worse after taking aspirin.
- Mild increase in PTT may be present.
- In type I vWD, levels of vWF are reduced.
- Low ristocetin cofactor activity.
- Normal number and morphology of platelets.

4. Management
- Avoid aspirin.
- In type I, treatment with DDAVP may be helpful.
- Infusion of plasma factor VIII concentrate containing vWF (e.g., Humate-P), or cryoprecipitate.
- Check bleeding time immediately before elective procedures.

C. Coagulopathy of Liver Disease

1. Etiology
- Damage to the liver may be caused by cancer, alcoholism, drugs, hemochromatosis, abscess, obstruction, viral hepatitis, ischemia.

2. Pathology
- **Reasons that liver dysfunction results in coagulopathy:**
  - The liver produces all coagulation factors except factor VIII and vWF.
  - Impaired hepatic synthetic function results in deficiencies of most clotting factors.
  - Liver macrophages remove activated factors (e.g., FSPs and fibrinolytic enzymes).
  - Liver produces antithrombin III, factors C and S.
  - Liver disease causes malabsorption of vitamin K.
  - Portal hypertension can lead to splenomegaly, mild thrombocytopenia, varices, peptic ulcer disease, bleeding.

3. Clinical Features
- Bleeding—classic finding.
- Assess for clinical signs of alcoholism (i.e., cardiomegaly, caput medusa, hepatomegaly, jaundice, scleral injection, and ecchymoses).

4. Diagnostic Studies
- Prolonged PT > PTT.
- Early liver disease is generally associated with prolonged PT only. Advanced liver disease may be associated with a prolonged PT and PTT.
- Elevated factor VIII level is often present in chronic liver disease.
- Mixing study (50:50 mix of normal plasma and patient plasma) corrects PT/PTT elevation completely.
- No response to vitamin K.
- Low fibrinogen level, decreased platelets may be present.
- Peripheral blood smear: Target cells, macrocytes may be present.

5. Management
- FFP may be given to replace deficient clotting factors if patient is bleeding or needs to undergo an invasive procedure.
- Cryoprecipitate contains concentrated form of fibrinogen and may be given to replace fibrinogen in a patient with severe hypofibrinogenemia if patient is bleeding or needs to undergo an invasive procedure.
- Vitamin K may be given in the setting of vitamin K deficiency; however, it does not typically correct the coagulopathy because patients with chronic liver disease often have significant impairment in hepatic synthetic function as well.
- Avoid alcohol consumption.
- Correct underlying disorder.

D. Vitamin K Deficiency

1. Etiology
- Vitamin K deficiency can be caused by poor diet, malabsorption, antibiotics, warfarin, biliary obstruction.
- Dietary sources of vitamin K present in leafy vegetables.

- Vitamin K is synthesized by intestinal bacteria.
- Body stores are small and may be depleted within <1 week.

2. **Pathology**
   - Vitamin K is necessary for γcarboxylation of the vitamin K–dependent clotting factors (II, VII, IX, X) in the liver.
   - These clotting factors, along with calcium and platelets, activate factors X and II in coagulation cascade.

3. **Clinical Features**
   - Bleeding.

4. **Diagnostic Studies**
   - Prolonged PT > PTT.
   - Early vitamin K deficiency is associated with elevated PT only; severe vitamin K deficiency is generally associated with prolonged PT and PTT.
   - Normal fibrinogen level, platelets.
   - Mixing study (50:50 mix of normal plasma and patient plasma) completely corrects PT/PTT abnormalities.

5. **Management**
   - Diet including consumption of green leafy vegetables.
   - Depending on the etiology of vitamin K deficiency and goal of treatment, management may differ. Depending on the clinical situation, patients with warfarin-induced vitamin K deficiency and an excessive elevation of PT/INR, who are not actively bleeding and will continue to require anticoagulation for treatment of an underlying hypercoagulable disorder, may not require complete correction of PT/INR, and smaller doses of vitamin K may be sufficient. Each case must be carefully evaluated on an individual basis.
   - Vitamin K replacement is typically given by oral or subcutaneous route, with subsequent correction of PT/PTT abnormalities generally within 12 to 24 hours. **NOTE:** Absorption of subcutaneous vitamin K may be less predictable in patients who are edematous.
   - For the treatment of vitamin K deficiency in the setting of active bleeding, or if the patient requires an invasive procedure, administration of FFP may be indicated.

V. Hypercoagulability

A. Antithrombin III Deficiency

1. **Etiology**
   - May be inherited as an autosomal dominant trait, or acquired (e.g., liver disease, nephrotic syndrome, in DIC, or from certain chemotherapy drugs).

2. **Pathology**
   - Antithrombin III inactivates surplus thrombin.
   - Its activity is potentiated by heparin.

- Deficiency of antithrombin III (25% to 60%) results in venous thrombosis.

3. **Clinical Features**
   - Patients may have a family history of thromboembolism or have recurrent deep venous thrombosis (DVT) or pulmonary emboli (PE).
   - First episode may occur at age 20 to 30 years.

4. **Diagnostic Studies**
   - Decreased levels of antithrombin III. **NOTE:** Functional antithrombin III assay should be done to allow evaluation of type I versus type II antithrombin III deficiency.
   - Resistance to heparin may be a clinical clue.

5. **Management**
   - Asymptomatic patients may require anticoagulation only before surgical procedures.
   - Patients who experience a thrombotic event receive IV heparin, then oral anticoagulation indefinitely.

B. Protein C Deficiency

1. **Etiology**
   - Autosomal dominant disorder.

2. **Pathology**
   - Protein C—vitamin K–dependent liver protein that stimulates fibrinolysis, clot lysis.
   - Deficiency of protein C causes recurrent DVT, PE.

3. **Clinical Features**
   - Patients may have a family history of thromboembolism, DVT.
   - Venous thrombosis may occur in unusual sites; arterial thrombosis is less common.

4. **Diagnostic Studies**
   - Decreased levels of protein C. **NOTE:** Functional protein C assay should be done for the diagnosis of protein C deficiency.
   - Normal PT, PTT, bleeding time.

   COMPLICATIONS
   - Coumadin-induced skin necrosis.
   - Newborns may have purpura fulminans or fulminant intravascular coagulation.
   - May result in cerebrovascular accident.

5. **Management**
   - Heparin, then oral anticoagulation for life.

C. Acquired Hypercoagulability

1. **Etiology**
   - Four major causes of acquired hypercoagulability need to be recognized and assessed if DVT or PE is suspected or diagnosed.
   - **Pregnancy:** results in increased venous stasis, hyperviscosity, decreased protein S and antithrombin III, decreased fibrinolysis.
   - **Malignancy:** in neoplastic diseases, tumor cells activate platelets. Approximately, 15% of patients with DVTs or PEs have cancer. In addition, 5% of patients without cancer who have had DVT or PE will have diagnosis of cancer within 1 year.

- **Oral contraceptive pills:** increased risk of stroke, DVTs, PEs especially in women older than 40 years and tobacco users.
- **Lupus anticoagulant:** immunoglobulin seen in patients with and without systemic lupus erythematosus, which causes increased risk of thrombosis and spontaneous abortions. Laboratory evaluation: PTT is often elevated; mixing study (50:50 mix of normal plasma and patient plasma) does not completely correct prolonged PTT.

2. **Management**
   - Good history, physical examination important.
   - Doppler U/S, impedance plethysmography study, CXR, ventilation/perfusion (V/Q) scans should be ordered, if indicated.
   - Thromboembolism can be treated with heparin, then Coumadin.
   - Greenfield filter may have to be placed to prevent recurrent PEs.
   - Women diagnosed with lupus anticoagulant (antiphospholipid antibody syndrome) and who have experienced multiple miscarriages previously are generally treated with low-dose aspirin, heparin, or a combination of both during pregnancy, and must be followed closely for the duration of the pregnancy.

VI. Other Disorders

A. Polycythemia Vera (Primary Erythrocytosis)
1. **Etiology/Pathology**
   - Acquired myeloproliferative disease resulting in overproduction of RBCs.

EPIDEMIOLOGY
   - Sixty percent of patients are men.
   - Rarely occurs before age 40; peaks at 50 to 60 years of age.

2. **Clinical Features**
   - Patients complain of headache, dizziness, blurred vision, pruritus (especially after a hot bath), fatigue, nosebleeds, tinnitus, LUQ pain, GI discomfort, chest pain, claudication. *Erythromelalgia* (burning/throbbing sensation in digits of the hands, feet) may be a prominent symptom.
   - Patients with polycythemia vera (PV) have an increased bleeding tendency, and hemorrhage due to GI bleeding, epistaxis, or gingival bleeding may occur.
   - Patients with PV have increased tendency of thrombosis, and may experience arterial and venous thrombotic events.
   - On physical examination, splenomegaly, plethora, and engorged retinal vessels may be noted.

3. **Diagnostic Studies**
   - Elevated RBC mass (nuclear medicine study using radiolabeled RBCs to determine RBC mass).

- EPO level is low.
- Elevated HCT.
- Elevated WBCs (10,000 to 20,000 per mm^3); neutrophilia and basophilia may be present.
- Elevated platelets; the platelet count may exceed 1,000,000 per mm^3 in some patients.
- Elevated serum B_{12} level, elevated LAP, and elevated serum uric acid level may be present.
- Normal arterial O_2 saturation.
- Pseudohyperkalemia may occur, because of elevated platelet count.
- Artificial prolongation of PT/PTT may occur in the presence of significantly elevated HCT.
- Genetic testing for *JAK2* mutation: (+) in approximately 95% of patients.
- Bone marrow—hypercellular with increased megakaryocytes, absent iron stores.

COMPLICATIONS
- Thrombosis, bleeding, splenic infarction, peptic ulcer disease, gout.
- Patients with PV are at increased risk for thrombotic and bleeding complications with surgery.
- Approximately, 15% of all patients with PV enter a "spent phase" characterized by hepatosplenomegaly, anemia, circulating immature WBCs in peripheral blood, and leukocytosis. The bone marrow shows myelofibrosis. Treatment of this phase is supportive, and median survival is approximately 2 years.
- May progress to secondary AML.

4. **Management**
   - The goals of treatment are to reduce blood volume to normal and to prevent complications such as thrombosis and hemorrhage.
   - Therapeutic phlebotomy is typically continued until HCT <45%. Repeated phlebotomy induces iron deficiency, gradually decreasing the frequency of phlebotomy necessary to maintain target HCT. Administration of iron supplementation, therefore, is not appropriate in these patients and may result in rapid recurrence of the elevated HCT.
   - Myelosuppressive therapy may be indicated instead of, or in addition to, therapeutic phlebotomy, depending on the clinical presentation of the patient. Hydroxyurea (Hydrea) is a commonly used myelosuppressive agent and does not appear to be associated with the increased leukemogenic potential associated with alkylating agents (e.g., chlorambucil). IFN-α is also used to treat PV.
   - For patients who require an additional agent for control of thrombocytosis, anagrelide may be a useful option. It inhibits megakaryocyte maturation, thereby decreasing the platelet count. This agent does not appear to be associated with increased leukemogenic potential.

- Treat gout with allopurinol.
- Acetylsalicylic acid (ASA) to reduce the risk of thrombosis; current studies evaluating the efficacy of low-dose aspirin in reducing thrombotic risk without increasing the risk of bleeding complications.
- Antihistamines are used for the treatment of pruritus.

B. Secondary Erythrocytosis

1. Etiology/Pathology
- **Three major causes:**
  - Reactive (physiologic) as response to hypoxia: high altitude, pulmonary disease, tobacco smokers, high-affinity Hgb, cyanotic heart disease.
  - Pathologic (underlying tissue hypoxia is absent): renal cell carcinoma, renal disease, uterine fibroids, hepatomas, cerebellar hemangiomas, elevated androgen levels.
  - Relative polycythemia characterized by normal RBC mass and decreased plasma volume. Patients are typically overweight, hypertensive men on diuretic therapy, with a history of cigarette smoking.

EPIDEMIOLOGY
- Major cause of increased red cell mass.

2. Clinical Features
- Patients may have a history of chronic obstructive pulmonary disease, smoking more than two packs of cigarettes a day, congenital heart disease, renal disease.
- On examination, heart murmur, cyanosis, hypertension, clubbing (pulmonary osteoarthropathy), ecchymoses, hepatosplenomegaly may be found.

3. Diagnostic Studies
- Elevated RBCs, HCT with normal WBCs, platelets.
- EPO may be normal or high.
- CT scan of abdomen, renal U/S, or IV pyelogram may be indicated in patients with possible renal tumor or other renal cause of secondary polycythemia.
- RBC mass is normal in relative polycythemia and elevated in secondary polycythemia because of pathologic or reactive conditions (see Section B1 above).
- Hgb electrophoresis.
- Oxygen saturation level.

4. Management
- Treat underlying disorder.
- Smoking cessation.

C. Hereditary Hemochromatosis

1. Etiology/Pathology
- Intestinal iron absorption inappropriately large, leading to increase in plasma iron and increased transferrin saturation.
- Excess iron then deposits in parenchymal cells of the heart, liver, pancreas, endocrine organs.

EPIDEMIOLOGY
- Familial genetic iron storage disorder.
- Clinical phenotype of skin pigmentation and organ damage occurs only in homozygotes.
- Among Caucasian population, 1/200 with homozygous C282Y *HFE* genotype.
- Five to 10 times more common in men than in women.

2. Clinical Features
- May be asymptomatic in early stages.
- Patients may then complain of fatigue, weakness, loss of libido, impotence, abdominal pain, arthritis.
- Diabetes may occur.
- On examination, one may find hepatomegaly in >95% of cases, splenomegaly in >50%.
- Skin may appear metallic or bronze.
- Cardiomyopathy with arrhythmias, congestive heart failure, heart block can occur.
- Testicular atrophy, synovitis, polyarthritis may be present.

3. Diagnostic Studies
- Increased plasma iron (>200 μg per dL).
- Increased transferrin saturation (>70% up to 100%).
- Increased SF, normal or low TIBC, increased liver iron, increased urinary iron after deferoxamine.
- Increased LFTs may be present.
- Increased hepatic iron content demonstrated on CT, MRI; not indicated for routine screening.
- Genetic testing for *HFE* gene mutations consistent with diagnosis.
- Gold standard—liver biopsy with parenchymal hemosiderin.

COMPLICATIONS
- Cirrhosis of liver can lead to liver cancer.
- Insulin-dependent diabetes.
- Peripheral neuropathy, nephropathy, retinopathy.
- Without treatment, life expectancy about 4 years after clinical symptoms; with treatment, about 15 years; full life expectancy if treated before clinical symptoms occur.

4. Management
- Phlebotomy to decrease body iron to normal.
- Phlebotomy is typically performed on a weekly basis initially, until depletion of iron is confirmed by laboratory studies (e.g., mild anemia, decreased ferritin, and transferrin saturation <30%). Maintenance phlebotomy regimen is then performed approximately three to four times per year, for the remainder of the patient's life.
- Chelating agents may be indicated if anemia occurs, thus restricting the use of therapeutic phlebotomy (IM injection of deferoxamine).
- Test blood relatives; genetic counseling should be made available.
- Treat complications.

- Dietary restrictions, no iron pills, no alcohol or vitamin C.
- Avoid other potential hepatotoxins.

SELECTED REFERENCES

Ahya SN, Flood K, Paranjothi S, eds. *Washington Manual of Medical Therapeutics*. 30th ed. New York, NY: Lippincott Williams & Wilkins; 2001.

Barker LR, Burton JR, Zieve PD, et al, eds. *Principles of Ambulatory Medicine*. 3rd ed. Baltimore, MD: Williams & Wilkins; 1991.

Berkow R, Fletcher AJ, eds. *The Merck Manual of Diagnosis and Therapy*. 15th ed. Rahway, NJ: Merck, Sharp & Dohme; 1987.

Braunwald E, Fauci AS, Kasper DL, et al, eds. *Harrison's Principles of Internal Medicine*. 17th ed. New York, NY: McGraw-Hill; 2008.

Braunwald E, Fauci AS, Kasper DL, et al, eds. *Harrison's Manual of Medicine*. 17th ed. New York, NY: McGraw-Hill; 2009.

Casciato DA. *Manual of Clinical Oncology*. 6th ed. Philadelphia, PA: Lippincott Williams & Wilkins; 2009.

Casciato DA, Lowitz BB, eds. *Manual of Clinical Oncology*. 4th ed. New York, NY: Lippincott Williams & Wilkins; 2000.

Cashen AF, Wildes TM, eds. *The Washington Manual Subspecialty Consult Series: Hematology and Oncology Subspecialty Consult*. 2nd ed. Philadelphia, PA: Lippincott Williams & Wilkins; 2008.

Dale DC, Federman DD, eds. *Web MD Scientific American Medicine*. New York, NY: WebMD; 2002.

Fauci AS, Braunwald E, Iselbacher KJ, et al, eds. *Harrison's Principles of Internal Medicine*. 14th ed. New York, NY: McGraw-Hill; 1998.

Ferri FF, ed. *Practical Guide to the Care of the Medical Patient*. 4th ed. St Louis, MO: CV Mosby; 1998.

Ferri FF, ed. *Practical Guide to the Care of the Medical Patient*. 5th ed. St Louis, MO: Mosby; 2001.

Fischbach F, Dunning MB, eds. *Manual of Laboratory and Diagnostic Tests*. 7th ed. New York, NY: Lippincott Williams & Wilkins, 2004.

Goroll AH, May LA, Mulley AG, eds. *Primary Care Medicine*. 3rd ed. Philadelphia, PA: JB Lippincott; 1995.

Govindan R, Arquette MA, eds. *The Washington Manual of Oncology*. New York, NY: Lippincott Williams & Wilkins; 2002.

Iselbacher KJ, Braunwald E, Wilson JD, et al, eds. *Harrison's Principles of Internal Medicine*. 13th ed. New York, NY: McGraw-Hill; 1994.

Kutty K, Schapira RM, Van Ruiswyk J, et al, eds. *Kochar's Concise Textbook of Medicine*. 4th ed. Philadelphia, PA: Lippincott Williams & Wilkins; 2003.

Lichtman MA, Beutler E, Kipps TJ, et al, eds. *Williams Manual of Hematology*. 6th ed. New York, NY: McGraw-Hill; 2003.

Lichtman MA, Kaushansky K, Kipps TJ, et al. *Williams Manual of Hematology*. 8th ed. New York, NY: McGraw Hill; 2011.

Mazza JJ, ed. *Manual of Clinical Hematology*. 3rd ed. New York, NY: Lippincott Williams & Wilkins; 2002.

McKenzie SB, ed. *Textbook of Hematology*. 2nd ed. Baltimore, MD: Lippincott Williams & Wilkins; 1996.

Pillot G, Chantler M, Magiera H, et al, eds. *The Washington Manual Subspecialty Consult Series: Hematology and Oncology Subspecialty Consult*. New York, NY: Lippincott Williams & Wilkins; 2004.

Tierney LM Jr, McPhee SJ, Papadakis MA, eds. *Current Medical Diagnosis and Treatment (Ambulatory and Inpatient Management)*. Stamford, CT: Appleton & Lange; 1998.

Tierney LM Jr, McPhee SJ, Papadakis MA, eds. *Current Medical Diagnosis and Treatment*. 42nd ed. New York, NY: Lange Medical Books/McGraw-Hill; 2003.

Wagner ND, Bartlett NL. Lymphoma. In: Govindan R, Arquette MA, eds. *The Washington Manual of Oncology*. New York, NY: Lippincott Williams & Wilkins; 2002:chap 14:278–296.

World Health Organization. Classification of neoplastic diseases of the hematopoietic and lymphoid tissues. *Manual of Clinical Oncology*. 4th ed. Philadelphia, PA: Lippincott Williams & Wilkins; 2000.

www.cancer.gov.

www.medscape.com.

Infectious Diseases

Rebecca Lovell Scott

I. Fungal (Mycotic) Infections

A. Aspergillosis

1. **Etiology**
   - *Aspergillus fumigatus*, the most common cause of aspergillosis, is a fungus capable of causing disease in healthy individuals as well as an opportunistic pathogen causing infection in immunocompromised hosts; other species also cause disease.
   - It is characterized by large septate hyphae that branch at a 45° angle.
   - *Aspergillus* is commonly found in garden and houseplant soil and compost.

2. **Pathology**
   - The immunologic status of infected hosts primarily determines the manifestations of the disease.
   - Routes of transmission include inhalation (most common), direct inoculation of the skin, or injection into the blood stream.

3. **Clinical Features**
   - Clinical features vary from a hypersensitivity reaction to life-threatening illness.
     - Allergic bronchopulmonary aspergillosis, found mainly in patients with asthma and also in patients with cystic fibrosis, is characterized by thick, brown, tenacious, mucus plugs in sputum.
   - Acute invasive *Aspergillus* sinusitis may occur in persons with normal or mildly suppressed immunologic function. Symptoms include fever, headache, toothache, epistaxis, and purulent nasal discharge.
   - Aspergilloma occurs when the fungus colonizes existing cavitary pulmonary lesions; it may be an incidental finding or present with hemoptysis because of its propensity for invading blood vessels.
   - Chronic necrotizing pulmonary aspergillosis, although rare, occurs in immunocompromised patients and produces nonproductive cough, dyspnea, and pleuritic chest pain.
   - Potentially fatal invasive or disseminated aspergillosis occurs in severely immunocompromised and neutropenic patients, who may have pleuritic chest pain, cough, necrotic skin lesions, tissue infarction, wound infections, and brain abscesses.

4. **Diagnostic Studies**
   - In an immunocompetent host, isolation of organism from sputum, burn eschar, ear canal debris, or other areas usually does not indicate disease or require treatment.
   - In allergic bronchopulmonary aspergillosis, transient or migratory upper lobe pulmonary infiltrates appear; patients have eosinophilia, markedly high levels of total serum immunoglobulin E, and high titers of anti-*Aspergillus* antibodies.
   - For sinusitis, diagnosis is usually based on histology following surgery.
   - Specific immunoglobulin G (IgG) antibody testing is not helpful for diagnosing disseminated *Aspergillus* in compromised hosts because of immunosuppression.
   - CT scanning of the chest may suggest invasive aspergillosis, but biopsy of lesions is the mainstay of diagnosis. Rounded nodular infiltrates are the most common finding on chest X-ray.
   - Invasive aspergillosis in immunocompromised patients is associated with elevated serum lactate dehydrogenase (LDH).

5. **Management**
   - Allergic bronchopulmonary aspergillosis responds to tapered corticosteroid therapy, postural drainage, and chest physiotherapy. Itraconazole may also be helpful.
   - Sinusitis requires a prolonged course of antifungal agents following surgical debridement in immunocompromised patients.
   - Surgical resection is the treatment of choice for symptomatic aspergilloma.
   - Chronic necrotizing pulmonary aspergillosis may require surgery in addition to antifungals.
   - Severe invasive or disseminated aspergillosis is treated with itraconazole or high-dose amphotericin B.
   - Any underlying disease should be treated.

6. **Prevention**
   - Elimination of environmental exposure and prophylactic antifungal therapy is indicated in immunosuppressed and neutropenic patients.

B. Blastomycosis

1. **Etiology**
   - *Blastomyces dermatitidis*, a dimorphic fungus, occurs as a mold in nature and as a yeast in tissue.
   - Infection usually occurs in immunocompetent men involved in outdoor activities in proximity to waterways.

- The fungus is endemic in southeastern, central, and midwestern United States and Canada, particularly the Mississippi and Ohio River basins.

2. **Pathology**
   - Infection is believed to occur from inhalation of fungus from rotting wood or soil.
   - Pulmonary infection is most common; hematogenously disseminated disease is most likely to affect bone, skin, and genitourinary system.
   - Infection rates are high in endemic areas, but symptomatic disease occurs in only about 50% of infected individuals.

3. **Clinical Features**
   - Disease may be acute or chronic.
   - Dry cough, dyspnea, headache, and fever may resemble influenza or pneumonia.
   - Symptoms may resolve or progress to productive cough, hemoptysis, pleuritic pain, weight loss, and prostration resembling a bacterial pneumonia.
   - Verrucous, crusted, or ulcerated cutaneous lesions expand and may leave a central scar with healing.
   - Ribs and vertebrae are most frequently involved in disseminated bone disease.
   - Symptoms suggesting prostatitis or epididymitis are common.

4. **Diagnostic Studies**
   - Nonspecific laboratory findings include leukocytosis and anemia.
   - Sputum, pus, cerebrospinal fluid (CSF), or tissue analysis reveals readily culture and grow thick-walled cells with single broad-based bud.
   - An available urinary antigen test has considerable cross-reactivity with *Histoplasma* so its utility is not clear.
   - Chest X-ray findings are variable and nonspecific.

5. **Management**
   - Itraconazole is the treatment of choice for most non-life-threatening blastomycosis.
   - Amphotericin B is used for severe or rapidly progressing illness, treatment failures, acquired immunodeficiency syndrome (AIDS) related, and central nervous system (CNS) disease.

6. **Prevention**
   - Patient education and awareness in endemic areas.

C. Coccidioidomycosis

1. **Etiology**
   - *Coccidioides immitis* or *Coccidioides posadasii*, soil molds that grow in arid regions of southwestern United States, Mexico, Central and South America.
   - *Coccidioides immitis* is a possible agent for bioterrorism.

2. **Pathology**
   - Inhalation of highly infectious arthroconidia, the hyphae of the mold form.
   - Coccidioidomycosis is a common opportunistic infection in human immunodeficiency virus (HIV) positive persons in endemic areas.

3. **Clinical Features**
   - Primary disease occurs in about 40% of infections and resembles respiratory tract infection with nasopharyngitis, bronchitis, fever, chills, cough, headache, and pleuritic pain.
   - Pain and swelling of the knees and ankles are common; erythema nodosum may also occur.
   - Persistent pulmonary cavitations, abscesses, nodules, or bronchiectasis occurs in about 5%.
   - Disseminated infection is most common in African Americans, Filipinos, and pregnant women, and can affect any organ system, most commonly skin, bones, joints, and CNS.

4. **Diagnostic Studies**
   - The mold form is highly contagious and must be clearly labeled, so laboratory personnel do not become infected.
   - Diagnosis is established by tube precipitin test and immunodiffusion test to detect immunoglobulin M (IgM) antibodies.
   - Serial serologic (complement fixation) titers assess dissemination of disease and treatment; in HIV-infected patients, the false-negative rate is high.
   - Meningitis is diagnosed with CSF complement-fixing antibodies; CSF also shows lymphocytosis and reduced glucose.
   - Imaging may show pulmonary infiltrates, cavitation, hilar or mediastinal lymphadenopathy, pleural effusions, and lytic bone lesions.

5. **Management**
   - Most cases are asymptomatic and self-limited; localized lung disease is treated symptomatically.
   - Use of amphotericin B, itraconazole, fluconazole, or ketoconazole depends on the severity of disease.
   - Fluconazole is used to treat most patients with CNS disease, although intrathecal amphotericin B, voriconazole, or posaconazole may be used.

6. **Prevention**
   - Patient education and awareness in endemic areas.

D. Cryptococcosis

1. **Etiology**
   - *Cryptococcus neoformans*, a large, thick-walled, encapsulated budding yeast.
   - *Cryptococcus gattii* also causes disease in humans, primarily outside North America.

2. **Pathology**
   - *Cryptococcus neoformans* is present in pigeon and other bird droppings and soil.
   - Infection is acquired through inhalation, causing lung disease that may be localized, self-healing, or disseminated.
   - Immunocompetent persons rarely develop clinical disease, but patients with hematologic cancer, Hodgkin disease, chronic steroid use, HIV infection, or other immunodeficiency states do. It is the most common life-threatening fungal infection in

AIDS patients and the third most common CNS infection in these patients.

3. Clinical Features
- Disseminated cryptococcosis may affect any organ system, but the CNS is most common.
- Onset may be acute or insidious; the more immunosuppressed the patient, the more rapid the onset.
- In cases of CNS involvement, headache is usually the first symptom of meningoencephalitis, followed by a varying course of confusion, irritability, or dizziness appearing over weeks or months without pattern.
- Behavioral changes, fever, seizures, cranial nerve palsies, papilledema, dementia, and decreased level of consciousness may appear later.
- Pulmonary infections are often asymptomatic with minimum sputum production.
- Skin and bone may be involved in disseminated disease.

4. Diagnostic Studies
- Ninety-five percent of patients with AIDS and solid organ transplant will show a positive result for a serum antigen test; the test is also 95% sensitive for cryptococcal meningitis in screening these patients.
- Lumbar puncture is essential and demonstrates increased opening pressure, variable pleocytosis, increased protein, and usually decreased glucose; demonstration of *C. neoformans* by direct examination or cultural isolation from CSF or other infected sites is definitive.
- CT or MRI of the head is indicated for papilledema or focal neurologic signs and may demonstrate cryptococcoma or hydrocephalus; MRI is more sensitive.

5. Management
- Owing to azole resistance, initial treatment with fluconazole is no longer recommended; amphotericin B followed by fluconazole is effective in about 70% of patients; flucytosine is associated with improved survival, but patients must be monitored for toxicity.
- Hydrocephalus or high CSF pressures require ventricular shunting or repeated lumbar punctures.
- Maintenance therapy with fluconazole prevents relapse.

6. Prevention
- Immunosuppressed patients should avoid dried bird droppings.

E. Histoplasmosis
1. Etiology
- *Histoplasma capsulatum* is a dimorphic fungus found in soil contaminated with bat or bird droppings in many areas of the world, especially Ohio and Mississippi River valleys.

2. Pathology
- Infection is acquired by inhalation of spores. Spores convert to budding cells in lungs, proliferate, and spread through the bloodstream and lymphatics.

3. Clinical Features
- Most cases in immunocompetent patients are asymptomatic or mild; primary histoplasmosis typically resembles influenza.
- Acute histoplasmosis, often epidemic, lasts 1 to 6 weeks and is characterized by fever and prostration. Findings on chest radiography may show diffuse pneumonia, but patients have few lung symptoms.
- Progressive disseminated histoplasmosis involves all body organs and is usually fatal. Findings include fever, dyspnea, weight loss, cough, prostration, hepatosplenomegaly, oropharyngeal ulcers, and bloody diarrhea. Adrenal involvement occasionally leads to adrenal insufficiency.
- Chronic progressive pulmonary histoplasmosis occurs primarily in older patients with chronic obstructive pulmonary disease.
- Disseminated disease in severely immunocompromised patients may resemble septic shock.
- Disseminated histoplasmosis is an AIDS-defining illness in persons with a positive HIV test.

4. Diagnostic Studies
- Anemia of chronic disease is common in patients with progressive lung disease.
- Pancytopenia and elevations of alkaline phosphatase, LDH, and transferrin occur in disseminated disease.
- Sputum culture is rarely positive in acute disease; antigen testing of fluid obtained by bronchoalveolar lavage may be helpful.
- In immunocompromised patients, bone marrow and blood cultures are usually positive.
- In AIDS patients with disseminated disease, a urine antigen assay is >90% sensitive; a combination of screening immunodiffusion and complement fixation titers is also helpful.

5. Management
- In limited disease, spontaneous resolution may occur.
- Itraconazole in oral solution is recommended for local or mild-to-moderate disseminated disease and for secondary prevention in those with AIDS.
- Amphotericin B is the treatment of choice for the severely ill, immunocompromised patient and patients with life-threatening or CNS disease.

6. Prevention
- Patient education and awareness in endemic areas; avoidance of areas with droppings.

II. Protozoal Diseases

A. Amebiasis

1. **Etiology**
   - *Entamoeba histolytica*; this must be distinguished from the nearly identical *Entamoeba dispar*, which produces only an asymptomatic carrier state.
   - *Entamoeba histolytica* exists as cysts and motile trophozoites; cysts remain viable in soil and water for weeks to months.
   - In the United States, most cases are in immigrants from and travelers to developing nations; US rates are higher in communal living facilities, daycare centers, and men who have sex with men.
   - Humans are the only hosts; person-to-person transmission can occur, and flying insects are vectors.

2. **Pathology**
   - The amoeba lives as a commensal in most infected persons, and the host serves as a carrier. Amebic dysentery is acquired by ingestion of cysts present in contaminated food or water; excystation occurs in the small intestine; trophozoites become established in the lumen of large intestine where they encyst.
   - Trophozoites invade intestinal epithelium, causing characteristic ulcers, most commonly found in the cecum, descending colon, and rectosigmoid area, but may occur anywhere in the colon or terminal ileum.
   - The liver is the primary site of extraintestinal amebic disease, where typically a single abscess up to 15 cm diameter may form, usually in the upper right lobe; trophozoites may disseminate into lung, pleural cavity, and pericardium, and through bloodstream to brain.

3. **Clinical Features**
   - Following an incubation period of 1 to 4 weeks, some patients have acute diarrhea; however, symptoms range from none or mild to severe colitis.
   - In dysenteric colitis, early stools are watery with streaks of blood, and later with blood and necrotic tissue; patient may have high fever, abdominal cramping and tenderness, nausea and vomiting, and tenesmus.
   - Hepatic amebiasis includes development of fever, pain, and tender enlargement of the liver.
   - Other areas are rarely involved, but include skin, lungs, brain, and genitalia.

4. **Diagnostic Studies**
   - Identification of *E. histolytica* in feces microscopically and stool antigen detection is standard; serologic assays are fairly sensitive after the initial stage of disease.
   - Colonoscopy (without bowel preparation) will identify characteristic ulcers and allow collection of exudates for identification of trophozoites.
   - Ultrasonography, CT, or MRI are all used to identify hepatic abscess.

5. **Management**
   - Choice of amebicides is based on location and severity of infection.
   - Metronidazole and tinidazole both eradicate amebiasis in the bowel lumen, the bowel tissue, and other tissues; diloxanide furoate, iodoquinol, and paromomycin eradicate disease in the bowel lumen.
   - Combination treatment is most effective.

6. **Prevention**
   - Adequate disposal of human feces, and water sanitation and careful hand-washing are essential.
   - Travelers can minimize infection risk by drinking bottled water and by avoiding consumption of unpeeled fruits and vegetables.
   - Amebic cysts are not killed by chlorine; boiling water or treating with iodine or filtering usually ensures the absence of amoebae.

B. Giardiasis

1. **Etiology**
   - *Giardia lamblia*, a large flagellated protozoan with both trophozoite and cyst forms.
   - *Giardia* is the most common cause of epidemic waterborne diarrheal disease in the United States, is the most frequently identified intestinal protozoan in the United States and Europe, and has a large reservoir in animals.
   - It is seen frequently in daycare centers, residential facilities, and, increasingly, in food-borne outbreaks.

2. **Pathology**
   - Cysts are transmitted by the fecal-oral route through contaminated food or water, person-to-person contact, and anal-oral sexual contact.
   - The trophozoites emerge in the duodenum and jejunum, and exist as a flagellated trophozoite or cyst in the stool.

3. **Clinical Features**
   - Most infected persons are asymptomatic and clear the infection spontaneously.
   - **Three symptomatic syndromes occur:**
     - Acute diarrhea, usually mild, with copious, frothy, greasy, foul-smelling stools without blood or pus.
     - Chronic diarrhea is similar, may be daily or recurrent, and may be accompanied by weight loss; growth and cognitive development may be slowed in children. Less common symptoms include loss of appetite, nausea, vomiting, cramping, belching, flatulence, and distension.
     - Malabsorption syndromes may develop with either chronic or acute diarrheal syndromes.

4. **Diagnostic Testing**
   - Obtaining three stool specimens at 2-day intervals increases the likelihood of detection of cysts and trophozoites by microscopy.

- Antigen assays are simpler and less expensive than serial stool examinations, but will not identify other pathogens.
- Occasionally, duodenal aspiration, endoscopic brush cytology, or duodenal biopsy is indicated.

5. Management
- In adults, either tinidazole or metronidazole is used initially; retreatment with albendazole or paromomycin may be needed; paromomycin is safest in pregnant women.
- In children, furazolidone or nitazoxanide is used.
- Follow-up stool studies should begin 2 weeks after treatment.

6. Prevention
- Filtration of water is necessary to eliminate cysts; boiling is also effective.
- Careful hand-washing and separation of food-preparation and diaper-changing tasks in daycare centers are needed.
- Education about safer sex practices.

C. Malaria
1. Etiology
- *Plasmodium falciparum, Plasmodium vivax, Plasmodium ovale*, and *Plasmodium malariae* all infect humans, with *falciparum* and *vivax* causing most disease; malaria is endemic in most tropical and subtropical areas.
- *P. falciparum* predominates in Africa, Haiti, and the Dominican Republic; it causes most deaths.
- Malaria is the most important tropical parasitic disease of humans with more than 1 million deaths annually.

2. Pathology
- Infected female anopheles mosquitoes transmit the disease from person to person; congenital and blood transfusion transmission also occurs.
- **The three typical courses of disease are explained by the protozoan's life cycle:**
  - The mosquito ingests human blood containing gametocytes of the parasite, which develop into sporozoites in the mosquito's salivary glands.
  - The mosquito inoculates humans with sporozoites, which travel to the liver (exoerythrocytic stage), where they transform into merozoites in the hepatic cells.
  - The merozoites are released into the bloodstream and infect red blood cells (erythrocytic stage).
  - In the red blood cells, the merozoites undergo schizogamy, resulting in two asexual and two sexual forms; mature sexual forms infect other red blood cells, repeating the cycle.
- Recurring asexual cycles occur until host immunity stops the erythrocytic cycle.
- In *P. vivax* and *P. ovale*, dormant hepatic sporozoites may resume intrahepatic multiplication, which leads to relapses or delayed primary infection for up to 6 to 8 months.
- Recrudescent disease is recurrence due to the failure of treatment to eradicate infected RBCs.
- *P. falciparum* does not produce a dormant liver stage and does not cause late relapse. *Plasmodium malariae* has no persistent liver stage; relapse occurs due to low-level persistence in the bloodstream.
- Malaria is curable if diagnosed promptly and treated adequately.

3. Clinical Features
- During an attack, a typical sequence over 4 to 6 hours includes the cold stage (shaking chills), hot stage (high fever), and sweating stage (marked diaphoresis). Patients feel well between attacks.
- Attacks may occur every other day or every third day; following the primary attack, latent periods and recurrences are common.
- Hepatosplenomegaly is common.
- *P. falciparum* causes the most serious infection, with high fever, changes in level of consciousness, agitation, prostration, bleeding, and hyperventilation; complications include hypotension, shock, headache, retinal hemorrhages, convulsions, delirium, coma, mental status changes, pulmonary edema, acute tubular necrosis, renal failure, jaundice, cardiac arrhythmias, hypoglycemia, dysentery, electrolyte imbalance, and disseminated intravascular coagulation (DIC).
- "Blackwater fever" refers to dark urine due to severe hemolysis following treatment with quinine.

4. Diagnostic Studies
- Thick and thin blood films from serial finger- or earlobe-stick blood specimens obtained every 8 hours for 3 days demonstrate parasites; repeated blood films confirm success of treatment.
- Rapid antigen detection methods are increasingly available and are nearly as sensitive and specific as blood smear analysis.
- During attacks, leukocytosis may develop, followed by leukopenia with increased monocytes. Patients may also have thrombocytopenia, anemia, and liver function abnormalities.

5. Management
- Successful treatment requires destruction of all forms of parasite.
- Chloroquine is the mainstay of treatment for nonfalciparum and for nonresistant falciparum malarias; quinine and quinidine remain effective for all malaria, but are poorly tolerated.
- In resistant areas, treatments include artemether-lumefantrine, artesunate-amodiaquine, artesunate-mefloquine, amodiaquine-sulfadoxine-pyrimethamine, and dihydroartemisinin-piperaquine.

- Combination therapy may slow spread of drug-resistant malaria; artemisinin derivatives are usually included.
- For *P. vivax* and *P. ovale*, primaquine prevents relapse; it eradicates dormant liver forms of all species.
- Other options include atovaquone plus proguanil (Malarone), tetracycline and doxycycline, clindamycin, azithromycin, halofantrine, and lumefantrine.

6. **Prevention**
   - Avoid contact with mosquito vector (protective clothing, insect repellent, avoidance of endemic areas, and mosquito netting).
   - Chemoprophylaxis depends on resistance patterns; chloroquine is preferred in nonresistant areas.
   - Malarone, mefloquine, or doxycycline in resistant areas, but no prophylaxis is 100% effective.

D. Toxoplasmosis

1. **Etiology**
   - *Toxoplasma gondii*, an obligate intracellular parasite, exists in three forms: the disease-causing trophozoite, the latent cyst, and the infective sporozoite-containing oocysts.
   - Cat species, the definitive hosts, excrete oocysts in feces; these remain infective in moist soil for months to years.

2. **Pathology**
   - Humans become infected by ingesting cysts from raw/undercooked meat, ingesting oocysts from contaminated food or water, handling cat litter carelessly, from transplacental, blood transfusion, or organ-transplantation transmission of trophozoites.
   - Once ingested, bradyzoites from cysts or sporozoites from oocysts invade different types of cells, propagate as trophozoites, and cause cell death and inflammation.
   - Incubation period is 7 to 14 days.

3. **Clinical Features**
   - Initial infection is usually asymptomatic; when symptoms appear, they vary with the type of host involved.
   - In a normal host, the most common manifestation is asymptomatic localized cervical lymphadenopathy; a mild infectious mononucleosis-like illness may occur.
   - Manifestations of congenital toxoplasmosis vary by trimester of infection; first trimester disease is often catastrophic, resulting in abortion or stillbirth. Live-born children may demonstrate microcephaly, hydrocephaly, convulsions, psychomotor retardation, fever, hepatitis, pneumonia, and skin rash. Those infected later in pregnancy demonstrate milder disease at birth, but months later

may develop epilepsy, retardation, strabismus, uveitis, or retinochoroiditis if untreated.
   - In the immunocompromised host, reactivated toxoplasmosis most often affects brain, lungs, and eye, but may affect heart, skin, gastrointestinal (GI) tract, and liver, or present as disseminated disease. Often fatal encephalitis, mass lesions, and diffuse intracerebral lesions are common in patients with AIDS.
   - Chronic latent infection persists in both symptomatic and asymptomatic hosts following initial infection.

4. **Diagnostic Studies**
   - Reliable and sensitive serologic tests of blood, bone marrow, CSF, sputum, placental tissue, and others are the mainstay of diagnosis; identification of parasites in tissue or body fluids using polymerase chain reaction (PCR) is also diagnostic.
   - Chest radiographs may show interstitial pneumonia.
   - In patients with HIV, CT or MRI images show multiple ring-enhancing lesions, primarily in the corticomedullary junction and basal ganglion.

5. **Management**
   - Mild disease in immunocompetent hosts is self-limiting.
   - Pyrimethamine plus sulfadiazine or clindamycin is used for severe or persistent disease; folic acid supplementation and maintenance of urinary output prevent bone marrow suppression and nephrotoxicity, respectively. Other combinations are possible.
   - In immunocompromised patients, prophylaxis is indicated if serology is positive; treatment of acute disease should be followed by continued prophylaxis.
   - Pyrimethamine is teratogenic and contraindicated in first trimester of pregnancy; spiramycin is the standard therapy in pregnancy to prevent transmission to the fetus.

6. **Prevention**
   - Careful hand-washing after handling uncooked meat or working in potentially infected soil.
   - Cook food to safe temperatures and clean food preparation areas and utensils thoroughly.
   - Peel or wash fruits and vegetables thoroughly.
   - Avoid handling cat feces, particularly changing kitty litter; scald litter pans regularly.
   - Wear gloves when gardening and handling cat waste, especially if pregnant.

III. Viral Infections

A. AIDS (Tables 14–1 to 14–3)

1. **Etiology**
   - HIV is a retrovirus. HIV-1 causes AIDS; the related HIV-2 virus, found primarily in West Africans, progresses more slowly.
   - HIV is transmitted between humans by blood and body fluids (e.g., semen; cervical secretions; breast

TABLE 14-1.   1993 Revised CDC HIV Classification System and Expanded AIDS Surveillance Definition for Adolescents and Adults

CD4 Cell Category[a]	Clinical Category			Clinical Category A	Clinical Category B	Clinical Category C
	A	B	C			
(1) ≥500/mm³	A1	B1	C1	Asymptomatic HIV infection	Symptomatic, not A or C conditions	Candidiasis: esophageal, trachea, bronchi
(2) 200–499/mm³	A2	B2	C2	Persistent generalized lymphadenopathy	Examples include, but not limited to:	Coccidioidomycosis, extrapulmonary
(3) <200/mm³	B3	A3	C3	Acute (primary) HIV illness	Bacillary angiomatosis	Cryptococcosis, extrapulmonary
					Candidiasis, vulvovaginal: persistent >1 mo, poorly responsive to treatment	Cervical cancer, invasive[b]
					Candidiasis, oropharyngeal	Cryptosporidiosis, chronic intestinal (>1 mo)
					Cervical dysplasia, severe or carcinoma in situ	CMV retinitis, or CMV in other than liver, spleen, nodes
					Constitutional symptoms, e.g., fever (38.5° C) or diarrhea >1 mo	HIV encephalopathy
						Herpes simplex with mucocutaneous ulcer >1 mo, bronchitis, pneumonia
						Histoplasmosis, disseminated, extrapulmonary
						Isosporiasis, chronic, >1 mo
						Kaposi sarcoma
						Lymphoma, Burkitt immunoblastic primary in brain
						Mycobacterium avium or *Mycobacterium kansasii*, extrapulmonary
						Mycobacterium tuberculosis, pulmonary or extrapulmonary
						Pneumocystis carinii pneumonia
						Pneumonia, recurrent (>2 episodes in 1 y)
						Progressive multifocal leukoencephalopathy
						Salmonella bacteremia, recurrent
						Toxoplasmosis, cerebral
						Wasting syndrome due to HIV

The above diseases must be attributed to HIV infection or have a clinical course or management complicated by HIV.
[a]There is a diurnal variation in CD4 counts averaging 60 per mm³ higher in the afternoon in HIV-positive patients and 500 per mm³ equivalence between CD4 counts and CD4 percentage of total lymphocytes is ≥500 = ≥29%, 200 to 499 = 14% to 28%, <200 = <14%.
From Hume HD, ed. *Kelley's Essentials of Internal Medicine.* 2nd ed. Philadelphia, PA: Lippincott Williams & Wilkins; 2001:601, with permission.

milk; CSF; synovial, pleural, peritoneal, pericardial, and amniotic fluids); through unprotected sexual contact; blood, blood product transfusion, or organ transplantation (before routine screening); needle sharing; transplacental or perinatal infection; and occupational exposure of health-care workers.

- HIV is also present in saliva, tears, and urine, but is not transmitted through these fluids.
- No evidence exists for spread through respiratory droplets, mosquito or other vector bites, or non-sexual contacts.
- Initially a disease of men who have sex with men, AIDS is now increasing most rapidly in women (primarily through heterosexual contact with an infected partner) and African Americans.

2. **Pathology**
- HIV causes immunodeficiency through viral replication within cells.
- HIV can attach to any cell with the T4 (CD4) antigen; chemokine receptors CCR5 and CXCR4 are important for viral entry.
- The CD4 (helper-inducer) cell is the primary site of infection, but HIV may also infect B lymphocytes and macrophages.
- Immunologic defects are related not only to decreasing numbers of CD4 cells, but also to their inability to respond normally; autoimmunity and allergic/hypersensitivity reactions also occur.
- HIV may also cause neurologic, renal, and GI problems by direct infection of these systems.

TABLE 14–2.	Frequency of Symptoms and Findings Associated with Acute HIV-1 Infection in Symptomatic Patients
Symptom or Finding	**Percentage of Patients**
Fever	>80–90
Fatigue	>70–90
Rash	>40–80
Headache	32–70
Lymphadenopathy	40–70
Pharyngitis	50–70
Myalgia or arthralgia	50–70
Nausea, vomiting, or diarrhea	30–60
Night sweats	50
Aseptic meningitis	24
Oral ulcers	10–20
Genital ulcers	5–15
Thrombocytopenia	45
Leukopenia	40
Elevated hepatic-enzyme levels	21

From Kahn JO, Walker BD. Acute human immunodeficiency virus type 1 infection. *N Engl J Med*. 1998;339:33–39, with permission; Copyright © 1998 *Massachusetts Medical Society. All rights reserved.*

TABLE 14–3.	Initial Evaluation of Asymptomatic HIV-Seropositive Patients

History and physical examination
Complete blood cell count with differential and platelet counts
Erythrocyte sedimentation rate
Serum chemistry profile
Urinalysis
Serologic tests
    Hepatitis B and C
    VDRL
    Toxoplasma gondii antibodies[a]
    CMV antibodies[a]
Stool studies for ova and parasites, if indicated
Chest radiograph
Tuberculin skin test
Glucose-6-phosphate dehydrogenase measurement[a]
Measurement of prognostic serologic markers
    Viral load by branched DNA or PCR
    CD4$^+$ lymphocyte count and percentage of total lymphocytes
    ß-Microglobulin concentration[a]

[a]Optional study.
From Hume HD, ed. *Kelley's Essentials of Internal Medicine*. 2nd ed. Philadelphia, PA: Lippincott Williams & Wilkins; 2001:603, with permission.

3. **Clinical Features (Figures 14–1 and 14–2)**
   - The mean time from exposure to HIV to development of symptoms suggesting AIDS is 10 years.
   - Acute HIV-1 infection presents most commonly with fever, fatigue, rash, headache, lymphadenopathy, pharyngitis, myalgias or arthralgias, nausea and vomiting or diarrhea, and night sweats; less common findings include aseptic meningitis, oral ulcers, genital ulcers, thrombocytopenia, leukopenia, and elevated hepatic enzymes.
   - Findings highly specific for HIV infection include hairy leukoplakia of the tongue, disseminated Kaposi sarcoma, and cutaneous bacillary angiomatosis.
   - Generalized lymphadenopathy is common in early HIV infection.
   - Many HIV-positive patients have persistent fever, night sweats, and weight loss even without the presence of opportunistic infection.

4. **Diagnostic Studies**
   - HIV enzyme-linked immunosorbent assay (ELISA) screens for HIV infection; 95% of infected persons test positive within 6 weeks of infection.
   - Results of HIV ELISA must be confirmed with Western blot testing; together these tests are 99.9% specific.
   - Rapid antibody testing produces results in 10 to 20 minutes and must be confirmed by ELISA and Western blot.

   - Anemia, neutropenia, and thrombocytopenia are common in advanced HIV infection.
   - The absolute CD4 lymphocyte count is used to predict HIV progression; <200 cells per μL strongly predicts the risk of opportunistic infection or malignancy in the absence of treatment.
   - CD4 lymphocyte <14% in the absence of treatment is also strongly predictive.
   - HIV viral load is the best test for the diagnosis of infection before seroconversion; it is also used to monitor disease progression and response to treatment.
   - Initially, HIV-positive persons may test positive for purified protein derivative (PPD), rapid plasma reagin (RPR), Venereal Disease Research Laboratory (VDRL), cytomegalovirus (CMV) and toxoplasma IgG serology, or hepatitis screening; Pap smears performed for women.

5. **Management**
   - Serial viral load assessment plus CD4 counts and percentages guide therapy.
   - Management includes antiretroviral treatment, treatment of opportunistic infections, prophylaxis of opportunistic infections (INH; Isoniazed for those with a positive PPD and negative chest radiograph; flu, diptheria tetanus (dT),

FIGURE 14–1. Spectrum of HIV (front view). CHF, congestive heart failure.

pneumococcal, hepatitis A and B, human papillomavirus, haemophilus influenzae type B vaccines), and hematopoietic stimulation.

- Initiation of antiretroviral agents is situation specific. Recommendations include treating all symptomatic patients; asymptomatic persons who have CD4 counts below 500 cells per μL or who

have rapidly dropping CD4 counts or rapidly rising viral loads or those coinfected with hepatitis B or C or who have risk factors for cardiac disease or non-AIDs related cancers.

- Effective highly active antiretroviral therapies (HAART) are combinations of drugs from four major groups:

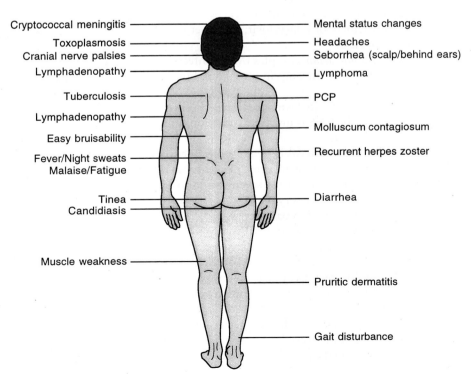

FIGURE 14–2. Spectrum of HIV (rear view). PCP, *Pneumocystis carinii* pneumonia.

- *Nucleoside and nucleotide reverse transcriptase inhibitors:* zidovudine, didanosine, stavudine, lamivudine, emtricitabine, abacavir, zalcitabine, and tenofovir; didanosine, zalcitabine, stavudine, and lamivudine are associated with peripheral neuropathy and emtricitabine with palmar/plantar discoloration.
  - *Protease inhibitors:* indinavir, nelfinavir, ritonavir, saquinavir, fosamprenavir, tipranavir, lopinavir, atazanavir, and darunavir; indinavir is associated with nephrolithiasis.
  - *Nonnucleoside reverse transcriptase inhibitors:* nevirapine, efavirenz, delavirdine, and etravirine.
  - *Entry inhibitors:* enfuvirtide and maraviroc.
  - *Integrase inhibitor:* raltegravir.
- Adherence and drug resistance are major challenges.
- Therapy for opportunistic infections and malignancies depends on specific problem, response to HAART, prior treatment, and the development of drug allergies.
- For *Pneumocystis pneumonia*, options include trimethoprim-sulfa, pentamidine, atovaquone, trimethoprim with dapsone, primaquine with clindamycin, and trimetrexate. Corticosteroid therapy improves the course of moderate to severe disease.
- Cryptococcal meningitis is treated with amphotericin B or fluconazole.
- CMV infection is usually treated with ganciclovir, valganciclovir, or foscarnet.
- Toxoplasmosis is treated with sulfadiazine or clindamycin with pyrimethamine plus folinic acid.
- Herpes simplex infections are treated with acyclovir, famciclovir, or valacyclovir; foscarnet is used in resistant cases.
- *Mycobacterium avium* complex (MAC) infection is treated with clarithromycin plus ethambutol or rifabutin.
- Lymphoma is treated with combination chemotherapy; if the CNS is involved, radiation plus dexamethasone.
- Esophageal candidiasis is treated with fluconazole.
- Prophylaxis for opportunistic diseases is based on CD4 count, the evidence of severe immunosuppression, and the history of prior infection.
- Epoetin alfa is used in patients with anemia (which may be due to zidovudine use) to decrease the need for blood transfusions; human Granulocyte colony-simulating factor (G-SCF) (filgrastim) and granulocyte-macrophage colony-stimulating factor (sargramostim) increase neutrophil counts.

6. **Prevention**
   - Primary prevention includes safer sexual practices, prevention of injective drug use and needle sharing, perinatal HIV prophylaxis, screening of blood products, and infection control processes in the health-care arena; zidovudine/lamivudine prophylaxis is recommended for health-care professionals who sustain needle sticks.
   - The variability in the viral envelope of various HIV strains hampers vaccine development.
   - Secondary prevention includes prophylaxis of opportunistic infections, PPD testing with appropriate follow-up, screening for syphilis, vaccination for pneumonia and hepatitis B, and avoidance of pathogens such as *Toxoplasma*.

B. **Hand-Foot-Mouth Disease**
   1. **Etiology**
      - Coxsackie A16 (an enveloped RNA virus) is the enterovirus implicated most frequently.
      - Coxsackie A5 and A10 and enterovirus 71 may also cause hand-foot-mouth disease (HFM).
   2. **Pathology**
      - Humans are major natural host; illness may represent host immunologic response to tissue injury by virus or to persistent viral antigens.
      - Transmission is by direct contact with nose, throat, discharge, or stools of infected person.
      - Most infections are subclinical.
      - HFM usually occurs in children younger than 5 years.
   3. **Clinical Features**
      - Mild fever, decreased appetite, rhinitis, and pharyngitis begin 3 to 5 days after exposure.
      - Vesicular lesions erupt in oral cavity (chiefly on the buccal mucosa and tongue) and on the distal extremities 1 to 2 days following initial symptoms.
      - Enterovirus 71 causes four stages of disease including HFM/herpangina, CNS disease (central hypoventilation, dysphagia, limb weakness), cardiopulmonary (pulmonary edema), and convalescence.
   4. **Diagnostic Studies**
      - Diagnosis is usually made clinically.
      - In acute phase of disease, diagnosis is most readily established by isolating virus from throat swabs and vesicles; enterovirus 71 may be isolated in the CSF.
   5. **Management**
      - Primarily supportive.
   6. **Prevention**
      - Careful hand-washing and sanitation.

C. **Infectious Mononucleosis (mono)**
   1. **Etiology**
      - Epstein–Barr virus (EBV), an enveloped DNA virus, found as two variants (EBV-1 and -2) of human herpesvirus 4.
      - EBV infection occurs worldwide among humans and usually occurs as a subclinical infection in early childhood; 80% of adults in the United States are seropositive for EBV. The virus persists for life.

- Infectious mononucleosis usually occurs in young adults 15 to 25 years of age, but can occur at any age.
- In the United States and Great Britain, seroconversion occurs in half the population before 5 years of age.

2. Pathology
- The primary mode of transmission appears to be saliva, but it may also be found in genital secretions; incubation is several weeks.
- Saliva may be infectious for 6 or months following onset of symptoms.
- Disease results from viral replication and host immune responses to viral antigens.
- EBV infects epithelial cells of oropharynx and nasopharynx and disseminates to the peripheral blood lymphocytes and plasma.

3. Clinical Features
- Most early infections are asymptomatic, but prodrome of headache, malaise, and fatigue may occur.
- In acute disease, patient has severe sore throat, fever, malaise, myalgia, and anorexia; signs include diffuse pharyngeal inflammation, edema, tonsillar exudates, and tender lymphadenopathy particularly in the posterior cervical chain; 50% of patients have splenomegaly.
- Petechiae on the soft palate may occur; 15% of patients have a maculopapular or petechial rash; this increases to 90% or more if ampicillin is given.
- Fever in adults may go as high as 101° to 102° F; children may be afebrile.
- Some patients develop hepatitis, renal failure, myocarditis, mononeuropathies, aseptic meningitis, encephalitis, dyspnea, or other manifestations.
- Complications include bacterial pharyngitis, splenic rupture, fulminant hepatitis, pericarditis, myocarditis, and, rarely, neurologic problems.

4. Diagnostic Studies
- Complete blood count initially shows granulocytopenia, followed within a week by lymphocytic leukocytosis with many atypical lymphs; thrombocytopenia and hemolytic anemia may rarely occur.
- Heterophil antibody tests become positive within 4 weeks of onset.
- During acute illness, IgM to EB virus capsid antigen (VCA) rises and falls; IgG to VCA rises and persists through life. IgG antibodies to EBV nuclear antigen appear after 4 weeks and persist. PCR analysis may help in detecting illness in children.
- Elevated hepatic aminotransferases and bilirubin are common.

5. Management
- In most cases, symptomatic treatment suffices.
- Corticosteroids are used if lymph node enlargement threatens the airway and for hemolytic anemia and thrombocytopenia.

- Ampicillin and amoxicillin should be avoided for the treatment of coexisting streptococcal pharyngitis; penicillin or erythromycin is preferred to avoid rash.
- Patients must avoid contact and collision sports for at least a month to prevent splenic rupture.

6. Prevention
- Avoidance of sources of infected saliva; careful dishwashing.

D. Mumps

1. Etiology
- Paramyxovirus, an enveloped single-stranded RNA virus, is spread by respiratory droplets and urine.
- Mumps occurs most often in children, in the spring.

2. Pathology
- Incubation period of 14 to 21 days (average 18) after entry into the respiratory tract and the local lymphoid tissue, where virus replicates and then disseminates to target tissues such as salivary glands, pancreas, testes and ovaries, and CNS.
- Tissue response is that of cell necrosis, inflammation, and mononuclear cell infiltration.

3. Clinical Features
- Tender swelling of salivary glands (particularly parotids) and facial edema are the most common findings.
- Swelling may be unilateral or bilateral and persist 7 to 10 days; the openings of Stensen's ducts may be swollen and red.
- Fever may be minimal in small children, but high with meningitis or orchitis.
- Orchitis, usually unilateral, is the most common extrasalivary manifestation in adults; sterility is rare. Oophoritis occurs in 5% of postpubertal women.
- Mumps is the most common cause of pancreatitis in children and is suggested by upper abdominal pain, nausea, and vomiting.
- CNS complications include encephalitis, Guillain–Barré syndrome, facial palsies, and transverse myelitis, but are rare.
- Eighth nerve neuritis is rarely associated with deafness.

4. Diagnostic Studies
- The diagnosis is usually clinical, without laboratory testing.
- Early in the illness, it is possible to isolate the virus from saliva, pharynx, CSF, or duct of the affected salivary gland for culture.
- Serum IgM elevations are diagnostic, although the rise may be delayed in persons who have been immunized.
- Serum amylase elevations are due to salivary gland involvement.
- More than half of patients have mild renal function abnormalities.

5. **Management**
   - For most patients, symptomatic treatment, light diet, and hydration suffice.
   - Patients are usually not contagious 9 days after the onset of parotid swelling and should be isolated until glandular swelling subsides; bed rest is advised until fever is gone.
6. **Prevention**
   - Live attenuated vaccine at 1 year of age with a booster before school.

E. **Rabies**
   1. **Etiology**
      - Rabies encephalitis is caused by a single-stranded RNA virus of the rhabdovirus group.
      - Primarily a viral infection of nonhuman carnivores; in the United States, it is most common in raccoons, skunks, bats, coyotes, and foxes; outside the United States, dogs.
      - The mortality rate exceeds 90%.
   2. **Pathology**
      - The virus gains entry to the body from saliva through a bite or open wound; the more extensive or severe the bite/wound, and the closer to the head and neck, the higher the mortality rate.
      - Incubation period is usually 3 to 7 weeks, but can be 10 days to many years.
      - The virus travels through the nerves to the brain where it multiplies, and then travels back through the efferent nerves to the salivary glands.
   3. **Clinical Features**
      - The prodromal stage begins as 2 to 10 days of pain at the wound site, sore throat, low-grade fever, malaise, headache, anorexia, nausea, and vomiting; hypersensitivity to temperature changes on the skin develops.
      - The CNS stage is most commonly encephalitic (delirium alternating with calm), but may be paralytic, resembling Guillain–Barré syndrome. Painful laryngospasm may occur with swallowing ("hydrophobia").
      - In most cases, coma, autonomic nervous system failure, and death ensue, even with supportive treatment.
   4. **Diagnostic Studies**
      - An apparently healthy biting animal must be observed in quarantine for 10 days; sick or dead animals must be tested for rabies.
      - Direct fluorescent antibody staining of biopsy or necropsy tissue is the standard for diagnosis. Skin biopsy from the back of the neck is 60% to 80% sensitive.
      - Reverse transcriptase–polymerase chain reaction (RT-PCR), nucleic acid sequence-based amplification, direct rapid immunohistochemical test, and viral isolation from CSF or saliva are definitive modalities.

5. **Management**
   - Thorough cleansing and flushing of wounds with soap and water are important; animal bites should not be sutured.
   - Rabies immune globulin (preferred) or antiserum should be infiltrated around the wound.
   - Inactivated rabies vaccine is given in the deltoid on 0, 3, 7, 14, and 28 days after exposure.
   - Symptomatic treatment includes respiratory support and anticonvulsants.
   - The Milwaukee protocol has been helpful in a handful of patients who survived; this includes induction of coma with ketamine, midazolam, and barbiturates, along with the administration of amantadine and ribavirin.
6. **Prevention**
   - Vaccination of domestic and wild animals and avoidance of animal bites.
   - Veterinarians, animal handlers, spelunkers, lab workers using rabies virus, and people planning to visit countries with a high prevalence of dog rabies should undergo preexposure prophylaxis.

F. **Respiratory Syncytial Virus Infection**
   1. **Etiology**
      - Pneumovirus within paramyxovirus family; enveloped virus with a single-stranded genome; produces characteristic fusion of human cells in tissue culture (syncytial effect).
      - Single most important etiologic agent in respiratory diseases of infancy (in infants, major cause of pneumonia and bronchiolitis).
      - Community outbreaks of disease usually occur from late fall to early spring.
   2. **Pathology**
      - Of the two subtypes identified, B is implicated in more severe clinical illness.
      - Transmission of virus to respiratory tract by way of contact with infective secretions (droplet, direct contact, and fomites). Infection is confined to respiratory epithelium with progression to middle and lower airways.
      - Mortality among infants hospitalized with respiratory syncytial virus (RSV) infection is 0.5% to 1%; percentage rises as high as 50 in immunocompromised children.
   3. **Clinical Features**
      - Two- to 8-day incubation period (average 5 days) followed by rhinorrhea and symptoms of common viral upper respiratory tract infection such as cough, pharyngitis, and hoarseness.
      - Progression of severity peaks within 1 to 3 days; fever is variable.
      - Infants may progress to bronchiolitis and pneumonitis with cough, wheezing, and respiratory distress.

- Tachypnea, hypoxemia, hypercapnia occur, along with interstitial infiltrates or pulmonary collapse on chest radiography.
- Milder illness in older children and adults includes rhinorrhea, pharyngitis, tracheobronchitis, and cough. RSV can cause acute flare-ups of chronic bronchitis and trigger asthma exacerbations.
- Symptoms usually resolve within 5 to 7 days.
- *Streptococcus pneumoniae* otitis media is a common complication.

4. Diagnostic Studies
- Immunofluorescent antibody (IFA) or ELISA tests detect viral antigen in the cytoplasm of nasopharyngeal epithelial cells; culture remains the gold standard, but PCR is used increasingly often.

5. Management
- Treatment includes hydration, humidification, and ventilatory support as needed.
- Corticosteroids, bronchodilators, and ribavirin are used in the majority of children, but controlled studies have shown that they are of limited or no benefit; pregnant women should avoid ribavirin.
- Palivizumab, a monoclonal RSV antibody, has replaced RSV immune globulin. Infants with high-risk conditions such as heart disease should receive palivizumab.

6. Prevention
- Good hand-washing, barriers to protect hands and conjunctivae in settings where high rates of transmission occur, and contact isolation are important.

G. Severe Acute Respiratory Syndrome

1. Etiology
- Caused by the virulent severe acute respiratory syndrome associated coronavirus (SARS-CoV).
- The primary mode of transmission appears to be respiratory droplet and fomite contact with mucous membranes of the mouth, nose, or eyes.
- SARS has been traced to a health-care worker in China in 2002, with rapid spread to Hong Kong, Singapore, Taiwan, Vietnam, and Toronto; now seen in 30 countries, including the United States.

2. Pathology
- SARS is an atypical pneumonia that may be asymptomatic, mild, moderate, or severe, and is found in persons of all ages.
- The incubation period is 2 to 7 days; spread to contacts of patients occurs for up to 10 days.

3. Clinical Features
- Persistent fever (>100.4° F) is usually accompanied by chills, rigors, cough, shortness of breath, rales, and rhonchi. Headache, malaise, myalgia, and sore throat are common.
- Watery diarrhea may occur late in the disease.
- In elderly patients, the only findings may be malaise and delirium.

4. Diagnostic Studies
- Chest radiographic findings may be normal or nonspecific; high-resolution computed radiography scan is likely to show ground-glass opacifications or focal consolidations.
- RT-PCR for SARS-CoV in urine, stool, and nasal secretion is often negative early in the disease, but variably positive by day 14. Stool is most likely to be positive; serum serologies may not be positive for 3 weeks.
- Leukopenia and lymphopenia are common; many patients have low-grade DIC.
- Arterial oxygen saturation is usually <95%.

5. Management
- Suspected cases should be reported to state health departments.
- Intensive supportive treatment may be required.
- Evidence for the use of corticosteroids, ribavirin, interferon 1, and systemic steroids is not definitive.

6. Prevention
- Clinicians evaluating suspected cases should use standard respiratory precautions.
- Family members and health-care workers caring for a SARS patient should use standard infection control precautions and respiratory isolation.

H. West Nile Fever

1. Etiology
- The West Nile virus (WNV) is a *flavivirus* (an arbovirus) which causes encephalitis in humans.

2. Pathology
- Infected mosquitoes are the primary vectors; birds are the main reservoir of infection.
- Person-to-person transmission may occur through blood transfusion, organ transplantation, transplacental transmission, and possibly breast milk.
- First reported in North America in 1999 in New York City area, WNV is found in the entire United States. The homeless appear to be particularly susceptible.
- Outbreaks tend to occur in late summer and early fall.

3. Clinical Features
- The incubation period is 2 to 14 days. Most infected people are asymptomatic; 20% develop a flu-like illness (fever, sore throat, headache, fatigue, malaise, nausea, and vomiting), typically lasting 3 to 6 days.
- Less than one-third of patients develop a roseolar or maculopapular rash on face and trunk.
- The most common neurologic signs are stiff neck and mental status changes; 10% of patients develop flaccid paralysis, about 5% seizures. Muscle weakness reminiscent of Guillain–Barré syndrome is common.

- Young patients tend to develop the febrile syndrome, adults aseptic meningitis, and elderly encephalitis. Elderly patients have the greatest mortality.

4. **Diagnostic Studies**
   - IgM capture ELISA can be done on serum or CSF for diagnosis.
   - Acute and convalescent IgM antibody titers may confirm acute infection.
   - PCR testing was introduced in 2003 for blood donor screening.

5. **Management**
   - Intensive supportive measures are the only treatment. Intravenous immunoglobulin or interferon α is possibly effective.
   - West Nile meningitis and encephalitis are reportable diseases.

6. **Prevention**
   - No human arbovirus vaccine is available.
   - Mosquito control is essential, including drainage of standing water.
   - Use of insect repellent with DEET (N, N-diethyl-meta-toluamide); wearing long-sleeved shirts, long pants, and socks; and avoiding outdoor activities between dusk and dawn when mosquitoes are most prevalent are helpful.

IV. Bacterial Diseases

A. Anthrax

1. **Etiology**
   - *Bacillus anthracis.*
   - Spore-forming, aerobic, gram-positive rod; the spores are infectious.
   - Naturally occurring disease, found in sheep and goats, cattle, horses, and pigs; human disease is rare, caused by inhalation or ingestion of spores, contact with infected animals or their products, or soil inoculation.
   - Anthrax is a category A bioterrorism threat.

2. **Pathology**
   - Spores germinate into bacteria that multiply locally in the skin or GI tract or disseminate; inhaled spores are carried to the regional lymph nodes before they germinate, causing hemorrhagic disease.
   - Sepsis occurs when the germs invade the blood stream.
   - Plasmid pXO1 encodes genes for lethal toxin, responsible for shock syndrome, and edema toxin, responsible for prominent edema in cutaneous anthrax. pXO2 encodes genes for capsule production, which protects bacteria from immune defenses.

3. **Clinical Features**
   - Cutaneous anthrax (most common) occurs within 2 weeks of exposure, beginning with a small, inflamed pruritic papule resembling an insect bite.

This ulcerates and necroses, developing a black painless eschar surrounded by edema and vesicles. In severe cases of cutaneous anthrax, regional tender lymphadenopathy, fever, headache, malaise, nausea, and vomiting may occur.
   - Inhalational anthrax (<5% of cases) has a biphasic clinical pattern with an initial 1- to 3-day period of fever, malaise, dry cough, substernal pressure beginning about 10 days after exposure. The second, fulminant phase begins suddenly, typically progressing to death from sepsis in 1 to 2 days.
   - GI anthrax has not been reported in the United States; it follows ingestion of insufficiently cooked contaminated meat. Patients have oral-pharyngeal or abdominal syndromes.

4. **Diagnostic Studies**
   - Culture of skin lesion, blood, pleural fluid, or CSF reveals typical organisms (chains of "box-car" encapsulated rods).
   - Other tests are available through the Centers for Disease Control and Prevention (CDC).
   - Mediastinal widening on chest radiography is a hallmark of inhalational disease.

5. **Management**
   - Ciprofloxacin is the drug of choice; doxycycline is also first line. Other agents include amoxicillin, penicillin G, rifampin, clindamycin, clarithromycin, erythromycin, vancomycin, and imipenem. Combination therapy is recommended in many cases.

6. **Prevention**
   - In case of an outbreak, prophylaxis consists of ciprofloxacin or doxycycline for 100 days or vaccination with an investigational agent and 40 days of antibiotic.
   - Existing stores of an approved vaccination are reserved for military personnel and others at high risk for exposure to spores.
   - Patients with draining lesions should be placed in contact isolation.

B. Botulism

1. **Etiology**
   - *Clostridium botulinum,* a spore-forming anaerobic bacillus found in soil, produces a neurotoxin that causes paralysis.
   - Toxin types A, B, E, and F cause human disease.
   - Botulism occurs in food-borne, infant, and wound forms; infant form is associated with ingestion of honey and wound form with injecting drug use.
   - The CDC has classified the toxin as a high-priority agent of terrorism because of its potency.

2. **Pathology**
   - The botulinum exotoxin binds to the synapses of motor neurons and inhibits the release of the neurotransmitter acetylcholine.

3. **Clinical Features**
   - Twelve to 36 hours following ingestion, diplopia, loss of accommodation, and other visual changes occur, followed by ptosis, cranial nerve palsies, and fixed, dilated pupils.
   - Most frequent symptoms in food-borne botulism are dysphagia, dry mouth, dysarthria, fatigue, upper-extremity weakness, constipation, lower-extremity weakness, dyspnea, nausea and vomiting, and dizziness; respiratory dysfunction may occur from upper airway obstruction or respiratory weakness.
   - Paralysis, respiratory failure, and death occur.

4. **Diagnostic Studies**
   - Presumptive diagnosis is made in the presence of rapidly descending paralysis in a patient with history of ingestion of home-canned food or honey.
   - Demonstration of botulinum toxin in the patient's serum or feces or in the suspected food source using a mouse toxin-neutralization test confirms the diagnosis.

5. **Management**
   - Patients should be admitted to an intensive care unit for intubation and monitoring and support of respiratory and cardiac function.
   - State or federal health officials can assist in obtaining antitoxin to neutralized unabsorbed toxin.
   - Prompt diagnosis decreases chance of death; full recovery may take 3 months to 1 year.

6. **Prevention**
   - Maintenance of food at an acid pH; storage at <4° C; thorough heating before serving.
   - Careful home canning.
   - Infants should not eat honey.

C. Brucellosis

1. **Etiology**
   - *Brucella* species (aerobic, slow-growing, non-motile, facultative intracellular gram-negative coccobacilli).
   - The most common animal vectors are cattle, hogs, and goats.
   - Rare in the United States, it is endemic in Mexico, the Mediterranean lands, Spain, and South America.
   - Pulmonary forms of brucellosis are a category B (see VIII) bioterrorist threat.

2. **Pathology**
   - Transmission to humans is usually from handling of infected tissues or ingestion of infected unpasteurized milk and cheese.

3. **Clinical Features**
   - Onset may be abrupt with fever, chills, and sweats.
   - Insidious onset is more common; patients experience low-grade fever, weakness, myalgia, arthralgia, headache, anorexia, weight loss, and easy exhaustion.

   - Undulant fever occurs in chronic disease with intermittent periods of normal temperature between episodes.
   - Hepatosplenomegaly and lymphadenopathy are common.
   - Complications include endocarditis, meningitis, encephalitis, epididymitis, orchitis, osteoarticular disease with septic arthritis, sacroiliitis, spondylitis, or osteomyelitis.

4. **Diagnostic Studies**
   - *Brucella* species may be recovered from the culture of blood, bone marrow, CSF, urine, and other sites.
   - Serum agglutination titer or rising serum titers are the usual means of diagnosis.

5. **Management**
   - Doxycycline plus rifampin and/or streptomycin and/or gentamicin is recommended.
   - Postexposure prophylaxis is reserved for cases of febrile illness or accidental veterinary vaccine inoculation.

6. **Prevention**
   - Eliminating livestock disease through vaccination, pasteurization of milk, and use of universal precautions are effective preventive measures.
   - No human vaccine is available.
   - Because brucellosis is the most common laboratory-acquired infection, laboratories should use BL-3 safety measures.

D. Campylobacter Dysentery

1. **Etiology**
   - *Campylobacter jejuni* is one of the most common causes of gastroenteritis worldwide.
   - Comma-shaped gram-negative rods are commonly occurring in pairs.

2. **Pathology**
   - Infection occurs with ingestion of contaminated water, raw milk, and food (especially poultry).
   - *Campylobacter jejuni* colonizes the jejunum where it elaborates an enterotoxin.
   - Three to 5 days after ingestion, overt disease occurs if organism penetrates and invades epithelial cells.

3. **Clinical Features**
   - Abrupt onset of watery diarrhea with occasional abdominal cramping relieved by defecation, plus pain, malaise, and fever.
   - Grossly bloody, loose, or watery stools occur in nearly half of patients.
   - Although frequently self-limiting, it can last more than 1 week in 10% to 20% of patients; relapse occurs in 5% to 10% of untreated patients.

4. **Diagnostic Studies**
   - Dark-field or phase contrast microscopy identifies gram-negative, S- or seagull-shaped bacteria in watery, bloody, leukocyte-filled feces.
   - Stool culture confirms the diagnosis.

5. **Management**
   - Course of disease may be shortened with treatment and is indicated in patients with high fevers, bloody stools, worsening symptoms, or unrelenting defecation.
   - Azithromycin and ciprofloxacin are both effective, although fluoroquinolone resistance is rising.
   - Fluid and electrolyte replacement is important.
6. **Prevention**
   - Cook food, especially poultry, thoroughly and wash hands frequently.
   - Ingest only pasteurized milk; wash fruits and vegetables before use.

E. **Cat-Scratch Disease**
   1. **Etiology**
      - *Bartonella henselae.*
   2. **Pathology**
      - Cat-scratch disease is primarily found in children and young adults.
      - The major arthropod vector is the cat flea, which is responsible for cat-to-cat transmission.
      - Transmission to humans occurs through scratch, bite, or other contact with infected secretions.
   3. **Clinical Features**
      - A papule or ulcer may develop within days at the inoculation site.
      - Low-grade fever, headache, and vague and generalized aches and pains follow in 1 to 3 weeks.
      - Enlarged tender regional nodes develop 1 to 7 weeks after inoculation and slowly regress within 2 to 4 months; some may suppurate.
      - In HIV-positive persons, disseminated disease (bacillary angiomatosis, peliosis hepatis) occurs.
   4. **Diagnostic Studies**
      - Diagnosis is usually based on history and physical examination.
   5. **Management**
      - Cat-scratch disease is usually self-limited in immunocompetent persons; macrolides or doxycyclines are used in the immunosuppressed.
   6. **Prevention**
      - Avoidance of cat scratches.

F. **Cholera**
   1. **Etiology**
      - *Vibrio cholerae* is a slightly curved gram-negative rod that elaborates an exotoxin (enterotoxin).
      - Only serogroups O1 and O139 are associated with cholera.
      - Cholera occurs in epidemics in conditions of poor sanitation and crowding in warm seasons.
   2. **Pathology**
      - Organisms that survive stomach and upper intestinal acidity attach to microvilli of brush border of epithelial cells of jejunum and ileum, where they multiply and liberate cholera enterotoxin and mucinase, but do not invade the mucosa.
      - The enterotoxin produces changes leading to massive hypersecretion of water and chloride ions, resulting in up to 15 L of diarrhea daily. Death results from hypovolemia.
   3. **Clinical Features**
      - Onset of symptoms is characterized by abrupt, painless, voluminous, watery diarrhea that may lead to several liters of fluid loss within a few hours; if uncontrolled, this may lead to profound shock; vomiting may follow or precede diarrhea; fever is rarely present.
      - Stools are gray and without fecal odor, blood, or pus ("rice water stool").
      - Patient may be cyanotic with sunken eyes and cheeks, scaphoid abdomen, poor skin turgor, thready or absent peripheral pulses reflecting hypotension and dehydration.
   4. **Diagnostic Studies**
      - Stool culture or agglutination studies.
   5. **Management**
      - Oral or intravenous fluid replacement is the basis of treatment.
      - Antibiotic administration will shorten the course of the disease, but multiple resistance occurs.
   6. **Prevention**
      - Avoidance of endemic areas.
      - A vaccine is available, but provides only short-term protection, and it is not useful in managing outbreaks.
      - Clean water and food and appropriate sanitation are the most effective prevention.

G. **Diphtheria**
   1. **Etiology**
      - *Corynebacterium diphtheriae*, a small pleomorphic gram-positive rod.
      - Rare in the United States.
      - Humans are the only known reservoir for *C. diphtheriae.*
   2. **Pathology**
      - The organism is spread by respiratory secretions and usually affects the respiratory tract, but may involve any mucous membrane or skin wound.
      - *C.* produces a potent exotoxin that causes an inflammatory response and the formation of a pseudomembrane on the respiratory mucosa; it is also absorbed by the circulatory system and distributed throughout the body.
      - Exotoxin also inhibits protein synthesis, which can damage the kidneys, heart, and nerves.
      - Death is due to either aspiration of membrane or diphtheria's toxigenic effect on heart.
   3. **Clinical Features**
      - Diphtheria occurs in nasal, laryngeal, pharyngeal, and cutaneous forms; pharyngeal is most common.

- After an incubation of 2 to 4 days, pharyngitis or tonsillitis, malaise, fever, and adenitis develop.
- Dense gray-white "pseudomembrane" in oropharynx may extend to larynx and trachea; scraping discloses intense underlying inflammation and edema.
- In mild cases, infection resolves and the membrane is coughed up after 5 to 10 days.
- Most common serious complications are myocarditis and neuropathies.

4. **Diagnostic Studies**
- Diagnosis is made clinically, but *C. diphtheriae* can be cultured on selective media from infected site.

5. **Management**
- Immediate administration of diphtheria antitoxin (available from the CDC) neutralizes the toxin.
- Removal of the membrane may be needed to alleviate airway obstruction.
- Hospitalization and isolation are needed until three cultures document elimination of organism.
- Erythromycin or penicillin eliminates the organism; azithromycin and clarithromycin are options; antibiotic therapy should not be substituted for antitoxin therapy.
- Manage complications of disease by supportive measures.

6. **Prevention**
- The diphtheria, pertussis, and tetanus (DPT) vaccine provides active immunity. However, antitoxin levels decline slowly over time, and booster doses of toxoid should be given at 10-year intervals.
- Contacts should receive erythromycin prophylaxis.

H. Disseminated *M. avium* Infection
1. **Etiology**
- MAC.
- This acid-fast, rod-shaped nonmotile organism is not communicable from person to person.

2. **Pathology**
- MAC produces a range of conditions from asymptomatic colonization to disseminated disease.
- Disseminated disease occurs in late HIV infection in patients with low CD4 counts.

3. **Clinical Features**
- Fever and weight loss are the most common symptoms.
- Other signs and symptoms depend on the site of infection.

4. **Diagnostic Studies**
- Blood cultures have a sensitivity of 98% and are the preferred diagnostic modality.
- MAC may also be cultured from the liver, lymph nodes, and bone marrow.

5. **Management**
- MAC is resistant to most conventional antituberculosis drugs; it also rapidly develops secondary resistance, so combination therapy is indicated.

- The treatment of choice is clarithromycin with ethambutol, with or without rifabutin; azithromycin is also effective.
- It is permissible to discontinue treatment in patients on HAART who have been treated for a year for disseminated MAC, who have no evidence of active disease, and whose CD4 counts exceed 100 cells per μL.

6. **Prevention**
- HIV-infected persons whose CD4 counts are <50 cells per μL should receive single-drug prophylaxis.

I. Erysipeloid
1. **Etiology**
- *Erysipelothrix rhusiopathiae* has a worldwide distribution in a variety of animals, especially hogs.

2. **Pathology**
- This occupational disease follows skin abrasion or puncture wound from contact with fish, shellfish, meat, and poultry.
- Infection is usually limited to skin (mainly hands, fingers).

3. **Clinical Features**
- Incubation period is 2 to 7 days.
- Patients experience severe pain described as burning, itching, throbbing; nonpitting edema; purplish erythema with sharp, irregular margins extending peripherally, but clearing centrally; absent or low-grade fever.
- Endocarditis occurs rarely.
- Erysipeloid is self-limiting and usually resolves without treatment in 3 to 4 weeks.

4. **Diagnostic Studies**
- Diagnosis is usually based on the typical clinical appearance in person with occupational exposure highly suggestive of infection.
- The organism may be cultured from biopsy material.

5. **Management**
- Penicillin G, cephalosporins, clindamycin, imipenem, and ciprofloxacin.
- Penicillin and imipenem are the most active agents in vitro.

J. Leprosy (Hansen Disease)
1. **Etiology**
- *Mycobacterium leprae* is an acid-fast gram-variable, rod-shaped obligate intracellular bacterium.
- It is endemic in tropical and subtropical areas of Africa, Asia, Central America, and South America, but is rare in the United States.

2. **Pathology**
- Leprosy is a chronic intracellular infectious disease unique to humans; its mode of transmission is thought to be respiratory.
- Development of disease requires prolonged childhood exposure.

- Two main types of disease occur: lepromatous and tuberculoid.
- Lepromatous is more malignant and progressive, and occurs in persons who lack cellular resistance.
- Tuberculoid is more benign and less likely to progress, and occurs in persons with intact immunity.
- Borderline or intermediate cases occur.
- Leprosy is usually not fatal and has predilection for cooler body areas (grows best at 37° C).

3. **Clinical Features**
- In lepromatous leprosy, patients have nodular skin lesions and slowly evolving, symmetrical nerve involvement.
- In tuberculoid leprosy, patients have macular lesions and sudden onset of sever asymmetric nerve involvement.
- Most deformity is due to trauma to, or secondary infection of, denervated tissues. Peripheral nerve damage is most common in ulnar nerve distribution (clawing of fourth and fifth fingers), posterior tibialis (clawing of toes and plantar anesthesia), and superficial peroneal (foot drop).
- Fine touch, temperature, and pain are impaired, whereas proprioception and vibratory sensation remain intact.
- Skin changes include symmetrically distributed macules, papules, plaques, nodules (lepromas); loss of eyebrows, eyelashes; rarely loss of scalp hair; leonine facies; thickened pendulous ears; spider telangiectasias; and edema of extremities.
- Eye changes include conjunctival and episcleral nodules; beading of corneal nerves; superficial punctate keratitis; interstitial keratitis with pannus formation of chronic plastic iridocyclitis.
- Upper respiratory changes include nasal stuffiness, coryza, epistaxis, and ulcers; ulcers of uvula, tonsils; loss of teeth; septal perforation, nasal collapse, hoarseness, stridor, asphyxia.
- Other organ/system changes may include hepatomegaly, splenomegaly, lymphadenopathy, testicular invasion and destruction, gynecomastia, cystic bone changes in distal phalanges, and skeletal muscle invasion. The kidneys are usually spared unless immune complex nephritis or amyloidosis occurs.
- Infection does not confer permanent immunity.

4. **Diagnostic Studies**
- Leprosy is usually diagnosed by the presence of the characteristic peripheral nerve abnormality or the demonstration of acid-fast bacillus in the affected skin or nerve tissue.
- Lepromin skin test, used primarily in research, is usually negative in lepromatous disease, but positive in tuberculoid.

- Biologic false-positive serologic tests for syphilis, antithyroglobulin antibody, and rheumatoid factor occur.

5. **Management**
- Lepromatous and borderline cases require combination therapy with dapsone, rifampin, and clofazimine for 2 to 3 years because of single-drug development of resistance.
- Tuberculoid leprosy is treated with dapsone and rifampin for 6 to 12 months followed by dapsone for 2 years.
- Prevention of disability from nerve damage and management of complications are essential.

K. Salmonellosis

1. **Etiology**
- *Salmonella enterica* is a motile gram-negative rod with many serotypes (~2,000); serotypes typhi, typhimurium, and choleraesuis cause almost all human infection.

2. **Pathology**
- Salmonella gastroenteritis is transmitted through the fecal-oral route; it has a large animal reservoir and is transferred to humans by contaminated food (especially poultry, dairy products, meat, and eggs) or through handling of exotic pets, especially reptiles.
- Enteric (typhoid) fever is caused by *Salmonella* species; "typhoid" is used only with serotype "typhi"; infection is transmitted by contaminated food and drink; the organisms cross the epithelium of the intestine and invade and replicate in macrophages in the mesenteric lymph nodes, spleen, and Peyer patches. The infection then localizes in the lymphoid tissues of the small intestine. Disseminated disease may occur in the lungs, gallbladder, kidneys, and CNS.

3. **Clinical Features**
- Gastroenteritis: after incubation of 6 to 48 hours, fever, chills, nausea and vomiting, cramping, abdominal pain and diarrhea, headache, and muscle aches; diarrhea may be bloody. The disease is usually self-limiting, but in patients with sickle cell disease, bacteremia and localization to joints and bones may occur.
- Enteric fever: the prodrome lasts 7 to 10 days with malaise, headache, cough, sore throat, abdominal pain, constipation, and stepwise fever. The patient then becomes much more ill with constipation or "pea soup" diarrhea, abdominal distension and tenderness, and possibly splenomegaly. The characteristic "rose spot" rash on the trunk appears in the second week; this is a 2- to 3-mm pink papule that fades with pressure. Improvement takes 1 to 2 weeks.
- Complications of enteric fever include intestinal hemorrhage, which may lead to death; rarer complications include urinary retention, pneumonia, thrombophlebitis, myocarditis, psychosis, cholecystitis, nephritis, osteomyelitis, and meningitis.

4. **Diagnostic Studies**
   - Gastroenteritis: isolation of organism from stool specimen; leukocytes in stool; serotyping in outbreaks.
   - Enteric fever: blood culture is preferred.
5. **Management**
   - Gastroenteritis: fluid and electrolyte replacement if uncomplicated; ciprofloxacin, trimethoprim/sulfamethoxazole (TMP/SMX), or ampicillin in severe cases, malnourished or severely ill patients, and those with sickle cell disease or HIV.
   - Enteric fever: intravenous or oral ciprofloxacin, levofloxacin, ceftriaxone, or other antibiotic suggested by sensitivity testing; ciprofloxacin is usually used for treating carrier state.
6. **Prevention**
   - Careful food handling, waste disposal, and water treatment.
   - For typhoid fever: immunization of household contacts, of travelers to endemic areas, and during epidemics.

L. Shigellosis

SHIGELLA DYSENTERY

1. **Etiology**
   - *Shigella sonnei* in majority of cases, followed by *Shigella flexneri*; *Shigella dysenteriae* in most serious cases.
   - Invasive nonmotile gram-negative facultative rod.
   - Shigellosis is the most communicable of the bacterial diarrheas.
2. **Pathology**
   - Shigellosis is transmitted by the fecal-oral route.
   - Bacteria invade intestinal mucosa producing local inflammation and ulceration.
   - An enterotoxin may cause watery diarrhea by inducing intestinal secretion.
3. **Clinical Features**
   - Following a 1- to 4-day incubation period, patients have abrupt onset of diarrhea mixed with blood and mucus, lower abdominal cramps, tenesmus, distention, malaise, and fever lasting an average of 7 days.
   - Sigmoidoscopy shows punctuate areas of ulceration and inflamed mucosa.
   - Some patients develop disaccharidase deficiency following shigellosis; occasional reactive arthritis occurs.
4. **Diagnostic Studies**
   - Fecal smear shows leukocytes and erythrocytes.
   - Stool culture is usually positive, but blood culture is not.
5. **Management**
   - Supportive care including hydration and electrolyte replacement may be required in elderly, young, or immunocompromised patients.
   - TMP/SMX or a fluoroquinolone is the treatment of choice in adults; ampicillin resistance is

common. Azithromycin has been used to treat multidrug-resistant *Shigella*.
   - Antibiotic treatment is important in limiting course of disease and may decrease the chance of complications and transmission.
6. **Prevention**
   - Good public health and education programs; hand-washing before handling food.
   - Refrigeration and proper cooking of potentially infected food.

M. Tetanus

1. **Etiology**
   - Neurotoxin tetanospasmin produced by *Clostridium tetani*.
   - Unvaccinated persons account for most cases, including newborns, elderly persons, injecting drug users, and migrant workers.
2. **Pathology**
   - Spores of *C. tetani* are found in the soil; they germinate when introduced into a wound.
   - Any wound may become colonized; puncture wounds are the most common.
   - The average incubation period is 8 to 12 days.
   - Tetanospasmin acts at the spinal of inhibitory neurons, where it cleaves a protein needed for the release of neurotransmitters.
3. **Clinical Features**
   - Diagnosis is suggested by a wound or recent history of wound without a clear history of tetanus immunization.
   - Pain and tingling occurs at the wound site, then muscle spasm of adjacent muscles.
   - Other early signs include jaw stiffness, dysphagia, stiff neck, and irritability.
   - Progression occurs usually over 2 weeks with hyperreflexia, spasms of the jaw muscles ("lockjaw" or trismus); other muscles may exhibit spasm and rigidity including facial, abdominal, neck, and back.
   - Minor stimuli precipitate painful tonic convulsions.
   - Death may occur because of spasms of the glottis and respiratory muscles.
   - Patients demonstrate clear mentation; sensory examination is normal.
4. **Diagnostic Studies**
   - This is a clinical diagnosis; however, patients will show moderate leukocytosis, normal CSF, and normal serum calcium.
   - Attempts to culture *C. tetani* from wounds are not useful in diagnosis.
5. **Management**
   - Supportive care until toxin is metabolized includes monitoring in quiet, nonstimulating environment; sedation; paralysis and mechanical ventilation as needed.

- Intramuscular administration of tetanus immune globulin neutralizes circulating toxin; the role of intrathecal administration is under study.
- Although the course of tetanus is not affected by debridement, appropriate wound care is essential.
- Intravenous penicillin is the drug of choice for eradication of *C. tetani*.
- Once well, the patient should have a full series of tetanus toxoid immunizations.

6. **Prevention**
   - DPT vaccine series in children; primary immunization in adults consists of two doses of tetanus toxoid 4 to 6 weeks apart and a third 6 to 12 months later.
   - Tetanus and diphtheria toxoids every 10 years throughout life or at the time of an injury if more than 5 years since the last dose.

V. Rickettsial Diseases

A. Ehrlichiosis

1. **Etiology**
   - Two forms exist in the United States: human monocytic ehrlichiosis (HME), caused by *Ehrlichia chaffeensis* and *Ehrlichia canis*; and human granulocytotropic ehrlichiosis (HGE), caused by *Anaplasma phagocytophilum* and *Ehrlichia ewingii*.
   - These are tick-borne gram-negative obligate intracellular organisms that exhibit tropism for either macrophages or granulocytes.
   - Ehrlichiosis occurs year-round in areas where ticks are active; incidence peaks in summer.

2. **Pathology**
   - The major vector of HME is the lone star tick and is endemic in the southeast, mid-Atlantic, and south central United States; vectors of HGE are deer ticks of the *Ixodes* species with the same geographic distribution as *Borrelia burgdorferi* (see Lyme disease).
   - Nonhuman hosts for HME-causing organisms include mice, dogs, and horses; for HGE-causing organisms, wood rats, deer mice, chipmunks, white-tailed deer, and white-footed mice.
   - Both types have a 7- to 10-day incubation period; the organism is present most commonly in blood, but can also be present in lymph nodes and bone marrow.

3. **Clinical Features**
   - Prodromal symptoms include rigors, malaise, and nausea, followed by abrupt onset of high fever, toxicity, myalgia, headache, and nausea.
   - Usually no rash; a few people develop maculopapular or petechial rash.
   - May progress to acute respiratory and renal failure and encephalopathy.
   - In case of HGE, fevers and malaise may occur for 2 years or more.

- Coinfection with Lyme disease or babesiosis may occur.

4. **Diagnostic Studies**
   - Leukopenia, lymphopenia, thrombocytopenia, and elevated liver transaminases are found.
   - For HME and HGE, nucleic acid amplification by PCR is sensitive and highly specific.
   - Serologic diagnosis by IFA in acute and convalescent serum is the most widely available technique.

5. **Management**
   - Oral or intravenous doxycycline is the treatment of choice.

6. **Prevention**
   - Avoidance of tick-infested areas, protective clothing, and use of tick repellent.

B. Rocky Mountain Spotted Fever

1. **Etiology**
   - *Rickettsia rickettsii*.
   - In the United States, most cases occur along the mid-Atlantic and southeastern seaboard and Mississippi River valley.
   - Most cases occur late spring and summer.

2. **Pathology**
   - The primary vector is *Dermacentor andersoni* (Rocky Mountain wood tick) in the west and *Dermacentor variabilis* (American dog tick) in the east.
   - *Rickettsia* multiplies within endothelial cells lining small blood vessels.

3. **Clinical Features**
   - Rocky Mountain spotted fever is the most serious rickettsial disease.
   - Incubation time between tick bite and onset of illness is 2 to 14 days (mean 7 days).
   - Fever, chills, headache, rash, toxicity, mental confusion, myalgias, nausea, and vomiting occur.
   - Fever rises rapidly; characteristically is high and spiking. Cough and pneumonitis may appear, as may delirium, lethargy, seizures, stupor, and coma.
   - Rash occurs between the second and sixth day of fever; initial lesions are small faint macules that blanch with pressure. Lesions rapidly become maculopapular, then petechial.
   - Rash appears first on wrists and ankles, spreading centrally but remaining more marked on extremities; palms and soles are typically involved; however, 10% have no or minimal rash.
   - Facial flushing and conjunctival injection are common.
   - Headache (beginning soon after onset) is extreme, intense, continuous, and intractable.
   - Some patients develop hepatosplenomegaly, jaundice, myocarditis, uremia, or necrotizing vasculitis.

4. **Diagnostic Studies**
   - Common findings include thrombocytopenia, elevated liver function tests, hyponatremia, and hyperbilirubinemia.

- IFA testing of serum is most commonly used to confirm the diagnosis, but patients may not demonstrate antibody response until week 2.
- Skin biopsy early in illness may demonstrate presence of *R. rickettsii*.

5. Management
- Doxycycline is the treatment of choice; chloramphenicol in pregnant women.

6. Prevention
- Avoidance of tick-infested areas, protective clothing, and the use of tick repellent.

VI. Spirochetal Diseases

A. Lyme Disease

1. Etiology
- *Borrelia burgdorferi.*
- Lyme is the most common vector-borne infection in the United States.
- The vector is a species of the *Ixodes* (deer) tick; the larvae feed in late summer, nymphs in spring and early summer, and adults in fall.
- The preferred host for the larvae and nymphs is the white-footed mouse; for adults, the white-tailed deer. Most infections occur in the spring and summer.

2. Pathology
- Lyme disease is transmitted through the bite of tick that injects spirochete into bloodstream; in most cases, the tick must be attached for at least 24 hours to transmit infection.
- Immune complexes accumulate in joints and attract enzyme-releasing neutrophils that attack antigen–antibody complexes. Enzymes also attack joints, eroding bone and cartilage causing arthritis-like symptoms.
- O-antigen (lipopolysaccharide) of *Borrelia* stimulates macrophages to secrete interleukin 1, which subsequently stimulates the production of collagenase and prostaglandin. Collagenase degrades collagen leading to pattern of erosion seen in severe cases.
- Prostaglandins promote pain.

3. Clinical Features
- Although three stages of the disease have been described, overlap is common.
- Early localized infection: usually about 7 days (range 3 to 30) after bite by an infected tick, erythema migrans rash develops typically in groin, axilla, or thigh; this expands from the site of the bite, may have central clearing or intensification, and may be up to 50 cm in diameter. About half of patients develop flu-like symptoms.
- Early disseminated infection: if bacteremia occurs, patients progress within days to weeks to disseminated disease involving most commonly the skin, CNS, and musculoskeletal systems. Smaller skin

lesions not associated with site of bite may develop; headache, stiff neck, and migratory joint, muscle, and tendon pain may occur. Persistent fatigue is common. Up to 10% of patients develop cardiac (myocarditis, pericarditis, dysrhythmias, and heart block) and up to 20% neurologic (aseptic meningitis, Bell palsy, encephalitis, personality changes, forgetfulness) symptoms. Ocular involvement may occur.
- Late persistent infection: months to years later, patients develop variable musculoskeletal problems including joint pain without objective changes, frank arthritis of the large joints, and chronic synovitis. Neurologic involvement most commonly manifests as memory loss, mood swings, and sleep disturbance.

4. Diagnostic Studies
- ELISA for serum antibodies confirmed with Western blot is the preferred methodology, but up to half of patients will be antibody negative in the first few weeks.
- Isolation of organism in culture from biopsy of skin lesions early in the disease is readily accomplished, but culture from other sites is difficult; PCR of skin biopsy is even more sensitive.

5. Management
- A tick bite is not usually treated in the absence of symptoms.
- Early disease responds readily to doxycycline or amoxicillin, and cefuroxime for patients unable to tolerate doxycycline or amoxicillin, all for 2 to 3 weeks.
- IV penicillin G, ceftriaxone, or cefotaxime for 2 to 4 weeks is used for CNS or cardiac disease; arthritis requires oral doxycycline or amoxicillin for up to 60 days or cefotaxime, cephotaxin, or penicillin G for up to 4 weeks.
- "Chronic Lyme" or "post-Lyme syndrome" is treated symptomatically.

6. Prevention
- LYMErix, the only licensed Lyme disease vaccine, was withdrawn from market due to lack of demand.
- Wearing protective clothing, avoidance of habitats of the deer tick, use of repellents and insecticides, and prompt removal of ticks prevent Lyme disease.
- In limited circumstances, a single dose of doxycycline following tick bite may be indicated.

VII. Helminthic Infestations

A. Ascariasis

1. Etiology
- *Ascaris lumbricoides* (roundworm).
- Most common intestinal helminth worldwide.

2. Pathology
- Adult ascarids inhabit the upper small intestine; females deposit eggs into intestinal lumen, which

are eventually passed in the feces; eggs must mature in soil 2 to 3 weeks before becoming infective.
- Following ingestion of contaminated food or water, eggs hatch into larvae in the small intestine, enter bloodstream, move to right heart then the lung, enter the alveoli, move up the bronchi, are swallowed, and return to the intestine.
- Cycle takes 60 to 75 days.

3. Clinical Features
- A small worm load is generally asymptomatic; heavier loads produce vague abdominal discomfort.
- In higher worm loads, adults may migrate to common bile duct, pancreatic duct, appendix, or diverticula, causing symptoms associated with site of migration; very heavy disease may cause obstruction, intussusception, or other serious disease. Worms may also be coughed or vomited up.
- Nutritional disorders can occur secondary to impaired digestion or absorption of dietary proteins, particularly in children.

4. Diagnostic Studies
- Recovery of characteristic egg in feces is usually sufficient for the diagnosis or identification of a large worm after it emerges from the mouth, nose, or anus.
- Abdominal films, endoscopic retrograde cholangiopancreatography, and ultrasound may demonstrate a worm mass.
- Pulmonary phase is diagnosed by finding larvae and eosinophils in sputum.
- Eosinophilia occurs in the pulmonary phase; oxygen desaturation and migratory pulmonary infiltrates may occur.

5. Management
- Mebendazole, albendazole, and pyrantel pamoate are the treatments of choice; in pregnant women, treatment should be delayed until after the first trimester.
- Stools must be rechecked at 2 weeks with re-treatment as needed until all worms are removed.
- Intestinal obstruction usually responds to conservative management while the antihelminthic agents work; surgery may be required for appendicitis.

6. Prevention
- Adequate sanitation facilities, frequent hand-washing, and avoidance of foods fertilized with human feces.

VIII. Pathogens with Bioterrorism Potential

- The Working Group for Civilian Biodefense compiled a list of characteristics of biologic agents that are most likely to be used as weapons of terror: high morbidity and mortality, potential for person-to-person spread, low infective dose, highly infectious when aerosolized, difficulty in making rapid diagnosis, lack of available effective vaccines, anxiety-producing potential, availability, feasibility of production, environmental stability, database of prior research and development, and potential to be "weaponized."
- **The CDC has classified potential biologic terrorism agents into three categories:**
  - Category A is the highest priority and includes anthrax, botulism, plague, smallpox, tularemia, and viral hemorrhagic fevers.
  - Category B, the second highest priority, includes brucellosis, epsilon toxin of *Clostridium perfringens*, food safety threats such as *Salmonella* species, glanders, melioidosis, psittacosis, Q fever, ricin toxin, staphylococcal enterotoxin B, typhus, viral encephalitis, and water safety threats.
  - Category C bioterrorism threats are the third highest priority and include emerging infectious diseases such as Nipah and hantavirus.

A. Anthrax
- See IV. A. for naturally occurring presentation.

1. Etiology
- *Bacillus anthracis.*

2. Pathology
- Owing to availability, the agent's hardiness, ease of dispersion, and ability to cause grave illness, anthrax is considered the preferred agent of biologic terrorists.

3. Clinical Features
- The form considered most likely to be used for biologic terrorism is inhalational anthrax.
- This form is characterized by rapid progression from flu-like syndrome to lymphadenitis and hemorrhagic mediastinitis and is usually fatal within days.
- Anthrax infection should be suspected when large numbers of patients have respiratory and flu-like symptoms outside of influenza season.

4. Diagnostic Studies
- See IV. A.
- A 1-hour DNA test for anthrax is available from the CDC.

5. Management
- Because no human-to-human cases have been found, standard precautions (routine use of gloves for skin lesions, hand-washing, and use of gowns, masks, and eye protection during procedures in which splashing can occur) are sufficient for hospitalized patients.
- Early initiation of ciprofloxacin is recommended in cases of biologic warfare because these strains may have been altered to resist standard antibiotics.

- Burn or steam-sterilize contaminated dressings to destroy spores.
- Notify local and state health departments, CDC, and appropriate law enforcement agencies immediately of suspected biologic terrorist attack.

6. Prevention
- Vaccination is available in limited supply for those at risk (such as military personnel) and following a known exposure.
- Chemoprophylaxis with doxycycline or ciprofloxacin may prevent the development of inhalational form if administered before disease onset.

B. Botulism
- See IV. B. for naturally occurring presentation.

1. Etiology
- *Clostridium botulinum.*

2. Pathology
- Botulinum toxin is the most poisonous substance known.
- It is a major threat because of extreme potency, degree of lethality, ease of production, and transport.

3. Clinical Features
- See IV. B.

4. Diagnostic Studies
- Send samples (serum, stool, gastric aspirate, vomitus) and/or suspicious foods before treatment to CDC or special state and municipal public health laboratories for analysis.
- Botulism is highly suspected if a large number of cases of acute flaccid paralysis with prominent bulbar palsies occur or in the presence of an outbreak of an unusual botulinum toxin type.
- Bioterrorism is also suggested in the case of an outbreak with common geographic factor but without a common dietary exposure or in multiple simultaneous outbreaks with no common source.

5. Management
- Effectiveness of treatment based on timely diagnosis; administration of antitoxin should precede microbiologic test results.
- Treat all those with suspected exposure and signs of illness with antitoxin and supportive measures.

6. Prevention
- Investigational pentavalent (ABCDE) botulinum toxoid is available to those at high risk for exposure to botulinum toxin and the military; a recombinant vaccine is in development.

C. Glanders
1. Etiology
- *Burkholderia mallei* (a small, bipolar, gram-negative, nonmotile, aerobic bacillus).
- Although glanders is a category B agent, it is believed that attempts are being made to develop an aerosolized form of antibiotic-resistant *B. mallei* that could become a biologic weapon as potent as anthrax.

- Eradicated in North America in 1938, glanders still occurs in Asia, Africa, and South America.

2. Pathology
- Ordinarily *B. mallei* infects horses, mules, and donkeys; pigs and cattle are resistant, but it rarely infects humans.
- Disease is transmitted from animal-to-human by way of nasal, oral, and conjunctival mucous membranes, by inhalation into lungs, or through the lacerated or abraded skin; in humans, inoculation usually is into the skin of the hand or arm.

3. Clinical Features
- After a 10- to 14-day incubation period, patients exhibit fever, rigors, night sweats, malaise, prostration, myalgia, headache, pleuritic chest pain, photophobia, lacrimation, diarrhea, and/or regional lymphadenitis.
- The bacterium causes nodules to form in the affected area; these enlarge, forming ulcers; crater-like ulcers on skin along course of lymph vessels of extremities commonly called *farcy*.
- Acute presentation ranges from localized suppurative infection to pulmonary infection to septicemia; patients with this form have fever, cervical adenopathy, splenomegaly, rash with generalized papular or pustular eruptions.
- Chronic indolent suppurative infection is associated with subcutaneous ulcers, lymphatic thickening, and lymphatic nodules.
- Aerosolized dissemination may lead to any of the above presentations.

4. Diagnostic Studies
- Serology is the preferred diagnostic modality; 16s rRNA gene sequencing is used for rapid identification.
- Chest radiography demonstrates miliary nodules, lung abscesses, lobar, or bronchopneumonia.

5. Management
- Long-term administration of a variety of drug combinations may be used in treatment including streptomycin and tetracycline or chloramphenicol and streptomycin.
- Abscesses need surgical drainage.

6. Prevention
- Standard precautions for laboratory exposures.
- No vaccine is available currently.
- Postexposure prophylaxis with TMP/SMX, ceftazidime, and doxycycline.

D. Plague
1. Etiology
- *Yersinia pestis*, a nonmotile, gram-negative rod demonstrating bipolar "safety pin" staining with Wright, Giemsa, or Wayson stain.
- Optimal growth on blood or MacConkey agar at 35° C.

2. **Pathology**
   - Patient is inoculated with thousands of organisms by plague-infected flea or by handling infected rodents in naturally occurring infection; person-to-person spread is through droplets.
   - Aerosol dissemination leading to pneumonic plague is most likely in a bioterrorist attack.
   - The incubation period is 2 to 10 days.
   - Organisms spread through the lymphatic system, then to all organs through the blood.
   - Plague-associated pneumonia and meningitis are often fatal.

3. **Clinical Features**
   - Onset of fever, chills, weakness malaise, tachycardia, intense headache, delirium, and severe myalgias is rapid.
   - Three forms of the disease exist: bubonic, septicemic, and pneumonic.
   - Bubonic is the most common form (95%); it presents with an acutely swollen, extremely painful lymph node (bubo), 2 to 10 cm in diameter, in the groin, axilla, or cervical region.
   - Septicemic refers to the subsequent DIC and gangrene in advanced disease. Septicemic plague denotes plague without the presence of a bubo. Patients become toxic and comatose with extensive purpura ("black death") on the distal extremities, nose, or penis.
   - Pneumonic symptoms include tachypnea, productive cough, frothy blood-tinged sputum, and cyanosis. This form is usually fatal within a few hours if untreated.
   - Bleeding from GI, respiratory, or genitourinary tracts is common ("red death").
   - Plague is highly contagious by airborne transmission and invariably fatal if antibiotic therapy is delayed by more than 1 day after illness onset.

4. **Diagnostic Studies**
   - Gram stain will demonstrate the bacillus in smears from buboes.
   - Cultures from aspirate, pus, and blood are positive.
   - For rapid diagnosis, direct immunofluorescence can be applied to smears of fluids or cultures.

5. **Management**
   - Notify hospital, local, state, or military laboratories or, as necessary, the CDC immediately to confirm diagnosis.
   - Streptomycin or gentamicin is the preferred treatment and must be begun immediately; doxycycline is an alternative.
   - Patients with a cough or pneumonic plague require strict respiratory isolation for at least 48 hours after starting antibiotic therapy.

6. **Prevention**
   - Doxycycline or tetracycline is used for postexposure prophylaxis.

E. **Q Fever**
1. **Etiology**
   - *Coxiella burnetii* is a proteobacterium (formerly thought to be a *Rickettsia*) that is transmitted to humans primarily by inhalation of contaminated aerosols from the infected animal tissues. Ingestion of raw milk or cheese is another route.
   - The animal reservoir of this zoonotic disease is primarily cattle, sheep, and goats; secondary reservoirs include cats, rabbits, pigeons, and dogs.
   - *Coxiella* is resistant to heat and drying and can survive in harsh environments for weeks to months because of the formation of spore-like structures.
   - Q fever is a category B bioterrorism threat.

2. **Pathology**
   - Disease in animals is mild or subclinical, whereas humans may develop more serious illness.
   - Person-to-person transmission is extremely rare, but maternal–fetal infection occurs.

3. **Clinical Features**
   - After a 7- to 21-day incubation period, the patient experiences fever, weight loss, severe headache, dyspnea, myalgias, nonproductive cough, and prostration.
   - More fulminant cases are associated with pneumonia, hepatitis, meningoencephalitis, or, rarely, endocarditis or osteomyelitis.
   - Culture-negative endocarditis is the most common finding in chronic disease.
   - Some patients develop chronic, relapsing disease.
   - Reactivation in pregnant women may cause spontaneous abortions, fetal death, fetal growth retardation, premature labor, and olgoamnios.

4. **Diagnostic Studies**
   - *Coxiella burnetii* is highly infectious and must be tested in specialized laboratories.
   - The diagnostic methodology of choice is indirect immunofluorescence; ELISA and complement fixation are also appropriate.
   - Rheumatoid factor, C-reactive protein, and erythrocyte sedimentation rate levels are high; liver function test may be elevated; leukocytosis may occur.
   - Chest radiography shows patchy pulmonary infiltrates.

5. **Management**
   - Tetracycline or doxycycline are used to treat acute infection, but may not eradicate disease; newer macrolides and the quinolones are alternatives.
   - Heart valve replacement may be needed in chronic disease.
   - In case of exposure in a bioterrorist attack, doxycycline or TMP/SMX should be given for prophylaxis.

6. **Prevention**
   - Detection, prevention, and avoidance of diseased animals is primary; milk should be pasteurized.

- A vaccine has been used and found effective for high-risk exposures in Australia; none is available in the United States.

F. Smallpox (Variola)

1. **Etiology**
   - Variola major is a DNA virus of the genus *Orthopoxvirus*, among the largest and most complex of all viruses.
   - The aerosolized form is extremely stable in cool temperatures, low humidity, and when protected from ultraviolet light.
   - Variola minor is less severe form.
   - Smallpox is a category A bioterrorism agent.

2. **Pathology**
   - The infectious dose is believed to be only a few virions.
   - Following implantation, the virus migrates and multiplies in the lymph nodes, spleen, and bone marrow.
   - The incubation period is about 12 days (7 to 17).

3. **Clinical Features**
   - The prodrome consists of abrupt onset of high fever and severe head- and backache; patients may have chills and rigors, coryza, and pharyngitis.
   - Skin eruptions begin 1 to 2 days after the development of an enanthem; these begin as macules and progress through papules, pustules, and crusting over about 2 weeks. Palmar and plantar lesions are common.
   - Skin lesions develop all at once, rather than in crops, as in varicella.

4. **Diagnostic Studies**
   - Laboratory confirmation is important; a vaccinated laboratory worker wearing gloves and a mask should collect specimens from vesicular or pustular fluid.
   - Laboratory confirmation is made by electron microscopic examination.
   - Use state or local laboratory with high-containment (BL-4) facility.

5. **Management**
   - Supportive therapy plus antibiotics in the case of secondary bacterial infection.
   - Persons in whom smallpox is suspected should be isolated and vaccinated within first few days of exposure.
   - Household and face-to-face contacts should be vaccinated, placed under surveillance, and monitored for fevers.
   - Smallpox must be treated as international health emergency (report to national officials through local and state health authorities).

6. **Prevention**
   - Vaccination is available in limited amounts for persons at risk; eczema, other dermatitides, and burns are contraindications.

- Standard precautions include using gloves, gowns, and masks; handling laundry and waste as biohazardous; and decontaminating rooms.
- Limited supplies of vaccinia immune globulin are available for treating severe cutaneous reactions occurring as a vaccination complication.

G. Tularemia

1. **Etiology**
   - *Francisella tularensis* is one of the most infectious pathogenic bacteria.
   - Category A agent for bioterrorism due to the ease of dissemination and virulence.
   - Humans become infected because of tick or insect bite or handling animal tissues; aerosol infection is also highly likely.

2. **Pathology**
   - The incubation period is 2 to 10 days.
   - Small, nonmotile aerobic gram-negative coccobacillus.
   - Hardy, non-spore-forming organism with thin lipopolysaccharide-containing envelope.

3. **Clinical Features**
   - Tularemia may be asymptomatic or begin with sudden onset of fever, headache, and nausea, and a papule develops at the site of inoculation with progression to ulceration.
   - Pneumonia may be primary following inhalation or the result of hematogenous spread.
   - After ingestion of infected meat or water, patients may develop GI symptoms, stupor, and delirium.
   - Tender splenomegaly is common, as are rashes, myalgias, and prostration.

4. **Diagnostic Studies**
   - Diagnosis is usually made serologically.

5. **Treatment**
   - Streptomycin is the recommended treatment; gentamicin or doxycycline is an alternative.

6. **Prevention**
   - Avoidance of ticks and deer fleas, use of insect repellents, and wearing gloves when handling animal carcasses prevent naturally occurring disease.
   - The CDC has an intradermal vaccine available.

H. Viral Hemorrhagic Fevers

1. **Etiology**
   - One of four families of viruses capable of causing febrile disease and a bleeding disorder.
   - These families pose particularly serious threats as biologic weapons, based on their infectious properties, morbidity and mortality, and transmissibility by way of aerosol dissemination: Filoviridae (Ebola and Marburg viruses), Arenaviridae (Lassa fever and the New World arenaviruses), Bunyaviridae (Rift Valley fever, Crimean–Congo hemorrhagic fever virus), and Flaviviridae (dengue, yellow fever, Omsk hemorrhagic fever, and Kyasanur Forest disease viruses).
   - None occurs naturally in the United States.

2. **Pathology**
   - Small RNA viruses with lipid envelopes act in varied ways; much is unknown.
   - Some illness results from the body's immunologic response to infection.
   - Direct and indirect cell damage leads to platelet dysfunction.
   - Filoviruses extremely virulent and cytotoxic to cells leading to necrosis of visceral organs.
   - Arenaviruses may induce secretion of inflammatory mediators from macrophages because few or absent cytopathic effects are present.
   - Infection with Rift Valley and yellow fever viruses leads to destruction of infected cells.

3. **Clinical Features**
   - Early symptoms of all these resemble influenza or gastroenteritis with headache, upper respiratory or GI symptoms, and myalgias; hepatitis is common.
   - Later manifestations are more specific to the particular virus; symptoms typically include organ failure, mental status changes, and hemorrhage.
   - Fatality rates are up to 90% with Ebola fever.

4. **Diagnostic Studies**
   - Variable clinical presentations present a major diagnostic challenge.
   - Clinical microbiology and public health laboratories are not equipped to make rapid diagnosis, so specimens must be sent to CDC or U.S. Army Medical Research Institute of Infectious Diseases.

5. **Management**
   - Early treatment with intravenous ribavirin may be useful in Lassa fever and hemorrhagic fever with renal failure.
   - No antiviral medications are currently approved, so early supportive care is essential.
   - Close and high-risk contacts must be identified and monitored for 21 days.
   - An effective vaccine is available for yellow fever, but is not useful following bioterrorist attack because of short incubation period.
   - Suspected cases must be reported to local or state health departments immediately.

6. **Prevention**
   - Avoidance of sick animals or people and arthropod bites is essential.
   - Rift Valley fever and Flaviviridae are not transmissible from person to person.
   - Airborne transmission is rare, but may be transmitted to laboratory personnel through aerosol generated during specimen processing.
   - Virus culture must occur in high-containment (BSL-4) laboratories.
   - Barrier precautions include strict hand hygiene plus double gloving, impermeable gowns, face shields, eye protection, and leg and shoe coverings.

SELECTED REFERENCES

American Academy of Pediatrics Subcommittee on Diagnosis and Management of Bronchiolitis. Diagnosis and management of bronchiolitis. *Pediatrics*. 2006;118(4):1774–1793.

Anderson H, Stryjewska B, Boyanton BL, et al. Hansen disease in the United States in the 21st century: a review of the literature. *Arch Pathol Lab Med*. 2007;131(6):982–986.

Blyth CC, Palasanthiran P, O'Brien TA. Antifungal therapy in children with invasive fungal infections: a systematic review. *Pediatrics*. 2007;119(4):772–784.

Centers for Disease Control and Prevention. Emergency preparedness and response: bioterrorism agents. http://www.bt.cdc.gov/agent/agentlist-category.asp. Accessed November–December 2011.

Franco MP, Mulder M, Gilman RH, et al. Human brucellosis. *Lancet Infect Dis*. 2007;7(12):775–786.

Griffith KS, Lewis LS, Mali S, et al. Treatment of malaria in the United States: a systematic review. *JAMA*. 2007;297(20):2264–2277.

Halperin JJ, Shapiro ED, Logigian E, et al; Quality Standards Subcommittee of the American Academy of Neurology. Practice parameter: treatment of nervous system Lyme disease (an evidence-based review): report of the Quality Standards Subcommittee of the American Academy of Neurology. *Neurology*. 2007;69(1):91–102.

Hankins DG, Rosekrans JA. Overview, prevention, and treatment of rabies. *Mayo Clin Proc*. 2004;79(5):671–676.

Ho W; Hong Kong Hospital Authority Working Group on SARS, Central Committee of Infection Control. Guideline on management of severe acute respiratory syndrome (SARS). *Lancet*. 2003;361(9366):1313–1315.

Hotez PJ, Molyneux DH, Fenwick A, et al. Control of neglected tropical diseases. *N Engl J Med*. 2007;357(10):1018–1027.

Hui DS, Chan PK. Clinical features, pathogenesis and immunobiology of severe acute respiratory syndrome. *Curr Opin Pulm Med*. 2008;14(3):241–247.

Jackson AC. Update on rabies diagnosis and treatment. *Curr Infect Dis Rep*. 2009;11(4):296–301.

Keiser J, Utzinger J. Efficacy of current drugs against soil-transmitted helminth infections: systematic review and meta-analysis. *JAMA*. 2008;299(16):1937–1948.

Longo D, Fauci AS, Kasper DL, et al, eds. *Harrison's Principles of Internal Medicine*. 18th ed. New York, NY: McGraw-Hill; 2011.

Mandell GL, Bennett JE, Dolin R. *Principles and Practice of Infectious Disease*. Amsterdam, The Netherlands: Elsevier; 2007.

McPhee SJ, Papadakis MA, Rabow MW, eds. *Current Medical Diagnosis and Treatment*. 50th ed. Stamford, CT: Appleton & Lange; 2011.

Panel on Antiretroviral Guidelines for Adult and Adolescents. Guidelines for the use of antiretroviral agents in HIV-1-infected adults and adolescents. Department of Health and Human Services. 2009;1–161. http://www.aidsinfo.nih.gov/ContentFiles/AdultandAdolescentGL.pdf. Accessed December 2011.

Skalsky K, Yahav D, Bishara J, et al. Treatment of human brucellosis: systematic review and meta-analysis of randomized controlled trials. *BMJ*. 2008;336(7646):701–704.

Walsh TJ, Anaissie EJ, Denning DW, et al; Infectious Diseases Society of America. Treatment of aspergillosis: clinical practice guidelines of the Infectious Diseases Society of America. *Clin Infect Dis*. 2008;46(3):337–360.

Wormser GT. Clinical practice. Early Lyme disease. *N Engl J Med*. 2006;354(26):2794–2801.

Zimmerman RK, Middleton DB, Burns IT, et al. Routine vaccines across the life span, 2007 [review]. *J Fam Pract*. 2007;56(2)(suppl vaccines):S18–S37, C1–C3.

Pediatric Care and Common Disorders

Susan M. Dubendorfer • Joseph Mileto

I. Evaluation and Care of the Newborn Infant

A. Perinatal Care

1. Antenatal evaluation must begin with a thorough history that should include the current and past medical history of the mother and father, obstetric history, and current pregnancy including the labor and delivery.
2. Newborns should have a brief examination at birth consisting of Apgar scores at 1 and 5 minutes; brief examination for congenital anomalies, measurements, vital signs–skin color; musculoskeletal examination for birth trauma, and examination of the umbilical cord (number of vessels—two arteries and one vein) and the placenta for abnormalities. A complete examination should take place later in the nursery within the first day of life.
3. Vitamin K should be administered within 4 hours of birth to prevent hemorrhagic disease of the newborn.
4. Erythromycin ophthalmic ointment should be administered at the time of delivery for prophylaxis against gonococcal ophthalmia neonatorum.

B. The Newborn Examination

1. **General Survey—A general inspection of the infant is the first and most important step in the examination and provides much information in a short time**
   - Gross anomalies.
   - Respirations—observe for grunting respirations, normal respiratory rate for term neonate is 40 to 60 breaths per minute.
   - Activity.
   - Cry.
   - Edema (may be generalized [hydrops] or localized).
   - State of maturity/gestational age (Dubowitz gestational age) (Table 15-1, Figures 15-1 and 15-2).
2. **Skin**
   - Color.
     - Cyanosis.
       - Localized cyanosis of the hands and feet, known as acrocyanosis, is normal and will usually disappear after several days of life.
       - Generalized cyanosis should prompt search for respiratory, cardiac, or metabolic disorder.
   - Pallor—may represent acute or chronic blood loss.
   - Plethora—seen in polycythemia.
   - Ecchymoses, purpura, or erythema may represent birth trauma. (Purpura may also represent congenital infection.)
   - Jaundice—always considered pathologic in the first day of life.
   - Harlequin color change—transient, striking, but normal sign of vasomotor instability and divides the body from head to pubis through the midline, into equal halves of pink and pale color.
   - Lanugo hair—may be present over back and shoulders.
   - Vernix caseosa—a soft creamy substance covering the skin in preterm infants, that decreases in amount as fetus approaches term.
   - Meconium staining of skin/umbilical stump.
   - Common abnormalities.
     - Mongolian spots—dark blue-to-black pigmented macules seen over the lower back and buttocks in 90% of darker pigmented babies.
     - Nevus simplex (salmon patch)—pink, macular hemangiomas, usually transient and noted on the back of the neck, eyelids, and forehead.
     - Capillary hemangiomas—benign, raised red lesions.
     - Cavernous hemangiomas—deeper, blue-colored benign masses. **NOTE:** Both capillary and cavernous hemangiomas increase in size after birth, only to resolve between 1 and 4 years of age.
     - Erythema toxicum—benign, erythematous rash characterized by erythematous macules, with central papule or pustule; very common in neonates and usually develops between 24 and 48 hours after birth.
     - Pustular melanosis—more common in infants with darkly pigmented skin; these consist of a small vesicle on a pigmented brown macular base. A scale forms as the vesicle ruptures.
     - Milia—yellow-white epidermal cysts that can be found on the nose.
3. **Head**
   - Head circumference.
   - Shape of the head and molding—resolves 2 to 3 days after birth.

TABLE 15–1.   External Characteristics of the Dubowitz Examination

External Sign	0	1	2	3	4
			Score		
Edema	Obvious edema of hands and feet; pitting over tibia	No obvious edema of hands and feet; pitting over tibia	No edema		
Skin texture	Very thin, gelatinous	Thin and smooth	Smooth; medium thickness; rash or superficial peeling	Slight thickening; superficial cracking and peeling, especially on hands and feet	Thick and parchment-like; superficial or deep cracking
Skin color (infant not crying)	Dark red	Uniformly pink	Pale pink; variable over body	Pale; only pink over ears, lips, palms, or soles	
Skin opacity (trunk)	Numerous veins and venules clearly seen, especially over abdomen	Veins and tributaries seen	A few large vessels clearly seen over abdomen	A few large vessels seen indistinctly over abdomen	No blood vessels seen
Lanugo (over back)	No lanugo	Abundant; long and thick over whole back	Hair thinning, especially over lower back	Small amount of lanugo and bald areas	At least half of back devoid of lanugo
Plantar creases	No skin creases	Faint red marks over anterior half of sole	Definite red marks over more than anterior half; indentations over less than anterior third	Indentations over more than anterior third	Definite deep indentations over more than anterior third
Nipple formation	Nipple barely visible; no areola	Nipple well defined; areola smooth and flat; diameter <0.75 cm	Areola stippled, edge not raised; diameter <0.75 cm	Areola stippled, edge raised; diameter >0.75 cm	
Breast size	No breast tissue palpable	Breast tissue on one or both sides <0.5 cm diameter	Breast tissue both sides; one or both 0.5 to 1.0 cm	Breast tissue both sides; one or both >1 cm	
Ear form	Pinna flat and shapeless, little or no incurving of edge	Incurving of part of edge of pinna	Partial incurving whole of upper pinna	Well-defined incurving whole of upper pinna	
Ear firmness	Pinna soft, easily folded, no recoil	Pinna soft, easily folded, slow recoil	Cartilage to edge of pinna, but soft in places, ready recoil	Pinna firm, cartilage to edge; instant recoil	
Genitalia male	Neither testis in scrotum	At least one testis high in scrotum	At least one testis down in scrotum		
Female (with hips half abducted)	Labia majora widely separated; labia minora protruding	Labia majora almost cover labia minora	Labia majora completely cover labia minora		

From Dubowitz L, Dubowitz V. *Gestational Age of the Newborn*. Saddle River, NJ: Prentice-Hall; 1977, with permission.

FIGURE 15–1. Neurologic characteristics of the Dubowitz examination. (From Dubowitz L, Dubowitz V. *Gestational Age of the Newborn.* Saddle River, NJ: Prentice-Hall; 1977, with permission.)

- Fontanels and suture lines should be palpated. Large fontanelles may signify hypothyroidism; Trisomy 13, 18, or 21; or bone disease.
- Craniotabes—slight indentation and recoil of parietal bones elicited by light pressure is normal in newborns.
- Cephalohematoma—a subperiosteal collection of blood caused by localized trauma that appears as a firm swelling on day 1 and does not cross suture lines. May take weeks to months to resolve.
- Caput succedaneum—edema of the presenting part of the scalp following a vertex delivery. Edema is soft and crosses the suture lines.
- Head tilt—congenital torticollis.

FIGURE 15–2. Both the external physical criteria score and that for the neurologic criteria are added together, and gestational age (±2 weeks) may be read off this graph. (From Dubowitz L, Dubowitz V. *Gestational Age of the Newborn.* Saddle River, NJ: Prentice-Hall; 1977, with permission.)

4. **Face**
   - Characteristic facies of disease (i.e., Down syndrome, fetal alcohol syndrome, and congenital hypothyroidism).
   - Facial hemiparesis—results from pressure on sacral promontory in utero, or forceps trauma.
5. **Eyes**
   - Lid edema is common.
   - Conjunctival, retinal, and sclera hemorrhage—present during birth trauma.
   - Pupil—papillary reflex should be present.
   - Retina—a red reflex should be present in ophthalmoscopic examination.
   - Chemical conjunctivitis is common in first 24 to 48 hours from erythromycin.
6. **Ears**
   - Low set ears—may be sign of genetic disorders (i.e., Down syndrome and Turner syndrome).
   - Preauricular skin tags or pits—may be associated with hearing loss.
   - Visualize tympanic membranes (TMs)—may be opaque in appearance with decreased mobility.
7. **Nose**
   - Check patency bilaterally—cyanosis that improves with crying is significant for choanal atresia.
   - Check for discharge.

8. **Mouth**
   - Cleft lip.
   - Cleft palate—check hard and soft palate.
   - Natal teeth—should be removed if mobile.
   - Epstein pearls—benign, white, beady papules on the hard palate (keratin cysts).
9. **Neck**
   - Mobility.
   - Masses—usually vascular malformations, dermoid cysts, or thyroglossal duct cyst.
   - Clavicles—the most common fracture resulting from birth trauma is to the clavicle.
10. **Chest**
    - Shape and symmetry.
    - Breast hypertrophy—breasts are palpable in mature males and in females.
    - Supernumerary nipples—bilateral and occasionally are associated with renal anomalies.
11. **Lungs**
    - Respiratory rate—typical rate should be 40 to 60 breaths per minute.
    - Character—breathing is abdominal.
    - Retractions—with tachypnea, may be a sign of respiratory distress syndrome.
    - Auscultation—diminished or absent breath sounds on one side may suggest a pneumothorax or a diaphragmatic hernia.
12. **Heart**
    - Heart rate—typical rate should be 90 to 160 beats per minute.
    - Rhythm—initially may be irregular.
    - Murmurs—transient murmurs are common and benign, but persistent murmurs or murmurs associated with other signs of cardiac disease need further evaluation.
    - Pulses—check both upper and lower extremity.
13. **Abdomen**
    - Shape and symmetry.
    - Diastasis recti—a normal finding that represents incomplete closure of the two rectus muscles.
    - Palpation—liver palpated 2 cm below right costal margin. The tip of the spleen may be palpable. Kidneys should be palpated bilaterally.
    - **Umbilical cord:**
      - Should have three vessels—two arteries and one vein.
      - Erythema of the cord may represent infection.
      - Oozing of blood—provides clue to bleeding disorder.
      - Umbilical or inguinal hernias.
    - Anus—check patency.
14. **Genitalia**
    - Edema is common.
    - Ambiguous genitalia should be ruled out.
    - Male.

- Testes—both testis should be descended.
- Scrotum—scrotal swelling may represent a transient hydrocele.
- Meatus—check for epispadias, hypospadias, or meatal stenosis.
- Foreskin—it is common for newborn to have congenital phimosis; do not forcibly retract foreskin.
    - Female.
      - Imperforate hymen may be visible.
      - A whitish discharge, with or without blood, may be present.
15. **Spine**
    - Midline lumbosacral lesions may represent spinal dysraphism and should have MRI or spinal ultrasound.
      - Myelomeningocele.
      - Lipomas.
      - Dimples.
      - Sinus tracts.
      - Hemangiomas.
      - Hypertrichosis.
    - Scoliosis—check for abnormal curvature of the spine.
16. **Extremities**
    - Symmetry and length.
    - Simian crease—present in Down syndrome.
    - Erb palsy—due to brachial plexus injury during delivery.
    - Deformities—clubfoot, polydactyly, syndactyly.
    - Hips—examine for signs of developmental dysplasia of the hip.
      - Barlow sign—"clunk" represents dislocatability in posterior-superior direction (Figure 15-3A).
      - Ortolani sign—"clunk" represents relocation into joint (Figure 15-3B).
      - Galeazzi sign—foreshortening of the affected limb (femur will appear shorter with knees flexed) (Figure 15-4).
      - Limited abduction at the hip.
      - Asymmetric subgluteal skin creases (nonspecific sign).
17. **Neurologic**
    - Assess muscle tone and strength.
    - Check primitive reflexes: Moro, Babinski, palmar grasp, sucking, rooting, stepping, and abdominal reflexes.

C. Care of the Normal Newborn

1. Following stabilization, the infant's vital signs, voiding, stooling, and feeding patterns should be recorded every 8 hours.
2. The normal term neonate passes meconium in the first 24 hours and voids within the first 12 hours. If there is a delay, 48 and 24 hours, respectively, there may be an obstruction.
3. Infants should be placed in the supine position to reduce risk of sudden infant death syndrome.

FIGURE 15–3. **Assessing for Barlow and Ortolani signs.** Place the child supine on a firm surface. Be gentle, not forceful. **A:** Barlow test is used to detect hip instability. The located hip is subluxed or dislocated during the maneuver. The examiner's fingers are placed over the child's greater trochanters. Holding the hips and knees at 90° of flexion, a backward pressure is applied while adducting the hips. The femoral head is felt slipping out of the acetabulum posterolaterally when the test is positive. **B:** Ortolani sign is present when the hip is dislocated. The maneuver relocates the femoral head. With the examiner's fingers on the child's greater trochanters, the hips and knees are flexed to 90°. The hips are then abducted while applying upward pressure over the greater trochanter. A positive sign is detected when a "clunk" is felt as the femoral head reenters the acetabulum. (From Nettina SM. *The Lippincott Manual of Nursing Practice.* 7th ed. Lippincott Williams & Wilkins; 2001, with permission.)

Unequal knee height

FIGURE 15–4. **Diagnosing developmental dysplasia of the hip (DDH).** Galeazzi sign—when knees are flexed and feet together, the knee on the affected side appears lower. Asset provided by Anatomical Chart Co.

4. State mandated newborn metabolic/genetic screening tests are typically performed at 24 to 48 hours of life, and typically include testing for in-born errors of metabolism, congenital hypothyroidism, sickle cell anemia, and cystic fibrosis (CF).
5. The decision to circumcise an infant should be made by the parents after consultation with a pediatrician.
6. Neonates and their mothers are routinely discharged after 24 to 48 hours.

7. Hepatitis B vaccination is typically administered before discharge.
8. Parental education on both routine infant care and signs/symptoms of concern to watch for (i.e., fever, jaundice, lethargy, irritability, poor feeding, and vomiting) should be given before discharge.

D. Feeding the Newborn
1. Breastfeeding
- One of the most important influences on children's health worldwide. The World Health Organization recommends exclusive breastfeeding for the first 6 months of life and continued breastfeeding with age appropriate supplementation through 2 years of life.
- Advantages of breastfeeding:
  - Numerous immunoactive immunologic factors are present in breast milk and provide protection against gastrointestinal and upper respiratory infections (URIs), allergic and atopic disease, and some chronic adult diseases.
  - Increased maternal–infant bonding.
  - Decreased cost.
  - Delayed return of maternal fertility.
  - Faster return to prepregnancy weight.
  - Decreased maternal incidence of ovarian and premenopausal breast cancer.

- Absolute contraindications to breastfeeding:
  - Human immunodeficiency virus (HIV) infection in developed countries where suitable formula preparations and safe water supply are available.
  - Active tuberculosis.
  - Use of some medications (lithium, radioactive iodine, antimetabolites, tetracycline, and antithyroid medications).
  - Maternal use of illicit drugs.
- Neonates should breastfeed on demand (typically every 2 to 3 hours with longer periods at night.) After 3 days of life, the infant should feed from 10 to 15 minutes on each side for every feed.
- Failure to pass several stools each day in the early weeks of life suggests inadequate milk intake and supply.
- Common problems.
  - Sore nipples may indicate improper positioning or improper latch on. It may be managed by correcting these, air drying nipples, and application of lanolin after feeds.
  - Breastfeeding jaundice should be managed by increasing the frequency of nursing or temporary formula feeding for 24 to 36 hours.
  - Maternal mastitis should be treated with β-lactam antibiotics and analgesics as necessary; breastfeeding should continue. Presence of an abscess requires temporary discontinuation of breastfeeding on the affected side.

2. **Formula Feeding**
   - The standard 20 kcal per oz infant formulas are adequate for use in newborns.
   - Soy protein formulas are indicated in infants with lactose intolerance.
   - Soy formulas may be substituted when cow's milk protein allergy is suspected; however, infants who are truly allergic to cow's milk protein are frequently allergic to soy protein as well.
   - Semielemental formulas are effective in feeding infants who cannot tolerate cow's milk or soy protein and are useful in infants with malabsorptive conditions.

II. Common Disorders/Diseases of the Newborn

A. Colic
1. **Etiology**
   - The etiology of colic is not well understood; some of the following factors may have a role and have been suggested as causes: gastrointestinal, behavioral, and parental.
2. **Clinical Features**
   - Characterized by the "Rule of 3s": prolonged bouts of crying for a total of >3 hours a day, for more than 3 days per week, for longer than 3 weeks in a previously well infant with no apparent underlying cause.
   - Crying spells are characterized by clenched fists, posturing with the knees drawn up, and minimal response to attempts to calm the infant.
   - Spells typically occur in the late afternoon or evening, but can occur at any time.
   - Typically occurs between 2 and 3 months of age.
3. **Management**
   - Careful history and physical examination to search for organic cause of fussiness—that is, URI, otitis media (OM), urinary tract infection, and GI disease.
   - If the evaluation discloses no underlying cause, conservative management is acceptable.
     - Supportive, sympathetic instruction to parents regarding colic and its benign nature.
     - Regular schedule for feedings and naps to avoid chaotic routines and over- or underfeeding.
     - Low-level sound in the infant's sleeping area, such as a radio or vacuum cleaner, may be soothing.
     - Gentle movement in a swing, or rides in an automobile.
     - A trial of a milk-free diet may help an infant with true cow's milk allergy, but avoid frequent formula changes.
     - Rest and assistance for the infant's caretakers is essential to prevent exhaustion.
   - Medications are only occasionally useful and include antihistamines, antispasmodics, and antacids.

B. Neonatal Jaundice
1. **Epidemiology**
   - Seen in up to 65% of neonates in the first week of life, with bilirubin levels of up to 6 mg per dL.
   - Eight percent to 10% of newborns develop excessive hyperbilirubinemia (>17 mg per dL), and 1% to 2% have levels above 20 mg.
   - Extremely high levels are rare, but potentially dangerous due to risk of kernicterus.
2. **Etiology**
   - Physiologic causes.
   - Increased bilirubin production:
     - Antibody-mediated hemolysis (maternal–infant ABO-incompatibility or RH-isoimmunization).
     - Nonimmune hemolysis (hereditary spherocytosis, G6PD deficiency).
     - Enclosed hemorrhage (i.e., cephalohematoma or excessive bruising from birth trauma).
     - Polycythemia.
   - Decreased conjugation:
     - Crigler–Najjar syndrome.
     - Gilbert syndrome.

- Unknown factors:
  - Prematurity.
  - Ethnicity (Asians have higher risk than Caucasian or African Americans).
- Breast milk jaundice.
- Congenital infection.

3. **Pathophysiology**
   - Hyperbilirubinemia may be conjugated (always pathologic) or unconjugated (may be physiologic or pathologic).
   - Most infants will develop a transient hyperbilirubinemia during the first week of life because of:
     - Increased bilirubin production secondary to increased red blood cell volume, decreased RBC survival time, and increased enterohepatic circulation.
     - Limited hepatic reuptake of bilirubin.
     - Inadequate conjugation and reduced bilirubin excretion.

4. **Clinical Manifestations**
   - Visible jaundice that progresses in a cephalocaudal direction, and total serum bilirubin (TSB) levels may be estimated by the extent of progression of visible jaundice:
     - Involving the face—TSB is approximately 5 mg per dL.
     - Involving the midabdomen—TSB is approximately 15 mg per dL.
     - Involving the feet—TSB is approximately 20 mg per dL.
   - Estimations should not be relied upon to guide management decisions; the use of transcutaneous bilirubinometry or serum levels is recommended.
   - Jaundice will typically appear after 24 hours of life peak at 3 to 5 days of life and resolve by 7 days (term infants) or 14 days (premature infants).
   - Breast milk jaundice is seen exclusively in breast-fed infants, and peak levels tend to be higher and last longer.
   - Signs of pathologic jaundice include:
     - Clinically evident jaundice in the first 24 hours of life.
     - Indirect hyperbilirubinemia lasting longer than 7 days (in a term infant)—suggests hemolysis.
     - Conjugated hyperbilirubinemia (direct fraction exceeds 2 mg per dL or 15% of TSB level).
     - Bilirubin levels increasing at a rate of >0.5 mg/dL/hour.
   - Severely elevated levels of bilirubin may result in kernicterus—which is characterized by bilirubin deposition and staining in the basal ganglia and hippocampus. Affected infants show spasticity, muscular incoordination, and variable degrees of cognitive impairment.

5. **Diagnostic Studies**
   - Total bilirubin is increased.
   - Indirect bilirubin (increased when unconjugated hyperbilirubinemia is the cause).
   - Direct bilirubin (increased when conjugated hyperbilirubinemia is the cause).
   - Complete blood count (CBC) with differential and RBC morphology.
   - Reticulocyte count (increased with hemolysis).
   - Blood type and Rh on mother and infant.
   - Direct coombs test on infant (if at risk for ABO or Rh incompatibility).

6. **Treatment (Table 15-2)**
   - Phototherapy.
   - Exchange transfusion.
   - Treat underlying cause if applicable.

TABLE 15–2.   Management of Hyperbilirubinemia in the Healthy Term Newborn

Age (h)	TSB Level, mg/dL (μmol/L)			
	Consider Phototherapy[a]	Phototherapy	Exchange Transfusion If Intensive Phototherapy Fails[b]	Exchange Transfusion and Intensive Phototherapy
=24[c]	—	—	—	—
25–48	= 12 (170)	= 15 (260)	= 20 (340)	= 25(340)
49–72	= 15 (260)	= 18 (310)	= 25 (430)	= 30(510)
>72	= 17 (290)	= 20 (340)	= 25 (430)	= 30(510)

[a]Phototherapy at these TSB levels is a clinical option, meaning that the intervention is available and may be used on the basis of individual clinical judgment.

[b]Intensive phototherapy should produce a decline of TSB of 1 to 2 mg per dL within 4 to 6 hours, and the TSB level should continue to fall and remain below the threshold level for exchange transfusion. If this does not occur, it is considered a failure of phototherapy.

[c]Term infants who are clinically jaundiced at <24 hours old are not considered healthy and require further evaluation.

TSB, total serum bilirubin.

From American Academy of Pediatrics. Practice parameter: management of hyperbilirubinemia in the healthy term newborn. *Pediatrics.* 1994;94(4):560, with permission.

C. Hyaline Membrane Disease (HMD)

1. Pathophysiology
- Deficiency or inactivation of pulmonary surfactant, leading to a decrease in surface tension in the alveolus.
- Decreased surface tension results in poor lung compliance and atelectasis.
- Leads to hypoxemia and ultimately respiratory failure.

2. Epidemiology
- Seen most commonly in preterm infants. Incidence is:
  - Five percent in infants born between 35 and 36 weeks of gestation.
  - Greater than 50% in infants born before 28 weeks.
- Other risk factors:
  - Caesarean delivery.
  - Birth asphyxia.
  - Infants of diabetic mothers.
  - Siblings with the history of HMD.

3. Clinical Features
- Cyanosis.
- Grunting with expiration.
- Tachypnea.
- Nasal flaring.
- Intercostal retractions.
- Progressive dyspnea.
- Respiratory failure.

4. Diagnostic Studies
- Pulse oximetry—hypoxemia.
- Chest X-ray (CXR).
  - Bilateral atelectasis with a "ground glass" appearance.
  - Air bronchograms.
  - Hypoinflation/doming of diaphragms.

5. Management
- Prevention.
  - Administration of steroids to mothers in preterm labor or conditions where preterm labor is likely.
  - Administration of artificial surfactant in the delivery room in infants born before 27 weeks.
- Treatment.
  - Supplemental oxygen.
  - Nasal CPAP.
  - Tracheal intubation and administration of artificial surfactant as rescue therapy if oxygen and CPAP ineffective.

D. Meconium Aspiration Syndrome

1. Etiology/Epidemiology
- Passage of meconium before delivery with subsequent aspiration of material.
- More common in term and postterm infants—up to 20% will pass meconium before delivery.

2. Pathophysiology
- Aspiration of the meconium leading to in utero asphyxia.

3. Clinical Features
- Signs of respiratory distress.
  - Tachypnea.
  - Retractions.
  - Nasal flaring.
  - Grunting.
- Barrel chest.
- Coarse breath sounds or rales.

4. Diagnostic Studies
- CXR.
  - Hyperinflation with patchy infiltrates.
  - Pneumothorax may be present in 20% to 50% of affected infants.

5. Management
- Amnioinfusion and intrapartum oro/nasopharyngeal suctioning are *not* recommended to prevent MAS.
- Infants who are covered with thick meconium at delivery should receive adequate tracheal suctioning.
- Management is otherwise symptomatic:
  - Humidified O_2.
  - Intubation/ventilation.
- Use of antibiotics is controversial.

E. Perinatal/Congenital Infections (TORCH)

1. Etiology
- "TORCH" represents a group of parasitic, bacterial, and viral pathogens producing congenital and perinatally acquired infections: *Toxoplasmosis, Other, Rubella, Cytomegalovirus* (CMV), and *Herpes simplex virus* (HSV).
- "Other" represents an increasing number of infections such as syphilis, gonorrhea, TB, HIV, parvovirus, varicella zoster, malaria, *Borrelia burgdorferi*, coxsackie virus, hepatitis B, C, or G, and other viruses.
- Infections may be acquired in utero, intrapartum, or postnatally.

2. Clinical Features
- Signs and symptoms vary slightly by etiologic agent, but classic presentation includes:
  - Intrauterine growth retardation.
  - Nonimmune hydrops.
  - Anemia.
  - Thrombocytopenia.
  - Jaundice (especially in the first 24 hours of birth).
  - Hepatosplenomegaly.
  - Chorioretinitis.
  - Congenital malformations.

3. Diagnostic Studies
- Isolate organism by culture—Rubella, HSV, CMV, Neisseria gonorrhoeae, *Mycobacterium tuberculosis*.
- Identify antigen—Hepatitis B, *Chlamydia trachomatis*.
- Identify fetal production of antibodies—immunoglobulin M, or increasing titer of immunoglobulin G for *Toxoplasma*, syphilis, HIV, *Borrelia*.

4. **Management**
   - Treat specific pathogen after it is confirmed.

F. **Apparent Life-Threatening Events of Infancy**
   1. **Episode that is frightening to the observer and involves any combination of apnea, color change, change in muscle tone, choking or gagging.**
   2. **Epidemiology**
      - Peak incidence between 1 and 2 months of age.
      - Male to female ratio is 2:1.
      - Known risk factors include:
        - Prematurity.
        - Respiratory syncytial virus (RSV) infection.
        - Anatomic abnormalities.
        - Known gastroesophageal reflux disease (GERD).
   3. **Etiology**
      - Fifty percent of cases have no identifiable cause and are classified as apnea of infancy.
      - Gastrointestinal (i.e., GERD).
      - Neurologic (i.e., CNS infection, seizure disorder, and central apnea).
      - Respiratory (i.e., bronchiolitis, pneumonia, and upper respiratory tract infection).
      - Cardiovascular (i.e., congenital heart disease, dysrhythmias, and cardiomyopathy).
      - Metabolic (i.e., hypoglycemia and electrolyte abnormalities).
      - Infectious (i.e., sepsis).
      - Nonaccidental injury/poisoning (i.e., shaken baby syndrome).
   4. **Clinical Features**
      - Apnea—defined as >20 seconds without breathing, or apneic period of any duration with associated change in color, tone, or heart rate.
        - Central apnea—associated with no chest wall movement.
        - Obstructive apnea (i.e., GERD and respiratory secretions)—associated with paradoxical chest wall movements.
        - Normal periodic breathing of infancy—pauses of several seconds interspersed with normal periods of breathing.
      - Color change—usually cyanosis or pallor.
      - Change in muscle tone—usually infant will be limp.
      - Choking or gagging.
   5. **Diagnostic Studies**
      - CBC.
      - Electrolytes.
      - Arterial blood gases (ABGs).
      - O_2 saturation.
      - Blood cultures.
      - CXR.
      - Other studies as guided by history and physical examination (i.e., lumbar puncture [LP], electroencephalogram [EEG], polysomnography, and esophageal pH).

6. **Treatment**
   - Based on the management of underlying cause (i.e., antireflux medications and antibiotics).
   - Caffeine or aminophylline are indicated in certain cases of apnea of infancy.
   - All caregivers should be trained in CPR before discharge from the hospital.
   - Use of home apnea monitors is controversial and has not been shown to reduce the incidence of sudden infant death syndrome.

G. **Sudden Infant Death Syndrome**
   1. **Definition**
      - Sudden, unexplained death of an infant, despite case investigation.
      - Investigation should include complete autopsy, review of clinical history, and evaluation of the death site.
      - Approximately, 20% of infant deaths will be explained by autopsy.
   2. **Epidemiology**
      - Incidence is 1/1,000 live births in the United States.
      - Peak number of deaths is between 2 and 4 months, with most being younger than 6 months.
      - Male to female ratio is 3:2.
      - Seen more commonly in African American or Native American race.
   3. **Risk Factors**
      - Prone/side sleeping position.
      - Male gender.
      - Low birth weight/IUGR
      - Prematurity.
      - Multiple gestation.
      - Pre- and postnatal exposure to cigarette smoke.
      - Lower socioeconomic status.
      - Young maternal age.
      - Use of soft bedding.
      - Warm sleeping environment.
      - Bottle feeding.
      - Family history of sudden infant death syndrome (SIDS).
   4. **Prevention—see Table 15-3 for possible approaches to the prevention of SIDS.**

H. **Failure to Thrive**
   1. **Definition**
      - Inadequate physical growth over time when measured against a standardized growth curve.
      - Weight <5th percentile, or weight crosses two major percentile lines over time.
   2. **Etiology**
      - Historically was categorized as inorganic (psychosocial or feeding issues) and organic (specific metabolic or medical condition as the cause).

TABLE 15–3.	Possible Approaches to Prevention of SIDS

Risk Reduction

Abandon recommendation of prone sleeping position for all infants (prone sleeping position still recommended for infants with specific clinical indication)
Recommend side-lying or supine sleeping position for healthy infants
Advocate better and more standardized policy concerning death scene investigation
Better educate public about dangers of over-the-counter remedies to young infants
Decrease parental smoking, before and after birth of child
Decrease parental drug use (e.g., crack cocaine smoking), before and after birth of child
Improve access to and use of postnatal medical care
Improve prenatal care (anemia, smoking, nutrition)
Improve recognition of and services for dysfunctional families at risk for intentional injury of infants
Improve services to young mothers living in poor socioeconomic conditions
Improve targeting of very high risk groups (e.g., Native Americans with very high maternal smoking rates)
Improve understanding of child care practices that may increase SIDS risk

Physiologic Component

Improve diagnosis of metabolic disorders leading to SIDS
Increase understanding of possible sources of postnatal vulnerability
Increase understanding of the role of infant sleeping position in increasing SIDS risk

Increase Efficacy of Home Monitoring

Improve compliance with monitor use
Improve monitoring technology
Improve selection of candidates for monitoring

- Newer classification system divides causes into:
  - Inadequate caloric consumption (incorrect preparation of formula, insufficient feedings, behavior problems, disturbance of parent–child relationship, neglect, mechanical feeding problems).
  - Inadequate absorption (celiac disease, CF, food allergy, liver disease, short gut syndrome).
  - Increased metabolism (hyperthyroidism, chronic infection, or hypoxemia).
  - Inadequate utilization of nutrients (genetic abnormalities, metabolic diseases).

3. **Evaluation**
  - History:
    - Dietary/feeding history.
    - Past and current medical history.
    - Social history of child and household members and caregivers.
  - Physical examination—general PE should be performed to:
    - Identify dysmorphic features.
    - Identify features of underlying disease.
    - Assess for abuse/neglect.
    - Assess the severity of malnutrition.
    - Review all anthropomorphic measurements.
    - Observe parent–child interactions.

- Laboratory diagnostics are not routinely done unless indicated by history or physical examination, but may include:
  - CBC.
  - Erythrocyte sedimentation rate (ESR).
  - Urinalysis (UA)/culture.
  - Renal function and electrolytes.
  - Sweat chloride test.
  - Fecal fat/reducing substances.
  - Purified protein derivative (PPD).
  - CXR.
  - Bone age.

III. Principles of Health Supervision and Preventive Care of Children

A. General Principles

1. Do history and physical examination at routine intervals from birth to age 21, including specific attention to height/length, weight, BMI (starting at 2 years), head circumference (up to 2 years), and compare with standardized growth charts.
2. Evaluate blood pressure (starting at 3 years), hearing, speech, neurologic findings, deformities, sexual development, and other parameters as outlined in the American Academy of Pediatrics (AAP) Bright Futures Guide to Preventive Services.

Recommended Immunization Schedule for Persons Aged 0 Through 6 Years—United States 2011
For those who fall behind or start late, see the catch-up schedule

Vaccine▼ Age ►	Birth	1 month	2 months	4 months	6 months	12 months	15 months	18 months	19–23 months	2–3 years	4–6 years	
Hepatitis B[1]	HepB	HepB				HePB						Range of recommended ages for all children
Rotavirus[2]			RV	RV	RV[2]							
Diphtheria, Tetanus, Pertussis[3]			DTap	DTap	DTap	see footnote[3]	DTap				DTap	
Haemophilus Influenza type b[4]			Hib	Hib	Hib[4]	Hib						
Pneumococcal[5]			PCV	PCV	PCV	PCV				PPSV		
Inacticated Poliovirus[6]			IPV	IPV		IPV					IPV	
Influenza[7]						Influenza (Yearly)						Range of recommended ages for certain high-risk groups
Measles, Mumps, Rubella[8]						MMR		see footnote[8]			MMR	
Varicella[9]						Varicella		see footnote[9]			Varicella	
Hepatitis A[10]						HepA (2 doses)				HepA Series		
Meningococcal[11]										MCV4		

FIGURE 15–5. Recommended immunization schedule for persons aged 0 to 6 years, 2011. Courtesy of Department of Health and Human Services, Centers for Disease Control and Prevention.

Recommended Immunization Schedule for Persons Aged 7 Through 18 Years—United States 2011
For those who fall behind or start late, see the schedule below and the catch-up schedule

Vaccine▼ Age ►	7–10 years	11–12 years	13–18 years	
Tetanus, Diphtheria, Pertussis[1]		Tdap	Tdap	Range of recommended ages for all children
Human Papillomavirus[2]	see footnote[2]	HPV (3 doses) (females)	HPV series	
Meningococcal[3]	MCV4	MCV4	MCV4	
Influenza[4]	Influenza (Yearly)			Range of recommended ages for catch-up immunization
Pneumococcal[5]	Pneumococcal			
Hepatitis A[6]	Hep A Series			
Hepatitis B[7]	Hep B Series			
Inacticated Poliovirus[8]	IPV Series			Range of recommended ages for certain high-risk groups
Measles, Mumps, Rubella[9]	MMR Series			
Varicella[10]	Varicella Series			

FIGURE 15–6. Recommended immunization schedule for persons aged 7 to 18 years, 2011. Courtesy of Department of Health and Human Services, Centers for Disease Control and Prevention.

3. Provide immunizations: See Figures 15-5 and 15-6, and Table 15-4. The *Red Book*, published by the AAP Committee on Infectious Diseases, is the widely accepted reference for immunizations. It contains guidelines for the many exceptions to the standard childhood schedule.

4. Survey developmental progression/milestones: See Figures 15-7 and 15-8.
5. Develop alliance with parent/caregiver through open ended discussion.
6. Increase caregiver competence in child care through age appropriate anticipatory guidance.

TABLE 15–4. Guide to Contraindications and Precautions to Immunizations, 2009

Vaccine	Contraindications	Precautions[a]	Not Contraindications (Vaccines May Be Given)
General for all vaccines (DTaP, IPV, MMR, Hib, pneumococcal, hepatitis B, varicella, hepatitis A, influenza)	Anaphylactic reaction to a vaccine contraindicates further doses of that vaccine	Moderate or severe illnesses with or without a fever	Mild to moderate local reaction (soreness, redness, swelling) after a dose of an injectable antigen
	Anaphylactic reaction to a vaccine constituent contraindicates the use of vaccines containing that substance	Latex allergy[b]	Low-grade or moderate fever after a previous vaccine dose Mild acute illness with or without low-grade fever Current antimicrobial therapy Convalescent phase of illnesses Prematurity (same dosage and indications as for healthy, full-term infants) Recent exposure to an infectious disease History of penicillin or other nonspecific allergies or fact that relatives have such allergies Pregnancy of mother or household contact Unimmunized household contact Immunodeficient household contact Breastfeeding (nursing infant *or* lactating mother)
DTaP	Encephalopathy within 7 days of administration of previous dose of DTaP/DTP	Temperature of 40.5° C (104.8° F) within 48 h after immunization with a previous dose of DTaP/DTP Collapse or shock-like state (hypotonic-hyporesponsive episode) within 48 h of receiving a previous dose of DTaP/DTP Seizures within 3 days of receiving a previous dose of DTaP/DTPc Persistent inconsolable crying lasting 3 hours, within 48 hours of receiving a previous dose of DTaP/DTP GBS within 5 weeks after a dose[d]	Family history of seizures[c] Family history of SIDS Family history of an adverse event after DTaP/DTP administration
IPV	Anaphylactic reactions to neomycin, streptomycin, or polymyxin B	Pregnancy	—
MMR[e,f]	Pregnancy	Recent (within 3 to 11 months, depending on product and dose) immune globulin administration[g]	Simultaneous tuberculin skin testing

Vaccine	Contraindications	Precautions[a]	Not Contraindications (Vaccines May Be Given)
	Anaphylactic reaction to neomycin or gelatin	Thrombocytopenia or history of thrombocytopenic purpura[g]	Breastfeeding
	Known altered immunodeficiency (hematologic and solid tumors, congenital immunodeficiency, severe HIV infection, and long-term immunosuppressive therapy)	Tuberculosis or positive PPD[h]	Pregnancy of mother of recipient Immunodeficient family member or household contact Infection with HIV Nonanaphylactic reactions to gelatin or neomycin
Hib	None	—	—
Hepatitis B	Anaphylactic reaction to baker's yeast	Prematurity[j]	Pregnancy
Pneumococcal	None	—	—
Varicella[c]	Pregnancy	Recent immune globulin administration	Pregnancy of mother of recipient
	Anaphylactic reaction to neomycin or gelatin Infection with HIV[k] Known altered immunodeficiency (hematologic and solid tumors, congenital immunodeficiency, and long-term immunosuppressive therapy)[l]	Family history of immunodeficiency[m]	Immunodeficiency in a household contact Household contact with HIV
Hepatitis A	Anaphylactic reaction to 2-phenoxyethanol or alum	Pregnancy	—
Influenza	Anaphylactic reaction to eggs	GBS within 6 weeks after a previous influenza immunization	Pregnancy

NOTE: This information is based on the recommendations of the Advisory Committee on Immunization Practices (ACIP) and the Committee on Infectious Diseases of the AAP. Sometimes these recommendations vary from those in the manufacturers' package inserts. For more detailed information, health-care professionals should consult the published recommendations of the ACIP, AAP, and the manufacturers' package inserts. These guidelines, originally issued in 1993, have been updated to give current recommendations as of 2003 (based on information available as of February 2003).

DTaP, diphtheria and tetanus toxoids and acellular pertussis; DTP, diphtheria and tetanus toxoids and pertussis; GBS, Guillain–Barré syndrome; Hib, *Haemophilus influenzae* type b; IPV, inactivated poliovirus; MMR, measles-mumps-rubella; PPD, purified protein derivative (tuberculin).

[a]The events or conditions listed as precautions, although not contraindications, should be reviewed carefully. The benefits and risks of administering a specific vaccine to a person under the circumstances should be considered. If the risks are believed to outweigh the benefits, the immunization should be withheld; if the benefits are believed to outweigh the risks (e.g., during an outbreak or foreign travel), the immunization should be given. Whether and when to administer DTaP to children with proven or suspected underlying neurologic disorders should be decided on an individual basis.

[b]If a person reports a severe (anaphylactic) allergy to latex, vaccines supplied in vials or syringes that contain natural rubber should not be administered unless the benefits of immunization outweigh the risks of an allergic reaction to the vaccine. For latex allergies other than anaphylactic allergies (e.g., a history of contact allergy to latex gloves), vaccines supplied in vials or syringes that contain dry natural rubber or latex can be administered.

[c]Acetaminophen given before administering DTaP and thereafter every 4 hours for 24 hours should be considered for children with a personal or family (i.e., sibling or parents) history of seizures.

[d]The decision to give additional doses of DTaP should be made on the basis of consideration of the benefit of further immunization versus the risk of recurrence of GBS. For example, completion of the primary series in children is justified.

[e]A theoretic risk exists that the administration of multiple live-virus vaccines within 30 days (4 weeks) of one another if not given on the same day will result in suboptimal immune response. No data substantiate this risk, however.

[f]An anaphylactic reaction to egg ingestion previously was considered a contraindication unless skin testing and, if indicated, desensitization had been performed. However, skin testing no longer is recommended as of 1997.

[g]The decision to immunize should be made on the basis of consideration of the benefits of immunity to measles, mumps, and rubella versus the risk of recurrence or exacerbation of thrombocytopenia after immunization or from natural infections of measles or rubella. In most instances, the benefits of immunization will be much greater than the potential risks and justify giving MMR, particularly in view of the even greater risk of thrombocytopenia after measles or rubella disease. However, if a previous episode of thrombocytopenia occurred in temporal proximity to immunization, not giving a subsequent dose may be prudent.

(Continued)

TABLE 15–4.   Guide to Contraindications and Precautions to Immunizations, 2003 (Continued)

[h]A theoretic basis exists for concern that measles vaccine might exacerbate tuberculosis. Consequently, before administering MMR to people with untreated active tuberculosis, initiating antituberculosis therapy is advisable.

[i]Measles immunization may suppress tuberculin reactivity temporarily. MMR vaccine may be given after, or on the same day as, tuberculin testing. If MMR has been given recently, postpone the tuberculin skin test until 4 to 6 weeks after administration of MMR.

[j]For preterm infants weighing less than 2 kg at birth and born to hepatitis B surface antigen (HBsAg) negative mothers, initiation of immunization should be delayed until just before hospital discharge if the infant weighs 2 kg or more, or until approximately 2 months of age, when other routine immunizations are given, to improve response. All preterm infants born to HBsAg-positive mothers should receive immunoprophylaxis (hepatitis B immune globulin and vaccine) beginning as soon as possible after birth, followed by appropriate postimmunization testing.

[k]Varicella vaccine should be considered for asymptomatic or mildly symptomatic HIV-infected children, specifically children in Centers for Disease Control and Prevention class N1 or A1, with age-specific T-cell percentages of 25 or higher.

[l]Varicella vaccine should not be administered to people who have cellular immunodeficiencies, but people with impaired humoral immunity may be immunized.

[m]Varicella vaccine should not be administered to a person who has a family history of congenital or hereditary immunodeficiency in parents or siblings unless the person's immune competence has been substantiated clinically or verified by a laboratory.

From Carroll JL, Loughlin GM. Sudden infant death syndrome. In: Johnson KB, Oski FA, eds. *Oski's Essential Pediatrics*. 2nd ed. Philadelphia, PA: Lippincott-Raven; 1997:174, with permission.

B. The First 5 Years—Well Care

1. Characterized by continuous changes in growth, acquisition of competence in interaction with environment including gross and fine motor skills, language acquisition, and emotional development.
2. Continue to monitor growth and development according to standardized charts, and developmental milestones according to the Denver II screening.
3. Engage in interaction in child to assess expressive and receptive language competence.
4. Provide anticipatory guidance for family/social relationships, diet, sleep, toileting, and injury prevention including car seats, gun safety, and bicycle helmets.

C. Middle Childhood—Ages 6 to 12 Years—Well Care

1. Characterized by increasing separation from parent/caregiver, development of self-awareness and perception of how others see them, greater interaction in the social environment beyond immediate family.
2. Assess language and development, noting:
   • Acquisition of attention skills.
   • Movement from egocentric to rule-based thinking.
   • Competence in social skills with family, schoolmates, and friends.
3. Perform survey of growth according to standardized growth curves, nutrition, hearing and vision.
   • Growth tends to occur in three to six irregularly spaced spurts each year.
   • Assess for sexual maturity and awareness.
4. Provide anticipatory guidance for family/social and school issues, diet/physical activity, sleep, bike helmet, seat belt/booster seat, gun safety, and injury prevention.

D. Adolescence—Ages 13 to 21—Well Care

1. Early years (10 to 13) characterized by progression through puberty.

2. Middle years (14 to 16) characterized by dramatic changes in sexual maturation.
3. Late years (17 to 21) characterized by adult-like characteristics.
4. Perform survey of growth according to standardized growth curves, nutrition, hearing and vision.
5. Record sexual maturity rating:
   • Tanner stages (Figures 15-9 to 15-11).
   • Record menses and note cycle length and characteristic of blood flow.
6. Explore issues with emotional relationship with parents, family, friends, and school.
   • Perform a "HEADSS" assessment addressing the following issues: *H*ome and Environment, *E*ducation and Employment, *A*ctivities, *D*rugs, *S*exuality, *S*uicidality/Depression.
7. Provide anticipatory guidance for risk behaviors, including drugs and alcohol, driving, counseling regarding sexual behaviors, and contraception.

IV. Genetic Abnormalities

A. Phenylketonuria

1. **Epidemiology**
   • Most common amino acid metabolism disorder.
   • 1:10,000 live births.
2. **Pathology**
   • Autosomal recessive chromosomal disorder.
   • Classic phenylketonuria (PKU) is due to a deficiency in phenylalanine hydroxylase in the liver.
   • Children with PKU are unable to metabolize phenylalanine because of the enzyme deficiency; therefore, with normal dietary intake of phenylalanine, there is a buildup of its toxic metabolites.
3. **Clinical Features**
   • Typically diagnosed through newborn metabolic screen, otherwise symptoms will not manifest until later in childhood.
   • Mental retardation.

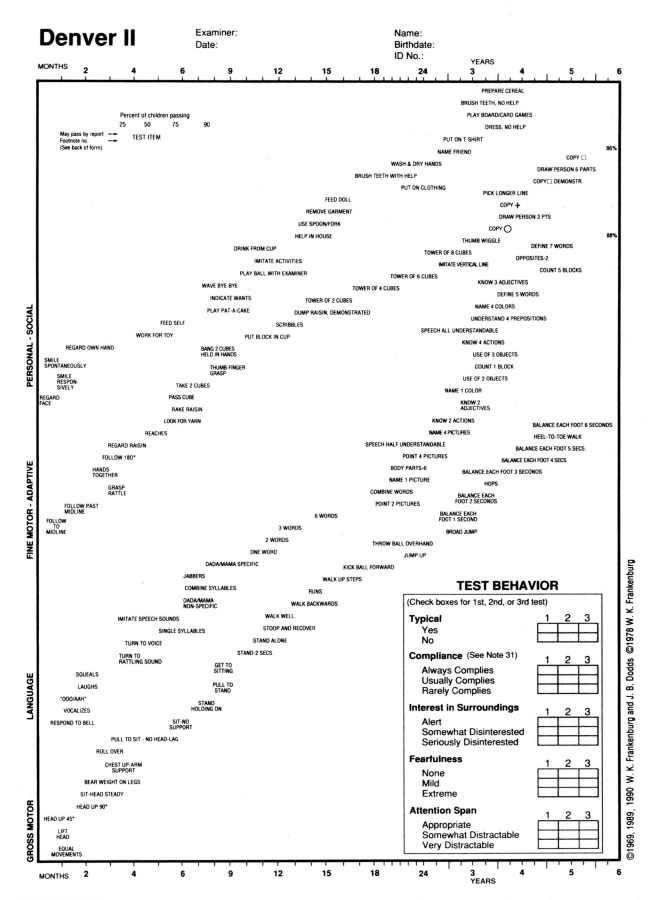

FIGURE 15–7. **Scoring form for the Denver II.** (From Frankenburg WK, Dodds JB. *Denver Developmental Screening Test.* 2nd ed. Denver, CO: Denver Development Materials, Inc.; 1990, with permission.)

DIRECTIONS FOR ADMINISTRATION

1. Try to get child to smile by smiling, talking or waving. Do not touch him/her.
2. Child must stare at hand several seconds.
3. Parent may help guide toothbrush and put toothpaste on brush.
4. Child does not have to be able to tie shoes or button/zip in the back.
5. Move yarn slowly in an arc from one side to the other, about 8" above child's face.
6. Pass if child grasps rattle when it is touched to the backs or tips of fingers.
7. Pass if child tries to see where yarn went. Yarn should be dropped quickly from sight from tester's hand without arm movement.
8. Child must transfer cube from hand to hand without help of body, mouth, or table.
9. Pass if child picks up raisin with any part of thumb and finger.
10. Line can vary only 30 degrees or less from tester's line.
11. Make a fist with thumb pointing upward and wiggle only the thumb. Pass if child imitates and does not move any fingers other than the thumb.

| 12. Pass any enclosed form. Fail continuous round motions. | 13. Which line is longer? (Not bigger.) Turn paper upside down and repeat. (pass 3 of 3 or 5 of 6) | 14. Pass any lines crossing near midpoint. | 15. Have child copy first. If failed, demonstrate. |

When giving items 12, 14, and 15, do not name the forms. Do not demonstrate 12 and 14.

16. When scoring, each pair (2 arms, 2 legs, etc.) counts as one part.
17. Place one cube in cup and shake gently near child's ear, but out of sight. Repeat for other ear.
18. Point to picture and have child name it. (No credit is given for sounds only.)
    If less than 4 pictures are named correctly, have child point to picture as each is named by tester.

19. Using doll, tell child: Show me the nose, eyes, ears, mouth, hands, feet, tummy, hair. Pass 6 of 8.
20. Using pictures, ask child: Which one flies?... says meow?... talks?... barks?... gallops? Pass 2 of 5, 4 of 5.
21. Ask child: What do you do when you are cold?... tired?... hungry? Pass 2 of 3, 3 of 3.
22. Ask child: What do you do with a cup? What is a chair used for? What is a pencil used for?
    Action words must be included in answers.
23. Pass if child correctly places <u>and</u> says how many blocks are on paper. (1, 5).
24. Tell child: Put block **on** table; **under** table; **in front of** me, **behind** me. Pass 4 of 4.
    (Do not help child by pointing, moving head or eyes.)
25. Ask child: What is a ball?... lake?... desk?... house?... banana?... curtain?... fence?... ceiling? Pass if defined in terms of use, shape, what it is made of, or general category (such as banana is fruit, not just yellow). Pass 5 of 8, 7 of 8.
26. Ask child: If a horse is big, a mouse is __? If fire is hot, ice is __? If the sun shines during the day, the moon shines during the __? Pass 2 of 3.
27. Child may use wall or rail only, not person. May not crawl.
28. Child must throw ball overhand 3 feet to within arm's reach of tester.
29. Child must perform standing broad jump over width of test sheet (8 1/2 inches).
30. Tell child to walk forward, ⚭⚭⚭⚭➤ heel within 1 inch of toe. Tester may demonstrate.
    Child must walk 4 consecutive steps.
31. In the second year, half of normal children are non-compliant.

OBSERVATIONS:

FIGURE 15–8. **Instructions for the Denver Development Screening Test.** Numbers are coded to scoring form (Figure 15-9). "Abnormal" is defined as two or more delays (failure of an item passed by 90% at that age) in two or more categories, or two or more delays in one category with one other category having one delay and an age line that does not intersect one item that is passed. A "suspect" or "questionable" score is given if one category has two or more delays or if one or more categories have one delay and in the same category the age line does not pass through one item that is passed. (From Frankenburg WK. *Denver Developmental Screening Test.* 2nd ed. Denver, CO: Denver Developmental Materials, Inc.; 1990, with permission.)

Sex Maturity Ratings in Boys

In assigning SMRs in boys, observe each of the three characteristics separately because they may develop at different rates. Record two separate ratings: pubic hair and genital. If the penis and testes differ in their stages, average the two into a single figure for the genital rating.

	Pubic Hair	Genital	
		Penis	*Testes and Scrotum*
Stage 1	Preadolescent—no pubic hair except for the fine body hair (vellus hair) similar to that on the abdomen	Preadolescent—same size and proportions as in childhood	Preadolescent—same size and proportions as in childhood
Stage 2	Sparse growth of long, slightly pigmented, downy hair, straight or only slightly curled, chiefly at the base of the penis	Slight or no enlargement	Testes larger; scrotum larger, somewhat reddened, and altered in texture
Stage 3	Darker, coarser, curlier hair spreading sparsely over the pubic symphysis	Larger, especially in length	Further enlarged
Stage 4	Coarse and curly hair, as in the adult; area covered greater than in stage 3 but not as great as in the adult and not yet including the thighs	Further enlarged in length and breadth, with development of the glans	Further enlarged; scrotal skin darkened
Stage 5	Hair adult in quantity and quality, spread to the medial surfaces of the thighs but not up over the abdomen	Adult in size and shape	Adult in size and shape

FIGURE 15–9. **Sex maturity ratings (SMRs) in boys.** (From Bates B, ed. Male genitalia and hernias. In: *Guide to Physical Examination and History Taking.* 6th ed. Philadelphia, PA: JB Lippincott; 1995:372, with permission.)

- Hypertonia.
- Tremors.
- Behavioral problems.
- Light complexion/hair.
- Eczema.
- Mouse-like odor to urine.

4. **Diagnostic Studies**
   - Neonatal screening demonstrates a hyperphenylal-aninemia (20 mg per dL or higher).
   - Diagnosis is confirmed by hyperphenylalaninemia in the presence of a normal or decreased level of plasma tyrosine.
   - Testing should be repeated as elevations may be transient in the perinatal period.

5. **Management**
   - Diet low in phenylalanine (lifelong).
   - Weekly monitoring of phenylalanine levels along with growth and development in the first year of life.

Sex Maturity Ratings in Girls: Pubic Hair

Stage 1
Preadolescent—no pubic hair except for the fine body hair (vellus hair) similar to that on the abdomen

Stage 2

Stage 3

Sparse growth of long, slightly pigmented, downy hair, straight or only slightly curled, chiefly along the labia

Darker, coarser, curlier hair, spreading sparsely over the pubic symphysis

Stage 4

Stage 5

Coarse and curly hair as in adults; area covered greater than in stage 3 but not as great as in the adult and not yet including the thighs

Hair adult in quantity and quality, spread on the medial surfaces of the thighs but not up over the abdomen

FIGURE 15–10. **SMRs in girls: pubic hair.** (From Bates B, ed. Female genitalia. In: *Guide to Physical Examination and History Taking.* 6th ed. Philadelphia, PA: JB Lippincott; 1995:388, with permission.)

Sex Maturity Ratings in Girls: Breasts

Stage 1
Preadolescent. Elevation of nipple only

Stage 2

Stage 3

Breast bud stage. Elevation of breast and nipple as a small mound; enlargement of areolar diameter

Further enlargement of elevation of breast and areola, with no separation of their contours

Stage 4

Stage 5

Projection of areola and nipple to form a secondary mound above the level of breast

Mature stage; projection of nipple only. Areola has receded to general contour of the breast (although in some normal individuals the areola continues to form a secondary mound)

FIGURE 15–11. **SMRs in girls: breasts.** (From Bates B, ed. The breasts and axillae. In: *Guide to Physical Examination and History Taking.* 6th ed. Philadelphia, PA: JB Lippincott; 1995:324, with permission.)

B. Cystic Fibrosis
1. Epidemiology
- Highest in Caucasians (1:3,000 live births).
2. Pathophysiology
- Autosomal recessive inheritance resulting in obstructive lung disease and exocrine gland dysfunction.
3. Clinical Manifestations
- May be diagnosed antenatally by screening or through state newborn screen.
- Meconium ileus at birth.
- Failure to thrive (FTT).
- Productive cough.
- Wheezing.
- Recurrent respiratory infections.
- Steatorrhea.
4. Diagnostic Testing
- Elevated immunoreactive trypsin (IRT) levels at birth.
- Elevated sweat chloride test associated with typical symptoms or family history.
- Genotypic analysis.
- Bronchiectasis on chest imaging.
- Sputum cultures typically show *Pseudomonas aeruginosa*, *Haemophilus influenzae*, or *Staphylococcus aureus*.
- Vitamin A, D, E, or K deficiency.

5. Management
- Children with CF should be managed at a facility that is accredited by the CF foundation if possible.
- Airway clearance therapy.
- Inhaled mucolytics (recombinant DNAse).
- Oral and inhaled antibiotics (antipseudomonal).
- Pancreatic enzyme supplementation.
- Supplementation of vitamins A, D, E, and K.
6. Prognosis
- Largely determined by progression of lung disease.
- Median life expectancy is 35.

C. Down Syndrome (Trisomy 21)
1. Epidemiology
- Most common chromosomal abnormality.
- Incidence (1:7,060 newborns).
- Higher incidence in newborns born to mothers >35 years old.
2. Etiology
- Presence of extra (complete or partial) chromosome. Twenty-one percent to 95% of these patients have 47 chromosomes with trisomy of 21 (sporadic), 4% translocation, 1% mosaic.

3. **Clinical Features**
   - Cognitive impairment, IQ is typically between 20 and 80.
   - Characteristic facies:
     - Brachycephaly.
     - Small dysplastic pinnae.
     - Upslanting palpebral fissures.
     - Epicanthal folds.
   - Limb abnormalities.
   - Hypotonia.
   - Associated conditions:
     - Hypothyroidism.
     - Cardiovascular defects—septal defects and endocardial cushion defect.
     - GI problems—esophageal/duodenal atresia, celiac disease, feeding problems, prolonged physiologic jaundice.
     - Leukemia.
     - Alzheimer dementia (average onset 35 years old).
     - Atlantoaxial subluxation.
4. **Diagnostic Studies**
   - Confirmed by chromosomal studies.
5. **Management**
   - Management of specific complications.
   - Goals of treatment are to have child develop to full potential.
   - Educational assistance.
   - Parents are encouraged to use support services.
6. **Prevention**
   - Genetic counseling for at risk population (advanced maternal age, parents with one child with Down syndrome).
   - Prenatal diagnosis through maternal serum α-feto protein levels, amniocentesis, chorionic villus sampling.

D. Trisomy 18
1. **Epidemiology**
   - Incidence 1 in 8,000 births.
   - Male to female ratio is 1:3.
2. **Etiology**
   - Additional copy of chromosome 18.
3. **Clinical Features**
   - Severe pre- and postnatal growth retardation.
   - Hypertonicity.
   - Dysmorphic facies—prominent occiput, micrognathia, cleft lip/palate.
   - Cardiac abnormalities—atrial septal defect, patent ductus arteriosus.
   - Limb abnormalities—Rocker bottom feet, overlapping fingers (clinodactyly).
   - Cognitive impairment.
   - Death usually occurs in infancy or early childhood from heart failure or pneumonia.
4. **Diagnostic Studies**
   - Confirmed by chromosomal studies.

5. **Management**
   - General support.
   - Grief counseling.
6. **Prevention**
   - Genetic counseling.
   - Prenatal diagnosis and decision to terminate pregnancy should be discussed with and left up to the parents.

E. Trisomy 13
1. **Epidemiology**
   - Incidence 1:12,000 births.
   - Male to female ratio is 3:2.
2. **Etiology**
   - Additional copy of chromosome 13.
3. **Clinical Features**
   - Usually associated with congenital anomalies incompatible with life; surviving infants usually die of congestive heart failure (CHF) or infection by the second year of life.
   - Characteristic facies: microcephaly, hypotelorism abnormalities of the ears, orbits, nose, and palate.
   - Omphalocele.
   - Polycystic kidneys.
   - Radial bone aplasia.
   - Polydactyly.
   - Skin abnormalities.
4. **Diagnostic Studies**
   - Confirmed by chromosomal studies.
5. **Management**
   - General support.
   - Grief counseling.
6. **Prevention**
   - Genetic counseling.
   - Prenatal diagnosis and decision to terminate pregnancy should be discussed with and left up to the parents.

F. Turner Syndrome (Gonadal Dysgenesis)
1. **Epidemiology**
   - 1:10,000 female live births.
2. **Etiology**
   - Chromosomal X monosomy.
3. **Clinical Features**
   - In the newborn—triangular facies, coarctation of the aorta, webbed neck, edema of the hands and feet.
   - In older children and adolescents—above symptoms, short stature, shield-shaped chest with widely spaced nipples, primary amenorrhea, absence of secondary sex characteristics, streak ovaries.
   - Patients with mosaic Turner syndrome—may only have short stature and primary amenorrhea.
4. **Diagnostic Studies**
   - Confirmed by chromosomal studies.

5. **Management**
   - Estrogen replacement therapy.
   - Growth hormone.
   - Fertility management.

G. Klinefelter Syndrome (XXY)

1. **Epidemiology**
   - 1:1,000 live male births.
2. **Clinical Features**
   - Normal appearance before the onset of puberty.
   - Variable cognitive impairment.
   - In postpubertal boys: microorchidism with otherwise normal external genitalia, gynecomastia, azoospermia, sterility, decreased facial hair, lack of libido/potency.
3. **Diagnostic Studies**
   - Confirmed by chromosomal studies.
4. **Management**
   - Testosterone replacement.
   - Psychosocial and educational counseling as needed.

H. Fragile X Syndrome

1. **Etiology**
   - Chromosome mutation of the *FMR1* gene.
2. **Clinical Features**
   - Variable degrees of intellectual difficulty.
   - Behavioral abnormalities: ranging from social anxiety and shyness to hyperactivity, ADHD, and autistic characteristics (primarily in males).
   - Characteristic facies with prominent ears and jaw, with oblong face.
   - Macroorchidism.
3. **Diagnostic Studies**
   - Confirmed by chromosomal studies.
4. **Management**
   - Management of behavioral and intellectual problems as needed.
   - Multidisciplinary team.
5. **Prevention**
   - Genetic counseling.

V. Cardiovascular System

A. Tetralogy of Fallot

1. **Epidemiology**
   - Most common form of congenital heart disease in infants.
2. **Pathology**
   - **Four classic clinical features:**
     - A large, unrestricted ventricular septal defect (VSD).
     - An aorta overriding the VSD.
     - Right ventricular hypertrophy (RVH).
     - Right outflow obstruction—infundibular pulmonary stenosis.
   - Anatomic abnormalities that may coexist include right aortic arch, atrial septal defect, absent pulmonary valve, pulmonary atresia, atrioventricular septal defect, and a left superior vena cava to the coronary sinus.
3. **Clinical Features**
   - Symptoms can range from the asymptomatic acyanotic child with a heart murmur ("pink tetralogy") to a severely hypoxic newborn infant.
   - The degree of right-to-left shunting determines whether the infant/child will be cyanotic or acyanotic.
   - Often, at birth, the infant is acyanotic.
   - After the first year of life, the infant is more likely to present with cyanosis.
   - Cyanosis can be exacerbated with exertion in acyanotic patients.
   - Squatting is a common posture in tetralogy of Fallot patients, especially after exercise.
   - Episodes of paroxysmal hypoxemia (tetralogy spells) may be seen.
   - Systolic ejection murmur.
   - Dyspnea on exertion.
   - Clubbing of the fingers may be present in the older cyanotic child.
4. **Diagnostic Studies**
   - Electrocardiogram (ECG) exhibits RVH and right axis deviation.
   - CXR, as seen in posterior-anterior view, shows a boot-shaped heart (caused by RVH) and a concavity of the upper left heart border (caused by absence of the main pulmonary artery segment).
   - Echocardiography showing right ventricle wall thickening, overriding aorta, and VSD confirms the diagnosis. In addition, pulmonary valve obstruction can be assessed.
   - Cardiac catheterization will show a right-to-left shunt at the ventricular level. The right ventricular pressure will be equal to the left ventricular pressure. A selective right ventriculogram confirms the diagnosis because it shows the thickened right ventricle, stenotic pulmonary valve, and VSD.
5. **Management**
   - Complete surgical correction involving the closing of the VSD and removing the right ventricular outflow is required if the patient is significantly symptomatic and hypoxemic.
6. **Prognosis**
   - Surgical mortality rate is <10%.
   - The earlier the complete surgical correction, the better the functional capacity as the child ages.

B. Ventricular Septal Defect

1. **Epidemiology**
   - The most common cardiac malformation.
   - More common in males.
2. **Pathology**
   - Congenital heart disease.
   - Range in size from "pinhole" to a virtual absence of septum.

- Membranous defects are more common than muscular defects.
- Most ventricular septal defects (VSDs) are small and close spontaneously or do not need repair.

3. Clinical Features
- Patients with small-to-moderate left-to-right shunts (most common) usually have no symptoms.
- Patients with larger shunts usually exhibit poor weight gain, frequent URI, and pneumonia in infancy.
- Dyspnea, poor exercise tolerance, fatigue, and CHF in childhood.
- Characteristic loud, harsh, holosystolic, high-pitched murmur heard best along the left sternal border, specifically the third to fifth intercostal spaces.
- A localized thrill may be palpated.

4. Diagnostic Studies
- CXR in small-to-moderate shunts—the findings are usually normal; larger shunts may show cardiomegaly, and the main pulmonary artery segment is dilated.
- ECG in small-to-moderate shunts—the ECG is normal; larger shunts may show left ventricular hypertrophy.
- Two-dimensional (2D) echocardiography— provides visualization of defects 2 mm or larger in about 75% of patients, and often can be used to pinpoint the anatomic location. Adding color Doppler can diagnose virtually all defects, including the smallest "pinpoint" lesion.

5. Management
- A significant number, estimated to be 30% to 70%, undergo spontaneous closure usually in the first 2 years of life.
- Small defects that do not close spontaneously require treatment rarely.
- Larger shunts should be surgically repaired before 2 years of age to prevent the possibility of pulmonary hypertension. Primary closure of the defect with a prosthetic patch is now used for nearly all isolated symptomatic defects.

6. Prognosis
- Adults with corrected defects have a normal quality of life.
- Functional exercise capacity and O_2 capacity are usually normal.
- Small asymptomatic VSDs that do not close spontaneously require subacute bacterial endocarditis prophylaxis.

C. Patent Ductus Arteriosus

1. Epidemiology
- Females outnumber males 2:1.
- More common in preterm infants weighing <1,500 g.
- May be seen with VSD and coarctation of the aorta.
- Common in children whose mothers contracted rubella in the first trimester of the pregnancy.

2. Pathology
- Patent ductus arteriosus (PDA) is persistence in extrauterine life of the normal fetal vessel that joins the pulmonary artery to the aorta.
- Normally closes by the fourth day of life.

3. Clinical Features
- The clinical finding and clinical course depend on the size of the shunt.
- Usually, no symptoms are associated with small patent ductus.
- **A large shunt:**
  - Apical pulse is prominent.
  - A loud, harsh, continuous murmur or a thrill heard maximally at the second left interspace is often present and may radiate toward the left clavicle and/or down the left sternal border.
  - Has a machine-like quality and is usually unaltered by postural changes.
  - May result in CHF.

4. Diagnostic Studies
- CXR in the small patent ductus shunt is normal, whereas the larger shunt may show findings of both left atrial and left ventricular hypertrophy, a prominent aorta, and prominent main pulmonary artery segment.
- ECG in the small patent ductus shunt is normal, whereas the larger shunt may show left ventricular or biventricular hypertrophy.
- Echocardiography with a small patent ductus shunt is normal, whereas the larger shunt may show enlargement of the left atrium, left ventricle, or both. Color Doppler and 2D echocardiography can show the turbulent blood flow in the pulmonary artery and usually eliminate the need for diagnostic cardiac catheterization.

5. Management
- Surgical correction when the ductus arteriosus is large (except in patients with pulmonary vascular obstruction).
- Transcatheter closure of small defects with a coil is becoming standard therapy.
- Although controversial, indomethacin may be used in premature infants to assist closure of the patent ductus.

6. Prognosis
- Patients with small-to-moderate PDA shunts do well even without surgery until their third or fourth decade of life. They may then begin to experience easy fatigability and dyspnea on exertion, at which point they require surgical correction.

D. Kawasaki Disease (Mucocutaneous Lymph Node Syndrome)

1. Epidemiology
- One of the most common causes of acquired heart disease and inflammatory arthritis.
- An acute, febrile, multisystem syndrome.

- Primarily occurs in children younger than 9 years (peak 13 to 24 months of age).
- Diagnosis is based entirely on clinical features.
- Males affected more than females (1.5:1).

2. **Etiology/Pathology**
   - Unknown.
   - May be related to bacterial toxins.
3. **Clinical Features**
   - The child appears ill.
   - Abdominal pain.
   - Carditis.
   - Arthralgia of large joints.
   - Desquamation beginning around the fingers and toes that occurs after the fever has dissipated (about 2 weeks).
   - **Diagnostic criteria:**
     - Acute onset of relentless fever (up to 104° to 105° F) lasting for at least 5 days.
     - **Presence of four of the following five conditions:**
       - Bilateral nonpurulent conjunctival injection.
       - Changes of the mucosa of the oropharynx, including pharyngeal injection, dry fissured lips, injected lips, and strawberry tongue.
       - Changes of the peripheral extremities, such as edema, erythema, or both of the hands or feet; desquamation, usually beginning periungually.
       - Rash, primarily truncal; polymorphous but nonvesicular.
       - Cervical lymphadenopathy.
       - Illness not explained by other known disease process.
4. **Diagnostic Studies**
   - Elevated white blood cells (WBCs).
   - Elevated ESR.
   - Elevated C-reactive protein.
   - Elevated platelets (late finding).
   - UA abnormal with elevated protein and pyuria.

   IMAGING FINDINGS
   - ECG abnormalities (peaked T waves, first-degree heart block, ST segment elevation or depression, and QT prolongation).
   - ECG discloses coronary artery aneurysms.
5. **Complications**
   - Coronary artery aneurysm.
   - Coronary artery thrombosis.
   - Myocardial infarction.
   - Myopericarditis.
   - CHF.
   - Pericardial effusion.
   - Hydrops of gallbladder.
   - Aseptic meningitis.
   - Polyarticular arthritis.
   - Uveitis.
   - Peripheral artery aneurysm.

6. **Management**
   - Intravenous (IV) β-globulin reduces the acute inflammation and also appears to reduce the frequency of coronary artery dilatation and aneurysm.
   - Aspirin at high doses initially to control inflammation, then low-dose antiplatelet therapy.
   - Disease is self-limited.
7. **Prognosis**
   - Cardiac damage sustained when the disease was active may be progressive; however, immediately beginning β-globulin and aspirin therapy can reduce the development of coronary artery aneurysms significantly.
   - Fatal in 0.1% to 3% of patients.

VI. Pulmonary System

A. Bronchiolitis

1. **Epidemiology**
   - Occurs within first 2 years of life, peak incidence 6 months of age.
   - Incidence is highest in the winter and early spring months.
   - May occur epidemically or sporadically.
   - Frequent cause of hospitalization.
   - Infants exposed to secondhand smoke are more likely to develop bronchiolitis than infants not exposed.
   - Infants who attend daycare centers are more likely to develop bronchiolitis than those who do not.
2. **Etiology**
   - RSV is the most likely pathogen; however, parainfluenza and influenza viruses, adenovirus, *Mycoplasma*, and *Chlamydia* are other causes.
3. **Pathology**
   - Bronchiolitis results from obstruction due to edema and accumulation of mucus and cellular debris and invasion of the small airways by RSV.
4. **Clinical Features**
   - Fever for 1 to 2 days.
   - Rhinorrhea.
   - Irritability.
   - Decreased appetite.
   - Cough.
   - Wheezing.
   - Tachypnea.
   - Intercostal retractions.
   - Nasal flaring.
   - Prolonged expiratory phase.
   - May be rales and/or rhonchi.
   - The liver and spleen may be palpable because of hyperinflation of the lungs.
5. **Diagnostic Studies**
   - CBC is normal.
   - CXR—typical findings are hyperinflation, peribronchial cuffing, and subsegmental atelectasis of the lungs with mild interstitial infiltrates.

- Viral culture or antigen assay from nasopharyngeal secretions may isolate RSV.
- Hypoxemia is common.

6. **Complications**
   - Children with bronchopulmonary dysplasia or certain congenital anomalies (i.e., congenital heart disease, neuromuscular disorders, malnutrition, and congenital or acquired abnormalities of immunologic function) have excessive morbidity and mortality.

7. **Management**
   - Most patients are readily managed as outpatients by supportive therapy.
   - Patients with respiratory distress and hypoxemia should be hospitalized.
   - Treated with humidified O_2 and supportive therapy.
   - An antiviral agent, ribavirin, may be of some benefit, especially in patients with respiratory distress or chronic cardiopulmonary disease. Its spectrum includes RSV, influenza, parainfluenza, and adenoviruses.
   - β_2-Agonist bronchodilators can be of some benefit, although controversy exists about their efficacy.
   - **Prophylaxis:**
     - Synagis (palivizumab) is indicated for prevention of serious lower respiratory tract disease caused by RSV in patients at high risk for RSV disease—that is, bronchopulmonary dysplasia and premature infants (<35 weeks gestational age).
     - The dosage of 15 mg per kg should be administered intramuscular (IM) on a monthly basis during RSV season.

8. **Prognosis**
   - Overall, the long-term prognosis is good.
   - Major concerns include acute effects of bronchiolitis and the development of chronic airway hyperreactivity (asthma).

B. Epiglottitis

1. **Epidemiology**
   - Most frequently seen in children 3 months to 6 years old, although reported in all age groups.
   - Males more than females, 2:1.
   - Occurs in any season.

2. **Etiology**
   - Usually due to bacteria—*H. influenzae* type B (HiB).

3. **Pathology**
   - An acute infection/inflammation of the epiglottis and edema of the surrounding soft tissue.
   - It is an immediate threat to life because complete upper airway obstruction may occur suddenly at any time.

4. **Clinical Features**
   - Sudden with rapid progression.
   - Pharyngeal pain.
   - Dysphagia.

- Odynophagia (pain on swallowing) is characteristic.
- Fever (approximately 104° F).
- Inspiratory stridor.
- Characteristic posture—TRIPOD-sitting leaning forward, elbows on legs, drooling.
- Tachypnea—the patient appears anxious.
- Do not examine the mouth or neck if you suspect epiglottitis—it may cause spasm, thereby exacerbating complete upper airway obstruction.

5. **Diagnostic Studies**
   - Obtain a lateral soft-tissue X-ray of the neck.
   - Epiglottis will be swollen and displaced posteriorly (thumb sign).
   - Blood cultures will often be positive.

6. **Management**
   - Immediate hospitalization.
   - Management of Airways, Breathing and Circulation is the first priority.
   - Consult an anesthesiologist for probable nasotracheal or orotracheal intubation.
   - IV antibiotics should be started with either cefotaxime (Claforan), ceftriaxone (Rocephin), or ampicillin with sulbactam (Unasyn).
   - Fluids and humidified O_2.

C. Laryngotracheitis (Croup)

1. **Epidemiology**
   - Most common in children 3 months to 3 years (but may occur at any age).
   - Life-threatening airway obstruction more likely to occur in the pediatric population because of the already narrowed airways.
   - Males affected more than females, 3:1.
   - Increased incidence from October to April.
   - One hundred to 1,000 times more common than epiglottitis.

2. **Etiology**
   - Almost always caused by viruses (usually parainfluenza types I to III).

3. **Pathology**
   - Infection/inflammation of the airway that involves the larynx and subglottic areas.

4. **Clinical Features**
   - Slow insidious onset.
   - Symptoms may persist up to 14 days (with the worst symptoms lasting 1 to 2 days).
   - Usually, a current or recent URI is noted.
   - Hoarseness.
   - "Barking," seal-like cough.
   - Stridor is common (both inspiratory and expiratory).
   - Symptoms usually worse at night or when child is agitated.
   - Fever (low-grade), rhinitis, pharyngitis, and wheezing may be present.

5. **Diagnostic Studies**
   - Performing diagnostic studies may agitate the patient; therefore, unnecessary invasive studies

should be avoided (an ABG may be needed in seriously ill patients).
- An anterior–posterior (AP) or lateral soft-tissue X-ray of the neck showing subglottic narrowing confirms the diagnosis.

6. **Management**
- Always ABCs first.
- Disturb the patient as little as possible.
- Cool air mist is the mainstay of therapy, although sitting in a steamed-up bathroom and/or taking the child for a ride with the windows slightly open are simple therapeutic measures.
- Antibiotics are not necessary.
- Observation and adequate hydration.
- Aerosolized racemic epinephrine may be required for severe cases.
- Dexamethasone IM improves symptoms, reduces the duration of hospitalization and frequency of intubations, and permits early discharge from the emergency department.
- Hospitalization is necessary for only the severe cases of croup.

D. Pertussis (Whooping Cough)

1. **Epidemiology**
- Mostly affects children younger than 5 years of age (mortality highest in infants younger than 1 year).
- Females affected more than males.
- Can occur in any season.

2. **Pathology**
- Predominantly caused by *Bordetella pertussis*, a gram-negative, pleomorphic bacilli.
- Highly contagious; transmission is by droplets released during intense coughing.
- It is postulated that the tracheal cytotoxin, dermonecrotic factor, and adenylate cyclase are responsible for local epithelial damage that produces respiratory symptomology and aids in absorption of pertussis toxin.

3. **Clinical Features**
- Incubation period ranges from 6 to 14 days.
- Illness lasts 6 to 8 weeks and is broken down into three stages:
  - **Catarrhal stage (1 to 2 weeks)—prodromal, preparoxysmal:**
    - Patients are most contagious during this stage.
    - Rhinorrhea.
    - Conjunctival injection.
    - Lacrimation.
    - Mild cough.
    - Low-grade fever.
    - Pertussis often overlooked during this stage because manifestations resemble those of a simple URI.
  - **Paroxysmal stage (2 to 4 weeks or longer):**
    - Episodes of cough increase in severity and frequency.

- Forceful coughs during expiration are followed by a sudden massive inspiration producing the whoop.
- Facial petechiae and redness.
- Cyanosis.
- Posttussive vomiting.
- Recurrent episodes are exhausting; patients appear apathetic.
- Attacks may be initiated by yawning, sneezing, eating, drinking, and physical exertion.
  - **Convalescent stage (1 to 2 weeks):**
    - Paroxysmal coughing and vomiting decrease in severity and frequency.
    - Chronic cough may persist for several months.

4. **Diagnostic Studies**
- Isolation of *B. pertussis* during early phase of illness by culture of nasopharyngeal swab on glycerin potato-blood agar medium (Bordet–Gengou), penicillin added to inhibit the growth of other organisms. PCR detection is replacing culture because of improved sensitivity, decreased time of diagnosis, and cost.

5. **Complications**
- The most frequent complication is pneumonia.
- OM and sinusitis are also common.

6. **Management**
- Erythromycin aborts or eliminates pertussis when administered in the catarrhal stage, but does not affect the duration of the paroxysmal stage.
- Clarithromycin or azithromycin are equally effective. Use azithromycin if erythromycin is intolerant and if infants are younger than 1 month.
- Erythromycin also shortens the period of communicability.
- Corticosteroid aerosols may be helpful in severe cases.
- Supportive care includes warm mist O_2, nasopharyngeal suctioning, and parenteral fluids.

7. **Prevention**
- The incidence of pertussis has decreased dramatically since the pertussis vaccine has been used.
- Immunization reduces the incidence and mortality rate of pertussis, but immunity is neither complete nor permanent.
- The pertussis vaccine carries with it side effects (seizures and neurologic effects), but a greater chance of mortality exists with pertussis than with the vaccine.

E. Sudden Infant Death Syndrome

1. Defined as the sudden death of an infant, unexpected by history, and unexplained by a thorough postmortem examination, which includes a complete autopsy, investigation of the scene, and review of the medical history.

2. **Epidemiology**
- The cause of sudden infant death syndrome (SIDS) is unknown.

- In the United States, SIDS occurs in 1/1,000 to 2/1,000 live births.
- Rare before 1 month, peaks at 2 to 4 months, and 95% occur before 6 months of age.
- Male gender (3:2).
- Most common cause of death in the neonatal period (before 1 year of age).

3. Pathology
- Suggests hypoxia (acute or chronic).
- Intrathoracic petechiae and mild inflammation and congestion of the respiratory tract may be present.

4. Risk Factors
- Ethnic and racial minorities.
- Low socioeconomic status.
- Low birth weight.
- Drug-addicted mothers.
- Maternal smoking during and after pregnancy.
- Sleeping in the prone position.
- Family history of SIDS.

5. Prevention
- See Table 15-5 for possible approaches to the prevention of SIDS.

VII. Gastrointestinal System and Nutrition

A. Infectious Gastroenteritis

1. Etiology
- Viruses: rotavirus, Norwalk virus, enterovirus, astroviruses.
- Bacteria: *Salmonella, Shigella, Yersinia, Campylobacter* spp.; pathogenic *Escherichia coli, Clostridium difficile,* tuberculosis.
- Parasites: *Giardia lamblia, Entamoeba histolytica, Cryptosporidium parvum.*

2. Pathology
- Acute inflammation of the intestinal epithelium lining.
- Produces watery and sometimes bloody stool.

3. Clinical Features
- Irritability.
- Vomiting.
- Diarrhea.
- Nausea.
- Abdominal pain.
- May have fever.
- Symptoms and signs of dehydration.

4. Diagnostic Studies
- Stool culture for rotavirus, bacteria, ova and parasites, and *C. difficile* if prolonged or clinically indicated.
- Electrolyte levels should be measured in moderately dehydrated children.
- Imaging studies and GI referral if anatomic abnormalities suspected.

5. Management
- Treatment of diarrhea is directed primarily by the degree of dehydration present.
- If mild, use oral rehydrating solution.
- Key to therapy is administering small volumes of glucose-electrolyte solution such as Pedialyte in 5-mL aliquots every 3 to 5 minutes for the first hour, then advance slowly.
- Wait 15 to 20 minutes after a vomiting episode to give fluid.
- IV solution is necessary to correct electrolyte imbalance or, when vomiting, prolonging BRAT diet (bananas, rice, toast, and applesauce) until solids are tolerated.
- Loperamide is not recommended to treat acute diarrhea in children.
- Anticholinergic agents are not recommended in the management of diarrhea in children.
- Bismuth subsalicylate is not recommended because of the possible absorption of salicylate and theoretical concern of Reye syndrome.

B. Intussusception

1. Epidemiology
- One of the most dangerous surgical emergencies in early childhood, and the most common cause of intestinal obstruction in the first 2 years of life.
- Most commonly seen in infants 3 months to 1 year of age.
- In 95% of the patients, no cause can be found.

2. Pathology
- Characterized by the telescoping of a proximal portion of the intestine into a more distal position. This "telescoping" results in impairment of the blood supply and necrosis of the involved bowel segment.
- In 95% of the patients, the telescoping involves the ileum into the colon (ileocolic).

3. Clinical Features
- Nearly, all affected infants present with an acute onset of episodic colicky pain and vomiting.
- Sausage-shaped mass may be palpated in the area of the hepatic flexure.
- Fever.
- Signs of dehydration may be present.
- Currant jelly stools (late finding).

4. Diagnostic Studies
- Barium enema discloses the intussusception outlined as an inverted cap, and an obstruction to the progression of the barium is noted.

5. Management
- IV rehydration should be instituted immediately, and a nasogastric (NG) tube is placed.
- Barium and air enema is the diagnostic test of choice and the treatment of choice; 75% of cases can be reduced successfully using a barium enema under fluoroscopy.

- **Contraindications to hydrostatic (barium) reduction:**
  - Free intraperitoneal air or peritoneal and systemic signs of compromised intestine.
  - These patients should be taken directly to surgery.
  - Surgical reduction or resection and anastomosis should be performed if barium enema reduction is unsuccessful.
6. **Prognosis**
  - Recurrence rate is near 5% and occurs shortly after reduction.

C. Volvulus (Malrotation)
1. **Epidemiology**
   - Accounts for about 10% of neonatal intestinal obstructions.
2. **Etiology**
   - Incomplete rotation of the intestine during fetal development.
3. **Pathology**
   - Most common type of malrotation is the failure of the cecum to move into the right lower quadrant. Here, the mesentery, including the superior mesenteric artery, may twist around itself, producing a midgut volvulus.
4. **Clinical Features**
   - Symptoms usually present within the first weeks of life (1 to 3 weeks).
   - Recurrent bile-stained vomiting.
   - Acute small bowel obstruction (i.e., irritability, distended, rigid abdomen, vomiting, and decreased stooling).
   - Older children may present with abdominal pain (25% to 50% may be asymptomatic) and may have an incomplete obstruction.
5. **Diagnostic Studies**
   - Abdominal plain film may demonstrate a "double bubble" sign.
   - Barium enema shows malposition of the cecum.
   - Upper GI series demonstrates malposition of the ligament of Treitz, confirming the diagnosis of malrotation. This is the procedure of choice in the nonobstructed patient.
6. **Management**
   - A surgical emergency.
   - Bowel necrosis results from occlusion of the superior mesenteric artery, and intestinal resection should be delayed until a second-look operation can be performed 24 to 48 hours later in anticipation that some bowel can be salvaged.

D. Constipation
1. **Etiology**
   - Beyond neonatal period, most common cause is fecal retention and withholding.
   - Prolonged fecal stasis in the colon with reabsorption of fluid.
   - Diet low in fiber.
   - Anal fissures.
   - Hemorrhoids.
   - Structural problems including tumor, inflammatory bowel disease.
2. **Pathology**
   - Subtypes—colonic inertia, obstructed defecation, generalized slow transit.
   - Rectal wall stretches.
   - Rectum habituates to stimulus of enlarging fecal mass.
   - Urge to defecate subsides.
3. **Clinical Features**
   - Parental concern of change in stool pattern.
   - Fecal soiling in children who are toilet trained.
   - Hard, painful stool.
   - Change in stool size and consistency.
   - Abdominal pain, cramps.
   - Fever, abdominal distention, anorexia, nausea, vomiting, weight loss or gain may indicate organic disorder.
   - Bloody diarrhea in the infant could be an indicative of enterocolitis complicating Hirschsprung disease.
4. **Diagnostic Studies**
   - Stool for occult blood in all infants.
   - Abdominal radiograph for selected patients.
   - CBC, ESR, thyroid panel, complete metabolic profile, celiac disease antibodies.
   - Sweat test to rule out CF for all infants and children with FTT.
   - If laboratory values are abnormal, refer to pediatric gastroenterologist.
5. **Management**
   a. **Management for Infants**
   - Rectal disimpaction with glycerin suppositories.
   - Avoid enemas.
   - Give juices that contain sorbitol; for infants <4 months, can add prune juice to formula—several teaspoons to 1 oz of formula or breast milk daily.
   - Avoid mineral oil and stimulant laxatives.
   b. **Management for Children**
   - Disimpaction with medication and/or enemas.
   - Balanced high-fiber diet.
   - Mineral oil and osmotic laxatives.
   - Short-term administration of stimulant laxatives.
   - Polyethylene glycol electrolyte solution PEG (MiraLax) given chronically in low dosage for usually 6 months of therapy.
   - Goal of treatment is two soft or runny stools per day.
   - Gradual return to one or two formed stools daily.

E. Pyloric Stenosis
1. **Epidemiology**
   - More apt to occur in firstborn infants.
   - More likely to occur in males than in females, 4:1.

2. Pathology
- Marked increase in the circular musculature of the pylorus, causing an obstruction of the lumen.

3. Clinical Features
- Signs and symptoms will likely occur between 2 and 12 weeks of age.
- Projectile vomiting that occurs within 2 hours of each feeding.
- Vomitus does not contain bile.
- Irritability; the child appears hungry.
- Weight loss, dehydration.
- Jaundice occurs in 2% to 5% of patients.
- An olive-shaped mass can be palpated in the right upper quadrant.
- Mass felt well immediately following vomiting.

4. Laboratory/Diagnostic Studies
- Ultrasonography demonstrates a hypertrophied pyloric muscle.
- Hypochloremic alkalosis with potassium depletion.

5. Management
- Rehydration and correction of electrolyte imbalance.
- NG tube insertion.
- Surgical intervention curative.

6. Prognosis
- Excellent following surgery.
- Recurrence unlikely.

VIII. Musculoskeletal System

A. Henoch–Schönlein Purpura

1. Epidemiology
- Occurs in children 4 to 10 years of age.

2. Etiology
- Cause unknown.
- An upper respiratory or other illness or allergy may precede Henoch–Schönlein purpura (HSP).
- Can affect the skin, GI tract, kidneys, and joints.

3. Pathology
- Vasculitis of the small blood vessels in children.
- An example of nonthrombocytopenic purpura.

4. Clinical Features
- Onset is acute.
- Cutaneous lesions are the hallmark of this disease.
- Circular purpuric lesions 2 to 3 mm in size, appearing first on the lower extremities.
- Nonpitting edema about the dorsum of the hands and feet may be present.
- Colicky abdominal pain.
- Melena.
- Ileus.
- Vomiting.
- Hematemesis.
- Arthritis (most commonly of the knees and ankles, but wrists, elbows, and fingers may be involved).
- Periarticular swelling.
- Joint tenderness.

5. Diagnostic Studies
- Platelets are normal to mildly elevated.
- Coagulation studies are normal.
- All other hematologic studies are normal.

6. Complications
- Nephritis.
- Intussusception.
- Anemia (secondary to GI bleeding).

7. Management
- Most children with HSP have a self-limited course.
- Most have a single exacerbation lasting about 4 weeks.

8. Prognosis
- Generally excellent, but depends on the extent of the disease and the age of the child.
- The younger the child, the better the prognosis.
- Less than 5% of children progress to end-stage renal disease.

B. Slipped Capital Femoral Epiphysis

1. Epidemiology
- Occurs in adolescence.
- Most common in obese males.

2. Etiology
- Unknown.
- Hypothesis.
  - Perichondrial ring stabilizing the epiphyseal area is weakened by hormonal changes during adolescence such that the overload of excessive body weight can produce a pathologic fracture through the growth plate.

3. Pathology
- Displacement of the proximal femoral epiphysis due to the disruption of the growth plate.
- Head of the femur is displaced medially and posteriorly relative to the femoral neck.

4. Clinical Features
- In small instances, it can occur with a fall or direct trauma.
- Most commonly, it is a healthy child who presents with pain and limp.
- Pain can be referred into the thigh or the medial side of the knee.
- On physical examination, limitation of internal rotation of the hip is found.

5. Diagnostic Studies
- Radiographic findings.
  - Osteoporosis of the head and neck on AP view early.
  - Indistinct epiphysis-widened.
  - Line along lateral edge of superior femoral neck on AP does not intersect epiphysis.
  - Metaphysis displaced laterally, so that it does not overlap posterior lip of acetabulum as normal.

6. Management
- Non–weight-bearing on crutches.
- Immediate referral to an orthopedic surgeon.

7. **Prognosis**
   - Due to the patient's continually being overweight, they have a high incidence of degenerative arthritis, even in those who do not develop avascular necrosis.
   - Development of avascular necrosis almost guarantees a poor prognosis.
   - Thirty percent of patients have bilateral involvement, which may occur as late as 1 or 2 years after the primary episode.

IX. Eyes, Ears, Nose, and Throat

A. Sinusitis

1. **Etiology**
   - Common pathogens include *Streptococcus pneumoniae*, *H. influenzae*, and *Moraxella catarrhalis*.
   - *Staphylococcus aureus* and anaerobic organisms are recovered more often in chronic sinusitis.

2. **Pathology**
   - Viral infection causes mucosal injury and inflammation which results in obstruction and hypersection.
   - Inflammation and sinus drainage obstruction of the paranasal sinuses.
   - Mucus thickening.
   - Acute—less than 30 days duration.
   - Subacute—90 days with resolution.
   - Recurrent acute—repeated episodes with resolution in between.
   - Chronic—more than 90 days with persistent respiratory symptoms such as cough, rhinorrhea, and nasal obstruction.

3. **Clinical Features**
   - Persistent respiratory symptoms.
   - Malodorous breath.
   - Headache and morning painless eye swelling.
   - Sometimes fever.
   - Frequent throat clearing.
   - Hyposmia (diminished smell) in older children.
   - Daytime cough worsening at night.
   - Facial pain when bending forward.

4. **Imaging**
   - Should be reserved for patients with complications, those not responsive to medications, or those who may undergo surgical management.
   - Coronal sinus computed tomography (CT) is the most often used study.

5. **Treatment**
   - Amoxicillin (90 mg/kg/day) for 10 to 14 days.
   - Amoxicillin/clavulanate (80 to 90 mg/kg/day of amoxicillin with 6.4 mg/kg/day of clavulanate in two divided doses for 14 days) if not improving on amoxicillin alone, daycare exposure, or recent antibiotic use.
   - Alternative therapies include cefdinir, cefuroxime, and cefpodoxime.

   - Highly allergic patients use clarithromycin, azithromycin, or clindamycin for penicillin-resistant *Streptococcus pneumoniae*.

6. **Complications**
   - Severe facial pain.
   - Orbital or intracranial invasion.

B. Otitis Media

1. **Epidemiology**
   - Accounts for 15% to 20% of all ambulatory visits.
   - Classified as acute otitis media (OM), OM with effusion, chronic OM with effusion, or chronic suppurative.
   - Recurrent OM is >3 episodes in 6 months, or >4 episodes in 1 year (occurs in 20% to 30% of pediatric population).

2. **Etiology**
   - *Streptococcus pneumoniae* 40% to 50%.
   - *Haemophilus influenzae* 20% to 30%.
   - *Moraxella catarrhalis* 10% to 15%.

3. **Pathology**
   - Antecedent event: URI.
   - Congestion of respiratory mucosa.
   - Obstruction of the isthmus portion of the tube.
   - Increased tube negative pressure.
   - Development of effusion.
   - Effusion colonization.

4. **Clinical Features**
   - Ear pain.
   - Cold symptoms.
   - Irritability.
   - May or may not have fever.
   - Red TM.
   - Bulging TMs.
   - Decreased TM mobility by pneumatic otoscopy.
   - Perforation with drainage.

5. **Management**
   - Eighty percent of untreated children resolve spontaneously in 7 to 14 days compared with 95% of treated.
   - Treatment prevents progression.
   - Amoxicillin 90 mg/kg/day is considered first-line therapy.
   - Azithromycin in allergic children.
   - For treatment failure, use amoxicillin/clavulanate (80 to 90 mg/kg/day of the amoxicillin component) and cefuroxime axetil, cefdinir, clindamycin, or ceftriaxone.
   - **Indications for tympanostomy tube placement:**
     - Chronic OM with effusion and associated conductive hearing loss of >15 dB.
     - Failed treatment for recurrent OM.
     - TM retraction with ossicular erosion or cholesteatoma formation.
   - **Risk factors:**
     - Male gender.
     - Recurrent OM in parents or siblings.

- Low birth weight or gestational age.
- Episode of OM before 6 months of age.
- Prone sleeping position.
- Pacifier use.
- Absence of breastfeeding.
- Group child care.
- Exposure to cigarette smoke.
- Congenital acquired immune deficiency.
- Down syndrome.
- Cleft palate.

C. Pharyngitis

- Primary goal is to distinguish viral from bacterial etiology.

1. Etiology

a. Viral

- Rhinovirus, adenovirus, enteroviruses, Epstein–Barr virus (EBV), CMV, HSV.

b. Bacterial

- Since the use of *H. influenzae* vaccine, incidence is <6 per million annually.
- Ten percent to 20% of patients with pharyngitis.
- Group A β-hemolytic streptococci (GABHS).
- Less than 2 years of age, GABHS is uncommon.
- GABHS is more common in children older than 5 years (5 to 15 years).
- *Mycoplasma* may be seen in adolescents and adults.

2. Pathology

- Inflammation of the throat.

3. Clinical Features

- Findings suggestive of GABHS:
  - Sudden onset of sore throat.
  - Fever.
  - Pain on swallowing.
  - Marked inflammation and erythema of pharynx and tonsils.
  - Tonsillar hypertrophy.
  - Patchy discrete exudate of tonsils.
  - Tender, enlarged anterior cervical nodes.
  - Scarlatina rash.
  - *Absence* of conjunctivitis, coryza, cough.
  - Winter, early spring.
  - History of exposure to documented case of GABHS.

4. Diagnostic Studies

- Except for the scarlatina rash, *none* of the above clinical findings is specific for GABHS; therefore, the positive predictive value of these findings is low. However, patients with acute pharyngitis whose clinical and epidemiologic findings do not suggest GABHS likely do not have streptococcal disease because the negative predictive value of such findings is high.
- Therefore, diagnosis can only be confirmed by throat culture or a rapid antigen detection test.
- **Throat culture versus rapid test:**
  - Throat culture is 90% to 95% sensitive (low rate of false negatives) and takes 2 to 3 days for results.
  - Rapid test is more expensive than culture, but results are acquired in 10 minutes. It has excellent specificity (95%), but sensitivity is low. Therefore, one may begin treatment on the basis of a positive result, but a negative result does not definitively rule out GABHS and must be confirmed by a throat culture.

5. Complications

a. Nonsuppurative Complications

- Acute rheumatic fever—can be prevented by eradication of GABHS from the pharynx.
- Poststreptococcal glomerulonephritis—*cannot* be prevented by antibiotic treatment.

b. Supportive Complications

- Tonsillar and peritonsillar abscess.
- Sinusitis.
- OM.

6. Management

- Supportive and symptomatic care only for viral pharyngitis.
- **For GABHS:**
  - Penicillin is currently recommended by the American Medical Association (AMA) and AAP. Ampicillin and amoxicillin are acceptable.
  - Continue treatment for 10 days.
  - May use IM benzathine penicillin as a one-time dose if compliance is uncertain.
  - If penicillin is allergic, use cephalosporin or macrolide.

X. Neurologic System

A. Cerebral Palsy

1. Etiology

- Cerebral injury before birth, during delivery, or in the perinatal period.

2. Types

- Spasticity.
- Ataxia.
- Choreoathetosis.
- Hypotonia without spasticity.

3. Clinical Features

- Motor deficits.
- Seizures.
- Mild to severe retardation.
- Disorders of language, speech, vision, hearing, and sensory perception.
- On physical examination, spasticity, hyperreflexia, ataxia, and involuntary movements.
- Microcephaly.
- Affected arm and leg may be smaller and shorter than the unaffected limbs.

4. Laboratory/Diagnostic Studies

- MRI.
- Genetic testing.

5. Management

- Goal is to attain the maximal physical functioning.
- Medications to treat seizures.

- Botulinum toxin to treat spasticity.
- Constraint-induced movement therapy.

6. **Prognosis**
   - Depends on the child's IQ, severity of the motor deficits, and degree of disability.

B. Bacterial Meningitis

1. **Epidemiology**
   - Incidence is highest between birth and 2 years of age, with peaks during the neonatal period and between 3 and 8 months.
   - Failure to make a prompt diagnosis and institute antibiotic treatment may result in significant illness and possibly death; examiner must have a high suspicion of meningitis.
   - Occurs more frequently in the winter and spring and in more males than females.
   - Less commonly, the result of hematogenous dissemination of microorganisms.

2. **Etiology**
   - In children 1 to 3 months old, the usual bacterial organisms that cause meningitis are group B *Streptococcus*, *E. coli*, *Listeria*, *H. influenzae*, *S. pneumoniae*, or *Neisseria meningitidis*.
   - In children 3 months to 6 years old, the usual organisms that cause bacterial meningitis are *S. pneumoniae*, *H. influenzae*, *N. meningitidis*, *Salmonella* species, and group A *Streptococcus*.
   - In children 7 years and older, the usual organisms are *S. pneumoniae*, *N. meningitides*, *Listeria monocytogenes*, and aerobic gram-negative bacilli.

3. **Pathology**
   - An inflammation of the leptomeninges.

4. **Clinical Features**
   - Preceded by several days of upper respiratory tract symptoms.

   a. **Infants**
   - May be nonspecific.
   - Fever.
   - Restlessness.
   - Irritability (especially increased irritability when being handled).
   - Inconsolable crying.
   - Poor feeding.
   - Emesis.
   - Diarrhea.
   - Lethargy.
   - Decreased tone.
   - Respiratory distress.
   - Full fontanelle (late finding).
   - Seizures.
   - Neck stiffness, Kernig and Brudzinski signs are not reliable in children (18 months old).

   b. **Children Older than 18 Months**
   - Fever.
   - Headache.
   - Nausea.

- Vomiting.
- Alterations of consciousness (due to increased intracranial pressure).
- Lethargy.
- Photophobia.
- Nuchal rigidity.
- Seizures.
- Positive Brudzinski sign (involuntary lower-extremity flexion elicited with passive neck flexion).
- Positive Kernig sign (pain elicited with passive knee extension).
- Focal neurologic signs.
- Petechial or purpuric lesions may be present.

5. **Diagnostic Studies**
   - Blood culture, CBC, and complete metabolic profile.
   - LP should be performed in every child if bacterial meningitis is suspected.
   - CT scan of head before LP if contraindications exist.
   - Relative contraindications to LP:
     - Hemodynamic instability (shock or respiratory difficulty).
     - Evidence of mass lesion or increased intracranial pressure, altered pupillary reactions, bradycardia, hypotension, apnea, or posturing.
     - Known bleeding disorder.
     - Infection overlying the LP site (cellulitis).
   - If a contraindication exists in a patient with clinical suspicion of meningitis, give antibiotics immediately.
   - Cerebrospinal fluid (CSF) examination should include cell count with differential, glucose level, protein level, culture, and Gram stain.
   - CSF findings: WBC, glucose, protein, positive Gram stain.
   - CT scan.

6. **Management**
   - ABCs always first.
   - O_2 (100% nonrebreather), ECG monitor.
   - IV access.
   - If truly bacterial meningitis, administer dexamethasone, 0.15 mg per kg IV either before or immediately after the initial antibiotic dose.
   - Administer antimicrobial therapy based on the child's age and the most likely pathogens.
   - Infants younger than 3 months, cefotaxime or ceftriaxone and ampicillin.
   - Infants older than 3 months, ceftriaxone, cefotaxime, or ampicillin plus gentamicin.
   - Treat seizures aggressively with anticonvulsants (specifically, lorazepam, phenytoin, phenobarbital).
   - Prompt hospitalization, ideally in an intensive care unit.

C. Febrile Seizure

1. Epidemiology

- Most common seizure disorder during childhood.
- Prevalence: 2% to 5% in the United States.
- Rarely occurs before 3 months or after 5 years (peak onset: 6 to 22 months of age).
- Spontaneously remits without specific therapy.
- Be careful—febrile seizures may represent a serious underlying acute infectious disease (i.e., sepsis and bacterial meningitis).

2. Etiology

- Always look for the underlying cause (i.e., URI, OM, and accidental overdose).

3. Risk factors for occurrence of a first febrile seizure—two or more of the following, and the patient has a 30% chance of a febrile seizure:

- First-degree relative with febrile seizures.
- Second-degree relative with febrile seizures.
- Slow development as judged by parents.
- Attendance at day care.

4. Clinical Features

- Febrile seizures seem to be associated with a rapidly rising temperature (core temperature to 39° C, or 102.2° F).
- **Febrile seizures may be:**
  - Simple:
    - Typically tonic–clonic lasting a few seconds to 10 minutes.
    - Usually benign and require no treatment.
    - Most common.
  - Complex:
    - Typically tonic–clonic lasting >15 minutes.
    - Usually denotes high-risk features (i.e., focal onset, postictal neurologic abnormalities, prior neurologic or developmental abnormalities, or family history of epilepsy).
    - Usually associated with a URI (i.e., viral syndrome, OM, pharyngitis, and adenitis).
    - Meningitis must be ruled out.

5. Diagnostic Studies

- Spinal tap should be performed on children younger than 2 years; close observation in the emergency department for older children may negate the necessity to perform a spinal tap on them.
- EEG for complicated/complex seizures.
- CBC may help rule in bacteremia.

6. Management

- Always ABCs first.
- **If active seizure:**
  - O_2.
  - Glucose <3 years old, 25% dextrose at 2 mL/kg/dose IV slowly.
  - Three years old or older, 50% dextrose at 1 mL/kg/dose IV slowly.
  - Naloxone (Narcan) 2 mg IV.

- **If currently febrile:**
  - Acetaminophen 10 to 15 mg per kg.
  - Ibuprofen 5 to 10 mg per kg.
  - Tepid baths.
  - Sponging.
  - Prophylactic anticonvulsants are not indicated in the uncomplicated febrile seizure patient.
  - Antiepileptics have no effect on febrile seizures.

7. Prognosis

- A uniformly excellent prognosis.
- Rarely develops into epilepsy.
- Children presenting with high-risk features (i.e., complex seizures) are at a greater risk for recurrent afebrile seizures or epilepsy.

XI. Genitourinary System

A. Urinary Tract Infection

1. Epidemiology

- Girls older than 6 months have UTIs far more commonly than boys.
- Uncircumcised boys younger than 3 months have more UTIs than girls. Circumcision reduces the risk of UTI in boys. The density of distal urethral and periurethral bacterial colonization with uropathogenic bacteria correlates with the risk of UTI in children.

2. Pathology

- Ascending infections are the most common.
- Adhesions present on the fimbria of uropathogenic bacteria allow colonization of the uroepithelium in the urethra and bladder.
- Uncoordinated relaxation of the urethral sphincter during voiding leads to incomplete emptying of the bladder, increasing the risk of bacterial colonization.

3. Etiology

- Most commonly *E. coli* (>85%).
- *Klebsiella*.
- *Proteus*.
- Less frequently, *Enterococcus* or coagulase-negative staphylococci.

4. Risk Factors

- Constipation.
- Neurogenic bladder.
- Poor perineal hygiene.
- Structural abnormalities of the urinary tract.
- Catheterization.
- Instrumentation of the urinary tract.
- Sexual activity.

5. Clinical Features

- Newborns and infants:
  - Fever, poor feeding, irritability, vomiting, FTT, and sepsis. Strong, foul-smelling or cloudy urine may be noted.

- Preschool children:
  - May have abdominal or flank pain, vomiting, fever, urinary frequency, dysuria, urgency, or enuresis.
  - School-aged children:
    - Frequency, dysuria, urgency, fever, vomiting, flank pain, and costovertebral tenderness.
6. **Laboratory/Diagnostic Studies**
   - UA and culture are difficult in children.
   - For toilet-trained, cooperative, older children, a midstream, clean-catch method is satisfactory.
   - For infants and young children, bladder catheterization or suprapubic collection is necessary.
   - Bagged urine specimens are helpful only if negative.
   - Gold standard for diagnosis remains the culture and sensitivity.
   - BUN and serum creatinine concentration should be measured to assess renal function.
   - Routine ultrasound of the kidneys.
     - To detect renal or perirenal abscesses or obstruction of the kidneys.
   - Voiding cystourethrogram.
     - Urologic abnormality due to weak stream, dribbling, or perineal abnormalities.
7. **Management**
   - Children with dehydration, toxicity, or sepsis should be admitted to the hospital and treated with parenteral antimicrobials.
   - Uncomplicated cystitis can be treated with amoxicillin, trimethoprim–sulfamethoxazole, or a first-generation cephalosporin for 7 to 10 days.
   - Seriously ill children are initially treated parenterally with a third-generation cephalosporin or aminoglycoside.
   - Sexually active teenagers use fluoroquinolones such as ciprofloxacin and levofloxacin for 3 days because it is cost-effective.

XII. Dermatologic System

A. Diaper Dermatitis ("Diaper Rash")
1. **Etiology**
   - *Candida albicans.*

2. **Pathology**
   - Inability of newborns to control candidal infections is related to relative impairment of specific and nonspecific host defense mechanisms.
3. **Clinical Features**
   - Found in the regions of the body where warmth and moisture lead to maceration of the skin or mucous membranes.
   - Beefy red erythema with elevated margins located in the skin folds.
   - Satellite red plaques.
   - Occasionally, pustules, erythematous papules, and vesicles may be seen.
   - Also seen in the axillary, neck, inguinal, and inframammary skin folds in adolescents.
4. **Diagnostic Studies**
   - Potassium hydroxide (KOH) examination—positive for budding yeast hyphae.
5. **Management**
   - Topical therapy using nystatin, miconazole (Monistat), or clotrimazole (Lotrimin) applied four times a day results in complete resolution within 3 to 4 days.
   - Educate the caregivers about proper hygiene (i.e., changing diapers more frequently and letting the patient "air out" between changings).

SELECTED REFERENCES

American Academy of Pediatrics Task Force on Sudden Infant Death Syndrome. The changing concept of sudden infant death syndrome: diagnostic coding shifts, controversies regarding the sleeping environment, and new variables to consider in reducing risk. *Pediatrics.* 2005;116:1245.

Goldenring JM, Rosen DS. Getting into adolescent heads: an essential update. *Contemp Pediatr.* 2004;21:64–90.

Hay W, Levin M, Deterding R, et al. *Current Diagnosis and Treatment Pediatrics.* 20th ed. New York, NY: McGraw-Hill; 2010.

Wessel MA, Cobb JC, Jackson EB, et al. Paroxysmal fussing in infancy, sometimes called colic. *Pediatrics.* 1954;14:421–435.

Surgery Disorders

William Demshok • Richard Fien • Debbi Hanson • Randi Beth Cooperman • Michael R. Arnold • Doreen Parkhurst • Keith Moore • Lee Dresden Goldberg

I. Skin Disorders

VASCULAR LESIONS

A. Hemangiomas

1. **Etiology**
   - Congenital; commonly seen in children as "birthmarks."
   - Most common benign vascular tumors of infancy.
   - **Types:**
     - Strawberry hemangioma is most common of the hemangiomas; most of these lesions resolve spontaneously.
     - Cavernous hemangioma persists.
   - **Associated syndromes:**
     - Kasabach–Merritt: sudden enlargement of existing hemangioma, thrombocytopenia, and/or coagulopathy—an acute syndrome with high mortality.

2. **Pathology**
   - Increased number of blood vessels (capillary); hyperplasia of endothelial cells.
   - Proliferate after birth, grow intermittently, and commonly involute.

3. **Clinical Features**
   - Involuting hemangiomas are common at birth.
   - Most hemangiomas are asymptomatic—cosmesis may be the primary concern.
   - Size and distribution are highly variable.
   - Associated syndromes must be kept in mind.
   - Complications include ulceration, bleeding, vision complications, thromboangiitis, and pulmonary embolism (PE); all mostly seen with large lesions.
   - History and physical examination usually suffice for diagnosis.
   - Presence at birth, size, location, and associated symptoms are important.
   - Lesions are purple, red, or pink; are raised, have irregular borders and thinned dermis, and vary in size.

4. **Diagnostic Studies**
   - Laboratory tests are indicated preoperatively to assess complications or associated illnesses. Platelet and red blood cell (RBC) count are most important.
   - Immunohistochemical marker: positive Glut-1 (glucose transporter protein) may help in the evaluation of biopsied tissue.
   - Angiography and other imaging studies (magnetic resonance imaging [MRI], computerized tomography [CT] scan) may be needed to define larger lesions, particularly when considering surgical resection or embolization.
   - Computer tomography angiography (CTA) to map lesion.
   - Ultrasound (U/S) and color Doppler imaging.

5. **Management**

   CONSERVATIVE TREATMENT
   - Observation indicated in childhood for asymptomatic and stable lesions.
   - The majority of hemangiomas involute, leading to ulceration in small percentage of patients.
   - In general, cosmetically acceptable hemangiomas do not need treatment.

   MEDICAL TREATMENT
   - Corticosteroids—first-line treatment for most complicated hemangiomas.
   - Propranolol—inhibits growth of severe infantile hemangiomas. May be rising as first-line, single agent therapy.
   - Vincristine—another alternative choice for lesions unresponsive to corticosteroids.
   - Interferon α-2a—no longer widely used because of complications—used only with failure of other drugs.
   - Local injection of sclerosing agents is risky, and its benefit is temporary.
   - Radiotherapy rarely used—it can cause acute and late complications, such as actinic dermatitis and malignant transformation.

   SURGICAL AND INTERVENTIONAL TREATMENT
   - Cryoablation: effective in treating small lesions; may leave scar.
   - **Laser:**
     - Pulsed dye laser (PDL) is most effective for ulcerated and superficial hemangiomas.
     - Neodymium: yttrium aluminum garnet (Nd:YAG) laser: recommended for deep or rapidly growing hemangiomas.
     - Surgical resection: ample indications; may involve major amputations, reconstructions, and tissue transfer.

- Embolization: mostly used as a last resort with failure of medical therapy and palliative method for inoperable lesions.

VASCULAR MALFORMATIONS

1. **Etiology**
   - Present at birth, but may not be clinically apparent until later.
   - Grow with child, never involute.
   - Soft, flat, easily compressible.
2. **Pathology**
   - Two common capillary vascular malformations are the salmon patch (nevus simplex) and port wine stain (nevus flammeus).
3. **Clinical Features**
   - **Salmon patch:**
     - Most common vascular malformation of infancy.
     - Made up of superficial capillaries.
     - When located at the nape of the neck, also called "stork bite."
   - **Port wine stain:**
     - Made up of superficial capillaries and deep vessels of skin and soft tissue.
     - Soft-tissue or bony hypertrophy.
     - Associated syndromes.
       - Sturge–Weber syndrome:
         - Port wine stain in ophthalmic branch of trigeminal nerve.
         - Associated with ocular (glaucoma) and neurologic (mental retardation, seizures, hemiplegia) abnormalities.
       - Klippel–Trenaunay–Weber syndrome:
         - Port wine stain over an extremity.
         - Associated bony or soft-tissue hypertrophy of extremity.
         - Termed *Parkes Weber syndrome* when arteriovenous fistula is noted.
4. **Diagnostic Studies**
   - Immunohistochemical marker: negative Glut-1 (glucose transporter protein).
   - MRI.
5. **Management**
   - Sclerotherapy.
   - Laser treatment.
   - Surgery excision.
   - **Sturge–Weber:**
     - CT or MRI.
     - Screen for eye and central nervous system (CNS) disease.
   - **Klippel–Trenaunay syndrome:**
     - Routine measurement of extremity to detect evolving extremity hypertrophy/leg length discrepancies.

C. Neurogenic Tumors (Benign)
1. **Etiology**
   - **Types:**
     - Neurofibroma: benign nonencapsulated tumor of nerve fibers.

- Schwannoma: benign tumor of nerve sheath (Schwann cells).
- May be solitary and sporadic, or multiple and associated with neurofibromatosis (NF), a hereditary disease.
- Schwannoma or neurilemmoma is a variant arising from the perineural sheath of Schwann cells.
- **NF (von Recklinghausen disease):**
  - Autosomal dominant inheritance.
  - Appears to be caused by mutation of a gene on chromosome 17.
  - New mutations occasionally occur in the germ line of unaffected parent and can be transmitted to more than one offspring.
2. **Pathology**
   - Solitary neurofibroma: oval to elongated nuclei on fibrocollagenous background.
   - Schwannoma: round, tan, yellow tumor on gross examination; spindle cells on light microscopy; entangled processes lined by continuous basal laminas on electron microscopy.
   - NF: diffuse neurofibroma, café-au-lait spots, freckling, bilateral acoustic nerve schwannomas, intestinal neuromas, and arterial wall thickening.
3. **Clinical Features**
   - Solitary neurofibroma: small (approximately 2 to 8 mm) sessile or pedunculated skin lesions.
   - Schwannoma: deep-seated tumors (retroperitoneum, mediastinum), may reach 10 to 15 cm in diameter without causing symptoms.
   - NF: seven types (NF1 through NF7) have been recognized, according to clinicopathologic characteristics:
     - Café-au-lait macules (hyperpigmentation) are noted in the first year of life.
     - Numerous neurofibromas of varying size throughout the skin.
     - Paraspinal and acoustic neuromas, and spinal cord meningiomas.
     - Axillary/inguinal freckling.
     - Rarely, adrenal or extra-adrenal pheochromocytoma is associated.
4. **Diagnostic Studies**
   - Solitary neurofibroma: firm, nontender, cutaneous, or subcutaneous nodule.
   - Schwannoma: cannot be distinguished from neurofibroma clinically.
   - NF: familial pattern is identifiable.
   - Histopathology is essential for definitive diagnosis of any of the variants.
5. **Management**
   - Most individuals with NF1 do not need treatment. Painful subcutaneous neurofibromas can be excised. Intra-spinal and -cranial tumors are typically benign and treated surgically.
   - NF is treated conservatively; lesions causing compression, pain, bleeding, or altered function may

need surgical resection; select lesions may be resected for cosmetic reasons.
- Removal of schwannomas and other tumors often is indicated for individuals with NF2 and early recognition is important for successful treatment of VIII nerve tumors.
- Solitary neurofibromas: Excisional biopsy is indicated to exclude malignancy. Surgical resection is indicated for patients with pain, neurologic deficits.
- Genetic counseling should be provided to all patients and families.

D. Decubitus Ulcer
1. Etiology
- Excessive prolonged pressure causing ischemia and eventual necrosis of skin and subcutaneous tissues, also known as "pressure ulcer" or "pressure sore."
- Risk factors include paraplegia, chronic illness, neuropathy, age, uremia, jaundice, diabetes, corticosteroids, cancer, chemotherapy, malnutrition, and inadequately fit casts or other means of immobilization, immunosuppression.

STAGE I
- Nonblanchable erythema of intact skin, the heralding lesion of skin ulceration. In persons with darker skin, discoloration of the skin, warmth, induration, or hardness also may be indicators.

STAGE II
- Partial-thickness skin loss involving epidermis, dermis, or both. The ulcer is superficial and appears clinically as an abrasion, blister, or shallow crater.

STAGE III
- Full-thickness skin loss involving damage to, or necrosis of, subcutaneous tissue that may extend down to, but not through, underlying fascia. The ulcer appears clinically as a deep crater with or without undermining of adjacent tissue.

STAGE IV
- Full-thickness skin loss with extensive destruction, tissue necrosis, or damage to muscle, bone, or supporting structures (e.g., tendon and joint capsule). Undermining and sinus tracts also may be associated with Stage IV pressure ulcers.

2. Pathology
- Necrosis, which may involve skin, subcutaneous tissues, and muscle.
3. Clinical Features
- Early stages: red or purple skin; late stages: necrosis (dark blue or black discoloration).
- Size is variable; area of necrosis is usually deeper than it appears externally because subcutaneous tissues and muscle are more sensitive to ischemia than skin.
- Patients who are bedridden, paraplegic, or unable to sense pain should be examined frequently for damaged skin in areas of pressure, especially bony prominences.

- Extent of necrosis is best determined by local exploration and debridement.
- Associated illness always present.
- Complications: cellulites, fasciitis, osteomyelitis, abscess, sepsis and, rarely, bleeding.

4. Diagnostic Studies
- Laboratory tests and imaging may be needed (e.g., to rule out osteomyelitis, to assess nutritional status, and preoperatively).

5. Management
MEDICAL TREATMENT
- When feasible, correct underlying disorders (e.g., diabetes).
- Pain management.
- Correct nutrition deficiencies if present.

LOCAL WOUND CARE
- Avoid local pressure; positional changes, pressure-relieving mattress, and cushion pads.
- Dressings, such as topical sulfadiazine (Silvadene) or adhesive colloids with hydrophilic particles (DuoDERM, Restore, J&J ulcer dressing).
- Drainage of any purulent collection and sharp debridement of necrotic tissue.
- Coverage with healthy tissue: skin grafts, and rotational or advancement flaps.

II. Endocrine Disorders
A. Thyroid Carcinoma
1. Etiology
- Most primary cancers of the thyroid can be classified into *papillary, follicular, medullary*, and *anaplastic. Squamous cell carcinoma, lymphoma*, and *metastatic carcinoma* also occur, but rarely.
- Thyroid cancer is usually a solid lesion and rarely secretes thyroid hormones.
- *Familial predisposition:* medullary carcinoma is transmitted as an autosomal dominant trait—50% chance of disease in the offspring.
- *Ionizing radiation*—radiotherapy, atomic bomb, and nuclear accident—is a high-risk factor; thyroid cancer develops 5 to more than 25 years after exposure.

2. Pathology
- *Papillary:* 50% to 80% of thyroid cancers. On histology, papillary fronds are characteristic, and laminated microcalcifications ("psammoma bodies") can be present; tumor may be multicentric; it metastasizes to regional lymph nodes.
- *Follicular:* 20%; characterized by follicles containing colloid; may be encapsulated or invasive; spread is hematogenous.
- *Medullary:* <10% of all thyroid tumors; arises from C-cells that produce calcitonin; cells grow with nesting pattern; amyloid deposits can be noted.
- *Anaplastic:* a most aggressive neoplasm; represents 5% to 10% of thyroid cancers; variable histologic appearance; spindle and giant cells are seen commonly.

3. **Clinical Features**
   - *Papillary:* appears as asymptomatic (nonfunctional) thyroid nodule; affects younger population; prognosis is generally good.
   - *Follicular:* slow-growing, tends to invade locally; disseminates through the bloodstream; bone metastases may cause pain. Most patients are in the fifth decade of life, and women-to-men incident ratio is 3:1.
   - *Medullary:* can be sporadic nonfamilial, or familial. The latter form may be associated with pheochromocytoma, parathyroid adenoma, and neuroma—Sipple syndrome or multiple endocrine neoplasia, type II (MEN-II).
   - *Anaplastic:* dismal disease; appears as painful enlargement of the thyroid; rapidly invades surrounding structures (e.g., trachea, recurrent nerves, and carotids) causing hoarseness, respiratory obstruction, dysphagia, bleeding, and other life-threatening complications.
   - Most thyroid cancers appear as a "silent" nodule; *anaplastic carcinoma* can have dramatic presentation, with pain, hoarseness, and respiratory trouble.
   - Physical examination does not distinguish between benign and malignant nodules; signs of hyperthyroidism do not exclude cancer; cervical adenopathy suggests malignancy.

4. **Diagnostic Studies**
   - Thyroid function tests are usually normal in thyroid cancer; radioimmunoassay for calcitonin is used in screening of medullary carcinoma.
   - U/S can differentiate between cystic and solid lesions.
   - Fine-needle aspiration (FNA) cytology is the most useful test to diagnose cancer; however, definitive diagnosis of thyroid follicular cancer requires histologic analysis.

5. **Management**

   MEDICAL TREATMENT
   - Radioactive iodine (^{131}I) can ablate residual tumor and metastases, particularly of follicular tumors.
   - Thyroid suppressive therapy with thyroxine is given.
   - Chemotherapy (e.g., doxorubicin or multidrug regimens) can be used for metastatic disease and anaplastic carcinoma, but cure is extremely rare.

   SURGICAL TREATMENT
   - *Papillary:* at least thyroid lobectomy plus isthmectomy is often recommended.
   - *Follicular:* near-total thyroidectomy is favored.
   - *Medullary:* total thyroidectomy should be performed (because of multicentricity).
   - *Anaplastic:* total thyroidectomy and radical neck dissection for resectable tumors; in most instances, surgery is palliative.

B. **Hypercortisolism**
   1. **Etiology**
      - *Cushing disease:* hypersecretion of adrenocorticotropic hormone (ACTH) by pituitary adenoma stimulating adrenal gland to produce cortisol.
      - *Cushing syndrome:* constellation of signs and symptoms from excess cortisol; may be secondary to Cushing disease, adenoma of the adrenal cortex, or exogenous corticosteroids.
      - *Ectopic ACTH syndrome:* hypercortisolism secondary to nonpituitary tumor; usually a paraneoplastic syndrome (e.g., lung cancer secreting ACTH).
      - The most common cause of hypercortisolism is exogenous corticosteroid use for treatment of a variety of diseases, including asthma, autoimmune disorders, and inflammatory bowel disease.
   2. **Pathology**
      - *Pituitary adenoma:* typically, small basophilic intrasellar tumor; however, can reach large sizes and cause local compression.
      - *Adrenocortical adenoma:* composed of lipid-rich cells arranged in clusters and cords resembling normal zona fasciculata.
      - *Adrenocortical hyperplasia:* zona fasciculata markedly thickened by enlarged cells with abundant lipid.
      - *Ectopic ACTH-producing tumors:* lung, thymus, and pancreas.
   3. **Clinical Features**
      - Truncal obesity, "moon" facies, "buffalo hump," atrophic muscles, fragile skin, ecchymoses, purple striae, supraclavicular fat pad fullness, cataracts, osteoporosis, menstrual dysfunction, hyperglycemia, recurrent candidiasis, hirsutism, acne, poor wound healing, and psychiatric disturbances.
   4. **Diagnostic Studies**
      - Increased levels of cortisol in blood and urine.
      - Sellar X-rays, CT scan, and MRI to evaluate pituitary tumors.
      - Abdominal imaging to evaluate adrenal tumors.
   5. **Management**

      MEDICAL TREATMENT
      - External radiation may be used for residual tumor after pituitary surgery.
      - Sodium valproate, opiate antagonists, bromocriptine, and other drugs can be considered in select patients.

      SURGICAL TREATMENT
      - Pituitary adenomas are preferably resected through transnasal transsphenoidal approach to the sella turcica.
      - Adrenal gland tumors can be resected by way of laparotomy, lateral or posterior (lumbar) incisions, or laparoscopy.

RISK FACTORS (MOST PATIENTS HAVE NO RISK FACTORS)
   - Age >50 years.
   - African American women have higher incidence before age 40 and are more likely to die from

breast cancer at every age compared with Caucasian women.

III. Disorders of the Breast

A. Mammary Dysplasia (Fibrocystic Disease—Fibrodysplasia)

1. **Etiology**
   - Most common benign condition or lesion of the breast.
   - Common in women between ages 30 and 50 years.
   - Decreased incidence in postmenopausal women.
2. **Pathology**
   - These lesions are benign and noted frequently in normal breasts and, therefore, thought to be a "normal variant."
   - Fibrous tissue and multiple cysts.
   - Believed to be related to ovarian activity.
   - Estrogen hormone as a causative factor.
   - Gross and microscopic findings include adenosis, cysts, papillomatosis, and fibrosis.
   - Ductal and lobular hyperplasia are considered risk factors for development of cancer.
3. **Associated Factors**
   - Early menarche.
   - Small breast size.
   - History of cyclic breast discomfort.
   - Irregular menses.
   - Premenopausal status.
   - Late menopause.
   - Normal or low body weight.
   - History of spontaneous abortions.
   - Possible relation to increased caffeine intake.
4. **Clinical Features**
   - Asymptomatic or minimal symptoms termed *fibrocystic changes*.
   - Typically, bilateral breast involvement with multiple smooth lumps.
   - Nipple discharge may be noted (usually green or brownish).
   - Sudden appearance or disappearance of cysts is common.
   - Symptoms are often exacerbated during premenstrual cycle.
   - Fluctuance in size and breast tenderness are common.
   - Physical examination demonstrates tender, nodular breast(s).
5. **Diagnostic Studies**
   - Imaging;
     - Ultrasound—pregnant women or <30 years-old, useful to distinguish between solid mass and cystic lesion.
     - Mammogram—women >30 and not pregnant.
   - Fine-needle aspiration (FNA) of "dominant" cyusts
   - If no fluid is aspirated or bloody fluid is discovered or if mass persists or recurs after aspiration, biopsy is warranted. When suspicious lesion does not resolve over several months, it must be excised.
   - Biopsy—definitive.
   - Biopsy of suspicious or "dominant" lesion must be performed to rule out carcinoma.
6. **Management**
   - Breast pain due to mammary dysplasia is treated conservatively.
   - Avoidance of breast trauma; wearing a brassiere to provide support and protection.
   - Nonprescription analgesics (nonsteroidal anti-inflammatory drugs [NSAIDs]) for pain.
   - Avoidance of caffeine and addition of vitamin E to diet may improve symptoms.
   - Smoking cessation is recommended because nicotine is thought to worsen breast pain.
   - Discontinuing hormone replacement and decreasing estrogen in oral contraceptive pills may improve symptoms.
   - Severe pain—treated with danazol, a synthetic, weak androgen that has many undesirable effects and should be reserved for patients whose severe pain is uncontrolled with more conservative treatment.

B. Intraductal Papilloma

1. **Etiology**
   - Most common cause of bloody (or blood-tinged) nipple discharge.
   - Rarely palpable (size 2 to 5 mm).
   - Usually solitary, noted close to nipple.
   - Mostly located beneath areola.
2. **Pathology**
   - Polypoid epithelial tumors arise in ducts of the breast.
   - These lesions typically have a long, slender stalk and are subject to torsion.
   - Rarely, diffuse papillomas can be present; these are typically multiple, involve breasts bilaterally, have a more "serous" discharge, and are associated with increased risk of cancer.
3. **Clinical Features**
   - Appears commonly with unilateral, spontaneous bloody, serous, or cloudy nipple discharge.
4. **Diagnostic Studies**
   - Guaiac test to differentiate between bloody and brownish nipple discharge.
   - Breast imagining: ultrasound for all women, plus mammogram for women >30 years.
   - Other imaging tests: Ductography, MRI, MR ductography.
   - Biopsy results of subareolar excision for treatment of nipple discharge distinguishes between intraductal papilloma and cancer.
   - Cytology of nipple discharge rarely helpful and not cost-effective.
5. **Management**
   - Nipple duct excision over a lacrimal duct probe or terminal duct resection.

C. Fibroadenoma

1. **Etiology**
   - Most common benign breast tumor.
   - Common in adolescents and young women (<30 years).
   - Usually appears suddenly.
2. **Pathology**
   - Hallmark of lesion—presence of stromal tissue with epithelium-lined, duct-like structures and absence of elastic tissue.
   - Typically consists of a mixture of proliferating epithelial and fibrous tissues.
3. **Clinical Features**
   - Does not change with menstrual cycle.
   - Typically painless, slow-growing mass.
   - Commonly noted on breast self-examination (BSE).
   - Palpable breast mass—round, smooth, rubbery, mobile.
4. **Diagnostic Studies**

   BREAST EXAMINATION
   - Well-circumscribed oval or round mobile mass with firm, but rubbery texture; typically 3 cm.
   - Older women may present with small, hard nodule.

   U/S
   - To distinguish between cyst and solid mass.
   - Preferred use in women younger than 30 years or pregnant.
   - Fibroadenoma is a well-marginated, homogenous mass.

   MAMMOGRAPHY
   - If lesion has degenerated, may demonstrate micro-characteristic calcifications; otherwise, findings are not uniformly characteristic for fibroadenoma.
   - Preferred use in women ≥ 30 years and not pregnant.

   "TRIPLE TEST"
   - Diagnostic mammography, clinical breast examination, and FNA for any persistent, palpable breast mass.
5. **Management**
   - **<30 years old with breast examination and U/S appearance of fibroadenoma:**
     - Observe, with excision of lesion upon change or enlargement.
   - **≥30 years old—fine-needle biopsy or aspiration:**
     - Excise with absence of cytologic confirmation of fibroadenoma.
     - Excise with change or enlargement of lesion.

D. Breast Abscess

1. **Etiology**
   - Relatively uncommon inflammatory process; purulent collection.
   - Two types: lactational and nonlactational.
2. **Pathology**
   - Staphylococcus aureus; *methicillin-resistant S. aureus* cases are increasing.

3. **Clinical Features**
   - Localized, painful, tender, erythematous, warm breast mass; breast edema.
   - Fever and chills may occur.
   - Subareolar—nipple abnormality (nipple inversion or retraction).
   - Fluctuance.
   - Axillary lymphadenopathy.
4. **Diagnostic Studies**
   - Ultrasound guided aspiration of the abscess sent for culture and sensitivity.
5. **Management**
   - If cellulitis is discovered without a palpable mass, antibiotic treatment is usually successful.
   - No need to stop breastfeeding.
   - Drainage: FNA or open surgical with adequate debridement.
   - Antibiotics based on culture and sensitivity results.
   - Recurrent or unresolved mass needs biopsy to exclude cancer.

E. Breast Carcinoma

1. **Etiology**
   - Most common cancer in women.
   - Three- to 6-fold increased risk to patient with family history of breast cancer.
   - Approximately, 11% of women in the United States develop breast cancer.
   - Most cancers are diagnosed as a result of abnormal mammograms.
   - Caucasian women have higher incidence of breast cancer than African American women after age 40.
   - African American women have higher incidence before age 40 and are more likely to die of breast cancer at every age compared with Caucasian women.

   RISK FACTORS (MOST PATIENTS HAVE NO RISK FACTORS)
   - Age >50 years.
   - Personal history of breast cancer.
   - BRCA1 and BRCA2 inherited susceptibility genes.
   - Family history (first-degree relatives).
   - Postmenopausal obesity.
   - Alcohol consumption.
   - Early menarche.
   - Late menopause.
   - Nulliparity or greater than 30 years old for first, full-term pregnancy.
2. **Pathology**
   - **Majority of breast cancers are invasive adenocarcinomas:**
     - Eighty percent are infiltrating, intraductal type (papillary, intraductal, medullary).
     - Approximately 10% are infiltrating lobular carcinomas.

- **Breast cancer spreads by both vascular and lymphatic routes:**
  - Adenocarcinomas (infiltrating, intraductal) spread to bones, lungs, liver, and brain.
  - Lobular spread to meninges, peritoneum, pleura, ovaries, mediastinal, and retroperitoneal lymph nodes.

3. **Clinical Features**
   - Early—tumor usually painless and may be mobile.
   - Most common—painless breast mass.
   - Most common sites—upper outer quadrant (first); beneath the nipple-areola complex (second).
   - As tumor grows, it becomes more fixed to ligaments and fascia and borders become less distinct.
   - Late—skin changes ("peau d'orange") and nipple discharge occur.

4. **Diagnostic Studies**
   - Complete history and physical examination.
   - Clinical breast examination.
   - Bilateral mammography.
   - MRI for high-risk patients.
   - FNA or core biopsy may be used initially.
   - Open biopsy definitive.
   - Staging: removal of primary tumor and ipsilateral lymph node resection.
   - CXR, bone scan, and CT for further diagnosis if there are symptoms, positive lymph nodes, or tumors >5 cm.
   - Presence of estrogen and progesterone receptor assessed in the specimen.

5. **Management**

   GOALS
   - Control of local disease; treatment of distant disease; improved quality of life.
   - Dependent on staging of disease and patient goals.

   TREATMENT
   - Lumpectomy and radiation therapy—standard for women with small tumors.
   - Mastectomy—used for large and multicentric tumors; when tumors are scattered, and suspicious microcalcifications throughout breast tissue are present; when patients are unable or unwilling to receive postoperative radiation.
   - Metastatic disease—treatment modified according to (1) menopausal status, (2) hormone receptor status, and (3) sites of metastases.
   - Radiation—used postlumpectomy to treat remaining breast tissue; used on axilla only for invasive disease and if no axillary dissection was performed; used if positive axillary lymph nodes were left behind during lumpectomy, used as palliative control of metastatic ulceration pain.
   - Chemotherapy—used in select patients after surgery, before resection of the primary tumor, and/or in metastatic disease.

- Hormonal—used in metastatic cancer or adjuvant therapy in early cancer for postmenopausal women (tamoxifen); used for premenopausal women with estrogen/progesterone receptors on the surface of tumor cells.
- Targeted therapy—used for breast cancer caused by overproduction of growth-promoting protein HER2. Trastuzumab is a monoclonal antibody that targets this protein. Lapatinib is a tyrosine kinase inhibitor that targets this protein and is used for patients who have failed treatment with Trastuzumab.
- Bisphosphonates (zoledronate or pamidronate)—decrease pain associated with bone metastasis and decreases fracture risk.

IV. Vascular Disorders

A. Compartment Syndrome
1. **Etiology**
   - Trauma of the extremity, with edema or hemorrhage in the interstitial space of a compartment (one or more muscles enveloped by fascia).
   - Common causes: reperfusion of ischemic tissue (revascularization of extremities), external compression, major vein ligation fractures.
   - Approximately 80% occur in the leg and 10% in the forearm.
2. **Pathology**
   - Increase in venous pressure, interstitial pressure, or both, leading to reduction of capillary blood flow and ischemia.
   - Peripheral nerve ischemia is the hallmark of the disorder.
3. **Clinical Features**
   - Pain, swelling, paresthesias, paralysis and tense compartment.
   - Tingling followed by sensory loss and paralysis of distal portions of the extremity involved—Volkmann contracture in the forearm, peroneal nerve injury, and foot drop in the leg.
   - Pain with passive flexion of involved extremity.
4. **Diagnostic Studies**
   - Distal pulses are usually present, although edema may impair palpation.
   - Compartment pressure can be measured by insertion of a needle connected to manometer; elevation >30 to 40 mm Hg indicates a need for decompression.
5. **Management**
   - Main goal is to avoid permanent nerve damage.
   - Fasciotomy of all compartments involved (four in the leg) should be performed, followed by wound care and delayed wound closure.

B. Arterial Disease
1. **Etiology**
   - Plaque formation within vessel.
   - Progressive stenosis of vessel.

- Embolism/thrombosis.
- Most common cause: atherosclerosis.
- Important risk factors: smoking, hyperlipidemia, diabetes.

2. **Pathology**
   - Changes in intima, media of arterial wall due to deposits of lipids, calcium, fibrin, inflammatory cells, hemorrhage.
   - Ischemia of tissue.

3. **Clinical Features**
   - Calf, hip, thigh claudication.
   - Impotence.
   - Ischemic rest pain.
   - Bruits.
   - Decreased/absent pulses (femoral, popliteal/pedal pulses).
   - Skin changes (coloration/pigmentation/ulcerations).

4. **Evaluation (6 Ps)**
   - Pulselessness.
   - Pallor.
   - Poikilothermia.
   - Paresthesias.
   - Pain.
   - Paralysis.

5. **Diagnostic Studies**
   NONINVASIVE
   - **Doppler U/S:**
     - Ankle/brachial (blood pressure [BP] ratio) (ABI = ankle pressure/brachial artery pressure rest or postexercise):
       - 1.2 to 2.0 or greater: medial calcinosis or noncompressible.
       - 0.95 to 1.2: normal.
       - 0.5 to 0.95: claudication.
       - 0.2 to 0.5: rest pain.
       - 0.0 to 0.2: tissue breakdown and threat to limb loss.

   INVASIVE
   - Angiography, anatomic description—only when reconstruction is planned.
   - CT angiography or MRA.
   - Cardiopulmonary, renal assessment, necessary pre-op evaluation.

6. **Management**
   SURGERY
   - Reserved for patients who fail medical therapy and have severe ischemia.
   - Amputation for patients with gangrene/extensive infection.
   - Aortoiliac occlusion: aortobifemoral or axillobifemoral bypass:
     - Endovascular stent percutaneous mechanical/laser atherectomy for high risk patients.
     - Synthetic material above the groin, if necessary, and autogenous vein below.

MEDICAL
   - Heparin (acute), but still needs surgical intervention.

7. **Carotid Disease**
   - **Indication:**
     - Transient ischemic attack—neurologic deficit.
     - CVA—neurologic deficit >24 hours.
     - Stenosis >70%, >69% to 50% if symptomatic.
   - **Treatment**
     - Carotid endarterectomy or angioplasty with stenting.
   - **Contraindication:**
     - Total occlusion.
     - Acute stroke.
     - Fixed severe stroke.
   - **Outcome:**
     - Stroke: 2% to 7%.
     - Transient cranial nerve injury 10%
     - Death: <1%.

C. **Aortic Aneurysm**
   - Weakness and dilatation of vessel wall, caused by genetic or atherosclerotic damage.
   - Most common cause is atherosclerosis—also syphilis, vasculitis, trauma, giant cell arteritis, and Marfan syndrome.
   - Aneurysms are 85% abdominal and 15% thoracic.
   - Rupture leads to death in 85%.
   - May be asymptomatic, pulsatile abdominal mass.
   - Rupture causes severe back, abdominal flank pain and hypotension.
   - Laboratory studies—abdominal U/S, CT; aortography is *not* a diagnostic study for aneurysms.
   - The treatment surgery with bypass graft or endovascular repair with endograft for elective cases.

D. **Prevention of Thromboembolic Events**
   - Use $CHADS_2$ score = **C**ongestive heart failure, **H**ypertension, **A**ge, **D**iabetes, **S**troke to determine risk.
   - Bridging anticoagulation for high risk patients on warfarin:
     - Stop warfarin 5 days before surgery and allow INR to return to near normal. If INR ≥1.5, give vitamin K.
     - Give bridging SQ low-molecular-weight heparin (LMWH) or IV unfractionated heparin (UFH). Give half of regular dose as last dose of LMWH 24 hours before surgery. Stop UFH 4 hours before surgery.
     - Restart warfarin in ~12 to 24 hours post-op if adequate hemostasis.
     - If bridging anticoagulation is continued, restart ~24 hours after surgery. If high risk for post-op bleeding, restart ~ 48 to 72 hours post-op.
     - If high risk of bleeding or contraindications to antithrombotic medications, use graduated compression stockings or intermittent pneumatoic compression.

V. Gastrointestinal Disorders

A. Esophagus

HIATAL HERNIA

1. **Etiology**
   - Portion of the stomach prolapses through diaphragmatic esophageal hiatus of the stomach into the chest.
   - Type I, sliding hernia: gastroesophageal (GE) junction is above the hiatus—most common type of hiatal hernia.
   - Type II, paraesophageal or "rolling" hernia: GE junction remains intra-abdominal; fundus of the stomach herniates.

2. **Pathology**
   - **Sliding hernias are often associated with GE reflux (heartburn), causing:**
     - Esophagitis: mucosal ulceration, neutrophils in epithelium.
     - Barrett esophagus: distal esophagus lined with heterotopic mucosa, with potential for cancer.

3. **Clinical Features**
   - Most hernias are asymptomatic.
   - GE reflux may cause heartburn and regurgitation.
   - Advanced cases may result in dysphagia, bleeding (chronic anemia), retrosternal pain, and respiratory symptoms (bronchoaspiration).
   - In paraesophageal hernia, part of the stomach can be strangulated, leading to necrosis and perforation. This acute syndrome carries high mortality if diagnosis and treatment are delayed.

4. **Diagnostic Studies**
   - Endoscopy also can identify hiatal hernias and allows biopsy of suspicious lesions.
   - Esophageal manometry and pH monitoring are used unclear.
   - Barium swallow is used if the diagnosis is unclear and clinically indicated

5. **Management**

   ### CONSERVATIVE
   - Postural adjustment, antacids after meals and at bedtime, histamine-2 (H_2) receptor blockers, proton-pump inhibitors diet modification.
   - Weight control.

   ### SURGICAL
   - Indicated for large hernias or persistent symptoms, stricture, bleeding, recurrent aspiration pneumonitis, and Barrett esophagitis.
   - Fundoplication (Nissen procedure): gastric fundus is wrapped around the intra-abdominal portion of the esophagus, and the hiatus is narrowed with sutures.

PERFORATION

1. **Etiology**
   - Spontaneous or strain-induced (Boerhaave syndrome).
   - Results in mediastinitis without prompt diagnosis and treatment.
   - Iatrogenic: esophagoscopy, dilation of strictures, intubation. Iatrogenic causes are the most common cause of perforation.
   - Traumatic: penetrating missile, swallowed foreign body, blunt chest or abdominal injury, surgical dissection, ingestion of caustic agents.
   - Intrinsic esophageal disease: peptic ulceration, carcinoma.
   - Anastomotic leak after esophageal surgery.

2. **Clinical Features**
   - Usually dramatic, irreversible sepsis may ensue within 24 hours.
   - Severe retching followed by acute pain.
   - "Mackler triad"—vomiting, lower chest pain, cervical subcutaneous emphysema.
   - Pain (chest or epigastric—depending on location of tear); respiratory symptoms (dyspnea, cyanosis); rarely, tension pneumothorax occurs (usually following endoscopy).
   - Cervical tear: pain in the neck; crepitus; dysphagia.
   - Thoracic tear: pain in the chest or epigastric area; tachypnea, dyspnea.
   - Fever, tachycardia, tachypnea, hypotension, and shock.
   - Hamman sign: "crunching" sound caused by heart beating against air-filled mediastinum.
   - Mediastinal and subcutaneous emphysema.

3. **Diagnostic Studies**
   - Chest X-ray (CXR): air in the mediastinum, pneumoperitoneum, and, less commonly, pneumothorax.
   - Esophagogram with water-soluble medium: extraluminal leak of contrast.
   - Esophagoscopy: assessment of location and extent of perforation; because of pneumothorax and pneumomediastinum, use minimal insufflation.
   - Thoracentesis—may demonstrate cloudy or purulent fluid.
   - CT scan—if esophagography is contraindicated or results are nondiagnostic.

4. **Management**
   - Prognosis depends on location and type of perforation and the time elapsed before treatment; mortality rates are 10% to 15% if treated within 24 hours, and >50% thereafter.
   - Rapid resuscitation with fluids and intravenous (IV) antibiotics is paramount.
   - Perforations of the cervical esophagus may respond to broad-spectrum antibiotics, elimination of all feeding, and total parenteral nutrition.
   - Drainage of the area of perforation, debridement, and closure are the basis of surgical therapy.

- Cervical esophagostomy with gastrostomy is an alternative when inflammatory changes preclude primary closure.

CARCINOMA

1. **Etiology**
   - Peak incidence in fifth and seventh decades; male:female ratio is 3:1.
   - **Squamous cell:**
     - Associated with smoking and alcohol use.
     - More common in African Americans than in Caucasians.
   - **Adenocarcinoma:**
     - Associated with GERD and increased body mass index.
     - More common in Caucasians than in African Americans.
     - Barrett esophagus is precursor.
   - Premalignant lesions: achalasia, reflux esophagitis, radiation esophagitis, caustic burns.
2. **Pathology**
   - Squamous cell carcinoma—most common type worldwide.
   - Adenocarcinoma—most common type in western hemisphere.
   - Rare types: anaplastic small cell carcinoma (oat cell carcinoma), adenoid cystic carcinoma, malignant melanoma, and carcinosarcoma.
   - Metastases to lymph nodes, liver, lungs, bone, and brain.
3. **Clinical Features**
   - Dysphagia and weight—loss most common presenting symptoms.
   - Odynophagia, chest pain, and hematemesis.
4. **Diagnostic Studies**
   - Barium esophagogram: demonstrates narrowing, mucosal changes, location and length of the lesion.
   - Esophagoscopy: allows biopsy, with definitive pathologic diagnosis.
   - Brush cytology has been used for screening in some regions.
   - Other studies (CT scan, bone scan) to rule out metastases.
5. **Management**
   - In majority of patients, local tumor spread or distant metastases preclude cure.
   - Palliation (i.e., restoring the patient's ability to swallow comfortably) is important. Palliative treatment using prosthetic stents and Laser can be used–the average 5 year survival is approximately 25%.
   - Chemotherapy and radiotherapy may also be used for palliation and as adjuvants to surgical treatment.
   - Surgical resection is the treatment of choice to attempt cure and stage. Surgery also provides good palliation.

- Types of resection include transthoracic esophagectomy (Ivor Lewis procedure) and transhiatal esophagectomy (cervical and abdominal incisions), which allows removal of the entire esophagus without thoracotomy.

B. Gallbladder Disease

CHOLELITHIASIS

1. **Etiology**
   - Gallbladder stones affect 10% to 25% of the population.
   - More common in females, in the forties, fertile, and obese (fat)—"the four Fs."
   - Also more common in Western Caucasian, Native American, Hispanics African Americans with sickle cell disease, patients with Crohn disease, and post-bariatric surgery patients.
2. **Pathology**
   - The gallbladder contains single or, more often, multiple stones and may have various degrees of inflammation (cholecystitis).
   - Types: cholesterol, pigmented (calcium), mixed.
   - Most common: cholesterol (>75%); pigment (15%).
3. **Clinical Features**
   - Majority of patients have no symptoms, or vague and occasional abdominal discomfort.
   - Symptoms are characterized by recurrent biliary colic attacks—right upper quadrant (RUQ) pain, diaphoresis, nausea, and vomiting, which last minutes to hours, subsiding spontaneously. Biliary colic may be precipitated by fatty food and rapid weight loss in obese patients.
   - Pain of biliary colic caused by obstruction of cystic duct.
4. **Diagnostic Studies**
   - U/S is the main diagnostic tool to determine the presence of stones, inflammation of gallbladder wall, and obstruction of the extrahepatic biliary ducts.
5. **Management**
   - Avoidance of offending foods.

   #### MEDICAL TREATMENT
   - Dissolution of gallstones through biliary lithotripsy and bile salt therapy (ursodeoxycholic acid), but has limited application and may only offer temporary relief.

   #### SURGICAL TREATMENT
   - Laparoscopic cholecystectomy is currently the treatment of choice for symptomatic cholelithiasis.
   - ERCP (endoscopic retrograde cholangiopancreatography) for removal of common bile duct stones in acute cholecystitis.
   - Open cholecystectomy needed in 1% to 2% of elective procedures and 5% to 10% of acute cholecystitis.

CHOLECYSTITIS

1. **Etiology**
   - Acute or chronic inflammation of the gallbladder.
   - Gallstones are present in 95% of cases (calculous cholecystitis), presumably causing obstruction of the cystic duct (gallbladder neck).
   - Less commonly, sepsis, prolonged fasting, vasculitis, and ischemia may cause acalculous cholecystitis.
   - Most of these cases occur in patients hospitalized for other causes.

2. **Pathology**
   - Acute: the gallbladder is tense and distended; may have areas of necrosis and contain purulent material. In acalculous cholecystitis, gangrene is the rule.
   - Chronic: the gallbladder wall is thickened and infiltrated with chronic inflammatory cells.

3. **Clinical Features**
   - Acute: mild-to-intense RUQ colicky/constant pain radiating to subcapsular area, nausea and vomiting, fever, leukocytosis, RUQ tenderness, and sometimes peritonitis. (+) Murphy sign; palpation of the gallbladder.
   - Pain may initially be epigastric, but rapidly advances to abdominal tenderness.
   - Chronic: ill-defined clinical picture with recurrent symptoms of biliary obstruction or vague abdominal pain and dyspeptic symptoms.

4. **Diagnostic Studies**
   - U/S—the test of choice.
   - CT/MRC scanning—have high sensitivity and specificity for acute cholecystitis; also useful for evaluating surrounding tissues.
   - Hepatobiliary scintigraphy scan (HIDA scan)—for negative U/S.
   - ERCP or endoscopic ultrasonography.

5. **Management**

   MEDICAL TREATMENT
   - Sixty percent of cases resolve with antibiotics and supportive care.
   - Calculous cholecystitis may be treated with antibiotics followed by surgery within a few days or in certain cases after 4 to 5 weeks when the inflammation is resolved.
   - Antiemetics and oral analgesics.

   SURGICAL TREATMENT
   - Cholecystectomy, laparoscopic or open, carries a low morbidity and overall mortality rate of <0.2%. Most deaths occur in elderly or severely ill patients undergoing emergency operation.
   - Acalculous acute cholecystitis requires emergent surgery.
   - Percutaneous cholecystostomy for drainage patients at high surgical risk until surgically stable.
   - Removed gallbladder should be evaluated for cancer in the OR.

C. Liver

CARCINOMA

1. **Etiology**
   - Primary hepatic carcinoma in the United States is uncommon.
   - Most malignancy in the liver is metastatic versus primary (20:1); the primary is usually in the gastrointestinal (GI) tract, breast, or lung.
   - Most common metastatic lesion from colorectal cancer.

   RISK FACTORS
   - Aflatoxins—food contamination by *Aspergillus flavus*.
   - Cirrhosis—particularly from hepatitis B and C, alcoholism.
   - Parasitosis—liver fluke *Clonorchis sinensis* (Asia).
   - Genetic—deficiency in α-antitrypsin.

2. **Pathology**
   - Hepatocellular carcinoma (HCC, hepatoma): single or multiple nodules with prominent vascularity.
   - Cholangiocarcinoma: a type of adenocarcinoma arising from intrahepatic or extrahepatic bile ducts.
   - Hepatoblastoma: the fetal variant of HCC with familial adenomatous polyposis; seen in infants.
   - Metastatic: more commonly multiple nodules; histology resembles that of the primary tumor; mostly GI tract adenocarcinoma.

3. **Clinical Features**
   - General: anorexia, fatigue, weight loss, abdominal mass (enlarged, hard liver, or other primary tumor).
   - RUQ tenderness; ascites.
   - Biliary obstruction: jaundice, pruritus.
   - Portal hypertension: ascites, splenomegaly, prominent abdominal veins ("caput medusae" represents periumbilical vein dilatation).

4. **Diagnostic Studies**
   - U/S: noninvasive, inexpensive, good resolution.
   - Liver function studies: α-fetoprotein (AFP) increased.
   - Helical multiphasic CT scan and MRI with contrast (CT preferred): provide precise location, extent of invasion of surrounding structures, and involvement of other organs.
   - Percutaneous or laparoscopic needle biopsy: definitive diagnosis.
   - PET scan for suspected metastasis to the liver.

5. **Management**

   MEDICAL TREATMENT
   - Metastatic liver cancer is usually treated with chemotherapy alone; exceptions include colon cancer and neuroendocrine tumors, which may respond better to resection.

SURGICAL TREATMENT

- Depending on location and number of lesions, primary and metastatic tumors can be removed by local excision, right or left hepatectomy (removal of half the liver), or various types of "segmentectomies."
- Liver transplantation for malignant tumors is evolving.
- Cryoablation (freezing with liquid nitrogen), alcoholization, and radiotherapy are used in select patients.

PORTAL HYPERTENSION

1. **Etiology**
   - Most common basic lesion: increased resistance to blood flow.
   - Most common cause: cirrhosis, due to chronic alcoholism (most common), posthepatitis, hemochromatosis.
   - Budd–Chiari syndrome: phlebitis or web obstructing suprahepatic veins.
   - Extrinsic compression: trauma, inflammatory process, tumor.
   - Schistosomiasis: common in tropical countries.

2. **Pathology**
   - Portal pressure >12 mm Hg, with associated complications: esophageal varices, encephalopathy, hypersplenism, ascites, and spontaneous peritonitis.
   - Variceal hemorrhage is most common complication.
   - Collateral circulation develops through:
     - Coronary vein (lesser curvature of the stomach and esophageal venous plexi).
     - Superior hemorrhoidal veins (tributaries of inferior mesenteric vein).
     - Anterior abdominal wall veins (from umbilical vein).
     - Plexus of Retzius (retroperitoneal anastomoses between mesenteric veins and inferior vena cava).
   - Ascites is the result of transudation from the liver capsule.

3. **Clinical Features**
   - History, symptoms, and signs of liver disease.
   - Abdominal distention from ascites (fluid wave on examination).
   - Esophageal varices often causing massive GI bleeding.
   - Caput medusae: dilated paraumbilical veins. Hemorrhoids and hemorrhoidal bleeding.
   - Other manifestations include primary peritonitis (infected ascitic fluid without visceral perforation), encephalopathy, hypersplenism (anemia, thrombocytopenia, leukopenia), and malnutrition.

4. **Diagnostic Studies**
   - Abnormal liver function tests (LFTs; bilirubin, transaminases), anemia, hypoalbuminemia.
   - U/S shows ascites, splenomegaly, and changes in liver parenchyma.
   - Duplex U/S may be useful to evaluate thrombosis of portal vein.
   - CT scan shows ascites, splenomegaly, dilated venous collaterals, associated intra-abdominal pathology (e.g., tumor), and portal vein thrombosis.
   - MRI/magnetic resonance angiography—similar result as CT scan.
   - Liver biopsy (percutaneous or laparoscopic) provides histologic diagnosis.
   - Peritoneocenteses to obtain ascitic fluid for biochemical and bacteriologic analysis.

5. **Management**

   MEDICAL TREATMENT
   - Mainstay of therapy for cirrhosis and portal hypertension.
   - Diuretics and nutritional measures to control ascites.
   - Endoscopic injection sclerotherapy or band ligation for bleeding esophageal varices.
   - Vasopressin with nitrates, octreotide, and propranolol to reduce portal pressure.

   SURGICAL TREATMENT
   - Control of ascites: paracentesis and peritoneovenous conduits (LeVeen and Denver shunts).
   - Decompression of the portal system:
     - Transjugular intrahepatic portosystemic shunt (TIPS).
     - Portosystemic shunts (splenorenal, mesocaval, portocaval) less commonly used, but still useful in select patients.
   - Direct control of variceal bleeding.
   - Devascularization procedures:
     - Splenectomy, GE devascularization (Sugiura procedure).
     - Direct suture-ligation of esophageal and gastric varices.
   - Liver transplantation.

D. **Small Bowel**

OBSTRUCTION

1. **Etiology**
   - Adhesions from previous surgery are the most common cause.
   - Without prior surgery, incarcerated or strangulated hernias are usually the cause.
   - Other causes include tumor, radiation enteritis, inflammatory stricture (e.g., Crohn disease), intestinal torsion, peritonitis (nonmechanical obstruction, or "ileus"), and ischemic disease.

2. **Pathology**
   - Adhesions are formed by fibrous tissue (bands) and may cause narrowing, kinking, twisting, or internal herniation of the bowel.
   - Inflammatory disorders such as TB and Crohn disease may cause thickening of the intestinal wall, perforation, and adhesions.

- Adenocarcinoma is the most common tumor obstructing the small bowel; and colon.

3. **Clinical Features**
   - Nausea and vomiting, obstipation, variable or crampy abdominal pain initially, followed by constant pain when necrosis or perforation is present.
   - Crampy abdominal pain has "crescendo-decrescendo" pattern.
   - Abdominal distention, increased bowel sounds or high-pitched, metallic sounds on auscultation; no stool in the rectum unless fecal impaction is the cause.
   - Peristalsis may be visible.
   - Incarcerated (nonreducible) hernia in the groin, epigastrium, umbilicus, or at site of scar from previous operation or trauma (incisional hernia).
   - Tumor or inflammatory mass may be felt on abdominal or rectal examination.
   - Insertion of nasogastric tube (NGT) disclosing fecaloid fluid usually reflects lower small bowel obstruction.
   - Strangulated (death of tissue).

4. **Diagnostic Studies**
   - Obstructive series (supine and upright abdominal, and CXRs): most important test following clinical evaluation; can show intestinal distention, air-fluid levels, free air under the diaphragm in the case of perforation, and suggest underlying cause of the obstruction (e.g., large tumor, gallstone ileus).
   - CT scan more sensitive with in showing tumor, abscess, or free air.
   - Blood tests may confirm dehydration, electrolyte disturbances, renal impairment, or suggest underlying cause.

5. **Management**

   MEDICAL TREATMENT
   - **Partial obstruction:**
     - Initial treatment is IV fluids and NGT decompression, antibiotics.
     - Most will spontaneously resolve with decompression.
   - **Complete obstruction:**
     - Initial treatment is IV fluids and NGT suction.
     - Antibiotics may be indicated preoperatively and for infectious causes.
     - Serial clinical examination, electrolytes, and imaging radiographic follow-up to rule out bowel ischemia or strangulation.

   SURGICAL TREATMENT
   - Indicated with (+) radiographic findings, increasing amylase, fever, leukocytosis, pain, and tachycardia or persistent partial obstruction.
   - Lysis of adhesions, transection of fibrous band, tumor excision, bowel resection or diversion (colostomy, ileostomy), insertion of gastrostomy

or jejunostomy tubes, and hernia repair may be needed.
   - Open and laparoscopic techniques may be used as indicated.

ILEUS
1. **Etiology**
   - Intestinal atony or hypotony due to nonmechanical cause; intestine is paralyzed, lacking peristaltic movements—"paralytic ileus."
   - Causes include peritonitis, electrolyte imbalance, postoperative and posttraumatic ileus medications (narcotics), and rare dysmotility disorders.
   - Most common cause of ileus medications (narcotics) is postsurgical procedures; spontaneously resolves over 1 to 3 days.

2. **Pathology**
   - Bowel distention, with intraluminal gas and fluid accumulation, without mechanical obstruction.
   - Nervous plexus cells may be absent in congenital dysmotility disorders.

3. **Clinical Features**
   - Distention, vomiting, and obstipation, mild-to-moderate abdominal discomfort unless peritonitis ensues.
   - Abdominal distention, hypoactive bowel sounds.

4. **Diagnostic Studies**
   - X-rays and CT scan show distention of both large and small bowel loops, and no "transition zone."

5. **Management**
   - The main goal is to correct any underlying pathology.
   - Supportive therapy includes NPO and NGT decompression, and replacement of fluid and electrolytes.
   - Consider selective opioid antagonists to prevent postoperative narcotic-induced ileus.
   - Surgery is reserved for complications, such as perforation with peritonitis or abscess, for chronic and intractable patients, and rarely for diagnosis.

NEOPLASMS
1. **Etiology/Pathology**
   - Relatively rare (2%); most common cancers are adenocarcinoma (30% to 50%).
   - Includes sarcomas and gastrointestinal stromal tumors and lymphomas.
   - Carcinoid tumors arise from neuroendocrine cells, appendix is most common site, terminal ileum second most common site.

2. **Clinical Features**
   - Typically asymptomatic in early stages.
   - Abdominal pain and weight loss—most common presenting symptoms.
   - Chronic colicky abdominal pain, chronic anemia or overt hemorrhage, small bowel obstruction, nausea, vomiting.

- Palpable mass.
- Carcinoid tumors may cause bronchospasm, cutaneous flushing, diarrhea, and right sided heart failure (B FDR) ("carcinoid syndrome").

3. **Diagnostic Studies**
   - Usually, the diagnosis is established during laparotomy for intestinal obstruction.
   - CT scan, enteroscopy, and laparoscopy may provide preoperative diagnosis in some patients.

4. **Management**
   - Surgical resection is indicated for all small intestinal tumors. Survival dependent on location. Adenomas unresponsive to chemotherapy. Imatinib reduces GIST tumors size in up to 60% of patients. Lymphoma is treated with abdominal radiation with or without chemotherapy. Carcinoid tumors are moderately responsive to chemotherapy.

   APPENDICITIS

1. **Etiology**
   - Obstruction of the vermiform appendix by foreign body, enlarged lymphatic tissue, parasites, or "fecalith."
   - Typically is present in second or third decade.
   - Most common nonobstetric surgical disease in pregnancy.
   - Perforation higher in elderly patients due to impaired blood flow (atherosclerosis) causing earlier perforation; atypical presentation.

2. **Pathology**
   - Early stages: vascular congestion, edema, neutrophilic infiltrates, mucosal necrosis, luminal occlusion (e.g., fecalith).
   - Late stages: gangrene, perforation, abscess formation, or diffuse peritonitis.
   - Cecum may be mobile; therefore, appendix may be located anywhere in the abdominal cavity, which may cause atypical presentation.

3. **Clinical Features**

   CLASSIC PRESENTATIONS
   - Periumbilical discomfort, anorexia, nausea, right lower quadrant (RLQ) pain, and fever.
   - Movement of pain from periumbilical area to RLQ.
   - Guarding, rigidity, + Rovsing and + psoas signs.
   - Vomiting.
   - RLQ tenderness (McBurney point) with rebound, right-sided tenderness on rectal examination.

   LESS COMMON PRESENTATIONS
   - Pain in other locations than RLQ; diarrhea; diffuse peritonitis (common in children and elderly patients); chronic recurrent appendicitis (poorly defined entity; other disorders must be excluded).

- Combination of history, physical examination, complete blood count (CBC), and plain abdominal films should provide correct diagnosis in >90% of patients.

4. **Diagnostic Studies**
   - CBC with differential demonstrates leukocytosis.
   - U/S and CT scan can be helpful in doubtful cases, particularly in children and elderly and in advanced appendicitis with abscess formation.

5. **Management**
   - Early appendicitis is best treated with urgent appendectomy with preoperative antibiotics.
   - Advanced cases, with rupture and localized abscess, may be treated with IV antibiotics and ultrasound-guided percutaneous drainage, followed by delayed ("interval") appendectomy.
   - Appendectomy can be performed through an oblique or transverse incision in the RLQ (McBurney and Rocky-Davis incisions), a midline incision, or by laparoscopy.

E. Colon, Rectum, and Anus

CARCINOMA

1. **Etiology**

   RISK FACTORS FOR COLORECTAL CANCER
   - Smoking, heavy alcohol use, obesity, lack of fiber, overconsumption of red meat.
   - Genetic: familial adenomatous polyposis, Gardner syndrome.
   - Others: inflammatory bowel disease (ulcerative colitis), neoplastic polyps (usually >2 cm), age >40.

   RISK FACTORS FOR ANAL CANCER
   - Human papillomavirus (HPV), prior radiation.

2. **Pathology**
   - Colorectal: >90% adenocarcinoma.
   - Anal: approximately 60% squamous cell carcinoma; approximately 20% cloacogenic.
   - Most common metastasis: regional lymph nodes.

3. **Clinical Features**
   - Abdominal pain, palpable mass.
   - Colorectal: obstruction/diarrhea, bleeding, chronic anemia, perforation.
   - Rectal: hematochezia, tenesmus, discharge, obstruction.

4. **Diagnostic Studies**
   - Fecal occult blood plus rectal examination are most cost-effective screening methods (rectal examination discloses ~20% of all colorectal tumors).
   - Proctosigmoidoscopy, colonoscopy, and barium enema can provide definitive diagnosis and location.
   - Blood levels of carcinoembryonic antigen are useful to detect recurrence after surgery.
   - CT scan of abdomen/pelvis/lung to evaluate metastasis.

5. **Management**
   - Patients at increased risk should undergo periodic early screening.
   - Colon: wide surgical excision and regional lymphatics.
   - Rectal: surgery with chemoradiation.
   - Depending on location, permanent colostomy may be necessary.

ANAL FISSURE
1. **Etiology**
   - Mechanical trauma, ischemia, and infection have all been postulated as causes of anal fissure.
   - Most common cause: passage of large, hard stools.
2. **Pathology**
   - Superficial tear in the anoderm.
   - Acute: sudden tearing pain, bleeding
   - Chronic: >6 weeks.
   - Most fissures are located on the posterior midline.
   - In the early phases, shallow ulceration with ill-defined edges; later, deeper ulcer, regular edges.
3. **Clinical Features**
   - Painful linear or elliptic ulceration in the anal canal.
   - Rectal pain, blood stools, mucoid discharge.
4. **Diagnostic Studies**
   - Digital examination discloses spasm of anal sphincter, and anoscopy confirms the presence of fissure—may require sedation to complete examination.
   - CBC to rule out anemia and infection.
   - Differential diagnosis: ulcerative colitis and Crohn disease, perirectal abscess, hemorrhoids, fistula-in-ano, squamous cell carcinoma, syphilis, TB, and ulcerations in immunosuppressed patients (leukemia, AIDS).
5. **Management**

   MEDICAL TREATMENT
   - WASH: **w**arm water baths (sitz baths), **a**nalgesics, **s**tool softeners, and **h**igh fiber diet resolve 90% of cases.
   - Majority of fissures resolve spontaneously.
   - Topical nitroglycerin to relieve anal spasm and promote healing.
   - Botulinum toxin injection.

   SURGICAL TREATMENT
   - Sphincterotomy of the internal sphincter reduces spasm and allows healing; the external sphincter must be spared to preserve anal continence.
   - Anal dilatation under anesthesia can provide pain relief in 80% to 90% of cases; however, recurrence occurs in approximately 10% and sphincter dysfunction in approximately 10%.

ISCHEMIC BOWEL DISEASE/MESENTERIC ISCHEMIA
1. **Etiology**
   - *Thrombosis:* hypercoagulable states, aortic dissection, atherosclerosis of visceral vessels (celiac trunk, superior mesenteric artery [SMA], inferior mesenteric artery [IMA] vasospasm).
   - *Embolism:* clot dislodged from the heart, atrial fibrillation, ventricular aneurysm.
   - *Low flow:* congestive heart failure (CHF), vasoconstrictive agents, shock.
2. **Pathology**
   - SMA syndrome: extensive ischemia or necrosis of small and large intestines, from ligament of Treitz to mid-transverse colon.
   - IMA syndrome: left colon and sigmoid involvement.
   - Celiac artery is usually narrowed or occluded.
3. **Clinical Features**
   - Acute event with rapid clinical deterioration: hypotension, shock, acidosis, renal failure, and death.
   - Manifestations more insidious in thrombosis and low flow; more abrupt in embolism.
   - Abdominal pain out of proportion with physical signs.
   - Abdominal distention, peritonitis, bloody stools later in course.
   - Severe acidosis, with high lactic acid in the blood.
   - High degree of suspicion when risk factors are present: old age, cardiovascular disease, and low flow states.
4. **Diagnostic Studies**
   - Plain X-rays show dilated loops with edema of the bowel wall ("thumbprinting").
   - Angiography can provide precise anatomic diagnosis and can be used for intra-arterial thrombolytic therapy in select patients.
   - CT scan can show aortic dissection, bowel distention and edema, arterial calcifications, and associated intra-abdominal pathology.
5. **Management**

   MEDICAL TREATMENT
   - Rapid fluid resuscitation, intensive care, anticoagulation, and thrombolysis—urokinase, streptokinase, tissue-type plasminogen activator (tPA)—as indicated.
   - NGT placement.

   SURGICAL TREATMENT
   - Visceral thromboembolectomy and revascularization when intestines are viable.
   - Most patients require extensive bowel resection, plus enterostomy.

PILONIDAL CYST AND ABSCESS
1. **Etiology**
   - Caused by hair and cellular debris finding entry into hair follicles (pit).
   - Cystic cavity containing keratin and hair in the subcutaneous tissues of the natal cleft (between the buttocks in the sacrococcygeal area).

2. Pathology
- Hyperkeratotic invagination, inflammation, granuloma, and sinus formation.

3. Clinical Features
- Acute presentation: abscess; red and warm swelling, sometimes fluctuance, in the upper intergluteal fold; may be paramedian.
- Chronic presentation: sinus felt in the natal cleft, with occasional discomfort or discharge.

4. Diagnostic Studies
- Physical examination is sufficient to make the diagnosis.
- Differential diagnosis includes hydradenitis, perirectal abscess with fistulas, and folliculitis.

5. Management

SURGICAL TREATMENT
- Abscess is treated with incision and drainage and removal of hair pit. Postoperative shaving and removal of hair from area have a 90% success rate.
- Chronic noninfected, symptomatic sinuses are best excised with open packing, marsupialization, or wound flaps; only complete excision prevents recurrence.

F. Pancreatic Cancer

1. Etiology
- Incidence has increased 3-fold in past 40 years.
- Approximately 34,000 deaths per year in the United States.
- Second most common GI tract malignancy.
- Fourth most common cause of cancer death.
- Incidence increases with age and peaks in fifth and sixth decade of life.
- Male to female incidence ratio 1:1.

2. Pathology
- Three types of tumors: (1) adenocarcinoma—arises from ductal epithelium, most common; (2) endocrine tumors; (3) cystic pancreatic neoplasms.
- Benign neoplasms are exceedingly rare.
- Half the lesions localized in the head; 20% in the body; <5% in the tail; 20% are multicentric.

3. Clinical Features
- Most commonly, painless; jaundice is presenting symptom.
- Severe weight loss, abdominal pain.
- Pruritus of hands/feet.
- Palpable nontender gallbladder (Courvoisier sign), due to neoplastic obstruction of common duct.
- Abdominal mass or supraclavicular node (suggestive of distant metastasis).

4. Diagnostic Studies
- Laboratory studies—often nonspecific, but usually support obstructive jaundice.
- Abdominal U/S—may show dilatation of biliary ducts and less commonly may disclose mass at the head of pancreas.
- CT scan—detects mass and ductal dilatation and is the test of choice for initial evaluation (helical or spiral CT).
- Endoscopic retrograde cholangiopancreatography (necessary if CT scan is negative)—may show duodenal or ampullary lesion, "double duct sign," irregular narrowing of both intrapancreatic common bile duct (CBD) and pancreatic duct, suggesting pancreatic cancer.
- Laparoscopy—may be used for staging, before laparotomy.
- Aspiration biopsy of pancreatic mass contradicted for resectable tumors secondary to risk of spreading tumor.

5. Management
- Resectable tumors (<25%) in the head of pancreas treated with pancreaticoduodenectomy (Whipple procedure) or duodenal sparing procedure (modified Whipple).
- Unresectable tumors (75%) treated with palliative biliary bypass, or endoscopic stenting of the CBD.
- Five-year survival rate after resection is <5%.
- Chemotherapy and radiotherapy have shown some short-term benefit, but do not improve long-term survival; clinical trials continue at some large medical centers.

VI. Genitourinary Tract Disorders—Male

A. Testicular Carcinoma

1. Etiology
- Most common solid tumors in male adolescents and adults (15 to 35 years).
- Risk for testicular malignancy is 1 in 500.
- Multimodality treatment has reduced mortality to <10%.

2. Pathology
- Almost all malignancies are of germ cell origin.
- Seminomas account for 60% of all germ cell tumors.

3. Clinical Features
- Most commonly, single, hard, nontender mass noted on testicle.
- Other symptoms related to metastasis may be present.

4. Diagnostic Studies
- U/S shows a hypoechoic area.
- Serum tumor markers—AFP, human chorionic gonadotropin (hCG)—aid in staging and identification of tumor.

5. Management
- Inguinal orchiectomy—mainstay of therapy.
- Retroperitoneal lymph node dissection.
- Chemotherapy and radiotherapy may be used dependent on type of tumor and stage of disease.

SEMINOMAS
- Low-stage disease treated with orchiectomy, followed by radiotherapy to the abdomen.
- High-stage disease warrants multiagent chemotherapy followed by surgery and radiotherapy.

NONSEMINOMATOUS GERM CELL TUMORS
- Low-stage disease, normal markers, treated with orchiectomy and retroperitoneal lymph node dissection.

RENAL CELL CARCINOMA
- Most common type of renal malignancy; 5% of all adult cancers.

WILMS TUMOR
- Nephroblastoma, most common renal tumor in childhood.
- Asymptomatic abdominal mass.
- Hypertension, hematuria, anemia.
- U/S, CT.
- Treatment: Nephrectomy. Radiation if tumor extends beyond renal capsule. Large tumors may require preoperative radiation and chemotherapy.

B. Bladder Carcinoma
1. Etiology
- Men affected more frequently than women.
- More common in smokers, occupational carcinogens, schistosomiasis, chronic infection.

2. Pathology
- Ninety percent of tumors of transitional cell origin.
- Squamous, adenocarcinoma less common.
- Transitional cell carcinoma has strong link to cigarette smoking.
- Transitional cell tumors classified as either superficial or invasive.

3. Clinical Features
- Most common presentation is painless microscopic hematuria.
- Other symptoms may include those of irritation (e.g., frequency and urgency).
- Ureteral obstruction common.

4. Diagnostic Studies
- Cystoscopy (can be diagnostic and therapeutic).
- Small lesions can be excised or fulgurated.
- Excretory urography for large masses used to evaluate renal pelvis and ureters because they are at risk for urothelial neoplasia.
- CT scanning of abdomen and pelvis is done to evaluate small tumors and metastasis.

5. Management
- Local noninvasive disease treated with endoscopic transurethral resection and close follow-up.

- Intravesical chemotherapeutic agents decrease recurrence.
- Invasive disease treated with cystectomy, urinary diversion.
- Chemotherapy, radiation reserved for invasive disease.
- Only 50% of patients with invasive disease are rendered tumor free.
- Radical cystectomy for recurrent cancer, diffuse transitional cell carcinoma combination chemotherapy.

C. Prostate Carcinoma
1. Etiology
- Most common cancer in men.
- Second most common cause of cancer-related mortality in men.
- Approximately 160,000 new cases are diagnosed each year.
- African Americans have higher mortality rates than Caucasians.
- Increased risk in men who have one or more relatives diagnosed before age 70.
- Only 3% of men with prostate cancer have clinically evident disease.
- Fifty percent of patients have advanced disease at time of diagnosis.

2. Pathology
- Ninety-five percent adenocarcinomas.
- Five percent transitional cell carcinoma of prostatic urethra, small cell carcinoma, sarcomas.
- Peripheral zone—area felt on digital rectal examination (DRE), most common site of origin.
- Transitional zone or periurethral-zone, next most common site (area removed by transurethral resection of prostate).

3. Clinical Features
- Asymptomatic until tumor invasion of bladder or bones, or obstruction of urethra.
- Prostate cancer rarely causes hematuria or obstruction when contained to gland.
- Early detection relies on DRE and prostate-specific antigen (PSA) testing.
- DRE—firm, nontender, fixed mass of prostate.
- All men aged 50 and older should undergo yearly DRE and serum PSA.
- African Americans and men with a family history of prostate cancer should begin testing at age 40.

4. Diagnostic Studies
- PSA level—elevated in prostate cancer.
- Men with abnormal DRE, PSA >4 ng per mL should undergo transrectal U/S (TRUS) and biopsy.
- TRUS may detect lesions in prostate, but is operator dependent; used in U/S-guided biopsy of prostate.
- PSA >10 ng per mL—radionuclide bone scan to rule out bony metastasis.

- PSA <10 ng per mL—low probability for metastatic disease.
- CT scan may not be reliable in detecting nodal involvement for prostate cancer.

5. **Management**

   ORGAN-CONFINED DISEASE
   - Negative bone scan, DRE not suggestive of extracapsular extension: local therapy with curative intent, radical prostatectomy, external beam radiation therapy.
   - Side effects of surgery include sexual impotence, urinary incontinence.
   - Morbidities of external beam radiation include sexual impotence, radiation cystitis, urethral stricture, and proctitis.

   ADVANCED AND METASTATIC DISEASE
   - Androgen ablation—either castration or medical alteration using luteinizing hormone—improved progression-free survival, but not overall survival.
   - Bone pain from metastatic disease may be treated with palliative, localized radiation therapy and analgesics.

VII. Genitourinary Tract Disorders—Female

A. Cervical Carcinoma

1. **Etiology**
   - Second most common malignancy in women.
   - Average age at diagnosis—50 years, although the very young as well as very old can be affected.
   - A bimodal distribution exists—peaks between 35 and 39 years, then between 60 and 64 years.

   RISK FACTORS
   - **Etiology is unknown; some risks factors include:**
     - Coitus at an early age.
     - Mutiple sexual partners.
     - HPV—type 16 and 18 account for 70% of all cervical cancers.
     - Male sexual partner participating in high-risk sexual behavior.
     - Smoking.
     - Use of birth control pills.
     - Immunocompromised patients.

2. **Pathology**
   - Seventy percent to 80%—squamous cell.
   - Ninety-five percent of squamous cell carcinoma occur within the transformation zone.
   - Twenty percent to 30%—adenocarcinomas, adenosquamous, undifferentiated carcinomas.
   - Cervical carcinoma spreads through cervical and paracervical lymphatics, through the parametria, and into regional lymph nodes.
   - Metastases—lungs, mediastinal, inguinal, axillary, and supraclavicular lymph nodes, bones, liver.

3. **Clinical Features**
   - Early disease—asymptomatic; routine Papanicolaou (Pap) smear indicative.
   - Intermenstrual bleeding—most common symptom of invasive cancer.
   - Postcoital bleeding or spotting.
   - Leukorrhea; typically sanguineous or purulent, odorous, and nonpruritic.

   ADVANCED DISEASE
   - Pelvic pain usually unilateral and radiating to the hip or thigh.
   - Involuntary loss of urine or feces through vagina (fistula formation).
   - Weight loss, anemia, weakness.

   PHYSICAL FINDINGS
   - Enlargement; irregularity; and fixed, firm consistency of cervix.
   - Friable, bleeding, cauliflower-like lesion within vagina.
   - Ulceration may be primary manifestation of invasive disease.
   - Unilateral leg edema, sciatic pain, and ureteral obstruction indicate advanced disease.

4. **Diagnostic Studies**
   - History and physical examination with Pap smear.
   - Cytologic (Pap smear) studies; suspect or positive Pap smears indicate the need for further studies.
   - Colposcopy and biopsy of lesions (staging of disease).
   - Conization if colposcopy is nondiagnostic.
   - MRI, CT scan, and/or pelvic lymphangiography may demonstrate involvement of pelvic or periaortic lymph nodes.
   - Advance disease cystoscopy, proctosigmoidoscopy.
   - CXR to rule out metastatic or primary disease.

5. **Management**
   - Dependent on staging and cell type, and may include patient's fertility desires.

   MICROINVASIVE CARCINOMA
   - When a thorough pathologic review of biopsy specimen demonstrates questionable invasion or early stromal invasion to 3 mm and no tumor or vascular space is involved, cone biopsy or simple or extended hysterectomy (without lymph node/extensive ureteral or bladder dissection) should be curative.

   INVASIVE CARCINOMA
   - Radial hysterectomy.
   - Fertility-preserving surgery preferred for young women of childbearing age or sexually active women (dependent on cancer stage).
   - Adjuvant radiation therapy or chemoradiation therapy for patients at risk for recurrence.

PALLIATIVE CARE OF CERVICAL CANCER
- Palliative chemotherapy and/or radiation therapy.
- Management of ulceration, vaginal hemorrhage, and pain control.

B. Vaginal Carcinoma

1. **Etiology**
   - One percent to 2% of primary gynecologic cancers located in the vagina.
   - Secondary carcinomas of the vagina are more common than primary.
   - Extension from cervix is the most common cause of secondary vaginal carcinoma.
   - HPV most common 16 or 18 subtype infection is a risk factor.
   - Typically affects postmenopausal women.

2. **Pathology**
   - Eighty-five percent are squamous cell carcinoma.
   - Remainder include adenocarcinomas, sarcomas, melanomas.
   - Route of metastasis is dependent on size and location of tumor within vagina:
     - Upper third—most common site of tumor metastases—similar to carcinoma of cervix.
     - Middle third—metastasize to inguinal nodes or directly to deep pelvic nodes.
     - Lower third—metastasize primarily to the inguinal lymph nodes.

3. **Clinical Features**
   - Most common symptom—abnormal, painless, bleeding or bloody vaginal discharge.
   - Postcoital bleeding.
   - Early—asymptomatic; typically discovered on routine vaginal cytologic examination; painless bleeding from ulcerated tumor.
   - Advanced—tumor causes vaginal discharge and vulvar pruritus.
   - Late—bleeding, pain, weight loss, swelling.

4. **Diagnostic Studies**
   - Diagnosis of primary vaginal carcinoma cannot be made until metastases from other sources are ruled out.
   - Biopsy establishes diagnosis; if positive, a search for metastatic disease is warranted.
   - Staged clinically including CXR, skeletal survey, cystoscopy, and proctoscopy.

5. **Management**
   - Treatment—may be surgery with or without radiotherapy, depending on location and stage of disease.
   - Prognosis—most important indicators: size and depth of tumor, and stage of disease at time of diagnosis.
   - Follow-up.
     - Early lesions: every 3 months for 2 years, then every 6 months for 3 years, and annually thereafter.
     - Advanced—as clinically indicated.

C. Vulvar Carcinoma

1. **Etiology**
   - Occurs in postmenopausal women.
   - Approximately 5% of gynecologic cancers.
   - Typically a slow-growing cancer.
   - Associated factors—HPV infection, sexually transmitted diseases, smoking, multiple sexual partners, prior history of cervical cancer, vulvar dystrophy.
   - High rate of recurrence.

2. **Pathology (Vulvar Intraepithelial Neoplasia [VIN])**
   - High-grade squamous lesions that have a high predilection for progression to severe dysplasia and continuing onto carcinoma.
   - Clinical presentations: vulvar pruritus, chronic irritation, development of raised mass lesions.
   - Treatment options include surgery, laser, and topical medications (imiquimod, topical 5-fluorouracil).
   - More than 90% of vulvar cancers are squamous cell with two subtypes that are frequently found on the labia or vestibule.
   - Keratinizing or differentiated type: more common, found in older patients, mostly associated with vulvar dystrophies.
   - Classic or warty type: found in younger women, mostly associated with HPV16, 18, and 33.
   - Less common types; melanoma, sarcoma, Paget disease, basal cell carcinoma, Bartholin gland adenocarcinoma.

3. **Clinical Features**
   - Most common presenting complaint: vulvar pruritus.
   - Patient has a long history of vulvar irritation with pruritus, local discomfort, bloody discharge.
   - Twenty percent are asymptomatic.
   - Lesion may appear erythematous, ulcerative, or leukoplakic; configuration—papular or macular.
   - Lesions are generally multifocal and occur on labia minora.
   - Appearance of early lesions similar to vulvar dermatitis.
   - Appearance of late lesions: cauliflower or hard, ulcerated area.

4. **Diagnostic Studies**
   - Colposcopic examination of vulva, vagina, cervix, perineum, perianal area.
   - Anoscopy to rule out disease in the anal canal.
   - Biopsy of vulvar mass or lesion.
   - If biopsy is positive for vulvar cancer, other studies may include:
     - CXR.
     - IV pyelogram.
     - Cystoscopy, proctoscopy, or both, indicated if lesion is located near the urethra or involves the anus or perineal regions.

5. **Management**
   - Complete laboratory evaluation to rule out metastases, primary or concurrent cancers.

- Surgical staging and management—mostly radical resection with inguinofemoral lymphadenectomy.
- Adjuvant radiation therapy for advanced stages.
- Chemotherapy for metastatic disease and recurrences.
- Follow-up—immediate postoperative period to detect recurrence or second primary cancer: every months for 2 years, then every 6 months thereafter.

D. Ovarian Carcinoma

1. Etiology
- Second most common cause of gynecologic cancer in women in the United States.
- Each year, epithelial ovarian cancer causes more deaths of American women than all other gynecologic malignancies combined.
- Seventy-five percent of ovarian cancers are still diagnosed at advanced stage (poor prognosis).
- Occurs in postmenopausal women (typically between ages 50 and 75 years).

RISK FACTORS
- Caucasian origin.
- Breast, uterine, or colorectal cancer.
- Nulliparity.
- Delayed childbearing.
- Family history of gynecologic cancer (first-degree relative).
- Genetics: *BRACA1* or *BRACA2* mutation, Lynch syndrome.
- Endometriosis.
- Increase with age.

PROTECTIVE FACTORS
- Oral contraceptive pills.
- Multiparity.
- Breast-feeding.
- Tubal ligation.

2. Pathology
- Three histopathologic categories (based on cell type):
  - Epithelial neoplasms (80% to 90%).
  - Stromal cell (5% to 15%).
  - Germ cell (5%)—occurs in young women and has a different course and treatment.
- Transperitoneal dissemination is most common type of extraovarian spread.
- Most common sites of spread include omentum, peritoneum, bowel surfaces, and retroperitoneal lymph nodes.

3. Clinical Features
- Typically asymptomatic until disease is widely disseminated.
- History of nonspecific abdominal or pelvic complaints (nausea/dyspepsia, change in bowel habits, urinary urgency/frequency).
- Abdominal bloating, vague abdominal discomfort.
- Pelvic mass palpated (although masses <10 cm are often undetected by routine examination). Malignant—solid, nodular, fixed.
- Enlarging mass.
- Advance disease: large pelvic mass causing obstructive symptoms; ascites; respiratory distress secondary to pleural effusion.

4. Diagnostic Studies
- Complete history and physical examination with emphasis on pelvis and adnexal areas.

RADIOGRAPHIC EVALUATION
- U/S (transabdominal and transvaginal examination).
- If U/S positive, CXR to rule out lung metastasis.

LABORATORY EVALUATION
- Serum level of CA-125 (a glycoprotein and antibody that reacts on a peritoneal cell antigen); increased or increasing levels of CA-125 indicate ovarian cancers and may be used as a monitor for known disease. *Not a screening test.*
- Serum hCG if pregnancy is a possibility.
- Exploratory laparotomy or laparoscopy.
- CT or MRI as needed.
- Barium enema or colonoscopy with patient complaints of change in bowel habits or positive guaiac stools.
- Mammography in patients with a breast mass.

5. Management
- Referral to gynecologic oncology specialist.
- Surgery—mainstay of therapy (to obtain complete surgical staging of disease).
- Post-op venous thromboembolism prophylaxis.

STAGES I AND II
- Laparotomy/total abdominal hysterectomy/bilateral salpingo-oophorectomy, and chemotherapy (dependent on grade).
- Unilateral salpingo-oophorectomy and staging biopsies if fertility is desired and determined to be Stage I/Grade 1.
- Follow-up every 2 to 4 months for 2 years, then every 6 months for 3 years, and then yearly: serial serum CA-125 level to detect the presence of ovarian recurrence. Pelvic examinations, CXR, CT scans as indicated.
- Serum CA-125 level to detect presence of ovarian recurrence.

STAGES III AND IV
- Cytoreductive surgery and chemotherapy.
- Chemotherapy only for patient unable to tolerate surgery.

E. Uterine Carcinoma

1. Etiology
- Endometrium carcinoma is the most common gynecologic malignancy in the United States.
- Seventy-five percent of patients presenting for initial diagnosis have disease confined to uterine corpus.
- Diagnosed primarily in postmenopausal women (mean age: 60 years); 30% occur premenopausal or <40 years of age.
- Incidence higher in Caucasian women.

RISK FACTORS
- **Classic triad of risk factors:**
  - Obesity.
  - Diabetes mellitus.
  - Hypertension.
- Long-term history of unopposed estrogen (either endogenously or by exogenous administration).
- Nulliparity.
- Uterine or ovarian cancer positive family history.
- Tamoxifen use.
- Lynch syndrome (hereditary nonpolyposis colorectal cancer).

2. **Pathology**
- Adenocarcinoma (Grade 1) is most common form.
- Other types—clear cell, secretory, squamous, and papillary serous endometrial carcinomas.

3. **Clinical Features**
- **Ninety percent complain of abnormal vaginal discharge:**
  - Ninety percent of these have abnormal bleeding after menopause.
  - Few have purulent vaginal discharge without bleeding (typically thin, elderly, and estrogen deficient).
- Painful or frequent urination (secondary to enlarging uterine mass).
- Premenopausal patient—prolonged, heavy menstrual periods; intermenstrual spotting.
- Advanced disease—feelings of pelvic pressure.

PHYSICAL EXAMINATION
- **Early:**
  - May have no abnormal findings.
- **Advanced:**
  - Abdominal examination: ascites with palpable hepatic or omental nodules.
  - Pelvic: uterine enlargement, boggy consistency.
  - Rectovaginal examination: to determine disease infiltration.

4. **Diagnostic Studies**
- Pregnancy test.
- Transvaginal U/S.
- Hysterosonography/hysteroscope for visualizing mass or abnormality.
- Endocervical curettage, biopsy, and sampling:
  - Endocervix.
  - Entire endometrial cavity.
  - Dilation and curettage, if office sampling is inconclusive.
- CT, MRI, or both.

5. **Management**
- **Search for metastatic disease:**
  - CXR.
  - MRI if a patient is staged clinically.
- Complete CBC, biochemical profile, including renal and LFTs, CA-125 (predicts extrauterine spread) measurement.
- Surgery—hysterectomy with bilateral salpingo-oophorectomy and surgical staging for most patients.
- Additional therapy depending on various factors (including staging and grade of tumor).
- Radiation—used in bulky pelvic disease and post-op in patients with invasion in the myometrium, positive lymph nodes, or adnexa involvement.
- Chemotherapy—for some stage III or IV carcinomas.
- Hormones—hydroxyprogesterone, medroxyprogesterone, or megestrol used when distant metastasis is present.

VIII. Hernia

A. Inguinal

1. **Etiology**
- Indirect hernia—a congenital defect; persistence of the processus vaginalis.
- Direct hernia—presumably degenerative; gradual weakening of transversalis fascia on the floor of the inguinal canal.

2. **Pathology**
- Indirect: intraperitoneal contents protrude through the internal ring, enter the spermatic cord, and may reach the scrotum.
- Direct: defect is medial to the internal ring and inside Hesselbach's triangle; protrusion usually does not reach the scrotum.
- Contents of hernia sac may include intestine, appendix, omentum, bladder, ovary, and fallopian tubes.

3. **Clinical Features**
- Indirect: more common in children and young adults.
- Direct: more common in older patients; rare in women.
- Incarceration: contents cannot be returned into abdominal cavity; usually painful.
- Strangulation: incarceration associated with compromise of blood supply (ischemia or gangrene), causing pain, fever, and leukocytosis.
- Clinical evaluation should establish the presence or absence of hernia (bulge), and of incarceration or strangulation.

4. **Diagnostic Studies**
- Rarely, X-rays, U/S, or CT scan may be necessary (e.g., in morbidly obese patients and when associated intra-abdominal pathology is suspected).

5. **Management**
- The treatment of hernias is surgical. Occasionally, patients with prohibitive risk, or having asymptomatic hernias with a wide neck (low risk of incarceration), may be managed conservatively with a supporter (truss).
- Incarceration requires urgent surgical reduction; strangulation is an emergency and may require resection of bowel or other strangulated structures.
- Most elective hernia repair is conducted on an ambulatory basis, under local-regional anesthesia.

- Open repair using synthetic mesh is the standard with fewer complications to laparoscopic repair.
- The use of synthetic mesh has decreased the recurrence of hernias by 50% to 75%.
- Laparoscopic repair takes longer to perform and is a more difficult procedure. Patients experience less short-term and long-term postoperative pain and have a faster return to activities.
- The rates of recurrence vary from 1-28% for direct and 0.6-3% for indirect hernias.
- Complications of surgery include nerve entrapment, damage to spermatic cord structures, ischemic orchitis, hematoma, chronic pain, and infection.

B. Femoral
1. Etiology
- Defect in the femoral canal, medial to the femoral vein (femoral anatomy—from lateral to medial: "NAV," nerve, artery, and vein).
2. Pathology
- Defect is small (approximately 0.5 to 2 cm); most common herniated structure is preperitoneal fat.
3. Clinical Features
- Bulge below the inguinal ligament, usually asymptomatic.
- The majority of cases occur in females.
- Differential diagnosis: lymphadenopathy, varicose saphenous vein, inguinal hernia.
- Physical examination: small bulge of the upper thigh; often nonreducible.
4. Diagnostic Studies
- Ultrasound or CT scan.
- Caution: needle aspiration or biopsy only if hernia is excluded with certainty; the term *wind abscess* was coined to denote puncture of a herniated ischemic bowel loop simulating abscess.
5. Management
- Surgical repair is indicated because of high risk of strangulation (narrow neck).

C. Umbilical
1. Etiology
- Congenital failure of umbilicus to close.
2. Pathology
- Large defects characterize "gastroschisis" and "omphalocele (>10 cm)," seen in newborns. Abdominal viscera protrudes out of the large defects.
- "Adult" umbilical hernias are usually small defects that become apparent when increased intra-abdominal pressure is present.
3. Clinical Features
- Pregnancy, intra-abdominal tumor, ascites, or bowel distention often precipitate clinical manifestation of small umbilical hernias.
- A round defect in the aponeurosis at the level of the umbilicus can usually be felt on palpation.
- Maneuvers to increase intra-abdominal pressure (coughing, straining) help in making the diagnosis.

4. Management
CONSERVATIVE TREATMENT
- Most small umbilical hernias in children resolve spontaneously before age 5.
SURGICAL TREATMENT
- Symptomatic or large hernias are best treated by surgical closure (sutures) of the defect; mesh repair may be needed for large defects.

D. Incisional
1. Etiology
- Any penetrating injury to the abdomen can eventually result in hernia.
- Physical examination; Hernia is often nonreducible. Most common cause is laparotomy, particularly midline incisions.
2. Pathology
- Defect in posterior fascial layers allowing passage of intra-abdominal contents.
3. Clinical Features
- Bulge in the region of previous scar from surgery or penetrating trauma.
- Incarceration and strangulation may occur except in large hernias.
4. Diagnostic Studies
- History of surgery (including laparoscopy) or trauma (commonly, stab wound).
- Physical findings consistent with fascial defect in the vicinity of a scar.
5. Management
- Most incisional hernias require surgical repair; experience is growing with laparoscopic approaches; mesh is often used and has a better outcome.

IX. Disorders of Bone
A. Osteosarcoma
1. Etiology
- Most common primary malignant bone tumor.
- Account for 20% to 30% of bone tumors; of these, 70% are metastatic or hematologic in origin.
- Male:female ratio is 3:2.
- Occurs predominantly in adolescents and young adults.
- Eighty percent occur in patients younger than 20 years.
- Secondary peak incidence occurs in patients 50 to 60 years old, with a history of radiation therapy for other types of malignancies.
- Paget disease—most common condition leading to osteosarcoma development.
- Pulmonary metastases—most common spread.
2. Pathology
- **Three common histologic subtypes:**
  - Osteoblastic (most common).
  - Chondroblastic.
  - Fibroblastic.

- Ninety percent noted in metaphyseal region of long bones; 50% of these are located around the knee area.
- Always contain osteoid and callus produced by abnormal, atypical anaplastic stromal cells.
- Malignant spindle cell produces the osteoid, deposited in thick masses between trabeculae of normal callus, which then destroys the compact bone and replaces it with abnormal callus and osteoid.
- Periosteal reaction—occurs when tumor lifts off the periosteum and makes bizarre patterns of new bone formation—seen on plain films.

3. **Clinical Features**
- Most common presenting symptoms—pain, swelling, palpable mass.
- Limitation of motion if mass is present near or within joint.
- May have tenderness, warmth, erythema, striae, or engorged veins around mass.
- Pain—initially mild and intermittent, but rapidly progresses in severity and duration; usually worse at night.
- May occasionally present as a pathologic fracture.

4. **Diagnostic Studies**
- Plain radiographs should demonstrate an extensive, poorly defined destructive bony lesion, usually with extraosseous component.
- Radionuclide bone scanning with technetium-99 (^{99}T) pyrophosphate to identify extent of primary lesion, as well as demonstrate bony metastases.
- CT scanning to assess degree of bony destruction, extent of soft-tissue involvement, relationship of tumor to neurovascular structures.
- Chest CT scan to rule out pulmonary metastases.
- MRI indicated for patients who qualify for limb-sparing surgery to assist in planning the procedure.
- Incisional biopsy to determine type of sarcomas and plan preoperative and postoperative chemotherapy.

5. **Management**
- Surgery—primary treatment.
- Limb-sparing resection—used for most patients with extremity sarcomas and no neurovascular involvement.
- Radical amputation for sarcomas involved with neurovascular structures.
- Preoperative chemotherapy—used to increase limb-salvaging excisions by decreasing the soft-tissue involvement.
- Serial scans (such as the thallium-201 scans) and serum alkaline phosphatase levels can be used to document preoperative response to chemotherapy.
- Postoperative chemotherapy—tailored to patient's response to preoperative chemotherapy and histologic determination from biopsy.

B. Osteochondroma

1. **Etiology**
- Most common primary benign bone tumor.
- Male:female ratio is 3:1.
- Most common sites—distal femur, proximal humerus, tibia, femur.

2. **Pathology**
- Aberrant cartilage growth (not neoplastic) resulting in bony mass.
- Begins in childhood and grows until completion of skeletal maturity.
- Arises in the area of growth plates of the long bones, pelvis, spine.

3. **Clinical Features**
- Appears as solitary mass, typically asymptomatic (unless nerve compression, mechanical irritation, or bursa formation are present).
- Complaint of pain or growth of lesion may indicate degeneration to malignancy.

4. **Diagnostic Studies**
- Plain films: lesion with peripheral rim of calcification and "stippled" calcification within lesion.
- CT scan to distinguish benign versus malignant indicators.

5. **Management**

   PREPUBERTAL PRESENTATION
- May be observed, but resected immediately upon growth of lesion or development of pain.

   ADULT PRESENTATION
- Observation if located on extremity.
- Resection if pelvis involved (most common site of malignant transformation).
- Resection only if symptomatic, or if growth occurs.

X. Shock

- An abnormality of the circulatory system that results in inadequate organ perfusion and tissue oxygenation.
- Shock can be divided into three categories: obstructive, hypovolemic, and distributive.

A. Obstructive

1. **Etiology**
- Intrinsic—myocardial infarction (MI) or contusion.
- Extrinsic—pericardial tamponade, tension pneumothorax, massive PE, air ambolus.

2. **Pathology**
- Decreased ability of the heart to pump secondary to heart muscle damage (intrinsic).
- Increased external pressure on the heart, or great vessels decrease heart's ability to pump (extrinsic).

3. **Clinical Features**
- Patients have pale, cool skin and slow capillary refill.
- May be quiet or apprehensive.
- **May have signs/symptoms consistent with MI:**
  - Chest, jaw pain, arm pain.

- Nausea.
- Shortness of breath.
- ECG changes—Q waves, ST segment elevation.
- **May have signs/symptoms consistent with pericardial tamponade (Beck triad):**
  - Jugular venous distention (JVD).
  - Muffled heart sounds.
  - Hypotension.
- **May have signs/symptoms consistent with tension pneumothorax:**
  - Tracheal deviation away from side of injury.
  - Decreased or absent breath sounds on side of injury.
  - Hyperresonance to percussion over affected side.
  - Subcutaneous emphysema.
  - JVD.
  - Shortness of breath, dyspnea.
  - CXR—mediastinal shift away from pneumothorax.
- **May have signs/symptoms of massive PE:**
  - Acute dyspnea.
  - Hemoptysis.
  - Pleuritic chest pain.
  - Cough.
  - Tachypnea.
  - ECG—right strain pattern, right arm deviation, $S_1Q_3T_3$ pattern.
  - Arterial blood gas—decreased partial pressure of oxygen (O_2) in arterial blood (PaO_2) <80 mm Hg.
  - Elevated alveolar-arterial (A-A) gradient.
  - Ventilation-perfusion scan—V/Q mismatch.
  - Pulmonary angiography—gold standard.
  - Low cardiac output, high peripheral resistance, high central venous pressure (CVP).

4. **Management**
   - O_2—given to all patients in shock.
   - Ensure adequate volume using isotonic IV fluids.
   - Inotropic support using dobutamine, amrinone, epinephrine, or intra-aortic balloon pump.
   - Early angioplasty or thrombolytic therapy in MI.
   - Needle decompression of tension pneumothorax (before chest X-ray).
   - Pericardiocentesis for pericardial effusion tamponade.
   - Heparin, thrombolytic therapy, embolectomy in PE.

B. **Hypovolemic**
   1. **Etiology**
      - Loss of circulating volume >20%.
      - Type of loss includes blood, plasma, extracellular, extravascular, or water.
      - Common causes include hemorrhage, dehydration, burns.
   2. **Pathology**
      - Loss of volume—followed by increased heart rate, vasoconstriction, and maintenance of BP (compensatory response).

- BP decreases if losses are not replaced, and causes are identified and treated.
- Low cardiac output.
- High peripheral resistance.
- Low CVP.

3. **Clinical Features**
   - Pale cool skin, slow capillary refill.
   - Apprehensive, restless.
   - Decreased mentation.
   - Hypotension, tachycardia.
   - Orthostatic hypotension.
   - Oliguria, anuria.

4. **Diagnostic Studies**
   - CBC—decreased hematocrit and hemoglobin (H&H) in hemorrhage (late sign); increased H&H in dehydration (hemoconcentration).

5. **Management**
   - Restoration of circulating blood volume with isotonic saline.
   - Transfusion with packed RBCs.
   - Source of hemorrhage must be identified and controlled.
   - Prevention of hypothermia.
   - Aggressive treatment of coagulopathy.

C. **Distributive**
   NEUROGENIC
   1. **Etiology**
      - Disruption, or alteration, of spinal cord function.
      - Spinal anesthesia.
      - Spinal cord injury.
   2. **Pathology**
      - Results from blockade of peripheral autonomic regulation.
      - Increase in overall vascular space without change in blood volume.
   3. **Clinical Features**
      - Hypotension.
      - Paralysis, paresthesia below level of injury.
      - Bradycardia or normal pulse instead of tachycardia because of autonomic dysregulation (no narrowed pulse pressure).
   4. **Management**
      - Isotonic IV fluids.
      - Vasopressors.
      - CVP monitoring.

   SEPTIC AND ANAPHYLACTIC
   1. **Etiology**
      - Overwhelming infection or sepsis.
      - Anaphylactic reaction.
   2. **Pathology**
      - **Decreased peripheral vascular resistance due to:**
        - Release of activated cytokines in sepsis.
        - Release of histamines in anaphylaxis.
      - Early, increased cardiac output is present.
      - Capillary leak.

3. **Clinical Features**
   - **Sepsis—search for septic focus:**
     - Central venous catheters.
     - Pneumonia.
     - Intra-abdominal, pelvic abscesses.
     - Urinary sepsis.
     - Physical examination findings:
     - Hypotension (decreased systolic pressure, and narrow pulse pressure).
     - Warm skin.
     - Rash.
     - Impaired urine output.
   - **Anaphylaxis:**
     - Bite or sting.
     - Previous reaction.
     - Food allergy.
     - Recent injection of IV contrast.
     - Physical examination findings:
     - Hives.
     - Angioedema.
     - Respiratory distress.
     - Stridor.
4. **Management**
   - **Sepsis:**
     - Isotonic IV fluids.
     - Vasopressors.
     - Pan culture before antibiotics.
     - Antibiotics.
     - Drainage of abscesses.
   - **Anaphylaxis:**
     - Airway management.
     - Epinephrine.
     - Antihistamines.
     - IV fluids.

XI. Trauma

A. Overview and General Management

1. **Etiology**
   - Sixty million injuries each year.
   - Thirty million injuries require medical care.
   - 3.6 million injuries require hospitalization.
   - Nine million injuries are disabling.
   - A total of 145,000 deaths each year.
   - Five million deaths per year worldwide.
   - Leading cause of death in 1 to 44 years of age.
   - Third leading cause of death, after cancer and atherosclerosis, in all age groups.

   TRIMODAL DISTRIBUTION OF MORTALITY
   - **First peak:**
     - Death in seconds to minutes.
     - Usually due to apnea from brain or spinal cord injury or cardiac/aortic rupture.
   - **Second peak:**
     - Death in minutes to hours.
     - Usually, these patients have devastating injuries, massive head trauma, or hemorrhage.
   - **Third peak:**
     - Death in days to weeks.
     - These patients succumb to complications of their injuries, brain injury, disseminated intravascular coagulopathy, multiorgan system failure, acute respiratory distress syndrome, and sepsis.
2. **Blunt versus Penetrating**

   BLUNT
   - Motor vehicle collisions (MVCs).
   - Rapid deceleration injuries.
   - Blast injuries.
   - Falls.

   PENETRATING
   - More common in urban settings.
   - Gunshots.
   - Stab wounds.
   - Blast injuries.
3. **Primary Survey**
   - Aims at diagnosis *and* treatment of immediately life-threatening conditions.

   ABCs OF TRAUMA
   - Airway (check patency; ensure passage of air) with cervical spine protection.
   - Breathing (check ventilation; provide assistance).
   - Circulation (check pulses, insert IVs; begin resuscitation and hemorrhage control).
   - Disability (assess eye opening and verbal and motor responses; treat brain swelling) neurologic status.
   - Exposure environmental control (expose patient to examine while preventing hypothermia).

   AIRWAY AND BREATHING
   - Protect or immobilize the cervical spine (C-spine).
   - All traumatized patients should be presumed to have a spinal cord injury until physical examination and X-rays have confirmed otherwise.
   - Assessment of airway patency (exclude obstruction by tongue; foreign body (e.g., teeth); blood; fractures; or swelling).
   - Assessment of ventilatory status (cyanosis, bilateral breath sounds).
   - Administration of O_2.
   - Intubation if necessary.
   - Cricothyrotomy if intubation is not feasible.
   - Pleural decompression.
   - Diagnosis of tension pneumothorax must happen early with prompt treatment to limit decompensation and death.
   - Immediate management: insertion of large-bore needle into pleural cavity (second intercostal space at midclavicular line).
   - Subsequent management: tube thoracotomy (placement of chest tube under water seal)—check with CXR.
   - C-spine radiograph.

- CXR—may disclose pneumothorax/hemothorax, widened mediastinum of aortic rupture or dissection, diaphragmatic herniation of abdominal contents, and free air below the diaphragm, signifying rupture of a hollow viscus.

CIRCULATION

- Assessment of circulatory status.
- Low levels of consciousness may indicate poor cerebral perfusion.
- Hypovolemic patients may have ashen, gray facial coloring and white extremities.
- Check for pulses (carotid/femoral), capillary refill (<2 seconds is normal), and BP.
- Stop exsanguinating hemorrhage.
- Bleeding from major arteries and scalp wounds can lead to exsanguination.
- Pericardiocentesis.
- Signs and symptoms of pericardial tamponade, Beck triad (JVD, hypotension, and muffled heart tones).
- Thoracotomy—mainly for penetrating injury of the heart or great vessels.
- Heart rate.
- Tachycardia, noted in hypovolemic shock.
- Bradycardia, noted in brain edema and spinal injury.
- **BP:**
  - Carotid BP >60 mm Hg.
  - Femoral BP >70 mm Hg.
  - Radial BP >80 mm Hg.

DISABILITY

- Brief neurologic examination noting best response from patient.
- Level of consciousness.
- Alert.
- Verbal.
- Pain.
- Unresponsive.
- Pupil size/reaction.
- Unequal or nonreactive pupils suggestive of increased intracranial pressure (ICP).
- **Glasgow Coma Scale (GCS) is useful for:**
  - Eye opening (1 to 4).
  - Verbal response (1 to 5).
  - Motor response (1 to 6).
  - GCS = (E + V + M); best possible score = 15 and worst possible score = 3.

EXPOSURE

- Patients need to be fully exposed and log-rolled (most missed injuries are secondary to the practitioner's failure to inspect the entire body).
- Full assessment of vital signs is then done, evaluating heart rate, BP, respiratory rate, and temperature.
- Care is taken to keep the patient warm and avoid hypothermia.

4. **History**
   - **A brief history is obtained focusing on the following (AMPLE):**
     - Allergies.
     - Medications.
     - Past medical history/pregnancy.
     - Last meal.
     - Events leading up to the injury.
     - Mechanism of action, including speed of vehicle, caliber of bullet, seat-belt use, deformity of vehicle, height of fall, and level of injury of others involved in trauma.
5. **Secondary Survey**
   - Complete head-to-toe physical examination performed after the primary survey, resuscitative efforts and stabilization of vital signs.

SKIN

- Decrease in skin color and capillary refill are signs of poor perfusion and occur early in hypovolemic shock.

HEAD

- Obvious trauma.
- Lacerations and hemorrhage can lead to rapid exsanguination.
- Fractures of the skull may allow passage of pathogens into the CNS, and damage to the brain itself.
- Battle sign (mastoid process ecchymosis) and raccoon eyes (periorbital ecchymosis) are seen in basilar skull fractures.

EYES

- Pupillary response—compression of the third cranial nerve causes pupillary dilation.
- Funduscopic examination—paying particular attention to papilledema, which often accompanies increased ICP.
- Visual acuity.
- Hemorrhage of conjunctiva or fundi, or discoloration of the lens.
- Ocular entrapment.

EARS

- Blood and CSF in the external auditory canals and hemotympanum are suggestive of basilar skull fracture.

NOSE

- Blood flowing from the nares may represent direct trauma to the tissues of the nose, but if CSF also is present, skull fracture is suspected. Blood from the ears or nose can be placed on a gauze pad, a halo sign or two distinct rings are noted if CSF also is present.
- Fracture.
- Septal hematoma may require drainage.

MOUTH

- Lacerations.
- Dental alignment and missing or loose teeth require rapid evaluation, so emergent treatment

can be undertaken. Teeth are best preserved in the patient's mouth, if no risk of aspiration is present, and reimplanted as soon as possible. Each minute the tooth is out of the mouth, tooth survival decreases 1%.

NECK

- Presence of JVD is suggestive of CHF, tension pneumothorax, or pericardial tamponade.
- Evaluation of the trachea for position and alignment—the trachea shifts away from a tension pneumothorax.
- C-spine point tenderness.
- Examine patient for subcutaneous air.
- Carotid bruits may indicate carotid artery injury.
- Placement of NGT or orogastric tube can be both therapeutic and diagnostic. Traumatized patients may swallow air or have large volumes of food or liquids in their stomachs, causing decreased pulmonary function. Evacuation of gastric contents is important before any surgical procedure to minimize the risk of aspiration.
- Penetrating injuries to the neck that extend through the platysma should not be explored or probed until in the OR.

THORAX

- Equal expansion—unequal expansion in pneumothorax/hemothorax.
- Deformities.
- Wounds.
- Flail segments—paradoxical movement of the flail segment leads to hypoventilation.
- Breath sounds—decreased or absent over pneumothorax and hemothorax.
- Heart sounds—muffled in pericardial tamponade.
- Chest X-ray to confirm the presence of pneumothorax, hemothorax, most rib fractures, or a widened mediastinum (aortic rupture).

ABDOMEN

- Obvious trauma—seat-belt sign, ecchymoses, or abrasion across the lower abdomen should alert the examiner to the possibility of bowel injury.
- Bowel sounds—decreased in abdominal trauma.
- Tenderness.
- Upright abdominal X-ray—evaluation for free air in hollow viscus rupture or CT scan of abdomen and pelvis.
- Frequent reevaluation of the abdomen, as these findings often change over time.

GENITALIA

- Rectal examination is performed to evaluate sphincter tone (distal neurologic function) and prostate position. A high-riding or mobile prostate, along with blood at the urethral meatus, is suggestive of urethral disruption.
- If urethral injury is not suspected, a Foley catheter is placed, urine obtained is evaluated, and urine output is measured. Adequate urine output is approximately 0.5 mL/kg/hour.
- Pelvic examination is performed to evaluate the female genitalia and bony pelvis for fracture.
- Mandatory pregnancy test for all women of childbearing age.

PELVIS

- Examination is aimed at assessment of stability of the pelvis. The pelvis is rocked and palpated, and a pelvic X-ray assessing for fracture is obtained. Massive quantities of blood can be lost into the pelvis after fracture.

EXTREMITIES

- Neurovascular examination.
- Splint obvious fractures to reduce the chance of nerve or vascular injury and blood loss. Femur fractures may cause accumulation of several units of blood in the thigh.

NEUROLOGIC

- Serial neurologic examinations (motor, sensory, papillary response and level of consciousness), assessing for changing neurologic status.

6. **Resuscitation**
   - O_2.
   - Cardiac monitor.
   - Two IVs of lactated Ringer (LR) or normal saline solution by way of large-bore catheters are established. In any hypotensive patient, 1 to 2 L of crystalloid is infused.
   - Blood is given as needed—"O"-negative is the *universal donor*.
   - Military antishock trousers (MAST)—use is controversial; may help to relocate blood from areas beneath the suit to vital organs. MAST are helpful in splinting of pelvic fractures, reducing movement of bone ends, and reducing blood loss and neurovascular injury.
   - Chest tubes—placed to relieve pneumothorax or hemothorax. Blood loss of >200 mL per hour for 2 to 3 consecutive hours is suggestive of the need for thoracotomy.
   - Definitive care for trauma is exploration and repair in the operating room.

B. Specific Disorders

HEAD TRAUMA

1. **Etiology**
   - Blunt trauma is more common than penetrating.
   - Injuries may be sustained from MVCs, falls, gunshot, and knife wounds.
   - GCS is objective clinical measure of severity of brain injury. GCS of 8 or lower is considered severe and requires intubation.

2. **Pathology**
   - Brain injury may result from axonal sheer; cerebral contusion; secondary edema; subdural, epidural, or subarachnoid hematoma.

SUBDURAL HEMATOMA
- More common in elderly individuals.
- Slow, insidious onset.
- Torn cortical vessels or cortical lacerations usually cause acute subdural hematoma.
- Torn bridging veins are associated with chronic subdural hematoma.
- Shape conforms to the contours of the brain.

EPIDURAL HEMATOMA
- Typically associated with a brief period of unconsciousness followed by a lucid interval, then rapid deterioration of mental status.
- Rapid hematoma collection from middle meningeal artery rupture leads to rapid rise in ICP that causes brain herniation.
- Biconvex or lenticular in shape.

3. **Management**
   - Airway maintenance with cervical spine protection, breathing and ventilation, circulation with hemorrhage control, disability (neurological evaluation), exposure and environmental control (ABCDEs).
   - Management of hypertension and/or hypotension.
   - Any patient who has had transient or persistent unconsciousness with evidence of head trauma or skull fracture should undergo CT scan of the head.
   - Patients who sustain minor concussion and can be monitored at home can safely be discharged; all other patients require admission.
   - Elevation of the head above the level of the heart (reverse Trendelenburg position) to reduce ICP.
   - Rapid evacuation of the hematoma to reduce ICP after evaluation of the head.
   - Keep $PaCO_2$ at 35 mm Hg or above. Brief periods of hyperventilation are acceptable, but should be for as limited a period as possible.
   - Hyperosmolar therapy using IV mannitol.
   - Seizure prophylaxis with phenytoin or fosphenytoin.

CHEST TRAUMA—SPONTANEOUS PNEUMOTHORAX
1. **Etiology**
   - Young, tall, thin adults 18 to 25 years of age are affected most commonly.
   - Older patients with asthma or chronic obstructive pulmonary disease also are affected.
2. **Pathology**
   - Rupture of subpleural bleb into pleural space.
   - Lung collapse results from leakage of air into pleural space.
3. **Clinical Features**
   - Chest pain, cough, dyspnea common.
   - Decreased breath sounds over the affected side.
   - Hyperresonance to percussion on the affected side.

4. **Diagnostic Studies**
   - CXR shows increased radiolucency over the affected side.
5. **Management**
   - Chest-tube drainage of affected pleural space.
   - Surgery for persistent pneumothorax: air leak for more than 7 to 10 days; incomplete lung expansion.

CHEST TRAUMA—TENSION PNEUMOTHORAX
1. **Etiology**
   - Usually traumatic from blunt or sharp trauma to the thorax.
2. **Pathology**
   - Air is trapped in the pleural space, causing collapse of the affected lung.
   - In the instance of tension pneumothorax, pressure in the pleural cavity increases and may cause mediastinal contents to be pushed away from the side of the injury, resulting in decreased lung function and impediment of blood return to the heart.
3. **Clinical Features**
   - A life-threatening emergency, requiring immediate care.
   - Decreased or absent breath sounds over the affected side.
   - Hyperresonance to percussion over the affected side.
   - Increased radiolucency on the affected side.
   - JVD.
   - Tracheal shift away from the side of the injury.
   - Diagnosis of tension pneumothorax should be made clinically, not by radiography.
4. **Management**
   - Immediate decompression.
   - ABCs of trauma resuscitation.
   - Pleural decompression by way of needle thoracotomy—may be lifesaving in the event of tension pneumothorax.
   - Chest tube insertion to evacuate air and blood from the pleural cavity.

CHEST TRAUMA—HEMOTHORAX
1. **Etiology**
   - Blunt or sharp trauma to the thorax.
2. **Pathology**
   - Blood in the pleural space causing collapse of the lung.
   - Chest wall, intercostal vessels, and pulmonary vasculature are sites of hemorrhage.
3. **Clinical Features**
   - Shortness of breath, dyspnea, cough.
   - Decreased breath sounds over the affected side.
   - Dullness to percussion over the dependent areas of the affected pleural cavity.
   - Evidence of fluid within the affected pleural space with decrease in lung volume.
4. **Management**
   - Supportive care.
   - ABCs of trauma resuscitation.

- Insertion of large-bore chest tube for evacuation of blood from the pleural cavity.
- Surgical intervention (thoracotomy) if hemorrhage is large or continuing.

CHEST TRAUMA—ATELECTASIS

1. **Etiology**
   - Postoperative patients—particularly thoracic and abdominal procedures.
   - Most common cause of fever in the first 24 hours after surgery.
2. **Pathology**
   - Usually due to decreased tidal volume and inability to clear secretions.
   - Bed rest and pain are the two most common predisposing factors.
   - Pain causes patients to breathe more shallowly, causing decreased tidal volume; for the same reason, patients do less coughing and are less effective in clearing secretions.
   - Mucus plugs create a one-way ball valve allowing air to escape but not enter the bronchus, causing collapse of the lung tissue.
3. **Clinical Features**
   - Shortness of breath and fever early (first 24 hours) in the postoperative course.
   - Tachypnea.
4. **Diagnostic Studies**
   - CXR shows areas of lung collapse.
   - If large areas of the lung are affected, hypoxia may be present, followed by respiratory failure.
5. **Management**
   - Management is aimed at prevention—early ambulation, use of incentive spirometry, frequent coughing and deep breathing, and aggressive pulmonary toilet.
   - Aggressive tracheal suctioning, postural drainage, and chest physiotherapy.
   - Bronchoscopy may be necessary to clear secretions.

ABDOMINAL TRAUMA

1. **Etiology/Pathology**

   BLUNT TRAUMA
   - Usually results in injury to the spleen and liver.
   - Knowledge of height of a fall, speed of an MVC, seat-belt or helmet use, air-bag deployment, extrication requirements, extent of damage to the vehicle, and condition of other victims are helpful in judging the potential extent of injuries. Patients who fall from a height of >15 ft have a 5% mortality rate.

   PENETRATING TRAUMA
   - Size and length of the knife, caliber and type of gun used aid in understanding potential injuries.
   - Damage from bullet wounds is determined by speed (velocity) and size (mass) of the projectile.
   - The faster and heavier the bullet, the greater the cavitation caused; pressure, not the bullet, creates an injury tract.

2. **Clinical Features**
   - Abdominal pain and tenderness are common findings.
   - Clinical index of suspicion needs to be high because many traumatized patients have associated head trauma, or have been using alcohol (ethyl alcohol), and their examination may be unreliable.
3. **Diagnostic Studies**
   - Abdominal X-rays may show free air in peritoneum or retroperitoneum, fractures, and abdominal fluid collections.
   - U/S is useful in evaluation of the heart, great vessels, kidneys, spleen, and liver. Organ disruption and fluid collections may be noted.
   - CT scanning for stable patients is appropriate and highly sensitive and specific.
   - Diagnostic peritoneal lavage (DPL) is used to determine the presence of blood, food particles, and pancreatic enzymes.
   - U/S, CT scan, and DPL are helpful in patients in whom a high index of suspicion for injury exists but who have a normal or minimally abnormal examination.
4. **Management**
   - Directed by the type and extent of injury.
   - Patients who are in shock unresolved by fluid administration, or who deteriorate, need emergent laparotomy and repair of specific damage.
   - After initial stabilization, transfer to a trauma center should be considered.

BURNS

1. **Etiology**

   FIRST DEGREE: SUPERFICIAL
   - Frequently caused by excessive exposure to sunlight (sunburn).

   SECOND DEGREE: PARTIAL THICKNESS
   - Frequently caused by short flash or scalding liquid exposure.

   THIRD DEGREE: FULL THICKNESS
   - Frequently caused by high electrical current, prolonged exposure to flame, immersion in scalding liquid chemicals.

2. **Pathology**

   FIRST DEGREE
   - Outer layer of the dermis.

   SECOND DEGREE
   - Superficial—upper portion of the dermis.
   - Deep—involving most, but not the entire dermis.

   THIRD DEGREE
   - Complete destruction of the dermis, may involve fat, muscle, bone.

3. **Clinical Features**

   FIRST DEGREE
   - Erythema, mild discomfort.

SECOND DEGREE
- Blister formation, tissue edema, plasma leakage.
- Exquisitely painful.

THIRD DEGREE
- Painless, leathery, charred appearance.

4. **Determining the Extent of Injury**

RULE OF NINES (FIRST DEGREE NOT INCLUDED IN CALCULATION)
- Head and neck—9%.
- Arm (each)—9%.
- Trunk (anterior)—18%.
- Trunk (posterior)—18%.
- Leg (each)—18%.
- Genitalia—1%.

5. **Management**

INITIAL MANAGEMENT OF ALL BURNS
- Remove patient from the source of injury.
- Stop burning.
- ABCs of trauma resuscitation.
- O_2 therapy if possibility of coexisting inhalation injury exists.
- Provide IV therapy for larger second-degree and all third-degree wounds.
- Provide analgesia if patient hemodynamically stable.
- Provide tetanus prophylaxis for all burn patients.
- Systemic antibiotics not indicated in initial management.

FIRST DEGREE
- Pain resolves in 48 to 72 hours.
- Acetaminophen and NSAIDs usually provide adequate analgesia.
- Local wound care and surveillance for infection; ice.

SECOND DEGREE
- Superficial—usually heals in 7 to 14 days:
  - Local wound care; debridement of nonviable skin.
  - Topical antibiotic.
  - Wound coverage with dressings that promote moisture retention.
  - PO analgesia (may require narcotics).
- Deep—wound healing may be slow and unpredictable:
  - Local wound care; debridement of blisters.
  - Topical antibiotics.
  - Skin grafting as necessary.
  - Wound coverage with dressings that promote moisture retention.
  - PO narcotic analgesia.
  - May require IV analgesia with narcotics, especially for dressing changes.

THIRD DEGREE
- Unable to heal by reepithelialization because of the loss of epidermal appendages within the dermal layer.

- Spontaneous healing results in burn scar contracture.
- Early skin grafting is used to replace devitalized tissue, reduce septic complications.
- Escharotomy is performed in patients with decreased peripheral circulation, ventilatory exchange.

THERAPY
- **Parkland formula—using LR solution:**
  - Adults: 4 mL per kg/% total burn surface area (TBSA) burned; half given over first 8 hours, and the other half given over next 16 hours.
  - Children: 3 mL per kg/% TBSA burned; half given over first 8 hours, and the other half given over next 16 hours plus maintenance.

ADMISSION CRITERIA
- Age 10 to 50 years with partial-thickness burns of >15% TBSA, or deep partial-or full-thickness burns of >5%.
- Age <10 years and >50 years with partial-thickness burns >10%, or deep partial- or full-thickness burns >3%.
- Any patient with partial- or full-thickness burns to hands, feet, face, perineum, circumferential, or across major joints.
- Chemical or electrical burns.
- Associated inhalation injury, other trauma.
- Coexisting medical conditions, immunocompromised.

XII. Nutrition Disorders
- Goals are to provide enough energy and nutritional reservoirs to enable the patient to maintain function, repair body, and recover from diseased or postsurgical states.

A. Carbohydrates
- The primary fuel source for the body; metabolized to the form of glucose and stored as glycogen.
- RBCs, CNS, and renal medulla metabolize only glucose.
- Glucose and glycogen stores from the muscle and liver are depleted within 24 to 36 hours of fasting.
- Fat and protein are then used for fuel.

B. Fats
- Fatty acids are the basic unit of fat.
- Linoleic and linolenic acids are the essential fatty acids.
- Fat metabolism yields fatty acids, glycerol, and ketone bodies.
- Ketone bodies are used as fuel during starvation.

C. Protein (Amino Acids)
- Primary function is to maintain cellular structure and function.
- Used as fuel during starvation.

D. Caloric Requirements

- Nonprotein calories (NPC): estimated to provide enough nonprotein energy to maintain function without breaking down protein and restore lost weight.
- 500 kcal per day above estimated needs = 1 lb per week weight gain; 60% of NPC should come from carbohydrates; 40% of NPC should come from fats.

NPC ESTIMATION

1. Harris–Benedict Equation

- Estimates basal energy expenditure (BEE) in kilocalories per day of a healthy, resting adult. Standard: 25 to 35 kcal/kg/day.
- Males: BEE = 66 + [13.7 × (weight in kg)] + [5 × (height in cm)]/[6.7 × (age in years)].
- Females: BEE = 65.5 + [9.6 × (weight in kg)] + [1.8 × (height in cm)]/[4.7 × (age in years)].
- Healthy, ambulating patients: 1.2 × BEE.
- Fever: 1.1 (for each ° C above normal body temperature) × BEE.
- Severely stressed patient: 1.6 × BEE.
- Burn patients: 2.3 × BEE.

2. Indirect Calorimetry

- The body uses O_2 and produces CO_2 in metabolism; therefore, BEE can be calculated based on their measurement. These measurements are taken by "metabolic carts," which either hook into a ventilator or isolate a patient within a tent. Not useful because of its expense, unavailability in general settings, and inaccuracy for nonventilating patients or patients inspiring >50% O_2.

PROTEIN REQUIREMENTS

- **Needs:**
  - Protein is used constantly and metabolized, therefore not typically stored.
  - Minimal requirement: 0.54 g/kg/day.
  - Standard healthy adult: 0.8 g/kg/day.
  - Stressed patients: 1.0 to 1.5 g/kg/day.
- **Losses:**
  - Reflected in urine as nitrogen.
  - Standard healthy adult: 0.05 to 0.08 g/kg/day.
  - Stressed patient: 5-fold increase from normal.

PROTEIN ESTIMATION

1. Laboratory Values

- Plasma proteins (e.g., albumin and transferrin).
- Typically decrease with decreased protein balance.
- Not an exact measurement of protein balance.

2. Nitrogen Balance

- Because nitrogen is 16% protein and primarily excreted through urine, it is reflective of protein balance. Therefore, measurement of nitrogen in urine can be used to calculate protein balance with the following formula: N balance (g) = [(protein intake in g/6.25)]/[(urinary N + 4)]. (**NOTE:** 4 reflects nonurinary nitrogen losses, and it increases to 6 in critically ill patients.)

E. Method of Delivery

1. Oral

- Ideal and preferred route.

2. Enteral Nutrition

BENEFITS

- Relatively inexpensive.
- Maintains mucosal structure and function.
- Protects against infection by maintaining the integrity of the mucosal lining of the small bowel.

MODES

- NGT used for short-term support; risks: aspiration, diarrhea, bronchial intubation.
- Gastrostomy tube: used for chronic nutritional support; allows for bolus feeding because stomach is used; good prophylaxis against gastritis; risks: aspiration and diarrhea.
- Jejunostomy tube: used for chronic support, patient with high aspiration risk, or both; must give continuous feedings; risk: diarrhea.

3. Total Parenteral Nutrition

- Used preoperatively for severely malnourished patients.
- Used for instances when patient's stomach or gut cannot be used (e.g., short-bowel syndrome, hepatic failure, enterocutaneous fistulas, major thermal injury, acute renal failure, and prolonged ileus).
- Requires primarily a central venous access.

RISKS

- Mechanical: due to line placement, pneumothorax, pleural laceration.
- Metabolic: due to nutritional deficits, resultant metabolic disorders, dehydration.
- Sepsis: line placement contaminants.

XIII. Wounds

A. Stages of Wound Healing

1. Physiology

- Surgical or traumatic tissue disruption.
- Trauma stimulates a series of events that lead to spontaneous wound closure.

2. Inflammation

- Initially vasoconstriction to reduce blood loss after injury.
- Hemostasis (clot formation), vasodilatation follow.
- Vasodilatation allows inflow of neutrophils and monocytes.
- Phagocytosis by macrophages occurs at wound.
- Chemotactic factors stimulate migration of fibroblasts to wound.

3. Epithelialization

- Restores denuded epithelial surface.
- Occurs 12 to 24 hours after injury.
- At 48 hours, waterproof covering achieved preventing migration of bacteria into wound.

- Wound dressings can be removed safely after 48 hours (uncomplicated surgical wounds).
4. **Proliferation Phase**
   - Fibroblastic synthesis (2 to 21 days)—fibroblasts responsible for collagen synthesis.
   - Collagen synthesis (2 to 21 days)—primarily regulated by macrophages by way of cellular mediators.
   - Angiogenesis (2 to 7 days)—formation of new vessels, increasing vascular supply to wound.
   - Contraction (2 to 20 days)—gradual reduction in wound size secondary to retraction of granulation tissue.
5. **Maturation Phase**
   - At 21 days, collagen deposition reduced.
   - Wound tensile strength continues to increase.
   - Prewound strength never achieved.
   - Patients advised to protect wound and avoid strenuous activity for at least 6 weeks after injury.

B. **Wound Closure**
   1. **Primary Intention**
      - Wound edges are brought together using suture, tapes, or surgical staples.
      - Used for clean wounds <6 hours old.
      - Wound may be debrided and converted to clean wound if minimally contaminated.
   2. **Secondary Intention**
      - Wound left open to close by contraction and epithelization.
   3. **Delayed Primary Closure (Tertiary Closure)**
      - Wound is closed (skin, subcutaneous tissue) 4 to 5 days after injury.
      - Delaying closure decreases risk in potentially infected wounds.
   4. **Contraindications to Wound Closure**
      - Wound older than 6 hours.
      - Wound older than 24 hours on face.
      - Wound infection present.
      - Heavily contaminated wound.
      - Excessive tension of wound.
      - Retained foreign bodies.
   5. **Classification of Wounds**
      CLEAN WOUNDS
      - Incision made during operative procedure.
      - Skin has been prepared adequately with appropriate disinfectant.
      - No contamination from GI, respiratory, or genitourinary (GU) tracts.
      - Infection rates <2%.

      CLEAN-CONTAMINATED WOUNDS
      - Similar to clean wounds, exception being entrance into GI, GU, or respiratory tracts.
      - GI tract prepped to minimize amounts of bacteria.
      - GU, respiratory tracts assumed to have no active infection.

      - Some examples—routine cholecystectomy, bladder surgery, surgery of colon after preparation.
      - Infection rates of 3% expected.

      CONTAMINATED WOUNDS
      - Major contamination of wound.
      - All traumatic wounds.
      - Examples—intestinal obstruction with enterotomy and spillage of contents, surgery for acute cholecystitis with spillage of pus.
      - Although contamination is high, infection rates are approximately 5%.

      INFECTED WOUNDS
      - Active infection present before wound is made in skin.
      - Some examples—skin laceration with active infection present, appendiceal abscess, perirectal abscess.
      - Infection rates as high as 50% expected.

6. **Wound Infection**
   SIGNS AND SYMPTOMS
   - Erythema (redness, rubor).
   - Calor (heat).
   - Tenderness (dolor).
   - Discharge for >24 hours after injury.
   - Purulent discharge.
   - Lymphangitis (red streaking).
   - Pain at injury site.
   - Fluctuance, induration.

   TREATMENT
   - Open suture lines to allow drainage.
   - Incise, drain closed areas.
   - Oral antibiotics for mild infection.
   - Parenteral antibiotics for moderate-to-severe infections.
   - Agent of choice should be guided by possible contaminates.
   - Example—Augmentin (amoxicillin, clavulanic acid) for human bite wounds and first-generation cephalosporin for skin flora.

7. **Tetanus**
   HISTORY
   - Tetanus immunization status.

   FOLLOWING PATIENTS MUST BE CONSIDERED TO HAVE INCOMPLETE IMMUNIZATION
   - Age >50 years.
   - Foreign-born patients.
   - Unavailable or unreliable history.

8. **Anesthesia for Wound Care**
   - Direct infiltration—placement of anesthesia into wound edges.
   - Field block—placement of anesthetic agent parallel to the wound edge.
   - Regional block—anesthetic agent in injected adjacent nerve proximal to the wound.

9. **Anesthetic Agents**
   - Amides—lidocaine, mepivacaine, bupivacaine.
   - Esters—procaine, tetracaine, benzocaine, and cocaine.

- Epinephrine—used to increase the time of anesthesia and reduce bleeding. Its use should be avoided in areas of terminal circulation, ears, fingers, toes, nose, and tip of the nose.
- Dosage of lidocaine is limited to 5 mg per kg without epinephrine and 7 mg per kg with epinephrine.
- Suture size and removal schedule.

SELECTED REFERENCES

Albanese CT, Sylvester KG. Pediatric surgery. In: Doherty GM, Way LW, eds. *Current Surgical Diagnosis and Treatment*. 12th ed. New York, NY: McGraw-Hill; 2006:1322–1323.

American College of Surgeons Committee on Trauma. *Advanced Trauma Life Support for Doctors (Atls) Student Course Manual*. 8th ed. Chicago, IL: American College of Surgeons; 2008.

Andreoli TE, Benjamin I, Griggs RC, et al, eds. *Andreoli and Carpenter's Cecil Essentials of Medicine*. 8th ed. Philadelphia, PA: Elsevier; 2011.

Boelaert K. Revised guidelines for the management of thyroid cancer. *Nat Rev Endocrinol*. 2010;6(4):185–186.

Cooper CS, Williams RD. Urology. In: Doherty GM, Way LW, eds. *Current Surgical Diagnosis and Treatment*. 12th ed. New York, NY: McGraw-Hill; 2006:1033–1051.

Glasgow SC, Herrmann VM. Surgical metabolism and nutrition. In: Doherty GM, Way LW, eds. *Current Surgical Diagnosis and Treatment*. 12th ed. New York, NY: McGraw-Hill; 2006:140–164.

Hunt TK. Wound healing. In: Doherty GM, Way LW, eds. *Current Surgical Diagnosis and Treatment*. 12th ed. New York, NY: McGraw-Hill; 2006:75–80.

Kasper DL, Braunwald E, Fauci A, et al, eds. *Harrison's Principles of Internal Medicine*. 17th ed. New York, NY: McGraw-Hill Professional; 2008.

Kinder BK, Burrow GN. The thyroid: nodules and neoplasia. In: Felig P, Frohman LA, eds. *Endocrinology and Metabolism*. 4th ed. New York, NY: McGraw-Hill; 2001:349–383.

Schwartz LR, Balakrishnan C. Thermal burns. In: Tintinalli JE, Kelen GD, Stapczynski JS, eds. *Emergency Medicine: A Comprehensive Study Guide*. 6th ed. New York, NY: McGraw-Hill; 2004:1220–1226.

Stewart PM. Treatment of Cushing's syndrome. In: Kronenberg HM, Melmed S, Polonsky KS, et al, eds. *Williams Textbook of Endocrinology*. 11th ed, Philadelphia, PA: Saunders Elsevier; 2008:475–477.

Geriatric Disorders

17

Matt Dane Baker • Florida Olivieri

I. Demography of Aging
- Life expectancy in the United States has increased remarkably in the past century.
- Average life expectancy in 1900 was 47 years; current life expectancy is about 78 years. In 1947, about 4% of the population was ≥65 years old; today it is approximately 13%; and by 2020 it is estimated to be 25%.
- The elderly population is growing rapidly as a proportion of the US population and is becoming more ethnically diverse.
- Fastest growing subgroup of the elderly population is the "oldest old," those older than 85 years.
- Women live 5 to 7 years longer than men.

II. Health Status of Seniors
- Majority of elderly individuals live in the community.
- Proportion of those ≥65 years old living in nursing homes is small, 5%.
- On average, older people visit a physician more often than the general population.
- Seniors are hospitalized three times as often as the younger population, and their hospital stays are longer.
- Heart disease is the leading cause of death, followed by cancer and stroke.
- The rate of injury rises with aging; especially fall-related injury.
- Older people use twice as many prescription medications as the general population.
- Many seniors have multiple chronic conditions: arthritis (49%), hypertension (40%), heart disease (31%), and hearing impairments (>28%).
- Most hospital admissions of older adults are for acute episodes of chronic conditions, such as heart failure.

III. Age-Related Changes
- Age changes the human body.
- Medical problems often present differently in seniors.

A. Physiologic Changes of Aging
- The rate of aging varies among individuals.
- Organs in the same person age at different rates.
  1. **Homeostasis**
     - Deficits associated with aging are more apparent when an elderly person is challenged.
     - Seniors have limited physiologic reserves and, thus, can rapidly develop complications when they sustain injuries, develop common illnesses such as the influenza, and are hospitalized.
  2. **Control of Body Temperature**
     - Increased susceptibility to hypothermia and hyperthermia.
  3. **Blood Pressure Regulation**
     - Higher risk for orthostatic (postural) hypotension (especially in those with hypertension who are being treated).
  4. **Volume Regulation**
     - Higher risk for both volume depletion and volume overload.
     - Decreased reserves of body water.
     - Decreased thirst drive.
     - Renal impairments associated with aging.
  5. **Renal System**
     - The number and size of nephrons and renal mass are decreased by 25% to 30% between ages 30 and 80 years.
     - Fat and fibrosis partly replace renal parenchyma.
     - Glomerular filtration rate (GFR) and creatinine clearance decrease with age (1 mL/minute/year after 40 years).
     - Serum creatinine does not change with age, but elderly people produce less creatinine because of decreased muscle mass. Therefore, serum creatinine is not a reliable measure of creatinine clearance, as it underpredicts renal function.
     - For the purposes of estimating renal function or prescribing drugs, it is best to use the Cockcroft–Gault equation to estimate creatinine clearance (see below) or the Modification of Diet in Renal Disease (MDRD) method to estimate GFR.
  - **Estimate of creatinine clearance:**

$$\frac{\text{Males } (140 - \text{age}) \times (\text{body weight in kg})}{(\text{stable serum creatinine}) \times (72)}$$

$$\frac{\text{Females } (140 - \text{age}) \times (\text{body weight in kg}) \times (0.85)}{(\text{stable serum creatinine}) (72)}$$

  - Estimate is valid in patients in stable renal state; can be misleading in severely ill elderly people.

6. **Respiratory System**
  - Partial pressure of oxygen in arterial blood (PaO_2) decreases with age. Estimate of PaO_2: $(100 - \text{age})/3$.
  - Decreased chest wall compliance.
  - Increased usage of abdominal muscles.
  - Enlarged alveolar ducts due to loss of elastic tissue result in decreased surface area.
  - Decreased forced vital capacity and forced expiratory volume.
  - Decreased maximum consumption of oxygen (VO_{2MAX}) with age reflecting cardiac, respiratory, and peripheral muscle changes; and decreased level of fitness.

B. Host Defenses
1. **Aging Skin**
  - Skin is thinner, more likely to sustain abrasions or pressure ulcers.
  - Skin changes can lead to infections or bacteremia.
2. **Respiratory**
  - Impairments in swallowing and cough reflex increase risk of aspiration and pneumonia.
  - Ciliary action is less effective. Decreased pulmonary functional reserves.
3. **Genitourinary**
  - Less prostatic fluid is present in urine, and prostatic fluid has fewer antibacterial antibodies.
  - Incomplete bladder emptying—permits bacterial overgrowth.
4. **Immune Responses**
  - Up to 25% of clinically septic seniors are afebrile.
  - Decreased response to vaccines.
  - Humoral antibody-mediated response is decreased.
  - Increased autoantibodies, not associated with autoimmune disease, which can cause false-positive tests for syphilis, rheumatoid arthritis, and lupus erythematosus.
  - Erythrocyte sedimentation rate increases with age.
  - Significant increase for women: $(\text{age} + 10)/2$; for men: $\text{age}/2$.

IV. Geriatric Assessment
  - Evaluation of biopsychosocial problems and functional disabilities to improve quality of life and functional status.
  - **Assessment:**
    - Medical status.
    - Medications.
    - Eyes.
    - Ears.
    - Nutrition.
    - Functional status.
    - Osteoporosis.
    - Falls.

  - Incontinence.
  - Dementia, delirium, and depression.
  - Social support.
  - Economic factors.
  - Quality of life.
  - Katz activities of daily living (ADLs)—six basic ADLs: bathing, dressing, toileting, transferring, continence, and feeding.
  - Instrumental activities of daily living (IADLs)—six intermediate activities involving executive function: ability to use telephone, prepare meals, do housework, take medicine, use transportation, and manage own money. These are impaired earlier in the disease process than ADLs in dementia.

V. Geriatric Syndromes
  - **Definition and description:**
    - Syndromes or diseases are associated with elderly adults.
    - These conditions may affect quality of life as well as treatment of other morbidities, and lead to loss of independence.
    - Management—geriatric syndromes are often due to several problems and require a multidisciplinary health-team approach to be treated with success.

A. Hearing Loss
1. **Presbycusis: "Elderly Hearing" Loss; Age-Related Hearing Loss**
  - Common health problem in geriatric medicine.
  - Twenty-eight percent to 40% of those aged 65 years or older have hearing loss. Prevalence increases with each decade.
  - Bilateral high-frequency sensorineural hearing loss and decreased ability to understand speech.
  - Hearing loss is associated with social and emotional problems.
2. **Hearing Loss Types**
  a. **Sensorineural**
    - Due to damage to cochlea or fibers of eighth cranial nerve.
    - **Causes:**
      - Presbycusis: most common in aging (loss begins in the higher frequencies).
      - Noise exposure related loss is also common.
      - Less common: viral infection, trauma, vascular event, neoplasm (acoustic neuroma), autoimmune, Ménière syndrome, and certain drugs (aminoglycosides, chemotherapy, nonsteroidal anti-inflammatory drugs [NSAIDs], etc.).
  b. **Conductive**
    - Sound transmission through external or middle ear space damage.
    - Cerumen impaction is most common external ear cause in aging and is often result of using cotton-tipped swabs to clean ear.

- Other causes are otosclerosis, otitis media, and otitis externa.
  c. **Central auditory dysfunction**
  - Less common (loss of speech understanding in excess of that from hearing loss).
  - Involves the central nervous system (CNS): seen in dementia, Alzheimer, stroke, and neoplasm.
3. **Evaluation**
  - Ask about hearing problems.
  - Examine ear canal and tympanic membrane.
  - Whisper test: stand behind patient, 2 ft from the ear, cover the ear that is not tested, fully exhale, and whisper a question easy to answer or two-syllable words to be repeated.
  - Weber and Rinne tests can help distinguish between conductive and sensorineural hearing loss.
  - Audiometry: helps establish type and degree of loss of hearing.
  - Hearing is evaluated in decibels (dB) across range of frequencies with tests of air and bone conduction.
  - Normal hearing (0 to 24 dB), mild hearing loss (25 to 40 dB), moderate loss (41 to 55 dB), severe loss (56 to 80 dB).
4. **Management**
  - Avoid loud noises.
  - Cerumen removal.
  - Refer to ear, nose, and throat (otolaryngology/ENT) department and/or audiology.
  - Hearing aids: amplification improves communication and reduces hearing handicaps.
  - Assistive listening devices: small, portable pocket amplifiers are helpful in medical situations, especially in hospital setting.
  - Telephone devices.

B. Vision and Aging
1. **Definition and Description**
  - Vision impairment: visual acuity of 20/40 or worse.
  - Legal blindness (severe impairment): visual acuity 20/200 or worse.
  - Aging is associated with increased prevalence of visual impairment.
  - **Leading causes of visual impairment:**
    - Presbyopia—inability to focus on near items. Commonly begins in the mid-40s.
    - Cataract.
    - Age-related macular degeneration (ARDM).
    - Diabetic retinopathy.
    - Glaucoma.
  - Vision impairment can cause loss of independence and decrease quality of life.
2. **Cataracts**
  - Definition: clouding and opacification of lens.
  - Seen on ophthalmoscopic examination.

- Initial symptoms: decreased glare tolerance.
- Eventual loss of color vision.
- Risk factors: age, sun exposure, corticosteroids, diabetes mellitus (DM).
- Management: refer to ophthalmology for surgical evaluation (extraction with intraocular lens implant).
3. **Age-Related Macular Degeneration**
  - Definition: damage and atrophy of cells in central (macular) region of retinal pigmented epithelium.
  - Prevalence: leading cause of blindness in elderly Caucasians.
  - Risk factors: age, sun exposure.
  - Results in loss of central vision.

  CLASSIFICATION
  a. **Dry or atrophic ARMD**
  - Eighty percent of cases.
  - Patients see blurry dark spot in the center of visual field.
  - Degree of loss variable.
  - Only 10% experience severe loss or legal blindness.
  - Dry ARMD may change to wet ARMD.
  b. **Wet or exudative ARMD**
  - Associated with more severe vision loss.
  - Due to subretinal neovascularization.
  - May lead to partial retinal detachment.
  - Suspect subretinal hemorrhage if individual with ARMD has sudden loss of vision, blurred vision, or new scotoma.
  c. **Management**
  - Refer to ophthalmologist.
  - Zinc and antioxidant supplements.
  - Wet type: photocoagulation.
4. **Glaucoma**
  - Definition: increased intraocular pressure (>21 mm Hg), cupping and atrophy of optic nerve head, and peripheral visual field loss.
  - Prevalence: leading cause of blindness in elderly African Americans.
  - Risk factors: age, African American race, and diabetes.

  CLASSIFICATION
  a. **Open-angle glaucoma**
  - Chronic low-level impairment to the drainage of aqueous flow from anterior chamber that leads to increased intraocular pressure and optic nerve damage.
  - More than 80% of cases of glaucoma.
  - Insidious disease.
  b. **Narrow-angle glaucoma (acute angle-closure)**
  - Aqueous humor outflow is obstructed by narrow anterior chamber angle between the iris and the cornea.
  - Ten percent of cases of glaucoma.

- Symptoms can include ocular erythema and pain, headache, nausea, visual distortion-halos, and steamy cornea.
- Ocular pressures can rapidly become very high. This is an emergency situation.
  - **Management:**
    - Open angle—Medical: β-adrenergic blockers, sympathomimetics, and carbonic anhydrase inhibitors (not recommended in renal failure).
    - Narrow angle—Emergency referral to ophthalmology. Surgical: laser trabeculoplasty, peripheral iridotomy, and iridectomy.

5. **Diabetic Retinopathy**
   - Definition: chronic disorder of retinal microvasculature.
   - **Types:**
     - Background retinopathy: microaneurysms, flame, and dot-and-blot hemorrhages.
     - Proliferative retinopathy (PDR): ischemia, neovascularization, retinal detachment, and vitreous hemorrhage.
   - **Management:**
     - Maximize long-term glycemic control.
     - Refer to ophthalmologist for annual checkup.
     - Prompt treatment of neovascularization with laser therapy.
     - Photocoagulation to avascular retinal areas to prevent neovascularization.

6. **Keratoconjunctivitis Sicca**
   - Definition: dry eyes.
   - Produces symptoms of burning, discomfort, or foreign-body sensation.
   - **Etiology:**
     - Tear secretion decreases with age.
     - Medications with anticholinergic side effects can cause dry eyes.
     - Connective tissue disorders, Sjögren syndrome, and lupus erythematosus are associated with dry eyes.
   - **Management:**
     - Discontinue unneeded medications with this adverse effect.
     - Adequate lubrication: artificial tears. Cyclosporine ophthalmic (Restasis) can be used.

C. Falls and Gait Disorder

1. **Definition and Description**
   - Falls: a person unintentionally descends to the ground or lower level; excludes falls associated with a major event such as a stroke or seizure.
   - Gait disorder: limitation in walking.
   - Falls and gait disorders are commonly caused by multiple factors.
   - Falls can be nonspecific presentation for an acute illness in an elderly person.
   - Seventy-five percent of falls occur in the home.
- Falls can lead to:
  - Death.
  - Fractures.
  - Immobility.
  - Subdural hematoma.
  - Nursing home admission.
  - Fear of falling and self-imposed functional limitations.
  - Soft-tissue injury.
  - Accidental hypothermia.

2. **Risk Factors for Falls**
   - **Medications:**
     - Taking more than four medications.
     - Psychotropics: medication class most associated with falls.
     - Class Ia antiarrhythmic medications.
     - Digoxin.
     - Diuretics.
     - Analgesics (especially narcotics).
   - **Risk factors other than medications:**
     - History of previous falls.
     - Balance and gait abnormalities.
     - Dementia.
     - Postural hypotension.
     - Lower-extremity disabilities.
     - Proprioceptive deficiency.
     - Medical diseases.
     - Syncope.
     - Vestibular dysfunction: vertigo.
     - Upper-extremity disabilities or weakness.
     - High anxiety or depression.
     - Arthritis.
     - B_{12} deficiency.
     - Type of task preformed.
     - Acute illness (e.g., sepsis).
     - Environmental issues.

3. **Evaluation**
   - History. All elderly patients should be screened.
   - Medications.
   - Vision and hearing.
   - Neurologic.
   - Cardiovascular.
   - Lower-limb joints.
   - **Gait disorder and functional ability:**
     - Observe patient's ability to get up from chair, turn, gait stability, mobility, and speed.
     - Tinetti gait evaluation and the "Get Up and Go Test" can be used: directly observe and time patient's ability to stand up from chair without using arms, walk 10 ft, turn, and then return to chair. Strong association between performing this task and person's ability to retain functional independence. Most adults can perform in 10 seconds or less.

4. **Management**
   - Decrease risk factors.

- Review medications; if possible, decrease number and dosages.
- Treat underlying diseases.
- Address vision and hearing impairment.
- Proper footwear.
- Initiate physical therapy: balance and gait training, proper usage of assistive devices, request home physical therapy if needed by patient.
- Exercise program: Tai Chi or a balance training exercise.
- Treat osteoporosis: strengthen bone.
- Hip protectors if necessary.
- Reduce environmental risks: Consider home safety evaluation by home care nursing or occupational therapy.
  - Assess and make appropriate changes, such as removing electrical cords from walking areas, adding grab bars, raising toilet seats, improving lighting, reducing use of restraints.
    - **NOTE:** Restraints *do not* prevent serious injuries from falls.
- The American Geriatrics Association has produced updated guidelines (http://americangeriatrics.org/health_care_professionals/clinical_practice/clinical_guidelines_recommendations/2010/).

D. Osteoporosis

1. Definition and Description

- Loss of bone mass and deterioration of microarchitecture of bone tissue, which lead to increased fragility and increased risk of fractures.
- Most common systemic skeletal disease. Up to two-thirds of patients may go undiagnosed.
- Huge public health problem, associated with approximately 1.5 million fractures annually, loss of independence, psychological distress, and increased morbidity and mortality.
- Bone is live tissue: we are always making bone (osteoblasts) and destroying bone (osteoclasts).
- Bone is strongest and least likely to fracture at age 30 (peak bone density).
- Rate of bone formation changes with age.
- **Two types of bone—trabecular and cortical:**
  - *Spine*—mostly trabecular bone.
  - *Wrist* (distal radius)—mostly trabecular bone.
  - *Hip (femur)*—trabecular and cortical bone.
  - **NOTE:** *Trabecular bone* is very sensitive to *estrogen loss.*

2. Two Types of Primary Osteoporosis (Clinically Overlap)

- Type I: postmenopausal (approximately age 50) rapid loss of trabecular bone 3% to 5% per year during first 10 to 15 years following menopause. First site of bone loss is spine and wrist—distal radius.
- Type II: aging-associated osteoporosis (less rapid bone loss)—0.5% to 3% per year in women and men approximately 65 years and older.
- Associated with fractures of the hip (trabecular and cortical bone).
- Mixed type I and II is common.

3. Clinical Presentation

- Osteoporosis is asymptomatic and does not cause pain until fractures occur.
  - **a. Spinal fractures**
    - Microfractures of spine—common, cause no pain or minimal pain.
    - Larger fractures can lead to collapse of vertebral bodies (compression fractures) and more pain.
    - Patients are rarely hospitalized for vertebral fractures.
    - Lead to loss of height of two or more inches.
    - Fractures heal irregularly—lead to dorsal kyphosis and scoliosis, and can cause discomfort or pain.
    - Cause gait abnormality, exhaustion, increased risk of falls; can decrease forced expiratory volume in 1 second (FEV1) and increase risk of lung disease.
  - **b. Wrist fractures**
    - Fracture after a fall.
    - Wrist usually has a deformity confirmed by X-ray.
    - Orthopedic referral.
  - **c. Hip fractures**
    - Usually associated with a fall, but some fractures occur with weight bearing only.
    - Associated with pain, usually in groin with radiation to buttock.
    - External rotation and shortening of involved lower extremity (LE) are common.
    - If clinically suspicious and negative X-ray, then magnetic resonance imaging (MRI) or computed tomography (CT) is indicated.
    - There is a 14% to 36% mortality rate 1 year after hip fracture.

4. Risk Factors

- Heredity: female gender, Caucasian/Asian, thin (low BMI), family history, postmenopausal, and early menopause (before age 45).
- Behavioral/environmental: heavy alcohol drinkers, smoking, excessive caffeine, excessive carbonated drinks (sodas), low calcium and vitamin D intake, malnutrition including anorexia, immobilization, and exercise-induced amenorrhea.
- Medications: anticonvulsants (phenytoin, phenobarbital), corticosteroids, thyroid hormone, isoniazid (INH), aluminum containing antacids, loop diuretics, vitamin A and D excess, and methotrexate.

- Medical conditions (secondary osteoporosis): diabetes, renal disease, hyperthyroidism, hyperparathyroidism, Cushing, liver failure, gastrointestinal (GI) malabsorption, multiple myeloma, and hypogonadism.

5. **Diagnosis**
   - Early recognition and prevention are important.
   - Conventional X-rays are insensitive—do not detect osteoporosis until 30% to 50% bone mass has been lost.
   - Bone mineral density (BMD) is the best predictor of future fracture risk.
   - BMD can diagnose asymptomatic osteoporosis in women with risk factors.
   - **Dual energy X-ray (DEXA) absorptiometry:**
     - Diagnostic measure of choice.
     - Very low dose of radiation is used to measure spine, hip, and forearm.
     - DEXA results are reported in T- and Z-score.
     - Usually lumbar spine and total hip are measured.
     - T-score defines osteoporosis and its severity.
     - Density is compared with peak bone density (young healthy adult, 30 years old), same gender, and race.
   - **For each standard deviation below the peak mean, there is an approximate 2-fold increase in fracture risk:**
     - Normal bone density—T-score −1 or more is better.
     - Mild osteopenia—T-score −1 to −2.5 is below normal.
     - Osteoporosis—T-score −2.5 or more is below normal (2.5 standard deviations below peak).
   - Z-score—comparison of any given patient's bone density with mean age-matched bone density (comparison with same age peers).
   - Z-score does not define osteoporosis, but if patient deviates from his or her same-age peers, may need further evaluation for secondary osteoporosis.
   - Quantitative CAT scan can also be used.
   - **Bone turnover markers:**
     - Examples: urine N-telopeptide, Pyridinium crosslinks, and serum osteocalcin.
     - Used to monitor response to therapy; should decrease at least 35% within 3 months.
   - Tests to exclude secondary cause of osteoporosis: electrolytes, BUN, creatinine, calcium, thyroid-stimulating hormone (TSH), liver function tests (LFTs), complete blood count (CBC), calcium, vitamin D, and alkaline phosphatase (ALP). If appropriate, serum and urine protein electrophoresis, parathyroid hormone (PTH).

6. **Management**
   - When possible, decrease risk factors (alcohol, tobacco).

- Diet: 1,500 mg of elemental calcium for women after menopause and men aged 65 years and older (includes food sources and calcium supplements if needed).
- Calcium food sources: milk (1 cup = 300 mg calcium), yogurt, cheese, canned fish, broccoli, soy, kale, tofu, turnip, greens, some beans, orange juice with calcium supplementation.
- **Calcium supplements:**
  - Dosage depends on dietary intake.
  - Recommended: 1,000 mg daily premenopausal and 1,200 to 1,500 mg daily postmenopausal of elemental calcium in divided doses of 500 to 600 mg per dose; with vitamin D—400 to 800 IU daily.
  - Do not give to patients with hypercalcemia or hyperparathyroidism.
- Vitamin D—Most multivitamins contain 400 IU of vitamin D.
- Exercise: weight-bearing and resistance exercises such as walking, dancing, running, jumping, and tennis.
- Sunlight 15 minutes, two times per week.

7. **Therapies**
   - **Hormone replacement therapy (HRT):**
     - Estrogen replacement decreases fracture risk—associated with adverse effects such as increased risk of deep venous thrombosis (DVT), stroke, endometrial cancer, breast cancer, etc.
     - Postmenopausal women taking estrogen and progesterone for 5 years have increased risk of DVT, stroke, invasive breast cancer, myocardial infarction, and pulmonary emboli (WHI—Women's Health Initiative).
     - Because of these risks, HRT is not generally recommended for this indication.
   - **Bisphosphonates:**
     - Examples: alendronate, risedronate, etidronate, ibandronate, pamidronate, and zoledronic acid.
     - Alendronate decreases fracture risk by 50% in women with preexisting fractures. Relatively contraindicated in gastroesophageal reflux disease (GERD). Adverse effects: nausea, heartburn, esophagitis, dysphagia, ulcers, constipation/diarrhea, atypical femur fractures, Bisphosphonate-Related Osteonecrosis of the Jaw (BRONJ), and question of increased risk of esophageal cancer. Many of the serious adverse effects are seen with the IV preparations (BRONJ) and with long-term use of 3 to 5 years or greater (BRONJ, atypical femur fractures, cancer of the esophagus).
   - **Salmon calcitonin:**
     - Available intranasally, intravenously, or subcutaneously. May have analgesic effect in osteoporosis. Intranasal—alternate nostrils daily. Adverse effects: rhinitis and epistaxis. Injectable—adverse effects: allergic reactions—skin test.

- **Selective estrogen receptor modulators (SERMS):**
  - Example: raloxifene. Does not stop hot flashes. Does not increase risk of breast cancer. Increases risk of DVT.
  - Effect on mortality or other risks is not yet known.
- **Teriparatide (Forteo):**
- Recombinant human PTH. Indicated for moderate to severe disease (second-line agent).
- Adverse reactions: nausea, HA, dizziness, leg cramps, hypercalcemia, and hypotension (seated first doses).
- Risk osteosarcoma-rats. Black box warning. Avoid in Paget, with increased ALP, children and prior X-radiation therapy (XRT).
- **Denosumab (Prolia):**
  - Monoclonal antibody.
  - Adverse reactions: back/MS pain, urinary tract infection (UTI), and increased cholesterol.
- **External hip protectors.**

E. Urinary Incontinence
1. Definition and Description
- Involuntary loss of urine.
- Prevalence increases with age 65 and above: 15% to 30% in community; 30% in hospital; 50% in nursing home.
- Can cause morbidity—cellulitis, sleep deprivation, falls, and UTI.
- Associated with psychological distress and embarrassment, which can lead to social isolation.
- Symptoms can range from occasional dribbling to continuous loss of urine.
- Aging predisposes to incontinence, but does not cause incontinence.
- **Age-related changes (present in both continent and incontinent elderly):**
  - Bladder capacity decreases.
  - Bladder (detrusor) contractility decreases.
  - Bladder residual volume increases.
  - Prostate increases.
  - Estrogen decreases.
  - Urine output at night increases.
  - Involuntary contractions (detrusor overactivity) are common.
  - Urethral length in women decreases.
- **Risks:**
  - Female gender.
  - Aging.
  - Hospitalization.
  - Nursing home.
  - Other diseases.
  - Impaired cognition, ADLs.
  - Chronic constipation.
  - Cigarette smoking.

- **Acute incontinence etiologies (pneumonic DI-APPERS, usually reversible and multifactorial):**
  - **D**elirium.
  - **I**nfection.
  - **A**trophic vaginitis (urethritis).
  - **P**sychiatric.
  - **P**harmacologic. Examples: diuretics and narcotics.
  - **E**xcess output or endocrine—DM, diabetes insipidus, congestive heart failure (CHF), LE edema, and hypercalcemia.
  - **R**estricted mobility.
  - **S**tool impaction.
2. Types of Incontinence (Alone or in Combination) and Symptoms
  a. **Stress incontinence (outlet incontinence, sphincter incompetence)**
  - Female gender, small amount of urine loss with sneeze, laugh, and cough; sphincter/pelvic relaxation (estrogen loss, parity).
  b. **Urge incontinence (detrusor instability, "overactive bladder," reflex or spastic incontinence)**
  - Urgency, frequency, moderate amount of urine loss, and abnormal stimulation.
  - Caused by inflammation, brain inhibitory dysfunction, and diuresis.
  - Most common type of incontinence.
  c. **Overflow incontinence**
  - Decreased detrusor contractility (atonic or hypotonic bladder) or bladder outlet/urethral obstruction.
  - Reduced stream, difficult void: benign prostatic hyperplasia (BPH), neuropathy, fecal impaction, neoplasm, and anesthesia.
  - A postvoid residual volume of more than 400 mL indicates overflow incontinence is likely.
  d. **Functional incontinence (inability or unwillingness)**
  - "Normal" genitourinary.
  - Mobility problems.
  - Delirium and dementia.
  - Medications or environmental factors.
3. Evaluation
- History—medical history, voiding record.
- Medications, including over the counter and alcohol.
- Environmental evaluation.
- **Physical:**
  - Mental status/mobility—ADLs.
  - Neurologic.
  - Abdominal/gynecologic/genitourinary/rectal.
  - Stress testing (standing with full bladder, single strain)—ask patient to cough.
  - Postvoid residual—bedside. Can be done by straight catheter or ultrasound methods.

- Laboratory—BUN, creatinine, electrolytes, glucose, calcium, urinalysis, B12, consider Prostate Specific Antigen (PSA).

4. **Management**
   a. **General management**
      - Treat transient causes first.
      - Avoid coffee, alcohol, and cigarettes.
      - Correct constipation.
      - **Kegel exercises—pelvic muscle exercises:**
         - Pelvic floor muscles are squeezed for 10 seconds, squeeze is released, and exercise is repeated 10 to 20 times.
         - Exercise is performed three times a day.
         - Effective treatment if done consistently.
         - Good for all menopausal and postmenopausal women.
         - Also may help men with urinary leakage after prostate surgery.
         - Decrease evening intake of fluids.
   b. **Management by type of incontinence**
      - **Stress incontinence:**
         - Kegel exercises—pelvic muscle exercises.
         - Drugs (be aware of side effects)— -adrenergics (pseudoephedrine) and estrogen.
         - Duloxetine (Cymbalta).
         - Imipramine (be aware of side effects—use low dose).
         - Pessaries—women with vaginal or uterine prolapse.
         - Surgery to reestablish angle.
      - **Urge incontinence:**
         - Behavioral—bladder training and scheduled toileting.
         - Biofeedback.
         - Treat UTI.
         - Drugs (anticholinergics)—be aware of side effects (e.g., confusion, constipation, and dry mouth).
         - Oxybutynin (Ditropan).
         - Tolterodine (Detrol).
         - Solifenacin succinate (Vesicare).
         - Darifenacin (Enablex).
         - Trospium (Sanctura).
         - Fesoterodine fumarate (Toviaz).
         - Tricyclic antidepressants—imipramine (low dose).
      - **Overflow/atonic obstruction incontinence:**
         - Discontinue offending agent.
         - Drugs for atonic bladder (be aware of side effects): α-antagonists and cholinergics—bethanechol (Urecholine).
         - Drugs for BPH: α-blockers and 5α-reductase inhibitors.
         - Catheter—as briefly as possible—can cause significant morbidity.
      - **Functional incontinence:**
         - Treat psychological/alcohol/medical/mobility problems.

- Pain relief if needed.
- Physical/occupational therapy—assistive device, commode, and lighting.

THE THREE Ds OF GERIATRIC PSYCHIATRY: DEMENTIA, DELIRIUM, AND DEPRESSION

F. Dementia and Memory Loss
1. **Definition and Description**
   - Significant decline in two or more areas of cognitive functioning.
   - **Alzheimer disease (AD) is the most common dementia:**
      - Constitutes 60% to 70% of dementias (including mixed).
      - Affects possibly 5.3 million US residents. By year 2040, number may rise as high as 14 million.
      - Disease prevalence increases after age 60.
      - Prevalence of 5% to 10% in people 65 years and older and nearly 50% in those 85 years and older.
      - Has a gradual onset and is slowly progressive.
      - Causes deterioration of memory, speech, judgment, and executive function.
      - Patient usually dies within 5 to 10 years: recent studies indicate survival of some up to 20 years.
   - **Vascular dementia is the second most common dementia:**
      - Due to multiple occlusions of small cerebral arteries causing small lacunar infractions.
      - Progresses in stepwise increments.
      - Often causes abnormal gait and other focal neurologic abnormalities.
   - **Cortical Lewy body disease is the third most common cause:**
      - Brain histology—Lewy bodies as seen in Parkinson disease.
      - Quicker onset.
      - Rigidity simultaneous with dementia.
      - Visual hallucinations and paranoid delusions.
      - Changes in alertness and cognition.
      - Wandering.
      - Treatment: avoid neuroleptics/antipsychotics.
   - **Other less common causes of irreversible dementia:**
      - Parkinson disease, Pick disease, Huntington chorea, and Creutzfeldt–Jakob disease.
   - **Mild cognitive impairment (MCI):**
      - Memory impairment that is mild, and patient is able to function well.
      - Most will develop full dementia. Some believe that this as an early stage of dementia.
      - Recognize and monitor for cognitive decline.
2. **Risk Factors for AD**
   - Increasing age, family history, past head trauma, past cerebrovascular accident (CVA), obesity, diabetes, APOE4 allele and several other recognized genetic mutations, and Down syndrome.

- Possible risk factors—female gender, head injury, lower education.
- APOE4 is associated with increased risk of late-onset AD, but also is present in many people without the disease.

3. **Evaluation of Dementia**
   - History.
   - Physical and neurologic examination.
   - Assessment of functional status.
   - Assessment of mental status and cognition.

   Examples:

   a. **Mini-mental status examination (MMSE)**
      - Thirty questions assess orientation, registration, attention, calculation, recall, and language.
      - Scores <24 of a possible 30 are highly correlated with cognitive loss.
      - MMSE results are influenced by prior educational level. If highly educated, patient will score higher than if lower level of education.

   b. **Animal naming test**
      - Name as many animals as you can in 1 minute.
      - Scoring equals number named in 1 minute.
      - Average performance is 18 in 1 minute.
      - Less than 12 is abnormal.

   c. **Clock drawing test**
      - Draw a 3-in circle and put numbers on clock.
      - Score by quadrants.
      - Ability to complete fourth quadrant is most sensitive for predicting dementia.

   d. **Seven-minute neurocognitive screen for AD**
      - Identifies patients with AD with MMSE of 24 or more as early AD.
      - Age and education are not significant factors. Screen for depression—common treatable morbidity in patients with dementia.
      - Laboratory testing to rule out reversible causes of dementia: CBC, B_{12}, TSH, serum calcium, ESR, RPR, electrolytes, and liver- and renal-function tests.
      - Neuroimaging: noncontrast CT or MRI scan.
      - Neuropsychological testing—referral can be helpful if diagnosis is not clear; for example, early dementia or to distinguish from depression.
      - Newer biomarkers for β-amyloid accumulation and neuronal degeneration involving PET scanning and lumber puncture, and genetic testing are available and used for investigation and predictive purposes, but are not yet widely recommended.

   e. **Signs and Symptoms of AD**
      - Cognitive dysfunction (memory impairment, apraxia, and agnosia), aphasia, functional impairment (incontinence and inability to perform ADLs), behavioral manifestations (hallucinations, delusions, and agitation).

4. **Management**
   - Goal—improve functional level, behavior, and mood.
   - Treat medical conditions to maximize functioning. Example: control hypertension and hypercholesterolemia.
   - **Cholinesterase inhibitors for mild-to-moderate AD—small average degree of benefit:**
      - Donepezil, galantamine, and rivastigmine.
      - Side effects increase with higher dosing.
      - Possible adverse effects: nausea/vomiting, diarrhea, dyspepsia, and anorexia.
   - **Memantine—for moderate to advanced AD:**
      - *N*-methyl-D-aspartate (NMDA) receptor antagonist.
      - Monotherapy or in combination with donepezil.
      - Possible adverse effects: dizziness, confusion, headache, and constipation.
      - Not recommended in patients with severe renal impairment.
   - Follow patients' cognitive and functional status by caregiver reports and by test scores—MMSE.
   - **Nonpharmacologic management:**
      - Moderate stimulation (overstimulation may cause confusion and agitation; understimulation may cause withdrawal).
      - Familiar surroundings—avoid changing residences.
      - Daily routines.
      - Scheduled toileting and prompted voiding to reduce urinary incontinence.
      - Soothing music.
      - Family members providing reassurance to patients.
      - Regular health maintenance visits.

5. **Behavior Problems**
   - Agitation—aggressive behavior, combativeness, and hyperactivity.
   - Almost half of patients will experience periods of agitation.
   - Less common is psychosis—paranoia, delusions, and hallucinations.
   - First try nonpharmacologic—environmental manipulation.
   - Always rule out delirium.
   - Antipsychotic, benzodiazapams, and antiseizure medications have been used. Need to use in very small doses, titrate up slowly, and watch for adverse reactions (extrapyramidal side effects, sedation, and CVA). Atypical antipsychotic agents (olanzapine and risperidone) may be better tolerated, but now carry an FDA black box warning that they are not approved for use in dementias and are to be used with caution because of possible increase in mortality from cardiovascular events and infection.
   - Antidepressants are used to treat patients with AD who have depressive symptoms.

6. **Caregiver Issues**
   - Work closely, communicate, and educate family caregivers.
   - Improve patient support services to avoid caregiver burnout. Refer to social worker if available.
   - Recognize caregiver stress—30% to 50% of caregivers for patients with dementia meet criteria for major depression as defined in *Diagnostic and Statistical Manual of Mental Disorders*, 4th edition (*DSM-IV*). (Most are daughters and spouses.)
   - Refer to AD support group.

G. Delirium

1. **Definition and Description**
   - Acute change in mental status characterized by inattention, fluctuating course in the day, altered level of consciousness, and disorganized thinking, confusion.
   - Fifteen percent to 41% of hospitalized elderly individuals have delirium.
   - Hospitalized patients with delirium have higher mortality rates than those without delirium.
   - Delirium is often not recognized in elderly patients.
   - Postoperative delirium is common among elderly patients (up to 50%).
   - Intraoperative meperidine increases risk of delirium compared with other opioids.
   - Delirium in an elderly person can be a nonspecific presentation of an acute problem or illness (e.g., UTI and acute myocardial infarction).
   - Increases hospital length of stay by 60%.
   - Increases rate of nursing home placement.

2. **Reversible Causes of Delirium**
   - Fever/infections.
   - Fluids/electrolyte imbalance.
   - Neurologic events: subdural hematoma and CVA.
   - Endocrine: diabetic ketoacidosis (DKA), hyperthyroidism, hypothyroidism, and Cushing.
   - Drugs: especially drugs with anticholinergic effects.
   - Organ dysfunction, for example, myocardial infarction, liver failure with hepatic encephalopathy, and uremia.
   - Nutrition: B_{12} and folate deficiency.
   - Trauma—fractures.
   - Sleep deprivation and environmental change.
   - Fecal impaction.
   - Urinary retention.
   - Hypoxia.
   - Perioperative hypotension.
   - Sensory deprivation and environmental change.
   - Alcohol—acute toxicity and withdrawal.

3. **Irreversible Risk Factors for Developing Delirium**
   - Dementia.
   - Advanced age.
   - Brain disease. Examples: stroke and Parkinson disease.

4. **Evaluation**
   - Recognition of syndrome is important.
   - **Obtain history:**
     - Ask family members or caregivers if there is an acute change in patient's mental status and behavior.
     - Obtain baseline cognitive and functional levels.
     - Check for alcohol and benzodiazepine use.
     - Ask family members to bring all pill bottles patient is taking.
     - Assess if pain management is sufficient, especially in postoperative elderly patient with dementia.
   - Physical examination—include neurologic evaluation and rectal examination (rule out fecal impaction).
   - Routine laboratory studies (CBC, chemistry panel), electrocardiogram, pulse oximetry, chest X-ray, and, if indicated, B_{12}/folate, TSH, CT (if suspect trauma or focal neurologic deficits), electroencephalogram, drug levels, and blood cultures.

5. **Management**
   - Treat underlying medical problem(s).
   - Keep patient in quiet, well-lit room.
   - Family members at bedside to provide reassurance.
   - Orientation—clock and calendar.
   - Use of personal eyeglasses and hearing aids.
   - **Pharmacologic:**
     - For agitation and psychosis, low-dose Haldol PO or IM.
     - Start with 0.5 mg PO for most elderly patients.
     - Sedation is rapid, but full antipsychotic effect takes longer.
     - May cause hypotension and extrapyramidal effects.
     - If delirium because of alcohol or benzodiazepine withdrawal, use of benzodiazepines, such as lorazepam, may be indicated (in addition to thiamine and folic acid if alcohol problem).
     - Benzodiazepines may themselves cause delirium, and therefore it is desirable to taper them off slowly.

H. Depression

1. **Definition and Description**
   - **Major depressive disorder**—*DSM-IV* criteria—depressed mood and loss of interest and pleasure and five or more associated symptoms almost every day for 2 weeks.
     - Loss of interest or pleasure.
     - Weight loss or gain (appetite).
     - Fatigue.
     - Guilt.
     - Psychomotor agitation or retardation.
     - Insomnia or hypersomnia.
     - Suicidal ideation.
     - Impaired ability to think or make decisions.

- Pneumonic SIGECAPS: **S**leep disturbance; **I**nterest—decreased (anhedonia); **G**uilt; **E**nergy—fatigue; **C**oncentration—reduced; **A**ppetite—anorexia; **P**sychomotor—retardation or agitation; **S**uicide.
- **Minor depressive disorder**—provisional category of *DSM-IV-TR* ("subsyndromal depression"—depressive symptoms, but not sufficient criteria for "major depressive disorder").
- Particularly common in persons older than 75 years.
- Clinical presentation may include medical complaints, preoccupation with poor health or functional disabilities, fatigue, poor concentration, and loss of interest or pleasure.
- Older people are less likely to report disability.
- **Dysthymic disorder**—chronic mild depressive disorder—present on more days than not for 2 years.
  - Less depressed mood and two associated symptoms: impaired ability to think or make decisions, fatigue, low self-esteem, appetite disturbance, insomnia or hypersomnia, or hopelessness.
- Lifetime risk for major depressive disorder is 10% to 25% for women and 5% to 12% for men.
- **Community-living older adults—15% have depressive symptoms:**
  - Major depressive disorder—2% to 4%.
  - Minor depressive disorder—10%.
  - Dysthymic disorder—remainder.
- Minor depressive disorder accounts for greatest percentage of depression in older persons.
- **Elderly depressed adults compared with younger depressed adults are more likely to:**
  - Not report depressed mood.
  - Not report feelings of guilt.
  - Express somatic complaints.
  - Suffer from comorbid conditions or cognitive disorder, which can interfere with the diagnosis and recognition of depression by health care providers.
- Caucasian males 60 years and older are the group with highest rate of successful suicide in the United States.
- One-third of older persons report loneliness as the main reason for considering suicide.
- **Medical conditions associated with increased incidence of depression:**
  - Cerebrovascular disease—left frontal lobe is the location of strokes most often associated with depression.
  - AD.
  - Parkinson disease.
  - Endocrine.
  - B_{12}/folate deficiency.
  - Autoimmune disorders.
  - Viral—HIV and hepatitis.
  - Chronic pain.
- **Drugs associated with increased incidence of depression:**
  - β-Blockers, CNS drugs, benzodiazepines, major tranquilizers, steroids, NSAIDs, cimetidine, and centrally acting α_2-agonists (clonidine, methyldopa).
  - Alcohol.
- Some elderly patients develop depression that mimics dementia ("pseudodementia") and improves completely or partially when depression is treated.
- In 3 years, 43% of patients with pseudodementia are truly demented.
2. **Diagnosis**
- History—include reports from family or caregivers.
- Ask patient if he or she often feels sad or depressed.
- Check if considered harming himself or herself.
- Assess support systems available to patient.
- **Physical:**
  - Include evaluation of cognition—MMSE.
    - Neuropsychological testing can help distinguish depression from dementia, especially early AD.
    - Patients can have both depression and dementia at the same time.
  - Functional assessment—ADL and IADL.
  - Depression—Geriatric Depression Scale (GDS)—15 questions, a score of 5 or more suggests depression.
- Review medications, including over-the-counter medication, medication borrowed from friends, and alcohol.
- Laboratory studies.
3. **Management**
- Treat comorbid conditions.
- Review and adjust drugs as necessary.
- If appropriate, bright light treatment.
- Exercise—example, aerobic exercise.
- Request physical therapy if appropriate.
- Social worker support services, evaluate need for home assistance, community centers.
- Psychotherapy.
- Pharmacotherapy (see Table 5-1, Chapter 5).
- Selective serotonin-reuptake inhibitors (SSRIs), mixed serotonin/norepinephrine inhibitors, and tricyclic antidepressants are equally effective for treating major depression, although SSRIs may have fewer side affects, may be safer in overdose, and may be easier to titrate. These are generally recommended as first-line therapy.
- Saint John's wort is more efficacious than placebo.

- Efficiency compared with tricyclic antidepressants needs to be established.
- This treatment is not approved by the U.S. Food and Drug Administration. Dosages may vary.
- Saint John's wort affects plasma concentration of drugs metabolized by cytochrome P450 system.
- Selection of antidepressant is based on side effects and tolerance.
- Adequate trial of an antidepressant in geriatric patient is 12 weeks of treatment.
- Titrate dose every 2 to 3 weeks.
- Tricyclic antidepressant therapy must be titrated more than SSRIs.
- If, however, patient shows no response or poor response at 6 weeks, antidepressant should be changed.
- Tricyclic antidepressant side effects (anticholinergic)—dry mouth, constipation, blurred vision, dizziness, tremors, urinary retention.
  - Rarer adverse effects: orthostatic hypotension, cardiac arrhythmias, neuroleptic syndrome, decreased seizure threshold.
- SSRI side effects—GI upset, nausea, vomiting, diarrhea, headache insomnia.
- Approximately 35% of patients who discontinue antidepressant therapy will relapse within 6 months.
- Antidepressant therapy should be continued at same dose for at least 4 months after patient improves to avoid relapse.
- Electroconvulsive therapy (ECT) indications: severe depression requiring rapid improvement, severe depression that does not respond to antidepressants, inability to tolerate antidepressants, previous positive response to ECT, psychotic depression, depression in patients with Parkinson disease.
- Possible adverse effects: memory loss and confusion, arrhythmias, falls, aspiration, bronchospasm.
- Contraindications: increased intracranial pressure or tumor, recent myocardial infarction or CVA.

I. Pressure Ulcers

1. Definition
- Lesions caused by contact of skin with furniture.
- Also called decubitus ulcers or bed sores (old terms).
- Decreased local blood flow to area of contact causing ischemia and eventual necrosis.
- Occurs in areas of bony prominences.

2. Etiology
- **Factors that impair normal tissue perfusion, repair, and regeneration:**
  - Pressure.
  - Friction.
  - Shear.
  - Moisture.
  - Time in same position.
  - Anaerobic waste products.

3. Epidemiology
- Hospitalized patients: 8% to 25% over 3 weeks in bed- or chair-bound patients. Up to 50% in hip fracture and ICU.
- Nursing facility residents: 1 year incidence of 13.2%, 2 year incidence of 21.6%. Mortality rate is two to six times greater than for a nursing home resident without a pressure ulcer.
- Seventy percent of lesions develop in patients older than 70 years.

4. Risk Factors
- Age.
- Immobility.
- Paralysis.
- CVA.
- Orthopedic problems.
- Malnutrition: protein and calorie.
- Dehydration.
- Iron and vitamin deficiency.
- Moisture: urinary incontinence, fecal incontinence, and perspiration.
- Sensory impairment: neuropathy and dementia.
- Depression.
- Thin body habitus.

5. Complications
- Cellulitis—*Pseudomonas aeruginosa*, *Providencia*, *Staphylococcus aureus*, *Bacteroides*.
- Osteomyelitis.
- Septicemia.
- Abscess.
- Sinus tracts and fistulas.
- Tetanus.
- Infestations.

6. Evaluation
- History and physical examination.
- Dietary history.
- **Ulcer:**
  - Location.
  - Size, diameter.
  - Exudate—serous, sanguineous, and purulent.
  - Tissue—epithelial, granulation, necrotic, and eschar.

7. Staging
- Stage I: Nonblanchable erythema of intact skin.
- Stage II: Partial thickness skin loss involving epidermis and/or dermis. Superficial. Vesicle, bulla, or abrasion.
- Stage III: Full-thickness. Damage or necrosis of subcutaneous tissue may extend down to, but not through, fascia. Deep crater. Eschar, exudate.
- Stage IV: Full-thickness skin loss with extensive necrosis or damage to muscle, tendon, or bone. Eschar. Exudate.

- Unstageable: Full thickness loss with base of ulcer covered by eschar.
- Suspected deep tissue injury: Intact skin with ecchymosis or blood-filled vesicle.

8. **Prevention**
   - *Reduce tissue pressure.*
   - Use lifting devices.
   - Patient positioning: change frequently, at least Q15 minutes sitting and Q2 hours supine.
   - Avoid direct trochanteric and heel pressure.
   - Do not drag, raise head of bed, massage, or use donut cushions.
   - Skin care—keep clean and dry.
   - Pressure-reducing devices: pillows—heel, sheepskin, wheelchair cushions, static flotation mattress—static, low air loss mattress—dynamic/alternating excellent, air fluidized mattress—dynamic excellent.

9. **Management**
   - Reduce pressure and shear forces.
   - Control infection.
   - Control moisture—prevent maceration of surrounding tissue.
   - Dressings: wet-to-dry, bio-occlusive, and others.
   - Debridement: all necrotic tissue and eschar should be debrided.
   - Avoid cytotoxic agents (Betadine, hydrogen peroxide).
   - Keep wound moist, but surrounding skin dry.
   - Protect skin, prevent infection, and promote granulation.
   - Dry gauze—protection and absorbs exudate.
   - Nutritional support: albumen >3.5 g per dL, 30 to 35 kcal/kg/day with 2 g protein. Vitamins: zinc and vitamin C. Tube feedings, TPN.
   - Antibiotics: only in infection. No routine culture.
   - Agency for Healthcare Research and Quality guidelines.

10. **Prognosis**
    - Stage I and II—good.
    - Stage III and IV—poor.

11. **Referral**
    - Ostomy or wound care RN.
    - Occupational therapy for preventative devices.
    - General surgeon for debridement. Plastic surgeon for grafting.
    - Wound care center.

SELECTED REFERENCES

Agency for Healthcare Research and Quality. Osteoporosis Guidelines. National Guideline Clearinghouse. Available at: http://www.guideline.gov. Accessed February 14, 2003.

Alexopoulous GS, Meyers BS, Young RC, et al. The course of geriatric depression with "reversible dementia" a controlled study. *Am J Psychiatry*. 1993;150:1693–1699.

American Geriatrics Society, British Geriatrics Society, and American Academy of Orthopedic Surgeons Panel on Falls Prevention: guidelines for prevention of falls in older persons. *J Am Geriatr Soc*. 2001;49(5):666.

Beckman AT, Copeland JR, Prince MJ, et al. Review of community prevalence of depression in later life. *Br J Psychiatry*. 1999;174:307–311.

Capezuti E, Stumpf NE, Evans LK, et al. The relationship between physical restraint removal and falls and injuries among nursing home residents. *J Gerontol A Biol Sci Med Sci*. 1998;53A:M47–M52.

Cassel CK, Leipzig RM, Carson EB, et al, eds. *Geriatric Medicine: An Evidence-Based Approach*. 4th ed. New York, NY: Springer-Verlag; 2003.

Doody RS, Stevens, JC, Beck C, et al. Practice parameter: management of dementia (an evidence-based review). Report on the quality standards subcommittee of the American Academy of Neurology. *Neurology*. 2001;56:1154–1166.

Fantl J, Fanti JA, Kaschaknenman D, et al, eds. *Urinary Incontinence in Adults: Acute and Chronic Management*. Clinical Practical Guideline No. 2. AHCPR Publication No 96-0682. Rockville, MD: U.S. Department of Health and Human Services, Public Health Service, Agency for Healthcare Policy and Research; 1996.

Folstein MF, Folstein SE, McHugh PR, et al. Mini-mental state: a practical method for grading the cognitive state of patients for the clinician. *J Psychiatr Res*. 1975;12(3):189–198.

Glass RM. Treating depression as a recurrent or chronic disease (Editorial). *JAMA*. 1999;281:83–84.

Hay-Smith EJC, Bø K, Berghmans LCM, et al. Pelvic floor muscle training for urinary incontinence in women (Cochrane Review). In: *The Cochrane Library*. Issue 3. Oxford, UK: Update Software; 2003.

Knopman DS, DeKosky ST, Cummings JL, et al. Practice parameter: diagnosis of dementia (an evidence-based review). Report on the Quality Standards Subcommittee of the American Academy of Neurology. *Neurology*. 2001;56:1143–1153.

Koenig HG, Meador KG. Dosing recommendations and prescribing patterns for depressed, medically ill, hospitalized older patients. *J Am Geriatr Soc*. 1997;45:1409.

Laveretsky H, Kumar A. Clinically significant non-major depression. *Am J Geriatr Psychiatry*. 2002;10(3):239–255.

Leipzig RM, Cumming RG, Tinetti MEI, et al. Drugs and falls in older people: a systematic review and meta-analysis: I. Psychotropic drugs. *J Am Geriatr Soc*. 1999;47:30-39.

Lonergan E, Luxenberg J, Colford J. Haloperidol for agitation in dementia (Cochrane Review). In: *The Cochrane Library*. Issue 3. Oxford, UK: Update Software; 2003.

Mathias S, Nayak USL, Isaacs B. Balance in elderly patients: the "get-up and go" test. *Arch Phys Med Rehab*. 1986;67:387–389.

Mulrow CD, Williams JW Jr, Trivedi M, et al. *Treatment of depression: newer pharmacotherapies*. Evidence Report/Technology Assessment No. 7. Rockville, MD: Agency for Health Care Policy and Research; February 1999. AHCPR Publication No. 99-E014. Available at: http://www.ahcpr.gov/clinic/depresumm.htm. Accessed February 14, 2003.

Nevitt MC. Falls in the elderly: risk factors and prevention. In: Masdeu JC, Sudarsky L, Wolfson L, eds. *Gait Disorders of Aging: Falls and Therapeutic Strategies*. Philadelphia, PA: Lippincott-Raven; 1997:13–36.

Petersen RC, Stevens JC, Ganguli M, et al. Practice parameter: early detection of dementia: mild cognitive impairment (an evidence-based review). Report on the Quality Standards Subcommittee of the American Academy of Neurology. *Neurology*. 2001;56:1133–1142.

Pfeffer RI, Kuroski TT, Harrah H Jr, et al. Measurement of functional activities in older adults in the community. *J Gerontol*. 1982;37:323–329.

Podiallo D, Richardson S. The timed "up & go": A test of basic functional mobility for frail elderly persons. *J Am Geriatr Soc*. 1991;39:142–148.

Reisberg B, Doody R, Stoffler A, et al. Memantine in moderate-to-severe Alzheimer's disease. *N Engl J Med*. 2003;348(14):1331–1341.

Reuben DB. *Geriatrics at Your Fingertips: 2001 Edition*. Belle Mead, NJ: Excerpta Medica, for the American Geriatrics Society; 2001.

Reynolds CF III, Frank E, Perel JM, et al. Nortriptyline and interpersonal psychotherapy as maintenance therapies for recurrent major depression: a randomized controlled trial in patients older than 59 years. *JAMA*. 1999;281:39–45.

Snow V, Lascher S, Mottur-Pilson C. Pharmacological treatment of acute major depression and dysthymia. ACP-ASIM Clinical Practice Guidelines. *Ann Intern Med*. 2000;132(9):738–742.

Solomon PR, Hirschoff A, Felly B, et al. A seven minute neurocognitive screening battery highly sensitive to Alzheimer's disease. *Arch Neurol*. 1998;55:349–355.

Steffens DC, Skoog I, Norton MC, et al. Prevalence of depression and its treatment in an elderly population: the Cache County study. *Arch Gen Psychiatry*. 2000;57:601–607.

Tennstedt S, Cafferata GL, Sullivan L, et al. Depression among caregivers of impaired elders. *J Aging Health*. 1992;4:58–76.

U.S. Census Bureau. *Population Projections for the United States by Age, Race, and Hispanic Origin: 1993–2050*. Washington, DC: U.S. Census Bureau; 1993.

Pharmacology

18

G. John DiGregorio • Reamer L. Bushardt • Lawrence Carey

I. Pharmacokinetics

A. Absorption

1. Definition
- Ability of a drug to cross biologic membranes and enter blood.

2. Mechanisms
- Passive diffusion (requires no energy)—primary method for most drugs.
- Active transport (requires energy)—carrier-mediated, energy-dependent; competition is possible.
- Facilitated diffusion—carrier-mediated, but does not require energy.

3. Factors Affecting Absorption
- Route of administration (oral, intramuscular, rectal, inhalation, topical, etc.)
- Concentration of drug.
- Chemical properties of the agent (e.g., pKa and lipophilicity).
- Physiologic factors (e.g., blood flow and surface area of the site of administration).
- Metabolism before reaching the systemic circulation; for oral administration occurs in intestines and liver (first-pass effect)—examples of agents with high first-pass metabolism: verapamil, morphine, propranolol, and nitroglycerin.

4. Quantification
- Bioavailability (F)—quantifies the amount of administered drug reaching the circulation.
- Bioequivalence.

B. Distribution

1. Definition
- Estimation of the extent of spread of total drugs throughout the body.

2. Factors
- Physiologic (e.g., blood flow to organs and disease states).
- Protein binding—binding to plasma (free US), proteins (e.g., albumin).
- Tissue binding—drugs can be sequestered in tissues (e.g., lipid-soluble drugs in adipose tissue).

3. Quantification
- Volume of distribution (Vd)—relates the amount of drug in the body to plasma concentration; large Vd drug is widely distributed, small Vd drug is primarily in plasma.
- Examples of agents with high Vd: meperidine, morphine, verapamil, propranolol, and quinidine.
- Examples of agents with low Vd: nifedipine, sulfamethoxazole, theophylline, tobramycin, and warfarin.

C. Metabolism (Biotransformation)

1. Definition
- Process of chemical alteration of drug molecules; primary purpose is to inactivate drugs and increase water solubility to enhance renal elimination.

2. Major Sites
- Liver—primarily by way of cytochrome P450 system.
- Lungs.
- Gastrointestinal (GI) tract.

3. Types
- Phase I—primarily cytochrome P450 system-mediated reactions such as oxidation, reduction, and hydrolysis; products are more polar.
- Phase II—conjugation with endogenous substances such as glucuronide; products are highly polar and totally inactivate drug.

D. Excretion

1. Definition
- Removal of a drug and its metabolites from the body.

2. Sites
- Kidney—primary site.
- Lungs.
- Sweat, breast milk.

3. Mechanism (Kidney)
- Glomerular filtration—drugs moved from blood to tubular fluid.
- Tubular reabsorption—lipid-soluble drugs reabsorbed from tubular fluid into the blood vessels supplying the nephrons.
- Tubular secretion—pumps in the tubules actively pump drugs from blood into the tubules.

4. Factors
- Chemical properties—pKa, polarity.
- Physiologic factors—renal blood flow, glomerular filtration rate (GFR), plasma protein binding.
- Drug interactions—active transport process at tubules can be subject to competition with other drugs (e.g., probenecid).

5. Quantification
- Clearance—measures rate of elimination of a drug from the body as it relates to drug concentration, includes all sites of elimination.
- Half-life ($t_{1/2}$)—time required to decrease the amount of drug in the body by 50%, useful in determining dosage regimens.
- Example $t_{1/2}$ values: morphine = 1.9 hours, warfarin = 37 hours.

II. Pharmacodynamics "What the Drug Does to the Body?"

A. Dose–Response Relationships

1. Definition
- Relationship between administered dose of a drug and the resultant effect, generally expressed as a log-dose response that results in an S-shaped curve. Drug responses are graded, quantal, and time action.

2. Features
- Maximum response (E_{max})—maximum possible response.
- Effective concentration 50—concentration of the drug producing 50% of maximal response.

B. Targets of Drug Action

1. Receptors
- Agonists—drugs that bind to a receptor and mimic the effect of the endogenous neurotransmitter (e.g., opioids).
- Antagonists—drugs that block receptors and prevent binding of endogenous neurotransmitter (e.g., β-blockers).

2. Enzymes
- Inhibitors—drugs that inhibit the activity of enzymes (e.g., angiotensin-converting enzyme inhibitors [ACEIs], inhibit angiotensin-converting enzyme).
- Activators—drugs that enhance the activity of enzymes (e.g., tissue plasminogen activator activates the enzyme plasminogen in the presence of fibrin).

3. Channels
- Blockers—drugs can prevent channels from opening (e.g., calciumchannel blockers).

III. Principles of Drug–Drug Interactions

A. Pharmacodynamics

1. Physiologic: Two Drugs Taken Simultaneously That Have Effects on the Same Organ System
- Antagonism—agents with opposite effects (e.g., central nervous system [CNS] stimulation of pseudoephedrine and CNS depression of diphenhydramine—used to offset the adverse effects).
- Synergism—agents with similar effects (e.g., CNS depression caused by barbiturates and alcohol can be fatal).

2. Pharmacologic: Two Drugs Taken Simultaneously That Have Opposing Effects on a Receptor
- Receptor agonist and antagonist administered together will antagonize each other (e.g., nonselective β-receptor antagonist and a β-receptor agonist).

B. Pharmacokinetics

1. Altered Absorption
- Changes in GI pH, motility, or blood flow to the site of administration can affect absorption.

2. Altered Distribution
- Main mechanism is by way of competition for plasma protein binding sites.

3. Altered Metabolism: Cytochrome P450 Isozymes (e.g., CYP1A2, CYP2C9, CYP2C19, CYP2D6, and CYP3A4)
- Inducers—promote the synthesis of P450 enzymes and thereby increase the metabolism of many drugs; may result in a lack of therapeutic effect (e.g., phenobarbital, phenytoin, and rifampin).
- Inhibitors—prevent the metabolism of other agents; can lead to toxicity (e.g., ketoconazole, cimetidine, erythromycin, and grapefruit juice).

4. Altered Renal Excretion
- Alteration in renal blood flow can affect GFR, that is, agents that decrease the renal blood flow such as vasodilators.
- Alteration in urinary pH can affect ionization and the degree of reabsorption.
- Drugs can compete for the tubular active transporters.

IV. Autonomic Agents

A. Muscarinic Agents

DEFINE: AGENTS AFFECTING MUSCRINIC RECEPTORS

1. Direct Agonists
- **Work directly on muscaric receptors sites**
  - Mechanism of action: mimic the effects of the parasympathetic nervous system (PNS) by way of direct stimulation of muscarinic receptors in RS ANS innervated by PNS.
  - Effects: Eye—decrease intraocular pressure by way of enhanced outflow, pupil constriction; CVS—decrease heart rate, pulmonary; bronchoconstriction; Smooth muscle—enhance tone of GI causing increased bowel movements and urinary smooth muscle causing increased urination and stimulation of salivary secretions.
  - Therapeutic uses: wide-angle glaucoma (pilocarpine), postoperative ileus (bethanechol), postoperative or postpartum urinary retention (bethanechol), dry mouth (cevimeline, pilocarpine, ecothiophate).

- Common adverse effects: bradycardia, diarrhea, nausea and vomiting (N/V), incontinence, blurred vision.
- Contraindications/cautions: patients with asthma, patients with cardiovascular diseases.
- Example agents: bethanechol (Urecholine), pilocarpine (Isopto Carpine), cevimeline (Evoxac), ecothiophate (Phospholine).

2. **Indirect Agonists**
   - Mechanism of action: mimic the effects of acetylcholine (ACH) by way of inhibition of plasma acetyl-cholinesterase (ACHE); increasing ACH at effector organsand effects occur at both nicotinic and muscarinic receptors.
   - Primary effects are stimulation of skeletal muscle; CNS, especially learning and memory; effects similar to muscarinic agonists also occur.
   - Therapeutic uses: myasthenia gravis (pyridostigmine), Alzheimer disease (donepezil, tacrine, rivastigmine, galantamine), glaucoma (echothiophate, demecarium), reverse effects of neuromuscular blocking agents (edrophonium, neostigmine), antidote atropine poisoning (physostigmine).
   - Common adverse effects: shortness of breath, muscle fasciculations, bradycardia, delirium, and hepatotoxicity (tacrine only).
   - Contraindications/cautions: sarin is an ACHE inhibitor that is a nerve gas; many insecticides are ACHE inhibitors; poisoning is common.
   - Example agents: pyridostigmine (Mestinon), edrophonium (Tensilon), donepezil (Aricept), tacrine (Cognex), rivastigmine (Exelon), galantamine (Reminyl); echothiophate (Phospholine), demecarium (Humorsol); neostigmine (Prostigmin).

3. **Muscarinic Antagonists (Blockers)**
   - Mechanism of action: inhibit muscarinic receptors of PNS.
   - Effects: bronchodilation, relief of atrioventricular (AV) block or vagus-induced bradycardia, anti-tremor effects, vestibular effects, mydriasis (dilated pupil), decreased contraction (constipation) of GI and genitourinary smooth muscle (anuresis).
   - Therapeutic uses: chronic obstructive pulmonary disease (COPD) (ipratropium), bradycardia (atropine), motion sickness (scopolamine), Parkinson disease (benztropine, trihexyphenidyl), incontinence (tolterodine, oxybutynin).
   - Common adverse effects: dry mouth, dilated pupils, blurred vision, dry skin, flushing, tachycardia, urinary retention, constipation, fever, delirium, and hallucinations (overdose).
   - Contraindications/cautions: glaucoma (especially narrow angle), geriatricpatients (especially elderly male, risk of urinary retention).
   - Example agents: ipratropium (Atrovent), atropine, scopolamine, benztropine (Cogentin),

trihexyphenidyl (Artane), tolterodine (Detrol), oxybutynin (Ditropan).

B. Adrenergic Agents

1. **Catecholamines**
   - Norepinephrine (Levophed): effects mediated primarily through activation of α-receptors; can be used mainly to elevate blood pressure.
   - Epinephrine (Adrenalin): activates α_1, α_2, β_1, and β_2 receptors.
   - Dopamine (Intropin): low dose produces renal vasodilation by way of stimulation of D1 receptors, higher dose produces cardiac stimulation by way of β_1-receptor stimulation and α_1 vasoconstriction, used in emergency management of shock and heart failure.

2. **α_1-Receptor Agonists**
   - Mechanism of action: stimulates α-receptors blood vessels, causes vasoconstriction that results in increased blood pressure, decreased bleeding, relief of nasal congestion, mydriasis.
   - Therapeutic uses: emergency treatment of hypotension to preserve cerebral and coronary blood flow, decongestants, production of mydriasis during eye examinations; midodrine is used to treat chronic orthostatichypotension.
   - Common adverse effects: hypertension leading to vascular accident (e.g., stroke), reflex bradycardia, syncope, stress reactions.
   - Contraindications/cautions: if extravasation occurs, local tissue damage is possible; overuse as a topical nasal decongestant leads to rebound hyperemia (inverse quantity of blood flow).
   - Example agents: phenylephrine, midodrine (ProAmatine), epinephrine.

3. **α_2-Receptor Agonists**
   - Mechanism of action: stimulate central α_2-receptors which cause a decrease of adrenergic activity in the CNS and result in a decrease in blood pressure and heart rate.
   - Therapeutic use: hypertension.
   - Common adverse effects: dry mouth, sedation, postural hypotension, inhibition of sexual function, autoimmune hemolytic anemia (methyldopa only).
   - Contraindications/cautions: do not discontinue rapidly, rebound hypertension can occur.
   - Example agents: clonidine (Catapres), methyldopa (Aldomet).

4. **Miscellaneous α-Agonists**
   - Oxymetazoline (Afrin), xylometazoline (Neo-Synephrine): used topically (nasally) for decongestant effect, activate α_1- and α_2-receptors.
   - Pseudoephedrine (Sudafed): used as decongestant in over-the-counter (OTC) cold preparations, CNS effects may produce anorexia, used in OTC weight-loss products, activate α and α_2-receptors.

- Methylphenidate (Ritalin), pemoline (Cylert): similar to amphetamine, promote release and stimulation of α-receptors of norepinephrine and epinephrine used for attention-deficit/hyperactivity disorder (ADHD).
- Amphetamine and derivatives used as an anti-obesity drug and for narcolepsy.

5. **α_1-Receptor Antagonists**
   - Mechanism of action: block α_1-receptors, effects are primarily on blood vasodilation, also relax the prostate and bladder neck.
   - Therapeutic uses: hypertension, benign prostatic hyperplasia (BPH).
   - Common adverse effects: postural hypotension resulting in syncope, dizziness, and possibly fainting, reflex tachycardia, nasal congestion, inhibition of sexual function.
   - Contraindications/cautions: hypotensive effects are more prominent with the first dose; patients should be warned to rise slowly.
   - Example agents: prazosin (Minipress), terazosin (Hytrin), doxazosin (Cardura), tamsulosin (Flomax).

6. **β_1-Receptor Agonists**
   - Mechanism of action: stimulate β_1-receptors in the heart and kidney, results in positive inotropic effect and release of renin.
   - Therapeutic uses: emergency management of heart failure.
   - Common adverse effect: tachycardia.
   - Contraindications/cautions: α-receptors stimulated at a high dose, increase blood pressure.
   - Example agent: dopamine, dobutamine.

7. **β_2-Receptor Agonists**
   - Mechanism of action: stimulate β_2-receptors; main effects are bronchodilation and relaxation of the uterus.
   - Therapeutic uses: asthma, COPD, delay premature labor (terbutaline).
   - Common adverse effects: muscle tremor, heart palpitations, nervousness.
   - Contraindications/cautions: blood glucose levels can rise in diabetic patients; for acute treatment of asthma sustained release agents should not be used (e.g., salmeterol).
   - Example agents: albuterol (Proventil), terbutaline (Brethine), salmeterol (Serevent), metaproterenol (Alupent).

8. **Miscellaneous β-Agonists**
   - Isoproterenol (Isuprel): stimulates β_1- and β_2-receptors, used in the emergency treatment of bradyarrhythmias and cardiac shock.

9. **β-Receptor Antagonists—selective β_1; nonselective β_1 and β_2 blockers.**
   - Mechanism of action: block β-receptors, resulting in cardiovascular effects including decreased cardiac output, decreased heart rate, decreased contractility, decreased renin secretion, reflex vasoconstriction, increased sodium and water retention, decreased post-myocardial infarction (MI) cardiac remodeling.
   - Therapeutic uses: hypertension, tachyarrhythmias (class II agents, see arrhythmia section), heart failure (see congestive heart failure [CHF] section), angina, acute MI, migraine prophylaxis, essential tremor, performance anxiety, thyrotoxicosis, wide-angle glaucoma.
   - Common adverse effects: bradycardia, heart block, bronchoconstriction, depression, hypotension, insomnia.
   - Contraindications/cautions: can mask signs of hypoglycemia in diabetics, should not be stopped abruptly, use with caution in patients with asthma/COPD, heart block.
   - Example agents: *nonselective* (block β_1 and β_2): propranolol (Inderal), timolol (Timoptic); *selective* (block β_1): metoprolol (Lopressor), atenolol (Tenormin), esmolol (Brevibloc—IV only for arrhythmias); *nonselective plus selective and blocker*: labetalol (Normodyne), carvedilol (Coreg).

C. **Neuromuscular Blocking Agents (Depolarizing)**
   - Mechanism of action: block nicotinic receptors in skeletal muscle and produce paralysis by producing persistent depolarization.
   - Therapeutic uses: produce muscle relaxation during surgery, intubation or other procedures.
   - Common adverse effects: hypotension, respiratory arrest.
   - Contraindications/cautions: drug interaction occurs with general anesthetics, results in enhanced effects.
   - Example agents: pancuronium (Pavulon), vecuronium (Norcuron), atracurium (Tracrium), succinylcholine (Anectine).
   - **NOTE**: Succinylcholine is a depolarizing neuromuscular blocking agent used as a paralytic. It produces stimulation of nicotinic receptors leading to depolarization and paralysis. Short acting, associated with risk of malignant hyperthermia.

V. Cardiovascular Agents and Antihypertensive Agents

A. **Antihypertensive Agents**
   1. **Diuretics**
      a. **Thiazide diuretics**
         - Mechanism of action: increase the urinary excretion of sodium and chloride in approximately equivalent amounts at distal renal tubule.
         - Therapeutic uses: hypertension, edema.

- Common adverse effects: hypokalemia, hyponatremia, hypomagnesemia, hypercalcemia, hyperuricemia, muscle cramps, glucose intolerance, dyslipidemia (usually transient and at high doses).
- Contraindications/cautions: anuria, lupus erythematosus, hypersensitivity to sulfonamides, photosensitivity; use with caution in patients with impaired renal function (increased risk of toxicity or azotemia, decreased diuretic effectiveness).
- Example agents: hydrochlorothiazide (Esidrix), metolazone (Zaroxolyn), and chlorthalidone (Hygroton).

b. Loop diuretics
- Mechanism of action: primarily inhibit absorption of sodium and chloride in the renal tubules (ascending loop of Henle, proximal and distal).
- Therapeutic uses: hypertension, edema.
- Common adverse effects: hyperuricemia, hypokalemia, hyponatremia, hypomagnesemia, hypocalcemia, muscle cramps, bladder spasm, loss of appetite.
- Contraindications/cautions: anuria, liver disease, photosensitivity, ototoxicity.
- Example agents: furosemide (Lasix), bumetanide (Bumex), torsemide (Demadex).

c. Potassium-sparing diuretics
- Some potassium-sparing diuretics (i.e., triamterene) inhibit reabsorption of sodium in exchange for potassium and hydrogen ions through direct effects on the distal tubule. Others (i.e., spironolactone and eplerenone) are renal competitive aldosterone antagonists, inhibiting the effect of aldosterone by competing for the aldosterone-dependent sodium–potassium exchange site in the distal tubule cells. Result is increased secretion of water and sodium, whereas decreasing potassium excretion.
- Therapeutic uses: edema, ascites, heart failure syndrome, primary aldosteronism, hypertension.
- Common adverse effects: hyperkalemia, GI upset, gynecomastia (spironolactone).
- Contraindications/cautions: serum potassium >5.5 mEq per L, patients currently receiving potassium supplementation; avoid large quantities of potassium rich food.
- Example agents: spironolactone (Aldactone), triamterene (Dyrenium), eplerenone (Inspra).

2. β-Adrenergic Blocking Agents
- Mechanism of action: inhibit interaction of epinephrine, norepinephrine, and sympathomimetic drugs with β-adrenergic receptor sites.

- Therapeutic uses: hypertension, angina pectoris, cardiac arrhythmias, MI, heart failure syndrome, pheochromocytoma, migraine, and essential tremor.
- Common adverse effects: bradycardia, fatigue, dizziness, dyspnea, sexual dysfunction.
- Contraindications/cautions: sinus bradycardia, second- or third-degree heart block, decompensated cardiac failure, cardiogenic shock; use with caution in diabetes, airway disease, and peripheral vascular disease (PVD). Do not discontinue medication abruptly.
- Example agents: atenolol (Tenormin), bisoprolol (Zebeta), metoprolol (Lopressor, Toprol XL), nebivolol (Bystolic), nadolol (Corgard), sotalol (Betapace), and propranolol (Inderal).

3. Calcium Channel Blocking Agents

a. Dihydropyridine calcium antagonists
- Mechanism of action: selectively blocks the movement of extracellular calcium ions into cardiac and vascular smooth muscle; lowers blood pressure by reducing peripheral vascular resistance by a direct action on vascular smooth muscle.
- Therapeutic uses: angina pectoris, hypertension, Raynaud phenomenon.
- Common adverse effects: headache, peripheral edema, dizziness, flushing, weakness.
- Contraindications/cautions: hepatic dysfunction, hypotension.
- Example agents: amlodipine (Norvasc), felodipine (Plendil), isradipine (Dynacirc), nifedipine (Procardia).

b. Nondihydropyridine calcium antagonists
- Mechanism of action: exert inotropic and chronotropic effects on the heart.
- Therapeutic uses: hypertension, angina pectoris, atrial fibrillation/flutter, paroxysmal supraventricular tachycardia (PSVT).
- Common adverse effects: GI upset, dizziness, headache, bradycardia.
- Contraindications/cautions: sick sinus syndrome or second- or third-degree AV block except with a functioning pacemaker, hypotension 90 mm Hg systolic, acute MI and pulmonary congestion documented by X-ray on admission, and renal/hepatic dysfunction.
- Example agents: diltiazem (Cardizem), verapamil (Calan SR).

4. Renin Angiotensin System Antagonists

a. Angiotensin-converting enzyme inhibitors
- Mechanism of action: prevent the conversion of angiotensin I to angiotensin II, a vasoconstrictor agent, which decreases vasopressor activity and aldosterone secretion.
- Therapeutic uses: hypertension, heart failure syndrome, MI, kidney disease.

- Common adverse effects: asthenia, cough, dizziness, hyperkalemia; other serious but less common side effects include angioedema, neutropenia, and acute renal failure.
- Contraindications/cautions: renal artery stenosis, history of angioedema, volume and/or salt depletion states; teratogenic.
- Example agents: captopril (Capoten), benazepril (Lotensin), enalapril (Vasotec), fosinopril (Monopril), ramipril (Altace), lisinopril (Prinivil).

b. Angiotensin II receptor antagonists
- Mechanism of action: selectively blocks the binding of angiotensin II to the AT1 receptors in tissues such as vascular smooth muscle and the adrenal gland.
- Therapeutic uses: hypertension, heart failure, and kidney disease.
- Common adverse effects: headache, dizziness, somnolence, and hyperkalemia; serious but less common side effect is acute renal failure and angioedema.
- Contraindications/cautions: renal failure; teratogenic.
- Example agents: valsartan (Diovan), candesartan (Atacand), irbesartan (Avapro), losartan (Cozaar).

c. Direct renin inhibitors
- Mechanism of action: directly inhibits renin which decreases plasma renin activity (PRA) and inhibits the conversion of angiotensinogen to angiotensin I.
- Therapeutic uses: hypertension.
- Common adverse effects: dizziness, headache, diarrhea; less common but serious effects include hyperkalemia and angioedema.
- Contraindications/cautions: severe renal impairment, history of angioedema, volume- or salt-depletion states; teratogen.

5. α_1-Adrenergic Blockers
- Mechanism of action: selectively blocks α_1-adrenergic receptors and decreases total peripheral resistance and venous return; α_1-blockers produce antihypertensive effects secondary to selective postsynaptic α_1-adrenoceptor blockade.
- Therapeutic uses: hypertension, BPH.
- Common adverse effects: hypotension, dizziness, somnolence, headache.
- Contraindications/cautions: "first-dose" hypotension, priapism.
- Example agents: prazosin (Minipress), terazosin (Hytrin), doxazosin (Cardura); limited for use with BPH tamsulosin (Flomax) and alfuzosin (Flomax).

6. α/β-Adrenergic Blocking Agents
- Mechanism of action: selective, competitive postsynaptic α_1-adrenergic blocking and nonselective, competitive β-adrenergic blocking activity.

- Therapeutic uses: hypertension, heart failure syndrome.
- Common adverse effects: hypotension, dizziness, fatigue.
- Contraindications/cautions: bronchial asthma, decompensated cardiac failure, second- or third-degree heart block, severe bradycardia, cardiogenic shock, abrupt withdrawal, hepatic dysfunction.
- Example agents: labetalol (Normodyne), carvedilol (Coreg).

7. Vasodilators
- Mechanism of action: direct relaxation of vascular smooth muscle.
- Therapeutic uses: hypertension.
- Common adverse effects: blood dyscrasias, rash, palpitations, tachycardia, peripheral neuritis, fluid and electrolyte imbalance, pericardial effusion (minoxidil), hypertrichosis (minoxidil).
- Contraindications/cautions: coronary artery disease (CAD), mitral valvular rheumatic heart disease, pheochromocytoma (minoxidil); use caution in patients with renal dysfunction and tartrazine sensitivity.
- Example agents: hydralazine (Apresoline), minoxidil (Loniten).

8. Neuronal Adrenergic Blockers
a. Peripherally acting: reserpine
- Mechanism of action: depletes stores of catecholamine and 5-hydroxytryptamine in many organs, including the brain and adrenal medulla.
- Therapeutic use: hypertension.
- Common adverse effects: nasal congestion, arrhythmias, lethargy, depression.
- Contraindications/cautions: mental depression or history of mental depression, active peptic ulcer, ulcerative colitis, patients receiving electroconvulsive therapy.

b. Centrally acting
(1) Clonidine (Catapress), Guanfacine (Tenex)
- Mechanism of action: central α-adrenergic stimulant that inhibits cardiac workload and vasoconstriction.
- Therapeutic uses: hypertension, ADHD.
- Common adverse effects: dry mouth, sedation, fatigue.
- Contraindications/cautions: rebound hypertension—do not discontinue therapy abruptly, ophthalmologic effects.

(2) Methyldopa (Aldomet)
- Mechanism of action: lowers arterial pressure by the stimulation of central inhibitory α-adrenergic receptors, false neurotransmission, and/or reduction of PRA.
- Therapeutic uses: hypertension, hypertensive crises.

- Common adverse effects: positive Coombs test/hemolytic anemia, edema, weight gain, bradycardia, hepatic dysfunction, hematologic disorders, sedation, urine discoloration, sulfite sensitivity.
- Contraindications/cautions: active hepatic disease, coadministration with monoamine oxidase inhibitors (MAOIs).

B. Heart Failure SyndromeAgents

1. **Inotropic Agents**
   - Mechanism of action: slow AV conduction, increased contraction.
   - Therapeutic uses: heart failure syndrome, atrial fibrillation.
   - Common adverse effects: nausea, diarrhea, visual disturbances, arrhythmias.
   - Contraindications/cautions: sinus node disease, AV block, renal impairment, elderly.
   - Example agent: digoxin (Lanoxin).
2. **Angiotensin-converting enzyme inhibitors (see Hypertension)**
3. **β-Adrenergic Blocking Agents (see Hypertension)**
4. **Diuretics**
   a. **Thiazide diuretics**
      - Mechanism of action: increase the urinary excretion of sodium and chloride in approximately equivalent amounts at distal renaltubule.
      - Therapeutic uses: hypertension, edema.
      - Common adverse effects: hypokalemia, hyponatremia, hypomagnesemia, hypercalcemia, hyperuricemia, muscle cramps, glucose intolerance, dyslipidemia (usually transient and at high doses).
      - Contraindications/cautions: anuria, lupus erythematosus, hypersensitivity to sulfonamides, photosensitivity; use with caution in patients with impaired renal function (increased risk of toxicity or azotemia, decreased diuretic effectiveness).
      - Example agents: hydrochlorothiazide (Esidrix), metolazone (Zaroxolyn), and chlorthalidone (Hygroton).
   b. **Loop diuretics**
      - Mechanism of action: primarily inhibit absorption of sodium and chloride in the renal tubules (ascending loop of Henle, proximal, and distal).
      - Therapeutic uses: hypertension, edema.
      - Common adverse effects: hyperuricemia, hypokalemia, hyponatremia, hypomagnesemia, hypocalcemia, muscle cramps, bladder spasm, loss of appetite.
      - Contraindications/cautions: anuria, liver disease, photosensitivity, ototoxicity.

- Example agents: furosemide (Lasix), bumetanide (Bumex), torsemide (Demadex).
   c. **Potassium-sparing diuretics**
      - Some potassium-sparing diuretics (i.e., triamterene) inhibit reabsorption of sodium in exchange for potassium and hydrogen ions through direct effects on the distal tubule. Others (i.e., spironolactone and eplerenone) are renal competitive aldosterone antagonists, inhibiting the effect of aldosterone by competing for the aldosterone-dependent sodium–potassium exchange site in the distal tubule cells. Result is increased secretion of water and sodium, whereas decreasing potassium excretion.
      - Therapeutic uses: edema, ascites, heart failure syndrome, primary aldosteronism, hypertension.
      - Common adverse effects: hyperkalemia, GI upset, gynecomastia (spironolactone).
      - Contraindications/cautions: serum potassium >5.5 mEq per L, patients currently receiving potassium supplementation; avoid large quantities of potassium rich food.
      - Example agents: spironolactone (Aldactone), triamterene (Dyrenium), eplerenone (Inspra).
5. **Calcium Channel Blocking Agents**
   a. **Dihydropyridine calcium antagonists**
      - Mechanism of action: selectively blocks movement of extracellular calcium ions into cardiac and vascular smooth muscle; lowers blood pressure by reducing peripheral vascular resistance by a direct action on vascular smooth muscle.
      - Therapeutic uses: angina pectoris, hypertension, Raynaud phenomenon.
      - Common adverse effects: headache, peripheral edema, dizziness, flushing, weakness.
      - Contraindications/cautions: hepatic dysfunction, hypotension.
      - Example agents: amlodipine (Norvasc), felodipine (Plendil), isradipine (Dynacirc), nifedipine (Procardia).
   b. **Nondihydropyridine calcium antagonists**
      - Mechanism of action: exert inotropic and chronotropic effects on the heart.
      - Therapeutic uses: hypertension, angina pectoris, atrial fibrillation/flutter, PSVT.
      - Common adverse effects: GI upset, dizziness, headache, bradycardia.
      - Contraindications/cautions: sick sinus syndrome or second- or third-degree AV block except with a functioning pacemaker, hypotension <90 mm Hg systolic, acute MI and pulmonary congestion documented by X-ray on admission, and renal/hepatic dysfunction.
      - Example agents: diltiazem (Cardizem), verapamil (Calan SR).

C. Antianginal Agents

1. Nitrates

- Mechanism of action: relaxation of vascular smooth muscle through dose-dependent dilation of both arterial and venous beds.
- Therapeutic uses: acute angina, angina prophylaxis.
- Contraindications/cautions: severe anemia, closed-angle glaucoma, postural hypotension, early MI, head trauma, or cerebral hemorrhage; tolerance develops to use.
- Common adverse effects: dizziness, headache, hypotension, brady- or tachycardia, contact dermatitis (transdermal), burning or tingling sensation of oral cavity (sublingual).
- Example agents: isosorbide mononitrate (Imdur); isosorbide dinitrate (Isordil); nitroglycerin, sublingual (Nitrostat); nitroglycerin, transdermal (Nitro-Dur); nitroglycerin, ointment (Nitro-Bid); nitroglycerin, sublingual spray (NitroMist); nitroglycerin for intravenous injection.

2. β-Blocking Agents (see Hypertension)

3. Calcium Channel Agents

a. Dihydropyridine calcium antagonists

- Mechanism of action: reduce vascular resistance, cardiac afterload, and produce arteriolar/coronary vasodilatation.
- Therapeutic uses: angina pectoris, hypertension.
- Common adverse effects: headache, peripheral edema, dizziness, weakness.
- Contraindications/cautions: hepatic dysfunction, hypotension.
- Example agents: amlodipine (Norvasc), nifedipine (Procardia).

b. Nondihydropyridine calcium antagonists

- Mechanism of action: exert inotropic and chronotropic effects on the heart.
- Therapeutic uses: hypertension, angina pectoris, atrial fibrillation/flutter, PSVT.
- Common adverse effects: constipation, dizziness, headache, bradycardia.
- Contraindications/cautions: sick sinus syndrome or second- or third-degree AV block except with a functioning pacemaker, hypotension <90 mm Hg systolic, acute MI and pulmonary congestion documented by X-ray on admission, and renal/hepatic dysfunction.
- Example agents: diltiazem (Cardizem), verapamil (Calan SR).

4. Aspirin

- Mechanism of action: potent inhibitor of both prostaglandin synthesis and platelet aggregation.
- Therapeutic uses: unstable angina, patients with previous MI, and reduce the risk of recurrent transient ischemic attacks or stroke in men who have had transient ischemia of the brain due to fibrin platelet emboli.
- Common adverse effects: dyspepsia, nausea, prolongation of bleeding time, hematologic disorders (e.g., iron deficiency anemia, leukopenia, and thrombocytopenia), hematoma.
- Contraindications/cautions: hypersensitivity to salicylates or nonsteroidal anti-inflammatory drugs (NSAIDs), Reye syndrome, caution in patients with chronic renal insufficiency, GI, and hematologic disorders.
- Example agent: aspirin (Ecotrin).

5. Ranolazine (Ranexa)

- Mechanism of action: mechanism is unknown; however, ranolazine can inhibit the inactivating component of the sodium current and inhibits the rapid inward rectifying current, which prolongs the ventricular action potential.
- Therapeutic uses: angina pectoris (chronic).
- Common adverse effects: constipation, nausea, dizziness, and headache; less common but serious effects include QT prolongation and syncope.
- Contraindications/cautions: hepatic dysfunction, prolonged QT interval, concomitant use with potent CYP3A inhibitors or inducers.

D. Antiarrhythmic Agents

One approach to classifying antiarrhythmic agents is based on their primary electrophysiologic action (see table below), but it is important to note that many agents will possess multiple effects that contribute to their clinical action.

Class	Primary Action
I	Sodium channel blockade
II	β-Blockade
III	Action potential prolongation
IV	Calcium channel blockade

1. Class I

a. Class IA

- Mechanism of action: decrease conduction velocity and prolong repolarization.
- Therapeutic uses: atrial and ventricular arrhythmias.
- Common adverse effects: torsades de pointes, hypotension, tinnitus, diarrhea, blurred vision, headache, lupus-like syndrome (procainamide), blood dyscrasias.
- Contraindications/cautions: skin eruption or febrile reactions, myasthenia gravis, digitalis intoxication manifested by arrhythmias, conduction disorders, history of long QT syndrome, complete AV block with an AV nodal or AV pacemaker, aberrant ectopic impulses and abnormal rhythms due to escape mechanisms, complete heart block, lupus erythematosus, torsades de pointes.
- Example agents: quinidine, procainamide.

b. **Class IB**
- Mechanism of action: decrease conduction velocity and shorten repolarization.
- Therapeutic uses: ventricular arrhythmias.
- Common adverse effects: dizziness, blood dyscrasias, nausea, paresthesias, tremor, vomiting, pulmonary fibrosis.
- Contraindications/cautions: Stokes–Adams syndrome, Wolff–Parkinson–White syndrome, severe degrees of sinoatrial, AV, or intraventricular block in the absence of an artificial pacemaker.
- Example agents: lidocaine (Xylocaine), tocainide (Tonocard).

c. **Class IC**
- Mechanism of action: decrease conduction velocity.
- Therapeutic uses: atrial and ventricular arrhythmias.
- Common adverse effects: visual abnormalities, nausea, negative inotrope, dyspnea, headache, metallic taste.
- Contraindications/cautions: preexisting second- or third-degree AV block, right bundle branch block when associated with a left hemiblock (bifascicular block) unless a pacemaker is present, recent MI, presence of cardiogenic shock, uncontrolled CHF, conduction disorders in the absence of a pacemaker, bradycardia, marked hypotension, bronchospastic disorders, electrolyte imbalances.
- Example agents: flecainide (Tambocor), propafenone (Rythmol).

2. **Class II**
- Mechanism of action: compete with β-adrenergic agonists to slow ventricular rate.
- Therapeutic uses: atrial flutter/fibrillation, PSVT, sometimes symptomatic premature ventricular contractions.
- Common adverse effects: bradycardia, hypotension, fatigue, sexual dysfunction.
- Contraindications/cautions: sinus bradycardia, greater than first-degree heart block; cardiogenic shock; use with caution in diabetes, asthma, COPD, and PVD.
- Example agents: propranolol (Inderal), esmolol (Brevibloc), acebutolol (Sectral), sotalol (Betapace).

3. **Class III**
- Mechanism of action: prolong repolarization.
- Therapeutic uses: atrial/ventricular arrhythmias.
- Common adverse effects: corneal deposits, nightmares, increased hepatic enzymes, photosensitivity, blue-gray skin discoloration, hypo/hyperthyroidism, pulmonary fibrosis, bradycardia, torsades de pointes, hypotension, exacerbation of heart failure.

- Contraindications/cautions: severe sinus-node dysfunction causing marked sinus bradycardia, second-and third-degree AV block, cardiogenic shock.
- Example agents: amiodarone (Cordarone), bretylium, dofetilide (Tikosyn); amiodarone is known to possess electrophysiologic actions from all four classes of antiarrhythmics.

4. **Class IV**
- Mechanism of action: decrease heart rate.
- Therapeutic uses: slow ventricular rate in atrial flutter/fibrillation and PSVT.
- Common adverse effects: constipation, dizziness, headache, bradycardia (verapamil), visual disturbances, anorexia, N/V, lethargy (digoxin), chest discomfort, dyspnea, flushing, asystole, headache (adenosine).
- Contraindications/cautions: sinus node disease or second- or third-degree AV block except with a functioning pacemaker.
- Example agents: verapamil (Calan SR), adenosine (Adenocard).

5. **Other Antiarrhythmics**
a. **Cardiac glycosides, digoxin (Lanoxin)**
- Mechanism of action: inhibits sodium-potassium ATPase, which increases intracellular sodium concentration then increased intracellular calcium; vagal activity and baroreceptor sensitization lead to positive inotropic action, reduced sympathetic response and decreased renin-angiotensin system output.
- Therapeutic uses: atrial fibrillation, heart failure syndrome.
- Common adverse effects: headache, loss of appetite, weight loss, visual changes; less commonly ataxia and cardiac toxicity may occur.
- Contraindications/cautions: sinus node disease, AV block, renal impairment, elderly.
- Example agent: digoxin (Lanoxin).

VI. Anticoagulants

A. Properties
- The coagulation pathway is a complex, multistep process involving thrombin, fibrin, clotting factors, and various other regulatory substances.
- Various conditions can cause the system to function inappropriately. The greatest risks are either clot formation (lack of anticoagulation) or bleeding (excessive anticoagulation).

B. Low-Molecular-Weight Heparins
- Mechanism of action: inhibit factor Xa and thrombin by way of antithrombin III activity.
- Therapeutic uses: thromboembolic complications after surgery or ischemic complications of unstable angina and MI.

- Monitor: complete blood count; may monitor anti-factor Xa in select patients.
- Common adverse effects: hemorrhage, anemia, thrombocytopenia.
- Contraindications/cautions: active bleed, use with caution in renal failure, obese, and elderly patients.
- Example agents: enoxaparin (Lovenox), tinzaparin (Innohep), dalteparin (Fragmin).

C. Glycosaminoglycan
- Mechanism of action: antithrombotic agent, prevents fibrin formation by way of thrombin of activated factor Xa.
- Therapeutic uses: prevention of deep vein thrombosis and pulmonary embolism.
- Common adverse effects: hemorrhage, rash, fever, GI problems.
- Contraindications/cautions: active bleed, sulfite-sensitive patients.
- Example agent: danaparoid (Orgaran).

D. Heparin
- Mechanism of action: inactivates factor Xa and inhibits conversion of fibrinogen to fibrin.
- Therapeutic uses: thrombosis, pulmonary embolism, coagulopathies, deep vein thrombosis, clot prevention.
- Monitor: activated partial thromboplastin time (APTT) or activated coagulation time, platelet count, hematocrit, occult blood in stool.
- Common adverse effects: hemorrhage, thrombocytopenia, hypersensitivity reactions, hyperkalemia.
- Contraindications/cautions: severe thrombocytopenia, uncontrolled bleeding.
- Treatment of heparin overdose: protamine sulfate that binds with heparin.

E. Antithrombin Agents
- Mechanism of action: inhibits the formation of thrombin and other activating factors.
- Therapeutic uses: treat thromboembolisms in patients with hereditary antithrombin III deficiency.
- Monitor: antithrombin III levels.
- Common adverse effects: nausea, dizziness, dysgeusia, hemorrhage.
- Example agent: antithrombin III (Thrombate III).

F. Thrombin Inhibitor
- Mechanism of action: inhibits human thrombin.
- Therapeutic uses: deep vein thrombosis, pulmonary embolism, atrial fibrillation (prevention of thromboembolism).
- Monitor: APTT, potential for allergic reactions.
- Common adverse effects: hemorrhage, hypersensitivity.
- Contraindications/cautions: active bleeding or irreversible coagulation disorder.
- Example agents: dabigatran (Pradaxa), desirudin (Iprivask), lepirudin (Refludan), argatroban (Argatroban), bivalirudin (Angiomax).

G. Selective Factor Xa Inhibitor
- Mechanism of action: inhibition of factor Xa mediated by antithrombin III.
- Therapeutic uses: prophylaxis of deep vein thrombosis, pulmonary embolism.
- Monitor: antifactor Xa if needed.
- Common adverse effect: hemorrhage.
- Contraindications/cautions: active bleeding, uncontrolled arterial hypertension, GI ulceration.
- Example agent: fondaparinux (Arixtra), rivaroxaban (Xarelto).

H. Warfarin (Coumadin)
- Mechanism of action: inhibits the synthesis of vitamin K–dependent clotting factors (e.g., factors II, VII, IX, and X).
- Therapeutic uses: venous thrombosis, pulmonary embolism, thromboembolic complications of atrial fibrillation/cardiac valve replacement, post-MI.
- Monitor: prothrombin time, international normalized ratio (INR).
- Common adverse effects: hemorrhage, necrosis, thrombocytopenia.
- Contraindications/cautions: protein C deficiency, NSAIDs, high risk for bleeding, numerous food and drug interactions.
- Treatment of excessive warfarin coagulation: oral or IV vitamin K1 or blood product.

I. Dabigatran (Pradaxa)
- An oral anticoagulant for stroke prevention in patients with nonvalvular atrial fibrillation, unlike Coumadin does not require measurement of blood thinning levels and monitor using INR.
- Mechanism of action: direct thrombin inhibitor.
- Contraindications: patients with active pathologic bleeding and patients with a known hypersensitivity.
- Common adverse effects: bleeding, dyspepsia, abdominal pain, epigastric discomfort, liver enzyme elevation.
- In vitro anticoagulants—chelating agents that prevents blood clotting outside the body (oxalate, citrate, EDTA).

VII. Neurologic Agents
A. Antiepileptics/Anticonvulsants
1. General Properties
- These medications have the ability to depress abnormal neuronal discharges within the CNS, thereby inhibiting seizure activity.
- Medication initiation and withdrawal should be done only with supervision and caution; avoid abrupt withdrawal of any of the medications.
- Individual medications have demonstrated varying degrees of efficacy, in part based on the classification type of the seizure.

2. **Hydantoins**
   - Mechanism of action: proposed to stabilize the neurons from hyperexcitability by controlling cellular sodium without causing general depression of the CNS.
   - Therapeutic uses: generalized tonic–clonic and complex partial seizures; treatment and prophylaxis of seizure during and following neurosurgery.
   - Monitor: complete blood counts, urinalysis, drug level.
   - Common adverse effects: rash, nystagmus, slurred speech, confusion, dizziness, hematologic complications, gingival hyperplasia.
   - Contraindications/cautions: cardiac conduction abnormalities, significant drug–drug interactions.
   - Example agent: phenytoin (Dilantin).

3. **Succinimides**
   - Mechanism of action: motor cortex depression and elevated stimulatory threshold by reducing low threshold thalamic Ca^{2+} currents.
   - Therapeutic uses: absence seizures.
   - Monitor: complete blood counts, urinalysis, liver function tests.
   - Common adverse effects: drowsiness, ataxia, dizziness, headache, rash, GI upset.
   - Contraindications/cautions: patients with renal or hepatic failure.
   - Example agents: ethosuximide (Zarontin), methsuximide (Celontin).

4. **Benzodiazepine**
   - Mechanism of action: proposed to potentiate the effects of γ-aminobutyrate (GABA), decrease seizure activity.
   - Therapeutic uses: absence, akinetic, and myoclonic seizures; status epilepticus.
   - Monitor: may lose effectiveness over time, may need to increase dose.
   - Common adverse effects: sedation, ataxia, paradoxical reactions.
   - Contraindications/cautions: multiple seizure types, suicide risk, dependence.
   - Example agents: clonazepam (Klonopin), diazepam (Valium).

5. **Carbamazepine (Tegretol)**
   - Mechanism of action: proposed to reduce response and potentiation of impulses.
   - Therapeutic uses: partial, generalized tonic–clonic, mixed pattern and generalized seizures.
   - Monitor: drug level, complete blood count, liver function tests, urinalysis, blood urea nitrogen.
   - Common adverse effects: aplastic anemia, agranulocytosis, severe dermatologic reactions.
   - Contraindications/cautions: bone marrow suppression, patients with hypersensitivity to tricyclic antidepressants, MAOIs, potential drug–drug interactions.

- Oxcarbazepine (Trileptal) a metabolite of carbamazepine appears to be as effective as carbamazepine in the treatment of epilepsy; severe adverse effects have occurred less often with oxcarbazepine in some studies.

6. **Valproic Acid**
   - Mechanism of action: varying proposed mechanisms of actions.
   - Therapeutic uses: absence seizures; complex partial epileptic seizure.
   - Monitor: drug level, complete blood cell count.
   - Common adverse effects: pancreatitis, thrombocytopenia, hepatotoxicity, GI problems, asthenia.
   - Contraindications/cautions: patients with hepatic dysfunction, urea cycle disorder.
   - Example agents: valproic acid (Depakene), divalproex sodium (Depakote).

7. **Additional Anticonvulsants**
   - A wide variety of additional agents are currently available.
   - Each of the agents has a unique pharmacologic profile and monitoring requirements.
   - Examples: felbamate (Felbatol), gabapentin (Neurontin), lamotrigine (Lamictal), levetiracetam (Keppra), primidone (Mysoline), tiagabine (Gabitril), topiramate (Topamax), pregabalin (Lyrica).

B. Antiparkinsonian Agents

1. **General Properties**
   - The biochemical basis is complex with the primary defect appearing to be an imbalance in neurotransmitters.
   - There is not a curative agent.
   - Available medications are aimed at correcting the neurotransmitter defects.

2. **Anticholinergics**
   - Mechanism of action: suppress central cholinergic activity, may prolong activity of dopamine.
   - Therapeutic uses: adjunctive therapy for parkinsonism and drug-induced extrapyramidal symptoms.
   - Monitor: blood pressure, monitor for mental status changes.
   - Common adverse effects: mental confusion, disorientation, memory loss, blurred vision, dry mouth, hypotension, appetite changes.
   - Contraindications/cautions: angle-closure glaucoma, prostatic hypertrophy.
   - Example agents: benztropine (Cogentin), biperiden (Akineton), diphenhydramine (Benadryl), procyclidine (Kemadrin), trihexyphenidyl (Artane).

3. **Amantadine (Symmetrel)**
   - Mechanism of action: may increase dopamine by facilitating dopamine release and block reuptake.
   - Therapeutic uses: parkinsonism, drug-induced extrapyramidal symptoms, influenza A infection.
   - Monitor: renal function, CNS, adverse reactions.

- Common adverse effects: dizziness, lightheadedness, insomnia, nausea, orthostatic hypotension, agitation.
- Contraindications/cautions: suicide attempt history, seizure history, untreated angle-closure glaucoma; avoid abrupt withdrawal.

4. **Bromocriptine Mesylate (Parlodel)**
   - Mechanism of action: stimulation of the dopamine receptors in the brain.
   - Therapeutic uses: Parkinson disease.
   - Monitor: blood pressure.
   - Common adverse effects: hypotension, nausea, headache, dizziness.
   - Contraindications/cautions: ischemic heart or PVD.

5. **Carbidopa (Lodosyn)**
   - Mechanism of action: inhibits decarboxylation of peripheral levodopa, does not cross blood–brain barrier.
   - Therapeutic uses: Parkinson disease.
   - Monitor: clinical improvement in parkinsonian symptoms.
   - Common adverse effects: neuroleptic malignant-like syndrome, dyskinesias.
   - Contraindications/cautions: avoid if on tricyclic antidepressant.

6. **Levodopa**
   - Mechanism of action: a precursor that crosses blood–brain barrier and is converted to dopamine.
   - Therapeutic uses: Parkinson disease.
   - Monitor: liver enzymes, complete blood count, renal function, symptoms of depression.
   - Common adverse effects: "on–off" phenomenon, abnormal body movements, anorexia, N/V.
   - Contraindications/cautions: narrow-angle glaucoma, MAOIs, can activate melanomas, history of MI, tartrazine sensitivity.
   - Example agents: combined use of levodopa plus a peripheral dopa decarboxylase inhibitor enhances efficacy and reduces dose requirements and some adverse effects of levodopa; levodopa is available in combination with carbidopa (Sinemet, Sinemet CR).

7. **Entacapone (Comtan)**
   - Mechanism of action: inhibits catechol-*O*-methyltransferase, thereby increasing levodopa concentrations.
   - Therapeutic uses: adjunct to levodopa/carbidopa in treating Parkinson disease.
   - Monitor: blood pressure, clinical improvement.
   - Common adverse effects: hypotension, syncope, diarrhea, nausea, hallucinations, dyskinesia.
   - Contraindications/cautions: MAOIs, hepatic impairment.

8. **Pergolide Mesylate (Permax)**
   - Mechanism of action: dopamine receptor agonist, directly stimulates postsynaptic receptors.

- Therapeutic uses: adjunct to levodopa/carbidopa in treating Parkinson disease.
- Monitor: electrocardiogram if signs/symptoms of cardiac dysrhythmia occur.
- Common adverse effects: hypotension, neuroleptic malignant syndrome, hallucinations, dyskinesia, nausea.
- Contraindications/cautions: cardiac dysrhythmias; avoid abrupt discontinuation.

9. **Selegiline Hydrochloride**
   - Mechanism of action: increases dopaminergic activity.
   - Therapeutic uses: adjunct to levodopa/carbidopa in treating Parkinson disease.
   - Monitor: blood pressure, clinical improvement, potential drug interactions.
   - Common adverse effects: nausea, hallucinations, headache, confusion, cardiac effects.
   - Contraindications/cautions: avoid use with meperidine and use other opioids with caution; avoid concomitant use with a MAOIs or dextromethorphan.
   - Example agent: selegiline (Carbex, Eldepryl).

10. **Dopaminergics**
    - Mechanism of action: proposed stimulation of dopamine receptors.
    - Therapeutic uses: Parkinson disease.
    - Monitor: blood pressure, clinical improvement.
    - Common adverse effects: orthostatic hypotension, syncope, hallucinations, dyskinesia.
    - Contraindications/cautions: retinal changes, avoid sudden discontinuation, use caution with other CNS sedative agents, extensive drug–drug interactions.
    - Example agents: pramipexole (Mirapex), ropinirole (Requip).

VIII. Psychotherapeutic Agents

A. Antidepressants

1. **General Properties**
   - All agents are considered equally effective in treating depression, but their side effect profiles and tolerability vary significantly.
   - Patients should receive a trial of appropriate length before being switched to a second agent; trial duration varies by class of antidepressant.
   - Discontinuation of treatment versus life-long therapy should be based on the patient's history.

2. **Tricyclic Compounds**
   - Mechanism of action: inhibits reuptake of norepinephrine and serotonin.
   - Therapeutic uses: depression, insomnia, neuropathy.
   - Monitor: complete blood count, liver function tests, signs of infection, possibly electrocardiogram, signs of clinical improvement.

- Common adverse effects: anticholinergic effects, sedation, weight gain.
- Contraindications/cautions: avoid use with MAOIs, seizure history, cardiovascular history especially recent MI; use with caution in elderly individuals; avoid abrupt withdrawal.
- Example agents: amitriptyline (Elavil), amoxapine (Asendin), clomipramine (Anafranil), desipramine (Norpramin), doxepin (Sinequan), imipramine (Tofranil), nortriptyline (Pamelor).

3. **Tetracyclic Compounds**
   - Mechanism of action: enhance central noradrenergic and serotonergic activity.
   - Therapeutic uses: depression.
   - Monitor: blood pressure, weight, signs of infection (rare).
   - Common adverse effects: sedation, dry mouth, constipation, weight gain, agranulocytosis.
   - Contraindications/cautions: drug–drug interactions, seizure history, avoid use with MAOIs, caution with history of cardiac problems.
   - Example agents: mirtazapine (Remeron).

4. **Trazodone (Desyrel)**
   - Mechanism of action: unknown; has effects on serotonin uptake and serotonin precursor.
   - Therapeutic uses: depression, insomnia; comparative efficacy is generally lower when compared with other classes of antidepressants; thus primary use for trazodone is for the treatment of insomnia.
   - Monitor: signs of clinical improvement.
   - Common adverse effects: priapism, hypotension, sedation, dizziness, blurred vision, syncope, dry mouth.
   - Contraindications/cautions: caution with history of cardiac problems, drug–drug interactions.

5. **Bupropion Hydrochloride**
   - Mechanism of action: inhibits weakly the neuronal uptake of dopamine and norepinephrine.
   - Therapeutic uses: depression, smoking cessation.
   - Monitor: blood pressure, weight, signs of clinical improvement.
   - Common adverse effects: seizures, agitation, anxiety, restlessness, weight loss, hypertension, headache.
   - Contraindications/cautions: seizure disorder, avoid abrupt withdrawal, bulimia, anorexia nervosa, MAOIs, patients undergoing drug or alcohol detoxification.
   - Example agent: bupropion (Wellbutrin, Zyban—marketed for smoking cessation).

6. **Venlafaxine**
   - Mechanism of action: potentiates the neurotransmitter activity in the CNS; inhibits neuronal serotonin, norepinephrine, and dopamine reuptake.
   - Therapeutic uses: depression; anxiety disorders.
   - Monitor: blood pressure, weight, electrolytes.
   - Common adverse effects: hypertension, weight loss, anxiety, agitation, dizziness insomnia, hyponatremia.
   - Contraindications/cautions: avoid use with MAOIs, use caution in renal and hepatic impairment, seizure history; avoid abrupt discontinuation.
   - Example agent: venlafaxine (Effexor, Effexor XR).

7. **Selective Serotonin-Reuptake Inhibitors**
   - Mechanism of action: inhibit the CNS reuptake of serotonin.
   - Therapeutic uses: depression; anxiety disorders.
   - Monitor: signs of clinical improvement, weight.
   - Common adverse effects: anxiety, nervousness, insomnia, serotonin syndrome, appetite and weight changes, sexual dysfunction.
   - Contraindications/cautions: MAOIs, drug–drug interactions.
   - Example agents: citalopram (Celexa), escitalopram (Lexapro), fluoxetine (Prozac), paroxetine (Paxil), sertraline (Zoloft), fluvoxamine (Luvox).

8. **MAOIs**
   - Mechanism of action: block breakdown of neurotransmitters by inhibiting monoamine oxidase.
   - Therapeutic uses: depression (refractory).
   - Monitor: blood pressure.
   - Common adverse effect: hypertensive crisis.
   - Contraindications/cautions: must avoid tyramine-containing foods.
   - Example agents: phenelzine (Nardil), tranylcypromine (Parnate), isocarboxazid (Marplan).

B. **Antipsychotics**
   1. **General Properties**
      - Antipsychotic medications are used in the treatment of a wide variety of psychiatric disorders and problems.
      - Agents differ significantly in their side effect profiles and tolerability, several agents carry black-box warnings.
      - Agents are typically classified as a classic or atypical antipsychotic based on chemical structure and profile of activity.
      - There are concerns about the development of tardive dyskinesia with long-term use.
      - Patient-specific information may help determine the best agent for a particular patient.
   2. **Phenothiazines**
      - Mechanism of action: related to the inhibition of dopamine receptors.
      - Therapeutic uses: psychotic disorders.
      - Monitor: electrocardiogram, blood pressure, clinical response.
      - Common adverse effects: extrapyramidal symptoms, neuroleptic malignant syndrome, sedation, hypotension.

- Contraindications/cautions: QT abnormalities, cardiac arrhythmias.
- Example agents: chlorpromazine (Thorazine), fluphenazine (Prolixin), mesoridazine (Serentil), perphenazine (Trilafon), prochlorperazine (Compazine), trifluoperazine (Stelazine), thioridazine (Mellaril).

3. **Thioxanthenes**
   - Mechanism of action: exact mechanism unknown, effects related to antagonistic actions on receptors.
   - Therapeutic uses: schizophrenia.
   - Monitor: abnormal involuntary movement scale, akathisia, complete blood count, electrocardiogram, liver function tests, blood pressure, and heart rate.
   - Common adverse effects: extrapyramidal symptoms, sedation, orthostatic hypotension.
   - Contraindications/cautions: consider electrocardiogram in cardiac patients, caution with elderly patients.
   - Example agents: thiothixene (Navane).

4. **Phenylbutylpiperadines**
   - Mechanism of action: exact mechanism unknown, effects related to antagonistic actions on receptors.
   - Therapeutic uses: psychotic disorders.
   - Monitor: abnormal involuntary movement scale, complete blood count, liver function tests.
   - Common adverse effects: extrapyramidal symptoms, hypotension.
   - Contraindications/cautions: Parkinson disease, anticoagulant use, severe cardiovascular disorders.
   - Example agents: haloperidol (Haldol).

5. **Dihydroindolones**
   - Mechanism of action: exact mechanism unknown, effects related to antagonistic actions on receptors.
   - Therapeutic uses: schizophrenia.
   - Monitor: liver function tests, observe for early symptoms of tardive dyskinesia/dystonia.
   - Common adverse effects: extrapyramidal symptoms, sedation.
   - Contraindications/cautions: allergy to sulfites, history of breast cancer, urinary retention, glaucoma, liver impairment.
   - Example agents: molindone (Moban).

6. **Dibenzapines**
   - Mechanism of action: exact mechanism unknown, effects related to antagonistic actions on receptors.
   - Therapeutic uses: psychotic disorders.
   - Monitor: weight, blood pressure, blood sugar, lipid profile, clinical response, complete blood count, liver function test, electrocardiogram.
   - Common adverse effects: extrapyramidal symptoms, increase prolactin levels, hyperglycemia, hyperlipidemia, increased weight.
   - Contraindications/cautions: diabetes.

- Clozapine risks: agranulocytosis, seizures, myocarditis, special monitoring complete blood count.
- Example agents: clozapine (Clozaril), loxapine (Loxitane), olanzapine (Zyprexa), quetiapine (Seroquel).

7. **Benzisoxazoles**
   - Mechanism of action: exact mechanism unknown, effects related to antagonistic actions on receptors.
   - Therapeutic uses: psychotic disorders.
   - Monitor: complete blood count, liver function test, electrocardiogram, weight, blood pressure.
   - Common adverse effects: extrapyramidal symptoms, increased prolactin levels, sedation.
   - Contraindications/cautions: QT abnormalities, cardiac arrhythmias, cardiovascular or cerebrovascular problems, Parkinson disease.
   - Example agents: risperidone (Risperdal), ziprasidone (Geodon).

8. **Quinolinones**
   - Mechanism of action: exact mechanism unknown, effects related to antagonistic actions on receptors.
   - Therapeutic uses: psychotic disorders.
   - Monitor: blood pressure, heart rate, blood chemistry.
   - Common adverse effects: extrapyramidal symptoms, agitation, insomnia, dizziness.
   - Contraindications/cautions: dehydration, Parkinson disease, elderly, cardiovascular or cerebrovascular problems.
   - Example agents: aripiprazole (Abilify).

9. **Lithium**
   - Mechanism of action: may be a result of increased norepinephrine reuptake and serotonin receptor sensitivity.
   - Therapeutic use: mania.
   - Monitor: serum creatinine, complete blood count, urinalysis, sodium, potassium, electrocardiogram, thyroid function test, lithium levels, hydration status (instruct patients to drink 8 to 12 glasses of water a day).
   - Common adverse effects: hypothyroidism, sodium depletion, electroencephalogram changes, neurologic toxicities, GI problems, headache.
   - Contraindications/cautions: renal failure, elderly, dehydration.
   - Agents: lithium (Eskalith, Lithobid, Lithonate).

C. Sedative/Hypnotics/Anxiolytics
1. **General Properties**
   - These agents are used both to facilitate sleep and for their sedative effects.
   - Each of the agents has a specific duration of action and approved indications.

2. **Benzodiazepines**
   - Mechanism of action: potentiate the effects of GABA by binding to the benzodiazepine receptor sites.
   - Therapeutic uses: anxiety disorders, sedation, insomnia, anticonvulsant, skeletal muscle relaxant.
   - Monitor: clinical response, excessive sedation, respiratory function, symptoms of drug abuse or dependence.
   - Common adverse effects: sedation, dizziness, depression, dependency, transient memory impairment, headache.
   - Contraindications/cautions: potential for abuse, dependency, sleep apnea, glaucoma, other CNS depressants, alcohol abuse.
   - Example agents: alprazolam (Xanax), clorazepate (Tranxene), chlordiazepoxide (Librium), clonazepam (Klonopin), diazepam (Valium), lorazepam (Ativan), oxazepam (Serax).
   - **NOTE:** The nonbenzodiazepine hypnotics such as zaleplon (Sonata), eszopiclone (Lunesta), and zolpidem (Ambien) that are indicated for insomnia have similar safety and efficacy profiles within patients with sleep disorders.

3. **Chloral Hydrate (Aquachloral)**
   - Mechanism of action: unknown; causes mild cerebral depression and deep sleep.
   - Therapeutic uses: nocturnal sedation.
   - Monitor: effectiveness, signs of abuse, hangover effect during the day.
   - Common adverse effects: dizziness, drowsiness; potential for abuse, dependency, efficacy may decrease over time.
   - Contraindications/cautions: hepatic or renal impairment, severe cardiac disease, gastritis.

IX. Analgesics

A. General Overview
   - A variety of agents are available to treat pain.

B. Nonsteroidal Anti-inflammatory Drugs
   - Mechanism of action: inhibition of prostaglandin synthesis by blocking both cyclooxygenase isoenzymes, COX-1 and COX-2 (nonselective) or COX-2 only (selective).
   - Therapeutic uses: pain.
   - Monitor: complete blood count, chemistry profile, occult blood test, liver function test.
   - Common adverse effects: GI ulcers, bleeding.
   - Contraindications/cautions: active GI bleed, renal insufficiency, anticoagulant use, aspirin allergy, liver dysfunction, asthma.
   - Example agents: etodolac (Lodine), ibuprofen (Motrin), indomethacin (Indocin), ketoprofen (Orudis), ketorolac (Toradol), naproxen (Naprosyn), nabumetone (Relafen), piroxicam (Feldene).

- **NOTE:** Agents such as celecoxib (Celebrex) block only COX-2 mainly used as AN ANALGESIC; therefore, the agents provide less GI toxicity. In 2005, Vioxx and Bextra were withdrawn from the market because of cardiovascular complications.

C. Opioids
   - Mechanism of action: activity at the opioid receptors in the CNS.
   - Therapeutic use: analgesia.
   - Monitor: clinical response, signs of abuse.
   - Common adverse effects: sedation, dizziness, constipation, N/V, allergic reactions, addiction.
   - Contraindications/cautions: potential for abuse, dependency, other CNS depressants, alcohol abuse, paralytic ileus, or GI obstruction.
   - Example agents: fentanyl patch (Duragesic), hydromorphone (Dilaudid), methadone (Dolophine), morphine (MS Contin), oxycodone (Roxicodone, OxyContin), hydrocodone (Hycodan), propoxyphene (Darvon-N) have been taken off the market because of cardiotoxicity.

D. Opioid-like agents
1. **Trahadol**
   - Centrally acting opioid analgesic, weak agonist actions on v opioid receptor and modulation with serotonin and norepinephrine.
   - Therapeutic uses: tramadol similar to Codeine to treat moderately severe pain.
   - Common adverse effects: N/V, sweating, itching, drowsiness and constipation.
   - Examples: tramadol (Ultram).
2. **Tapentadol**
   - Centrally acting analgesic, working at the v receptor and has properties of norepinephrine reuptake inhibitor.
   - Therapeutic uses: treatment of moderate to severe acute pain.
   - Common adverse effects: nausea, dizziness, constipation, and sedation.
   - Schedule II drug, same category as morphine.
   - Examples: tapentadol (Nucynta).
   - **NOTE:** Many of the opioids are available commercially in combination products containing aspirin, acetaminophen, or an NSAID.

X. Pulmonary Agents

A. Asthma and Chronic Obstructive Pulmonary Disease
1. **Quick-Relief Agents**
   a. **Short-acting β_2-agonists**
      - Mechanism of action: relax airway smooth muscle by stimulating β_2-receptors.
      - Therapeutic uses: bronchodilation (asthma, COPD, exercise-induced bronchospasm).

- Common adverse effects: palpitations, tachycardia, tremor, nervousness, headache, N/V.
- Contraindications/cautions: cardiac arrhythmias, angina, organic brain damage, narrow-angle glaucoma.
- Example agents: albuterol (Ventolin), levalbuterol (Xopenex), metaproterenol (Alupent).

b. Anticholinergics
- Mechanism of action: inhibit vagally mediated reflexes by antagonizing the effects of ACH resulting in bronchodilation.
- Therapeutic uses: additive benefits to inhaled β_2-agonists in severe exacerbations or an alternative bronchodilator in patients who do not tolerate inhaled β_2-agonists.
- Common adverse effects: dry mouth, headache, dyspnea, bronchitis, upper respiratory tract infection.
- Contraindications/cautions: hypersensitivity to soya lecithin or related food products such as soybean or peanut (inhalation aerosol).
- Example agents: ipratropium bromide (Atrovent); tiotropium bromide (Spiriva) is indicated for the maintenance of symptoms in COPD patients.

c. Systemic corticosteroids
- Mechanism of action: reduce pulmonary inflammation.
- Therapeutic uses: bronchial asthma (including status asthmaticus).
- Common adverse effects: weight gain, increased appetite, mood swings, weakness, blurred vision, slow healing of cuts and bruises, hyperglycemia, moon face, stomach irritation.
- Contraindications/cautions: systemic fungal infections, IM use in idiopathic thrombocytopenic purpura, administration of live vaccines in patients receiving immunosuppressive doses, use of caution with prolonged therapy due to adrenal suppression, ocular effects (glaucoma, cataracts), peptic ulcer disease, osteoporosis and fluid/electrolyte imbalances.
- Example agents: prednisone (Deltasone), methylprednisolone (Medrol).

2. Long-Term Control Agents
a. Inhaled corticosteroids
- Mechanism of action: reduce pulmonary inflammation.
- Therapeutic uses: asthma.
- Common adverse effects: cough, sore throat, stomach irritation, upper respiratory tract infections, nasal congestion.
- Contraindications/cautions: relief of acute bronchospasm, primary treatment of status asthmaticus or other acute episodes of asthma when intensive measures are required; use

caution when withdrawing from oral steroids, monitor children for reduction in growth velocity; and rare instances of glaucoma, increased intraocular pressure, and cataracts have been reported.
- Example agents: budesonide (Pulmicort), flunisolide (AeroBid), fluticasone (Flovent).

b. Long-acting β_2-agonists
- Mechanism of action: relax airway smooth muscle by stimulating β_2-receptors.
- Therapeutic uses: bronchodilation (asthma, COPD, exercise-induced bronchospasm); used in combination with another maintenance therapy, such as an inhaled corticosteroid, by patients with asthma because of increased asthma-related deaths in studies with long-acting β_2 agonist agents as monotherapy.
- Common adverse effects: palpitations, tachycardia, tremor, nervousness, headache, N/V.
- Contraindications/cautions: cardiac arrhythmias, angina, organic brain damage, narrow-angle glaucoma; use of a long-acting β_2 agonist without current long-term asthma treatment (such as an inhaled corticosteroid).
- Example agents: formoterol (Foradil), salmeterol (Serevent).

c. Methylxanthines
- Mechanism of action: directly relax the smooth muscle of the bronchi and pulmonary blood vessels. The exact mode of action is unclear.
- Therapeutic uses: asthma, COPD.
- Common adverse effects: N/V, palpitations, irritability, insomnia, headache.
- Contraindications/cautions: active peptic ulcer disease, seizure disorders, cardiac arrhythmias.
- Example agents: theophylline, aminophylline.

d. Leukotriene modifiers
- Mechanism of action: inhibit inflammation, edema, mucus secretion, and bronchoconstriction.
- Therapeutic uses: asthma, seasonal allergic rhinitis.
- Common adverse effects: headache, dyspepsia, nausea, liver enzyme elevations, hypersensitivity reactions.
- Contraindications/cautions: acute liver disease or transaminase elevations greater than or equal to three times the upper limit of normal; patients instructed not to use for acute asthma attacks.
- Example agents: montelukast (Singulair), zafirlukast (Accolate), zileuton (Zyflo).

e. Mast cell stabilizers
- Mechanism of action: reduce bronchial inflammation by inhibiting the release of mediators,

histamine, and SRS-A (the slow-reacting substance of anaphylaxis, a leukotriene).
- Therapeutic uses: asthma, prevention of bronchospasm, allergic rhinitis.
- Common adverse effects: cough, dysgeusia, headache, sneezing, nasal congestion.
- Contraindications/cautions: agents have no role in acute asthma and may cause bronchospasm.
- Example agents: cromolyn sodium (Intal), nedocromil sodium (Tilade).

f. Monoclonal antibody agent
- Mechanism of action: inhibits the binding of immunoglobulin E to the surface of mast cells and basophils, and therefore limiting the release of mediators of the allergic response.
- Therapeutic use: asthma.
- Common adverse effects: site reactions, viral infections, upper respiratory tract function, sinusitis, headache, pharyngitis.
- Contraindications/cautions: use has been associated with malignant neoplasms (rare), and patients should be observed after injection for possible anaphylaxis reactions.
- Example agent: omalizumab (Xolair).

XI. Gastrointestinal Agents

A. Gastrointestinal

1. Histamine H₂ Antagonists
- Mechanism of action: inhibit gastric acid secretion by blocking the histamine-2 receptors in the gastric parietal cells.
- Therapeutic uses: duodenal ulcers, gastric ulcers, gastroesophageal reflux disease (GERD), erosive esophagitis, pathologic hypersecretory conditions, upper GI bleeding, heartburn.
- Common adverse effects: drowsiness, confusion, rash, constipation, psychosis, headache.
- Contraindications/cautions: use with caution in patients with renal/hepatic dysfunction.
- Example agents: cimetidine (Tagamet), ranitidine (Zantac), nizatidine (Axid), famotidine (Pepcid).

2. Proton Pump Inhibitors
- Mechanism of action: suppress gastric acid secretion by specifically inhibiting the hydrogen/potassium (H^+/K^+) ATPase enzyme at the secretory surface of the gastric parietal cell; this inhibition blocks the final step of acid production.
- Therapeutic uses: duodenal ulcers, gastric ulcers, GERD, pathologic hypersecretory conditions.
- Common adverse effects: dizziness, rash, headache, nausea, diarrhea, upper respiratory tract infection.
- Contraindications/cautions: use with caution in patients with hepatic dysfunction.
- Example agents: omeprazole (Prilosec), esomeprazole (Nexium), lansoprazole (Prevacid),

dexlansoprazole (Dexilant), rabeprazole (Aciphex), pantoprazole (Protonix).

B. Antidiarrheals
- Mechanism of action: slow intestinal motility.
- Therapeutic uses: acute diarrhea, chronic diarrhea.
- Common adverse effects: abdominal discomfort, dry skin, dry mouth and mucous membranes, constipation, sedation, rash, tinnitus (bismuth only), blackened tongue (bismuth only).
- Contraindications/cautions: obstructive jaundice, bloody diarrhea, diarrhea associated with pseudomembranous enterocolitis or enterotoxin-producing bacteria, body temperature >101° F; monitor for dehydration.
- Example agents: diphenoxylate with atropine (Lomotil), loperamide (Imodium A-D), bismuth subsalicylate (Pepto-Bismol, Kaopectate).

C. Laxatives

1. Saline Agents
- Mechanism of action: attract/retain water in the intestinal lumen, which increases intraluminal pressure.
- Therapeutic uses: constipation, rectal/bowel examinations.
- Common adverse effects: diarrhea, N/V, perianal irritation, fainting, bloating, flatulence, cramps.
- Contraindications/cautions: signs/symptoms of appendicitis, fecal impaction, intestinal obstruction, undiagnosed abdominal pain. Do not use in patients with megacolon, bowel obstruction, imperforate anus, or CHF.
- Example agents: magnesium hydroxide (milk of magnesia); monobasic sodium phosphate, and dibasic sodium phosphate (Fleet Phospho-soda).

2. Stimulant or Irritant Agents
- Mechanism of action: exhibit direct action on intestinal mucosa or nerve plexus.
- Therapeutic uses: constipation, rectal/bowel examinations.
- Common adverse effects: diarrhea, N/V, perianal irritation, fainting, bloating, flatulence, cramps, urine discoloration.
- Contraindications/cautions: signs/symptoms of appendicitis, fecal impaction, intestinal obstruction, undiagnosed abdominal pain.
- Example agents: sennosides (Ex-Lax, Senokot), bisacodyl (Dulcolax).

3. Bulk-Producing Agents
- Mechanism of action: retain water in the stool to increase bulk-stimulating peristalsis.
- Therapeutic uses: constipation, irritable bowel syndrome, diverticular disease.
- Common adverse effects: diarrhea, N/V, perianal irritation, fainting, bloating, flatulence, cramps.

- Contraindications/cautions: signs/symptoms of appendicitis, fecal impaction, intestinal obstruction, undiagnosed abdominal pain.
- Example agents: psyllium (Metamucil), polycarbophil (FiberCon).

4. **Emollient Agents**
   - Mechanism of action: retard colonic absorption of fecal water and soften the stool.
   - Therapeutic uses: constipation, soften stool following surgery/MI, fecal impaction.
   - Common adverse effects: diarrhea, N/V, perianal irritation, fainting, bloating, flatulence, cramps, anal seepage, perianal discomfort.
   - Contraindications/cautions: signs/symptoms of appendicitis, fecal impaction, intestinal obstruction, undiagnosed abdominal pain, concurrent docusate sodium administration (increase mineral oil absorption).
   - Example agent: mineral oil.

5. **Fecal Softeners/Surfactant Agents**
   - Mechanism of action: facilitate admixture of fat and water to soften stool.
   - Therapeutic uses: constipation, soften stool following surgery/MI.
   - Common adverse effects: diarrhea, N/V, perianal irritation, fainting, bloating, flatulence, cramps.
   - Contraindications/cautions: signs/symptoms of appendicitis, fecal impaction, intestinal obstruction, undiagnosed abdominal pain, concurrent mineral oil administration (increase mineral oil absorption).
   - Example agent: docusate sodium (Colace).

6. **Hyperosmotic Agents**
   - Mechanism of action: retain fluid in the colon, lower the pH and increase the colonic peristalsis.
   - Therapeutic use: constipation.
   - Common adverse effects: diarrhea, N/V, perianal irritation, fainting, bloating, flatulence, cramps.
   - Contraindications/cautions: signs/symptoms of appendicitis, fecal impaction, intestinal obstruction, undiagnosed abdominal pain, use caution in brittle diabetic patients and monitor electrolytes in elderly patients on long-term therapy (>6 months).
   - Example agents: glycerin, lactulose.

D. Antiemetic Agents

1. **Antidopaminergics**
   - Mechanism of action: block the effect of dopamine in the vomiting center of the brain.
   - Therapeutic uses: N/V, motion sickness.
   - Common adverse effects: drowsiness, diarrhea, restlessness.
   - Contraindications/cautions: comatose or greatly depressed state, blood dyscrasias, bone-marrow depression, preexisting liver disease; use with

caution in patients with seizure disorder, cardiovascular disease (history of MI, heart failure, ischemic heart disease, conduction abnormalities). Monitor for any signs/symptoms of tardive dyskinesia or extrapyramidal symptoms.
   - Example agents: prochlorperazine (Compazine), metoclopramide (Reglan).

2. **Antihistamines/Anticholinergics**
   - Mechanism of action: act on the brain center that controls N/V and dizziness; act on nerves affecting balance in the inner ear (scopolamine).
   - Therapeutic uses: N/V, motion sickness, vertigo.
   - Common adverse effects: drowsiness, constipation, blurry vision, dry mouth, nose, or throat.
   - Contraindications/cautions: narrow-angle glaucoma, symptomatic prostatic hypertrophy, bladder neck obstruction, MAOI use.
   - Example agents: diphenhydramine (Benadryl), meclizine (Antivert), scopolamine (TransdermScop).

3. **5-Hydroxytryptamine (5-HT3) Antagonists**
   - Mechanism of action: selective blockade of 5-HT3 receptors located in the vagal nerve terminals, GI tract, and centrally in the chemoreceptor trigger zone thus antagonizing nausea and emesis.
   - Therapeutic uses: prevention of N/V associated with cancer chemotherapy, postoperative sequelae, or radiotherapy.
   - Common adverse effects: constipation, fever, headache, diarrhea.
   - Contraindications/cautions: markedly prolonged QTc or AV block II to III (dolasetron); patients receiving class I or III antiarrhythmic agents (dolasetron).
   - Example agents: dolasetron (Anzemet), granisetron (Kytril), ondansetron (Zofran), palonosetron (Aloxi).

E. Benign Prostatic Hyperplasia

1. **α_1-Adrenergic Blockers**
   - Mechanism of action: block α_1-adrenergic receptors located in the prostate and bladder neck reducing urethral resistance, improving urine flow and BPH symptoms.
   - Therapeutic uses: hypertension, BPH.
   - Common adverse effects: hypotension, dizziness, somnolence, headache.
   - Contraindications/cautions: "first-dose" hypotension, priapism.
   - Example agents: terazosin (Hytrin), doxazosin (Cardura), tamsulosin (Flomax).

2. **Androgen Hormone Inhibitor**
   - Mechanism of action: inhibits enzyme known as type II 5-α reductase that converts testosterone into dihydrotestosterone; this inhibition decreases the size of theprostatein patients with BPH.
   - Therapeutic uses: BPH, androgenic alopecia.

- Common adverse effects: erectile dysfunction, decreased libido, breast tenderness and enlargement.
- Contraindications/cautions: use caution in patients with hepatic dysfunction and monitor for prostate cancer (e.g., digital rectal examinations).
- Example agent: finasteride (Proscar).

XII. Endocrine Agents

A. Antidiabetic Agents

1. Insulin

- Mechanism of action: stimulates peripheral glucose uptake and inhibits hepatic glucose production; this mechanism is based on each insulin's individual time to onset and duration of activity.
- Therapeutic uses: diabetes mellitus (DM) (types I and II), hyperkalemia.
- Common adverse effects: hypoglycemia, injection site reactions, lipodystrophy.
- Contraindications/cautions: do not use during episodes of hypoglycemia, use caution when changing insulin and when patients become ill.
- Example agents: insulin regular (Novolin R, Humulin R), isophane insulin suspension (Novolin N, Humulin N), insulin lispro (Humalog), insulin aspart (Novolog), insulin detemir (Levemir), insulin glargine (Lantus), insulin glulisine (Apidra).

2. Sulfonylureas

- Mechanism of action: stimulate pancreatic β cells to release insulin.
- Therapeutic use: DM (type II).
- Common adverse effects: hypoglycemia, diarrhea, weakness, nausea, allergic skin reactions.
- Contraindications/cautions: diabetes complicated by ketoacidosis with or without coma, sole therapy of type I DM, diabetes complicated by pregnancy, use caution in patients with renal/hepatic dysfunction.
- Example agents: glyburide (Diaβeta), glipizide (Glucotrol), glimepiride (Amaryl).

3. α-Glucosidase Inhibitors

- Mechanism of action: delay the absorption of complex carbohydrates, thereby resulting in a smaller rise in blood glucose concentration after meals.
- Therapeutic uses: DM (type II).
- Common adverse effects: flatulence, diarrhea, abdominal pain, elevated serum transaminase levels.
- Contraindications/cautions: diabetic ketoacidosis or cirrhosis, inflammatory bowel disease, colonic ulceration, partial intestinal obstruction or predisposition to intestinal obstruction, chronic intestinal diseases associated with marked disorders of digestion or absorption or with conditions that may deteriorate as a result of increased gas formation in the intestine.

- Example agents: acarbose (Precose), miglitol (Glyset).

4. Biguanides

- Mechanism of action: decrease hepatic glucose production and intestinal absorption of glucose, and improve insulin sensitivity.
- Therapeutic use: DM (type II).
- Common adverse effects: diarrhea, N/V, flatulence, abdominal discomfort.
- Contraindications/cautions: renal disease or dysfunction (serum creatinine level >1.5 mg/dL in males or >1.4 mg/dL in females); hepatic disease; acute MI; septicemia; cardiovascular shock; CHF requiring pharmacologic treatment; discontinue use of metformin before undergoing radiologic studies involving administration of iodinated contrast materials, reevaluate renal function 48 hours after procedure before reinstituting metformin; acute or chronic metabolic acidosis, including diabetic ketoacidosis with or without coma. Patients should be informed about the risk of lactic acidosis, its symptoms and conditions that predispose to its development; monitor renal function closely.
- Example agent: metformin (Glucophage).

5. Meglitinides

- Mechanism of action: nonsulfonylurea agent that stimulates the release of insulin from the pancreas.
- Therapeutic use: DM (type II).
- Common adverse effects: hypoglycemia, nausea, upper respiratory tract infection, headache.
- Contraindications/cautions: diabetic ketoacidosis with or without coma; type I diabetes.
- Example agents: nateglinide (Starlix), repaglinide (Prandin).

6. Thiazolidinediones

- Mechanism of action: improve sensitivity to insulin in muscle and adipose tissue and inhibit hepatic glucose production.
- Therapeutic uses: DM (type II).
- Common adverse effects: edema, weight gain (edema and weight gain can be precursor to rapid development of heart failure), myalgia, fatigue.
- Contraindications/cautions: not recommended in patients with symptomatic heart failure; is contraindicated in patients with NYHA heart failure class III or IV; use caution in patients with edema (e.g., CHF); liver enzymes must be monitored.
- Example agents: pioglitazone (Actos), rosiglitazone (Avandia).

7. Dipeptidyl Peptidase-4 Inhibitors

- Mechanism of action: slow the inactivation of incretin hormones released from the intestine; this inactivation allows incretin to remain active longer, thereby increasing insulin release and decreasing glucagon levels.

- Therapeutic uses: DM (type II).
- Common adverse effects: nasopharyngitis, headache, upper respiratory infection, hypoglycemia.
- Contraindications/cautions: monitor for development of pancreatitis; consider dose adjustment in moderate or severe renal impairment; assess for hypersensitivity reactions.
- Examples: sitagliptin (Januvia), saxagliptin (Onglyza), linagliptin (Tradjenta).

B. Oral Contraceptives

- Mechanism of action: inhibit ovulation by suppressing gonadotropins, follicle-stimulating hormone, luteinizing hormone; thicken cervical mucus to inhibit sperm penetration, slow movement of the ovum through the fallopian tubes, and alter the endometrium.
- Therapeutic uses: contraception, emergency contraception, acne vulgaris.
- Common adverse effects: breast tenderness, headache, N/V, breakthrough bleeding, spotting, edema, cramping.
- Contraindications/cautions: thrombophlebitis; thromboembolic disorders; history of deep vein thrombophlebitis; cerebral vascular disease; MI; CAD; known or suspected breast carcinoma or estrogen-dependent neoplasia; carcinoma of endometrium; hepatic adenomas/carcinomas; undiagnosed abnormal genital bleeding; known or suspected pregnancy; acute liver disease; cholestatic jaundice of pregnancy/jaundice with prior pill use; use with caution in patients who smoke and those with gallbladder disease.
- Example agents: ethinyl estradiol/norethindrone (Ortho-Novum), ethinyl estradiol/levonorgestrel (Triphasil), norgestrel (Ovrette), levonorgestrel (Plan B).

C. Thyroid Disorders

1. Hypothyroidism Agents

- Mechanism of action: exact mechanism is not known; however, it is believed that the agents listed below restore thyroid hormone that the body may be lacking.
- Therapeutic uses: hypothyroidism, pituitary TSH suppressant, diagnostic use, myxedema coma/precoma (injection only).
- Common adverse effects: palpitations, tachycardia, tremors, headache, weight loss, increased appetite, excessive sweating, muscle weakness.
- Contraindications/cautions: uncorrected adrenal cortical insufficiency; untreated thyrotoxicosis; patients with acute MI; untreated subclinical hypothyroidism; use caution when switching from one brand to the next.
- Example agents: thyroid desiccated (Armour Thyroid), levothyroxine sodium (Synthroid), liothyronine sodium (Cytomel).

2. Hyperthyroidism Agents

- Mechanism of action: inhibit the synthesis of thyroid hormones.
- Therapeutic use: hyperthyroidism.
- Common adverse effects: rash, pruritus, paresthesias, agranulocytosis (see Contraindications/cautions).
- Contraindications/cautions: monitor for hepatotoxicity with propylthiouracil; consider propylthiouracil in pregnant patients as methimazole is associated with fetal abnormalities; monitor patients closely for possible bone marrow suppression—white blood cell count for at the least the first 3 months of therapy, then follow closely for any other signs/symptoms of suppression (e.g., hay fever, sore throat, skin eruptions, fever, headache, or general malaise).
- Example agents: methimazole (Tapazole), propylthiouracil.

D. Hyperlipidemia

1. Bile Acid Sequestrant Agents

- Mechanism of action: bind bile acids in the intestine to form an insoluble complex excreted in the feces. The increased fecal loss of bile acids leads to increased oxidation of cholesterol to bile acids and a decrease in low-density lipoproteins (LDL) and serum cholesterol levels.
- Therapeutic uses: hyperlipidemia, biliary obstruction.
- Common adverse effects: constipation, abdominal pain, cramping, headache, bloating, flatulence.
- Contraindications/cautions: agents may interfere with normal fat absorption and digestion and may prevent absorption of fat-soluble vitamins such as A, D, E, K, and folic acid.
- Example agents: cholestyramine (Questran), colestipol (Colestid), colesevelam (WelChol).

2. HMG Co-A Reductase Inhibitors

- Mechanism of action: inhibit cholesterol biosynthesis by inhibiting the enzyme HMG Co-A reductase.
- Therapeutic uses: hyperlipidemia, hypertriglyceridemia, primary prevention of cardiovascular disease in patients with multiple risk factors, secondary prevention of cardiovascular events in patients with clinically evident heart disease.
- Common adverse effects: myalgia, dyspepsia, diarrhea, arthralgia.
- Contraindications/cautions: active liver disease or unexplained persistent elevated liver function tests, pregnancy (all statins are category X), lactation; monitor liver function tests as recommended by each product.
- Example agents: lovastatin (Mevacor), simvastatin (Zocor), pravastatin (Pravachol), fluvastatin

(Lescol), atorvastatin (Lipitor), rosuvastatin (Crestor), pitavastatin (Livalo).

3. **Fibric Acid Derivatives**
   - Mechanism of action: inhibit peripheral lipolysis and decrease the hepatic extraction of free fatty acids, thus reducing hepatic triglycerides production.
   - Therapeutic uses: hypertriglyceridemia, reduce coronary heart disease risk.
   - Common adverse effects: fatigue, dyspepsia, abdominal pain, taste perversion, diarrhea.
   - Contraindications/cautions: hepatic or severe renal dysfunction, primary biliary cirrhosis, pre-existing gallbladder disease; monitor for development of pancreatitis; use with caution in patients who are concurrently receiving HMG Co-A reductase inhibitors as skeletal muscle effects may be enhanced.
   - Example agents: gemfibrozil (Lopid), fenofibrate (Tricor, Trilipix).

4. **Niacin (Nicotinic Acid)**
   - Mechanism of action: decreases serum levels of apolipoprotein B-100, the major component of very low-density lipoprotein (VLDL) and LDL fractions; however, the exact mechanism is not entirely understood.
   - Therapeutic uses: hyperlipidemia, niacin deficiency, pellagra.
   - Common adverse effects: flushing, headache, pruritus, GI distress, activation of peptic ulcer disease, hyperuricemia, hyperglycemia.
   - Contraindications/cautions: hepatic dysfunction, active peptic ulcer, atrial bleeding, frequently monitor liver function tests due to its ability to cause hepatotoxicity; monitor for development of myopathy, especially with concurrent HMG-CoA reductase inhibitors; use caution when switching from immediate-release to extended-release products, as severe hepatoxicity may result because of nonequivalency of dosage forms.
   - Example products: extended-release niacin (Niaspan).

5. **Cholesterol Absorption Inhibitor**
   - Mechanism of action: acts at the brush border of the small intestine to inhibit the absorption of cholesterol.
   - Therapeutic uses: hyperlipidemia (often in combination with a HMG Co-A reductase inhibitor).
   - Common adverse effects: diarrhea, abdominal pain, back pain, arthralgia, sinusitis.
   - Contraindications/cautions: same as HMG Co-A reductase inhibitors when used together; use not recommended in moderate/severe hepatic impairment.
   - Example agent: ezetimibe (Zetia).

XIII. Anti-infective Agents

A. General Properties
- Anti-infective agents take advantage of unique features of bacteria and viruses to selectively destroy those organisms while causing minimal toxicity to the host.
- Resistance to anti-infective agents is a major clinical concern.
- Risk of superinfection is a concern (e.g., yeast infections and pseudomembranous colitis).
- Common adverse effects include allergic reactions and organ-specific toxicity of certain agents.

B. Antibacterial Agents
1. **Cell Wall Synthesis Inhibitors**
   a. **Mechanism of action**
      - Inhibit synthesis of cell walls, which are unique to bacteria; mammalian cells have membranes, not cell walls.
   b. **Spectrum of activity**
      - Penicillin G: gram-positive organisms, *Streptococcus, Pneumococcus, Meningococcus,* anthrax, *Clostridium, Bacteroides, Neisseria.*
      - Ampicillin and amoxicillin: broad spectrum, including gram-positive and gram-negative organisms including *Escherichia coli, Salmonella, Haemophilus influenzae, Listeria,* and gram-positive organisms susceptible to penicillin G.
      - Nafcillin, oxacillin: penicillinase resistant, used in cases of resistance to other penicillins, particularly *Staphylococcus aureus.*
      - Ticarcillin and piperacillin: effective against *Pseudomonas aeruginosa,* used in combination with β-lactamase inhibitor to decrease resistance (e.g., ticarcillin + clavulanic acid—Timentin; piperacillin + tazobactam—Zosyn).
      - First-generation cephalosporins (cefazolin [Ancef], cephalexin [Keflex]): primarily useful against gram-positive organisms such as *Staphylococcus* and *Streptococcus.*
      - Second-generation cephalosporins (cefaclor [Ceclor], cefoxitin [Mefoxin]): increased gram-negative activity, includes *E. coli, Klebsiella, Proteus, H. influenzae.*
      - Third-generation cephalosporins (ceftazidime [Fortaz], ceftriaxone [Rocephin]): primarily gram-negative activity, includes *P. aeruginosa, Enterobacter,* and *Serratia.*
      - Fourth-generation cephalosporins (cefepime [Maxipime]): broad gram-positive and gram-negative activity, including resistance to β-lactamase.
      - Fifth-generation cephalosporins (ceftaroline [Teflaro]): effective versus selected *Staphylococcus* species (including MSSA in skin infections

only), selected *Streptococcus* species, and selected gram-negative organisms (*H. influenzae, Klebsiella, E. coli*).

- Monobactam (aztreonam [Azactam]): activity against gram-negative rods including *P. aeruginosa, Serratia*, and *Klebsiella*.
- Carbapenems (imipenem [Primaxin], meropenem [Merrem], ertapenem [Invanz]): broad spectrum including anaerobes, particularly useful in penicillin-resistant pneumococci and *Enterobacter*; imipenem administered with cilastatin to ensure clinical activity.
- Vancomycin: active against gram-positive organisms, particularly staphylococci, main use is against methicillin-resistant staphylococci (MRSA) and *Clostridium difficile*–caused diarrhea.

  c. **Common adverse effects**
  - Allergic reactions, nephrotoxicity (mainly penicillins and cephalosporins); disulfiram reaction (second-and third-generation cephalosporins); chills,fever, and Redman syndrome (vancomycin); nausea/vomiting with rapid infusion, headache (carbapenem).

  d. **Cautions**
  - Resistance with β-lactamase producing bacteria is common.

2. **Protein Synthesis Inhibitors**
  a. **Mechanism of action**
  - Bind to ribosomes and prevent protein synthesis, results in cell death or decreased replication.

  b. **Spectrum of activity**
  - Aminoglycosides: active against gram-negative enteric bacteria, in particular *E. coli, Proteus, Mirabilis, Klebsiella, Serratia*, and *Enterobacter*; commonly used in combination with penicillins to provide broad empiric coverage.
  - Tetracyclines: gram-positive and gram-negative coverage, including *Mycoplasma pneumoniae, Chlamydia, Rickettsia*, and Lyme disease.
  - Macrolides: active against gram-positive organisms, useful in Legionnaires disease, *M. pneumoniae, Chlamydia, Helicobacter pylori* (clarithromycin).
  - Chloramphenicol: broad spectrum including *Salmonella*, resistant *H. influenzae* meningitis.
  - Clindamycin: gram-positive anaerobic infections such as Bacteroides.

  c. **Common adverse effects**
  - Aminoglycosides: nephrotoxicity, ototoxicity, neuromuscular junction blockade (possible drug interaction with anesthetics and paralytics).
  - Tetracyclines: nausea, diarrhea, superinfections, photosensitivity, inhibition of bone growth and teeth discoloration, teratogenic.

- Macrolides: GI distress, hepatotoxicity, pseudomembranous colitis.
- Chloramphenicol: bone marrow suppression, gray-baby syndrome.
- Clindamycin: pseudomembranous colitis.

  d. **Cautions**
  - Aminoglycosides must be given parenterally, monitoring of plasma levels is required to prevent toxicity; certain macrolides (erythromycin, clarithromycin) arepotent inhibitors of cytochrome P450; macrolides may cause QT prolongation.

  e. **Example agents**
  - Amikacin (Amikin), gentamicin (Garamycin), tobramycin (Nebcin); tetracycline (Achromycin V), minocycline (Minocin), doxycycline (Vibramycin); erythromycin (E-Mycin), clarithromycin (Biaxin), azithromycin (Zithromax); chloramphenicol (Chloromycetin); clindamycin (Cleocin).

3. **Antimetabolites**
  a. **Mechanism of action**
  - Block enzymes involved in the synthesis of purine or pyrimidine bases; prevent growth of microorganisms.

  b. **Spectrum of activity**
  - Sulfonamides: gram-positive and gram-negative, particularly useful for *E. coli, Salmonella, Shigella*, and *Enterobacter*.
  - Trimethoprim: used in combination with sulfonamides to treat urinary tract infections (UTIs), *Pneumocystis jiroveci* (*formerly carinii*) pneumonia, *Shigella, Salmonella*, and upper respiratory tract infections.

  c. **Common adverse effects**
  - Allergic reactions (Stevens–Johnson syndrome), blood dyscrasias, crystalluria, erythema multiforme, hematuria.

  d. **Cautions**
  - Monitor for development of blood dyscrasias (agranulocytosis, aplastic anemia) and or skin rash—consider discontinuation of drug if occurs as these may be early signs of severe adverse reactions.

  e. **Example agents**
  - Mainly combination products: Bactrim (sulfamethoxazole + trimethoprim).

4. **Inhibitors of DNA Gyrase**
- Mechanism of action: inhibit DNA synthesis in bacteria by way of inhibition of DNA gyrase involved with preventing supercoiling of DNA during replication.
- Spectrum of activity: Quinolones/Fluoroquinolones: aerobic gram-negative rods, including *Pseudomonas* and *Neisseria*, active against anthrax.

- Common adverse effects: nausea, may cause tendinitis and tendon rupture in all ages.
- Cautions: should not be used during pregnancy, norfloxacin can be used only in UTIs; may exacerbate muscle weakness in patients with myasthenia gravis-avoid concurrent use in this population.
- Example agents: ciprofloxacin (Cipro), gemifloxacin (Factive), moxifloxacin (Avelox) norfloxacin (Noroxin), ofloxacin (Floxin), levofloxacin (Levaquin).

C. Selected Antimycobacterial Agents
1. **Isoniazid (INH)**
   - Mechanism of action: inhibits synthesis of mycobacterial cell walls by way of inhibition of mycolic acid synthesis.
   - Spectrum of activity: bactericidal for actively growing *Mycobacterium tuberculosis*.
   - Common adverse effects: allergic reactions, drug-induced lupus, rare (1%) drug-induced hepatitis (mild increases in aminotransferases are common, but usually asymptomatic), neuropathy (high doses).
   - Contraindications/cautions: pyridoxine given in patients at risk for neuropathy, can be used as monotherapy for prevention, but generally used in combination for treatment of active disease.
2. **Rifampin (Rifadin)**
   - Mechanism of action: inhibits RNA synthesis.
   - Spectrum of activity: bactericidal for tubercle bacilli, many gram-positive and gram-negative organisms are susceptible.
   - Common adverse effects: rash, thrombocytopenia, nephritis.
   - Contraindications/cautions: orange discoloration of urine, sweat, tears; cytochrome P450 inducer; generally used in combination for treatment of active disease.
3. **Miscellaneous Agents Used for TB**
   - Ethambutol (Myambutol).
   - Pyrazinamide.
   - Streptomycin.

D. Selected Antiviral Agents
1. **Nucleoside Reverse Transcriptase Inhibitors**
   - Mechanism of action: inhibit HIV reverse transcriptase.
   - Common adverse effects: zidovudine (AZT)—myelosuppression (anemia and neutropenia), GI intolerance, headache, insomnia; didanosine (ddI)—peripheral neuropathy, pancreatitis, diarrhea, hyperuricemia, lactic acidosis, hepatomegaly with steatosis; lamivudine (3TC)—nausea, headache, fatigue, lactic acidosis, hepatomegaly with steatosis; stavudine (d4T)—peripheral neuropathy, oral ulcers lactic acidosis, hepatomegaly with steatosis.

- Contraindications/cautions: resistance is common to monotherapy—use in combination with other retrovirals, drug interactions common.
- Example agents: zidovudine (AZT, Retrovir), didanosine (ddI, Videx), lamivudine (3TC, Epivir), stavudine (d4T, Zerit).

2. **Nonnucleoside Reverse Transcriptase Inhibitors**
   - Mechanism of action: inhibit reverse transcriptase.
   - Common adverse effects: nevirapine and delavirdine—skin reactions, including Stevens–Johnson (nevirapine only), fulminant hepatitis, fever, nausea, headache, fatigue; efavirenz—dizziness, drowsiness/insomnia, headache, confusion, skin rash.
   - Contraindications/cautions: drug interactions common, resistance common with monotherapy.
   - Example agents: Nevirapine (Viramune), delavirdine (Rescriptor), efavirenz (Sustiva).
3. **Protease Inhibitors**
   - Mechanism of action: inhibit production of mature virions, inhibit replication.
   - Common adverse effects: hyperlipidemia, redistribution of fat, truncal obesity and buffalo hump, GI distress, paresthesias (ritonavir), nephrolithiasis, urolithiasis, hyperbilirubinemia (indinavir).
   - Contraindications/cautions: resistance common with monotherapy, drug interactions common.
   - Example agents: atazanavir (Reyataz), saquinavir (Invirase), ritonavir (Norvir), indinavir (Crixivan), nelfinavir (Viracept), amprenavir (Agenerase).

XIV. Cancer Chemotherapeutic Agents

A. General Principles
- Goal of chemotherapy is to selectively kill cancer cells.
- Generally chemotherapeutic agents target cancer cells as rapidly dividing cells.
- Common adverse effects include bone-marrow suppression, hair loss, and GI distress, all of which are result of lack of specificity of the agents and targeting of rapidly dividing cells.
- Many of these intravenous agents are considered irritants or vesicants, which can cause significant skin damage, local tissue necrosis, and extravasation; take proper precautions upon ordering and administration.
- Resistance to cancer chemotherapeutic agents is a common clinical concern.
- This section provides an overview of major classes of agents; however, therapeutics within oncology is rapidly changing and many experimental agents are used. Therefore, specific protocols are not discussed. Most agents are used in combination in protocols for specific types of cancers.

B. Alkylating Agents

- Mechanism of action: in general, agents transfer an alkyl group to DNA, disrupting DNA replication that can include strand breakage.
- Therapeutic uses: leukemias, lymphomas, myeloma, breast, ovarian, testicular, genitourinary, brain cancers.
- Common adverse reactions: bone-marrow suppression, alopecia, N/V, hemorrhagic cystitis (cyclophosphamide), renal dysfunction (cisplatin), local reactions at injection site.
- Example agents: cyclophosphamide (Cytoxan), busulfan (Myleran), carmustine (BCNU), cisplatin (Platinol), carboplatin (Paraplatin).

C. Antimetabolite Agents

- Mechanism of action: in general, inhibit enzymes in the replication pathway for cells.
- Therapeutic uses: lymphomas, gastric, breast, colorectal, and skin cancers.
- Common adverse reactions: bone-marrow suppression, N/V.
- Example agents: cytarabine (ara-C), gemcitabine (Gemzar), fluorouracil (5FU), methotrexate (MTX), thioguanine (6-TG).
- Leucovorin is a specific agent that can be given to "rescue" patients from high-dose MTX administration.

D. Inhibitors of Mitosis

- Mechanism of action: in general, agents bind to tubulin and prevent normal mitosis results in disruption of cell division.
- Therapeutic uses: lymphomas, ovarian, breast, and lung cancer.
- Common adverse reactions: alopecia, muscle weakness, bone-marrow suppression.
- Cautions: do not administer vinblastine intrathecally as death can result; only give vinblastine intravenously.
- Example agents: vincristine (Oncovin), vinblastine (Velban), paclitaxel (Taxol), docetaxel (Taxotere).

E. Hormone Regulators

- Mechanism of action: block receptors (estrogen receptors for tamoxifen), inhibit cytokine production (glucocorticoids such as prednisone), or mimic the effects of gonadotropin-releasing hormone (leuprolide).
- Therapeutic uses: breast cancer (tamoxifen), prostate cancer (flutamide and leuprolide), used to induce remission in leukemia (prednisone).
- Common adverse effects: related to inhibition of hormone (e.g., hot flashes with tamoxifen).
- Example agents: tamoxifen (Nolvadex), flutamide (Eulexin), prednisone, leuprolide (Lupron).

F. Intercalating Agents

- Mechanism of action: bind to DNA and prevent the synthesis of RNA or DNA.
- Therapeutic uses: leukemias, squamous cell carcinoma (bleomycin), lymphomas, testicular cancer.
- Common adverse effects: GI distress, cardiotoxicity (doxorubicin), alopecia, bone-marrow suppression, allergic reaction (bleomycin).
- Cautions: as doxorubicin use can lead to heart failure, monitor lifetime cumulative amount given and do not exceed these limits.
- Example agents: daunorubicin (Cerubidine), doxorubicin (Adriamycin), Bleomycin (Blenoxane).

SELECTED REFERENCES

Bourne HR, von Zastrow M. Drug receptors & pharmacodynamics. In: Katzung BG, ed. *Basic and Clinical Pharmacology*. 8th ed. New York, NY: Lange Medical Books/McGraw-Hill; 2001:chap 2:9–34.

Brown JH, Taylor P. Muscarinic receptor agonists and antagonists. In: Hardman JG, Limbird LE, eds. *Goodman & Gilman's the Pharmacological Basis of Therapeutics*. 10th ed. New York, NY: McGraw-Hill; 2001:chap 7:155–183.

Chambers HF. Aminoglycosides & spectinomycin. In: Katzung BG, ed. *Basic and Clinical Pharmacology*. 8th ed. New York, NY: Lange Medical Books/McGraw-Hill; 2001:chap 45:784–792.

Chambers HF. Antimycobacterial drugs. In: Katzung BG, ed. *Basic and Clinical Pharmacology*. 8th ed. New York, NY: Lange Medical Books/McGraw-Hill; 2001:chap 47:803–807.

Chambers HF. Beta-lactam antibiotics & other inhibitors of cell wall synthesis; Chapter 43. In: Katzung BG, ed. *Basic and Clinical Pharmacology*. 8th ed. New York, NY: Lange Medical Books/McGraw-Hill; 2001:754–773.

Chambers HF. Chloramphenicol, tetracyclines, macrolides, clindamycin, & streptogramins. In: Katzung BG, ed. *Basic and Clinical Pharmacology*. 8th ed. New York, NY: Lange Medical Books/McGraw-Hill; 2001:chap 44:774–782.

Chambers HF. Sulfonamides, trimethoprim, & quinolones. In: Katzung BG, ed. *Basic and Clinical Pharmacology*. 8th ed. New York, NY: Lange Medical Books/McGraw-Hill; 2001:chap 46:793–802.

Chobanian AV, Bakris GL, Black HR, et al. The seventh report of the Joint National Committee on Prevention, Detection, Evaluation, and Treatment of High Blood Pressure: The JNC 7 report. *JAMA*. 2003;289:2560–2571.

Connolly SJ, Ezekowitz MD, Yusuf S et al. Dabigatran versus warfarin in patients with atrial fibrillation. *N Engl J Med*. 2009;361:1139–1151.

Correia MA. Drug biotransformation. In: Katzung BG, ed. *Basic and Clinical Pharmacology*. 8th ed. New York, NY: Lange Medical Books/McGraw-Hill; 2001:chap 3:51–63.

Cytochrome P450 Interactions Page. Indiana University Department of Clinical Pharmacology Website. http://medicine.iupui.edu/clinpharm/ddis/table.aspx. Accessed July 9, 2011.

Decherney A, Nathan L, Goodwin T, et al. *Current Obstetrics and Gynecology*. 10th ed. New York, NY: McGraw-Hill; 2007.

Drugs at FDA. US Food and Drug Administration Website. http://www.accessdata.fda.gov/scripts/cder/drugsatfda/index.cfm?fuseaction=Search.Search_Drug_Name.Accessed July 9, 2011.

Executive Summary of the Third Report of the National Cholesterol Education Program (NCEP) Expert Panel on Detection, Evaluation, and Treatment of High Blood Cholesterol in Adults (Adult Treatment Panel III). *JAMA*. 2001;285:2486–2497.

Facts and Comparisons E-Answers. Facts and Comparisons Website. http://online.factsandcomparisons.com/index.aspx. Accessed July 9, 2011.

Global Initiative for Chronic Lung Disease. Available at: http://www.gold-copd.com.

Global Initiative for Chronic Obstructive Lung Disease (GOLD). Global strategy for the diagnosis, management, and prevention of chronic obstructive pulmonary disease. Bethesda,MD: Global Initiative for Chronic Obstructive Lung Disease (GOLD); 2010.

Hoffman BB. Adrenoceptor-activating & other sympathomimetic drugs. In: Katzung BG, ed. *Basic and Clinical Pharmacology*. 8th ed. New York, NY: Lange Medical Books/McGraw-Hill; 2001:chap 9:120–137.

Hoffman BB. Adrenoceptor antagonist drugs. In: Katzung BG, ed. *Basic and Clinical Pharmacology*. 8th ed. New York, NY: Lange Medical Books/McGraw-Hill; 2001:chap 10:138–154.

Holford NHG. Pharmacokinetics & pharmacodynamics: rational dosing & the time course of drug action. In: Katzung BG, ed. *Basic and Clinical Pharmacology*. 8th ed. New York, NY: Lange Medical Books/McGraw-Hill; 2001:chap 3:35–50.

Jackson CW, Cates ME, Feldman JM. Major depressive disorder. In: Chisholm-Burns MA, Schwinghammer TL, Wells BG, et al. eds. *Pharmacotherapy Principles & Practice*. 2nd ed. New York, NY: McGraw Hill Medical; 2010:chap 38:653–668.

Katzung BG, ed. *Basic and Clinical Pharmacology*. 10th ed. New York, NY: McGraw-Hill; 2007.

Kelly DL, Weiner E, Wehring HJ. Schizophrenia. In: Chisholm-Burns MA, Schwinghammer TL, Wells BG, et al. eds. *Pharmacotherapy Principles & Practice*. 2nd ed. New York, NY: McGraw Hill Medical; 2010:chap 37:631–652.

Koda-Kimble MA, Young LY, Alldredge BK, et al. eds. *Applied Therapeutics: The Clinical Use of Drugs*. 9th ed. Philadelphia, PA: Wolters Kluwer Health/Lippincott Williams &Wilkins; 2009.

McEvoy GK, Miller JL, Snow EK, et al. eds.*AHFS Drug Information*. Bethesda, MD; American Society of Health-System Pharmacists; 2011.

McPhee S, Papadakis M, Rabow M. *Current Medical Diagnosis and Treatment*. 46th ed. New York, NY: McGraw-Hill; 2007.

National Asthma Education and Prevention Program (NAEPP). Expert panel report 3: guidelines for the diagnosis and management of asthma. Bethesda (MD): National Heart, Lung, and Blood Institute; 2007:213–276.

National Institutes of Health. National Heart, Lung, and Blood Institute. *Expert Panel Report 2: Guidelines for the Diagnosis and Management of Asthma*. Publication 97-4051. Bethesda, MD: National Institutes of Health; 1997:1–146.

Pappano AJ. Cholinoceptor-activating & cholinesterase-inhibiting drugs. In: Katzung BG, ed. *Basic and Clinical Pharmacology*. 8th ed. New York, NY: Lange Medical Books/McGraw-Hill; 2001:chap 7:92–106.

Pappano AJ, Katzung BG. Cholinoceptor-blocking drugs. In: Katzung BG, ed. *Basic and Clinical Pharmacology*. 8th ed. New York, NY: Lange Medical Books/McGraw-Hill; 2001:chap 8:107–119.

Safrins S. Antiviral agents. In: Katzung BG, ed. *Basic and Clinical Pharmacology*. 8th ed. New York, NY: Lange Medical Books/McGraw-Hill; 2001:chap 49:823–844.

Salmon SE, Sartorelli AC. Cancer chemotherapy. In: Katzung BG, ed. *Basic and Clinical Pharmacology*. 8th ed. New York, NY: Lange Medical Books/McGraw-Hill; 2001:chap 55:923–958.

Straka RJ, Parra D, Birkeland KT. Hypertension. In: Chisholm-Burns MA, Schwinghammer TL, Wells BG, et al. eds. *Pharmacotherapy Principles & Practice*. 2nd ed. New York, NY: McGraw Hill Medical; 2010:chap 5:51–78.

Taylor P. Anticholinesterase agents. In: Hardman JG, Limbird LE, eds. *Goodman &Gilman's the Pharmacological Basis of Therapeutics*. 10th ed. New York, NY: McGraw-Hill; 2001:chap 8:175–191.

Vardeny O, Ng TMH. Heart failure. In: Chisholm-Burns MA, Schwinghammer TL, Wells BG, et al. eds. *Pharmacotherapy Principles & Practice*. 2nd ed. New Ysork, NY: McGraw Hill Medical; 2010:chap 6:79–108.

Wagner ML. Parkinson's disease. In: Chisholm-Burns MA, Schwinghammer TL, Wells BG, et al. eds. *Pharmacotherapy Principles & Practice*. 2nd ed. New York, NY: McGraw Hill Medical; 2010:chap 32:553–566.

Welty TE, Faught E. Epilepsy. In: Chisholm-Burns MA, Schwinghammer TL, Wells BG, et al. eds. *Pharmacotherapy Principles & Practice*. 2nd ed. New York, NY: McGraw Hill Medical; 2010:chap 30:521–540.

Ethical and Legal Considerations

19

Vicki D. Lachman • F. J. Gino Gianola

I. American Academy of Physician Assistants (AAPA) Guidelines for Ethical Conduct for the PA Profession

A. Statement of Values of the PA Profession

1. PAs hold as their primary responsibility the health, safety, welfare, and dignity of all human beings.
2. PAs uphold the tenets of patient autonomy, beneficence, nonmaleficence, and justice.
3. PAs recognize and promote the value of diversity.
4. PAs treat all persons who seek care equally.
5. PAs hold in confidence the information shared in the course of practicing medicine.
6. PAs assess their personal capabilities and limitations, striving always to improve their medical practice.
7. PAs actively seek to expand their knowledge and skills, keeping abreast of advances in medicine.
8. PAs work with other members of the health care team to provide compassionate and effective care of patients.
9. PAs use their knowledge and experience to contribute to improvement in the community.
10. PAs respect their professional relationship with physicians.
11. PAs share and expand knowledge within the profession.

B. PA and the Patient

1. **PA Role and Responsibility**
   a. PA practice is a three-way relationship that involves the PA, physician, and patient: PA–patient; PA–supervising physician; patient–PA–physician.
   b. Although being sensitive to a patient's beliefs and expectations, PAs are not expected to ignore their own personal values, scientific or ethical standards, or the law.
   c. In cases of conflict because of personal moral, religious, or ethical beliefs, the patient should not be abandoned:
      • Refer the patient to another qualified provider that does not restrict his or her access to care.
      • In emergency situations, responsibly transfer the patient after stabilization.

2. **Cost Containment**
   a. Cost containment and resource allocation policies can present particular ethical challenges to clinicians. PAs should always act in the best interests of their patients and as advocates when necessary.
   b. PAs should actively resist policies that restrict free exchange of medical information.
   c. PAs should inform patients of financial incentives to limit care, use resources in a fair and efficient way, and avoid arrangements or financial incentives that conflict with the patient's best interests.

3. **The PA and Diversity**
   a. PAs should respect the culture, values, beliefs, and expectations of their patients.

4. **Discrimination**
   a. PAs should not discriminate against patients in the delivery of needed health care based on gender, color, creed, race, religion, age, ethnic or national origin, political beliefs, nature of illness, disability, socioeconomic status, physical stature, body size, gender identity, marital status, or sexual orientation.

5. **Initiation and Discontinuation of Care**
   a. Provide care in emergency situations and arrange proper follow-up.
      • Contracts with health insurance plans might define a legal obligation to provide care to certain patients.
   b. Professional relationship with an established patient may be discontinued as long as proper procedures are followed:
      • Provide adequate notice, offer to transfer records, and arrange for continuity of care.
      • Discontinue the professional relationship only after a serious attempt has been made to clarify and understand the expectations and concerns of all involved parties.
   c. If the patient terminates the relationship, they are entitled to access appropriate information contained within their medical record.

6. **Informed Consent**
   a. Provide adequate information comprehensible to a competent patient or patient surrogate.
   b. PAs should be committed to the concept of shared decision making, which involves assisting patients in making decisions that account for medical, situational, and personal factors.

c. In caring for adolescents:
- Understand all the laws and regulations related to the ability of minors, including emancipated or mature minors, to consent to or refuse health care.
- Encourage adolescents to involve their families in health care decision making.

d. When a patient's surrogate, family member, or other legally authorized representative is giving consent:
- Assure the decisions made are consistent with the patient's best interests and personal preferences.
- If there is a conflict, work to resolve it, and this may require the use of additional resources, such as an ethics committee.

7. Confidentiality

a. Patients are more likely to seek medical care and discuss their problems candidly when they are confident that their privacy is protected.

b. By maintaining confidentiality, patient privacy is respected and discrimination based on medical conditions is prevented.

c. In cases of adolescent patients:
- Family support should be balanced with the patient's need for confidentiality and the PA's obligation to respect the patient's emerging autonomy.
- Adolescents may not be of age to make independent decisions about their health, but providers should respect that they soon will be.
- Allow them to participate as fully as possible in decisions about their care.
- Be familiar with and understand the laws and regulations in the applicable jurisdictions that relate to the confidentiality rights of adolescent patients.

d. Be aware that communication about a patient in the written, electronic, and verbal form may be intercepted or overheard.

e. Choose methods of storage and transmission of patient information that minimize the likelihood of data becoming available to unauthorized persons or organizations.

f. Advocate for policies and procedures that secure the confidentiality of patient information.

8. The Patient and the Medical Record

a. Information should be released only with the written permission of the patient or the patient's legally authorized representative, although specific exceptions to this general rule may exist (e.g., worker's compensation, communicable disease, human immunodeficiency virus [HIV], knife/gunshot wounds, physical/sexual abuse, and substance abuse).

b. Be familiar with and understand the laws and regulations that relate to the release of information. For example, stringent legal restrictions on release of genetic test results and mental health records often exist.

c. The medical chart is legally the property of the practice or institution, but information in the chart is the property of the patient.

d. Most states have laws that provide patients access to their medical records. Facilitate patient access to the information.

9. Disclosure

a. Errors do not always constitute improper, negligent, or unethical behavior, but failure to disclose them may.

b. Disclose errors made in the course of caring for a patient to the supervising physician.

10. Care of Family Members and Coworkers

a. Treating oneself, coworkers, close friends, family members, or students whom the PA supervises or teaches may be unethical or create conflicts of interest.

b. PA's judgment may be less than objective in cases involving friends, family members, students, and colleagues.

c. Providing informal care may sway the individual from establishing an ongoing relationship with a provider.

d. If it becomes necessary to treat a family member or close associate, a formal patient–provider relationship should be established. Consider transferring the patient's care to another provider as soon as it is practical.

e. There may be exceptions to this guideline (e.g., running an employee health center or working in occupational medicine).

11. Genetic Testing

a. Be informed about the benefits and risks of genetic tests.

b. Testing should be undertaken only after proper informed consent is obtained.

c. Assure appropriate pre- and posttest counseling is provided.

d. Patients should understand the potential consequences of undergoing genetic tests—impact on themselves, possible implications for other family members, and potential use of the information by insurance companies or others who might have access to the information.

e. Be aware of the need for confidentiality concerning genetic test results because of the potential for discrimination by insurers, employers, or others.

12. Reproductive Decision Making

a. Patients have a right to access the full range of reproductive health care services, including fertility treatments, contraception, sterilization, and abortion.

b. Provide balanced and unbiased clinical information about reproductive health care.

c. When personal values conflict with providing a patient full disclosure or certain services such as sterilization or abortion, the PA need not become involved in that aspect of the patient's care. By referring the patient to a qualified provider who is willing to discuss and facilitate all treatment options, PAs fulfill their ethical obligation to ensure the patient access to all legal options.

13. **End-of-Life Care**
    a. Recognize that dying is a personal experience and part of the life cycle.
    b. Discuss advance directives, living wills, durable power of attorney, and organ donation during routine patient visits.
    c. Assure terminally ill patients that their dignity is a priority and relief of physical and mental suffering is paramount, and that they will not be abandoned.
    d. To the extent possible, honor patient or surrogate preferences, using the most appropriate measures consistent with their choices, including alternative and nontraditional treatments.
    e. Explain and facilitate access to palliative and hospice care.
    f. End-of-life care should include assessment and management of psychological, social, and spiritual, or religious needs.
    g. Although respecting patients' wishes for particular treatments when possible, PAs must also weigh their ethical responsibility, in consultation with supervising physicians, to withhold futile treatments and to help patients understand such medical decisions.
    h. Involve the supervising physician in all near-death planning. Withdraw life support with the supervising physician's agreement and in accordance with the policies of the health care institution.

C. PA and Individual Professionalism
1. **Conflict of Interest**
   a. Place service to patients before personal material gain and avoid undue influence on clinical judgment.
      • Trust can be undermined by even the appearance of improper influence.
      • Disclose any actual or potential conflict of interest to patients.
   b. Acceptance of gifts, trips, hospitality, or other items is discouraged.
2. **Professional Identity**
   a. Skills, training, professional credentials, or identity should not be misrepresented.
   b. Uphold the dignity of the PA profession and accept its ethical values.
3. **Competency**
   a. Provide competent medical care and extend to each patient the full measure of one's

professional ability as a dedicated, empathetic health care provider.
   b. Strive to maintain and increase the quality of one's health care knowledge, cultural sensitivity, and cultural competence through individual study and continuing education.
4. **Sexual Relationships**
   a. Issues such as dependence, trust, transference, and inequalities of power may lead to increased vulnerability on the part of current or former patients or major third parties (individuals who have influence over the patient, e.g., spouses or partners, parents, guardians, or surrogates).
   b. It is unethical to become sexually involved with patients because of the provider's position of authority and inherent imbalance of knowledge, expertise, and status.
   c. It may be unethical to become sexually involved with former patients or major third parties.
5. **Gender Discrimination and Sexual Harassment**
   a. It is unethical to engage in or condone any form of gender discrimination; defined as any behavior, action, or policy that adversely affects an individual or group of individuals because of disparate treatment, disparate impact, or creation of a hostile or intimidating work or learning environment.
   b. It is unethical to engage in or condone any form of sexual harassment; defined as unwelcome sexual advances, requests for sexual favors, or other verbal or physical conduct of a sexual nature.
   c. Gender discrimination and sexual harassment have the purpose or effect of:
      • Interfering with an individual's work or academic performance.
      • Creating an intimidating, hostile, or offensive work or academic environment.

D. PA and Other Providers
1. **Team Practice**
   a. Work collegially with other members of the health care team to assure integrated, well-managed, and effective care of patients.
   b. Cooperate with other health care professionals, their organizations, and the general public.
2. **Illegal and Unethical Conduct**
   a. Do not participate in, or conceal, any activity that will bring discredit or dishonor to the PA profession.
   b. Report illegal or unethical conduct by health care professionals to the appropriate authorities.
3. **Impairment**
   a. "Impaired" means being unable to practice medicine with reasonable skill and safety because of physical or mental illness, loss of motor skills, or excessive use or abuse of drugs and alcohol.
   b. Be able to recognize impairment in physician supervisors, PAs, and other health care providers.

c. Seek assistance from appropriate resources to encourage impaired providers to obtain treatment.

4. **PA–Physician Relationship**
   - Supervision should include ongoing communication between the physician and PA regarding patient care.
   - Consult the supervising physician whenever it will safeguard or advance the welfare of the patient.
   - Seek assistance in situations of conflict with a patient or another health care professional.

5. **Complementary and Alternative Medicine**
   a. Gain a basic understanding of alternative therapies being considered or being used and how the treatment will affect the patient.
   b. If the treatment would harm the patient, the PA should work diligently to dissuade the patient from using it, advise other treatment, and perhaps consider transferring the patient to another provider.

E. PA and the Health Care System

1. **Workplace Actions**
   a. Potential harm to patients should be weighed carefully against the potential improvements to working conditions and patient care that could result when workplace actions (e.g., strikes, sick-outs, slowdowns) occur.
   b. Work to find alternatives to workplace actions when addressing workplace concerns.

2. **Managed Care**
   a. Oppose managed care policies that restrict free exchange of medical information (e.g., withholding information about treatment options simply because the option is not covered by a particular managed care plan).
   b. Inform patients of financial incentives to limit care.
   c. Use resources in a fair and efficient way.
   d. Avoid arrangements or financial incentives that conflict with the patient's best interests.

3. **PAs as Educators**
   a. Share knowledge and information with patients, other health professionals, students, and the public.

4. **PAs and Research**
   a. Assure subjects' informed consent, follow treatment protocols, and report findings accurately.
   b. Report fraud and dishonesty, so the appropriate authorities can take action.
   c. Disclose any conflict of interest. The patient's welfare takes precedence over the desired research outcome.
   d. Report information honestly and accurately. Include sources of research funding in published reports.
   e. Cite appropriate sources for any portion of a document when submitting for publication.

5. **PAs as Expert Witnesses**
   a. Testify to what is believed to be the truth.
   b. Review of medical facts should be thorough, fair, and impartial.
   c. Compensation should be for the time spent preparing, appearing, and testifying.
   d. Personal or professional favor should not be gained from being an expert witness.

F. PA and Society

1. **Lawfulness**
   a. Respect the law and work for positive change to laws that will enhance the health and well-being of the community.

2. **Executions**
   a. Participation in executions violates the ethical principle of beneficence.

3. **Access to Care/Resource Allocation**
   a. Use health care resources in an appropriate and efficient manner, so that all patients have access to needed health care.
   b. When participating in policy decisions about resource allocation, consider medical need, cost-effectiveness, efficacy, and equitable distribution of benefits and burdens in society.

4. **Community Well-Being**
   a. Uphold and enhance community values, be aware of the needs of the community, and use the knowledge and experience acquired as a professional to contribute to an improved community.
   b. Work for the health, well-being, and best interest of both the patient and the community.
   c. There can be conflict between the well-being of the community and the individual patient, which is not always resolved easily.

II. Essence of Clinical Ethics

A. Definition of Ethics

1. The word "ethics" originates from the Greek *ethike tekne*, meaning the moral art.
   - Ethics is a subset of philosophy; philosophy is metaphysical, meaning it cannot be sensed physically.
2. Ethics assumes reflective thinking and critical judgments about acts and beliefs; an examination of morality, conduct, and social practices.
3. Bioethics is a critical examination of the moral dimensions of decision making in health-related and biologic science contexts.
4. Interpretative and analytical—why should I do X? What reasons do I have to justify my action?

B. Definition of Morality

1. From the Latin word *mores*, meaning character, custom, or habit.
2. Social conventions about right and wrong human conduct so widely shared that they form a stable, communal consensus.

3. Normative or prescriptive—what should I do in this situation and similar situations?

C. Definition of Law

1. The minimum good behavior is the law, but it is not the same as the ideal behavior reflecting the highest standard of morality.
   - Behavior that people have agreed should be mandatory or prohibited.
   - The more severe the penalty for breaking the law, the more strongly the law is enforcing an ethical value.
2. Law will either mandate (prescribe), that is, something must be done, or prohibit (proscribe), that is, something must not be done (e.g., parents must take care of and not abuse their children).

D. Ethical Dilemma

1. Moral obligations exist on both sides of the choice to either perform or refrain from performing the actions involved, and ethical reasons support choosing both alternatives (i.e., abortion and withdrawing artificial nutrition and hydration).
2. Deliberation on dilemmas is primarily problem solving, where individuals or groups struggle to determine their beliefs and reach a decision; they consider which among the possible courses of action is morally justified.
   - Our actions express what we believe is the right course of action.
   - The justification is showing that one has sufficient reasons for one's belief and is able to explicitly state what warrants this belief.
3. Primarily, ethical dilemmas occur in (1) choices in diagnoses or treatment (giving artificial hydration by way of a percutaneous endoscopic gastrostomy tube, or allowing the severe stroke patient to die) and (2) conflicts in basic obligations to patients (duty to tell the truth, but the truth will cause pain because the patient is dying).

E. Bridging Ethical Principles and the Clinical Situation

1. Balance between Benefits and Harms in Patient Care
   - Clinicians must use their knowledge to determine what treatments will maximize benefits and minimize harm to the patients.
   - Obligations of clinicians include preserving life; healing, restoring, or maintaining bodily functions and mental capacities; preventing disease and injury; relieving suffering; and curing when possible.

2. Disclosure, Informed Consent, and Shared Decision Making
   - Clinicians cannot determine what is in the best interest of the patients without discussing all options, disclosing benefits and burdens, and sharing in the decision-making process.
   - It is the right of all competent adults to determine what treatment they are willing to accept.

- An ongoing dialog between clinician and patient assures the shared decision-making process.

3. Families Are Part of the Process
   - Most individuals face medical decisions as members of a family.
   - A clinician must consider the moral dimension of family life.

4. Relationship between Clinician and Patient
   - Patients are partners in the process of making health care decisions; therefore, clinicians must be responsible for communicating effectively and eliciting the patient's participation.

5. Professional Integrity of Clinicians
   - Patients are free to refuse treatment, but they are not entitled to receive whatever treatment they want.
   - Clinicians violate their integrity by providing medically inappropriate treatments (i.e., futile care).
   - If a disagreement occurs between clinicians and patients or family, an ethics consultation is indicated.
   - Clinicians are not obligated to provide treatment they oppose for reasons of consciousness. They must transfer care, but not abandon the patient.

6. Cost-Effectiveness and Allocation
   - Distributive justice is a fair distribution of resources. Practice guidelines and managed care focus the clinician on cost considerations in making decisions about treatment.
   - Clinicians cannot avoid the need to select which patients receive scarce medical resources.

7. Issues of Culture and Religion
   - Family members, rather than the patient, may be in charge of health care decisions in some cultures.
   - Some religions forbid certain practices (i.e., abortion for Catholics and blood transfusions for Jehovah's Witnesses).
   - Religious or cultural consultation may be necessary to respond appropriately.

8. Considerations of Power
   - Illness can render patients in a dependent, vulnerable position.
   - Respecting the patient's autonomy through shared decision making helps reduce the power differential.

F. The Virtues of Ethical Clinicians

1. Definition of Virtues
   - Virtues are dispositions of character and conduct.

2. Plato's Four Highest Virtues
   - Justice (fairness), temperance (moderation), prudence (sensibility), and fortitude (courage, endurance).

3. Objectivity
   - Plato's justice (fairness).
   - Detachment from the troubling circumstances of clinical practice, yet compassionate toward the patient.

4. **Caring**
   - Plato's temperance (moderation), indicating the need for calmness.
   - Emotional relationship with the patient that helps clinician individualize his or her interactions with the individual.
   - Use the relationship with the patient as a means to promote healing and relieve suffering.
5. **Reflective Intelligence**
   - Plato's prudence (sensibility).
   - By using critical thinking, the clinician can anticipate problems, set goals of care, evaluate outcomes, and adjust interventions.
   - Recognizes the need for clinical judgment under conditions of uncertainty that characterize medicine.
6. **Courage**
   - Plato's fortitude (courage).
   - Willingness to take the risks to act ethically in a situation that may be seen as contrary.
   - Meet and cope with cost of caring, when it would be easier to become detached.
7. **Technical Competence**
   - A good clinician has mastered the knowledge and techniques for practice and is committed to continuing education to maintain competence.
8. **Humility**
   - Clinician recognizes his or her fallibility and the limits of medical knowledge.

III. Ethical Theories

A. Principles
1. Four-principle approach to biomedical ethics is derived from common morality and medical tradition (Beauchamp and Childress).
2. Principles are general guides that leave room for judgment in specific cases and provide guidance for development of policies.
3. A morality theory that is pluralistic, not relying on one absolute principle.
4. The four principles are autonomy, beneficence, nonmaleficence, and justice.
   a. Autonomy—a norm of respecting the decision-making capacities of other persons; self-determination.
      - Paternalism—describes acting in a paternal way toward patients, where clinicians assume they know what is best for the patient in making their decisions.
   b. Beneficence—acts in the patient's best interest and prevents harm from occurring.
      - Malpractice law enforces the value of beneficence.
   c. Nonmaleficence—do no harm; do not impose unnecessary burdens on the patient.
   d. Justice—fairness, equitable treatment; patients in similar circumstances should receive similar care.
   e. Distributive justice—a group of norms for distributing benefits, risks, and costs fairly.
5. **The principles are used to make judgments in particular circumstances. Therefore, it is necessary to leave room for interpretation and a balancing of the principles in the presence of conflict.**

B. Utilitarianism
1. The most famous exponents of utilitarianism were Jeremy Bentham and John Stuart Mill.
2. Utilitarianism is one of the consequentialism theories and holds that an action is right or wrong according to the balance of the good or bad consequences (outcomes) of the action.
3. "The Principle of Utility" states an action is right when it produces the greatest good (happiness or pleasure) for the greatest number.
4. Utilitarianism lays stress on the effects of an action; if an action produces more beneficial effects than harmful ones, it is the right action.
5. An objection to this theory is we can only judge the rightness or wrongness of an act after we know all its effects; therefore, we would have to wait indefinitely to declare an act right or wrong.
6. Another objection to utilitarianism is the belief that our actions cannot be evaluated properly apart from examining the motives from which they are done.
   - A person may be morally good and yet do something that has undesirable effects.
7. Utilitarianism is often used in a formation of public policy—maximize good outcomes for the most people (i.e., Oregon's Medicaid Program).

C. Kantian Ethics
1. Ethical thought of Immanuel Kant, often called deontological theory, states that the intention of actions, in addition to consequences, makes actions right or wrong.
2. Kant's focus was on determining the difference between a moral action and an immoral one. He believed the answer to this lies in distinguishing between acts done from "inclination" and those done from a sense of duty (obligation).
   - A good person is one who acts from a sense of duty (i.e., he or she repays debts, not to avoid punishment, but because it is the right thing to do).
3. One is acting morally only when one suppresses one's feelings and inclinations and does that which one is obliged to do; one is doing one's duty, fulfilling one's obligation.
4. The categorical imperative states that one should judge every act by whether one would choose the same behavior for everyone else in the world.
   - Do only what you would have others do to you.
   - One must always behave as if one's course of conduct were to become a universal law.
   - To behave morally, one must behave consistently (i.e., one should always honor an advance directive).

- Another formulation of categorical imperative is that human beings are ends in themselves and not the means to an end.
- To treat a person as merely a means is to treat a person as a thing, which disregards his or her humanity.

5. Kant takes an absolute stance on always telling the truth and never breaking promises.
   - A maniac armed with a knife asks me if a relative he wants to kill is at home—telling the truth would cost the relative her life.
   - I promise to keep a secret and then someone else asks me about it. I cannot both tell the truth and keep my promise.

D. Communitarianism
1. Aristotle, Hegel, and Hume were all exponents of this theory.
2. Everything fundamental in ethics is derived from communal values, the common good, traditional practices, and cooperative virtues.
3. Social order or morality rests on historically developed norms and moral rules, which derive their correctness from shared conventions.
4. The focus is not on liberal individualism or protecting individuals' rights of autonomy, but on expressing communal values and examining what effect the actions will have on the community.
5. Communitarians would support "presumed consent" laws for organ transplant (laws that assume individuals will donate unless they have registered dissent).

E. Rights Theory
1. John Locke and John Stuart Mill were proponents.
2. The Bill of Rights in the American Constitution uses rights language as a basic terminology for expressing a moral point of view.
   - Statements of rights provide vital protection of life, liberty, expression, and property.
   - Rights protect the individual in a democratic society.
   - The language of rights has promoted social reform, secured legal protection, and secured freedom (of press and of religious expression).
3. Political decisions normally advance communal interests, but rights language constrains communities from acting at the expense of the individual.
4. Rights are justified claims that individuals or groups can make upon others in a just society. If a person possesses a right, others are constrained from interfering when he or she exercises that right.
5. A positive right is the right to be provided with a particular good or service by others. This entails another's obligation to do something for that person (i.e., right to health care services).
6. A negative right is the right to be free to hold a belief or pursue a course of action without interference by some action taken by others. This entails another's obligation to refrain from doing something (i.e., right to health, therefore, Occupational Safety and Health Administration protection against unhealthy workplace).
7. If a state has an obligation to provide food or health care to needy citizens, any citizen who meets the criteria of need can claim entitlement to food or health care.

F. Ethics of Caring
1. Noddings' caring ethics reflects an image of human connectedness.
   - Grounded in the sentiment of caring.
2. In caring for others, we aspire to be our highest self.
3. It does not focus on universal rules or principles, but on forming a relationship with this particular individual, and through this caring relationship, you act in a moral way.
   - The way we manage the details (particulars) in a relationship matters.
   - Fosters reciprocity in caring.

G. Casuistry
1. It is a system of justification that moves from cases to principles; it focuses on practical decision making in particular cases.
2. By examining the historical record of similar cases, one can reach an understanding of a particular case.
3. The casuist would attempt to identify particular features in a case and then identify the relevant precedents in previous cases, in an effort to determine how similar and different this case is from other cases.
4. Moral belief and knowledge evolve incrementally through reflection on cases.
   - The analogy is the doctrine of precedent—social ethics develop from a social consensus formed around cases.
   - It is a common law ethics model.
5. The problem is the cases do not often speak for themselves or inform moral judgment by the facts alone. Interpretation of cases is essential for moral judgment.
6. Paradigm end-of-life cases (such as *Quinlan*, *Cruzan*, and *Schiavo*) form a shared resource and become an important way we think and draw conclusions.

H. Pragmatism
1. Pragmatists William James, Charles Peirce, and John Dewey believed their method could be of value in solving problems.
2. A method for solving or evaluating problems and a theory about the kinds of knowledge we are capable of acquiring.
3. According to James, we "think" only to solve our problems, and therefore, ethical theories should be judged in terms of their success in performing this function.

4. Pragmatists contend the only reason people have for calling one view true and another false is that one works in human experience and the other does not.
   - No fixed world to be uncovered through experience, but rather a continuous quest for workable solutions to difficulties.

IV. Primary Ethical Obligations

A. Privacy and Confidentiality

1. **American Hospital Association Patients' Bill of Rights**
   - Patients have the right to have all information about their illness and care treated as confidential.
2. **Health Insurance Portability and Accountability Act (HIPAA)**
   - Federal law defines who can share what information with whom, and what type of approval must be secured before sharing information.
3. **Privileged Communication**
   - May not be disclosed by a clinician in a court proceeding without consent of the patient who provided it.
   - Human subjects' research is governed by federal regulations for protection of privacy and confidentiality.
   - Institution should limit access to only the particular information that a certain category of clinician might need.
4. **Legitimate Breaches of Confidentiality**
   - Necessary when the public's interest, or the patient, or a third party is at risk for harm (i.e., child abuse and neglect, contagious diseases, or criminally inflicted injuries).
   - *Tarasoff v. Regents of the University of California*—psychotherapist failed to inform a former girlfriend of his patient's threat to kill her. Psychotherapist was unsuccessful in detaining the patient in temporary custody. The family sued the therapist when the woman was killed. California Supreme Court established the duty to warn as a responsibility of the psychotherapist.
   - Since *Tarasoff*, the U.S. Supreme Court has upheld the responsibility of the therapist to warn when violence is foreseeable. Foreseeability is determined by the following three factors: (1) history of violence, (2) threat to a named or clearly identifiable victim, and (3) plausible motive.
   - *Tarasoff* has been widely discussed as a threat to confidentiality, as it is argued that civil commitment of a potentially violent patient is preferable to warning an identified victim. However, the Court has upheld the duty to warn if two of the three factors above are present.
   - *Behringer v. The Medical Center at Princeton*—a case in which the hospital breached the confidentiality of a positive HIV test and the result of a bronchoscopy, with a subsequent loss of the surgeon's (the patient's) hospital surgical privileges.
   - Competing privacy interests of the infected clinician against the patient's right to adequate disclosure by clinician is a complex issue in informed consent.
   - Both the American Psychiatric Association and the American Medical Association take a stand that when the physician is aware that a seropositive individual is endangering a third party, the physician should (1) attempt to persuade the infected patient to cease endangering the third party; (2) if persuasion fails, notify authorities; and (3) if the authorities take no action, notify the endangered third party.

B. Veracity—Duty to Tell the Truth

1. **Historical Perspective**
   - St. Augustine, and later Kant, held that a lie is wrong, even when based on benevolent motives, because it degrades the person who lies and violates the universal social duty to tell the truth.
   - Casuists counter this position by stating that "concealing the truth was considered permissible when a person was questioned unjustly or when revealing it could cause great harm to another person."
   - In the past 50 years, there has been a shift in attitude toward truth telling by physicians because of increased attention to the patient's right to be informed, fear of malpractice suits, and the multidisciplinary approach to delivery of health care.
2. **Deception**
   - The President's Commission for the Study of Ethical Problems in Medicine (1982) (now called President's Council on Bioethics) concluded that there is strong evidence that disclosure of information is beneficial to the patient in making decisions, regardless of how bad the news may be. This focus on truth telling has been emphasized in codes published by all major medical specialties.
   - The four forms of deception to be avoided by clinicians are (1) obscuring the facts with medical jargon; (2) dodging the futility or hopelessness of a situation with optimistic falsification; (3) remaining silent, where omission is a form of lying; and (4) evading telling the truth out of clinician's inability to communicate effectively or fear.
3. **Disclosure**
   - Clinician's duty is to tell the patient what is meaningful, important, and useful to the patient and not maintain the charade that medicine is more certain than we know it to be.
   - The patient's questions, responses, and actions guide the clinician's decision about how much information he or she wants to be given.
   - If the patient chooses to have a family member be the primary conduit for information, when

the physician has determined that the "patient chooses to not know," the physician is justified in not disclosing information to the patient. Patients determine the level of detail of information they choose to have.

4. **Buckman's Model for Communicating Bad News**
   - Step 1. Create a conducive environment and ensure the right people are present. Plan what you will say to confirm the medical facts. Turn off beeper, sit down, and talk to patient eyeball to eyeball.
   - Step 2. Find out what the patient knows. Establish what the patient already knows and assess his or her ability to comprehend new bad news.
   - Step 3. Determine how much does the patient want to know. Recognize patient preferences on how to handle information.
   - Step 4. Share the information in a caring, but straightforward manner. Do not minimize the severity of the situation.
   - Step 5. Respond to the patient's feelings by being prepared for emotions and giving the patient time to react.
   - Step 6. Plan for the next steps (i.e., what further tests, how to treat symptoms, and other sources of support).

C. **Participation in Decision Making**
   1. **Capacity Standards**
      - Capacity is the ability to make decisions. However, there is no universally accepted legal definition, but there are a variety of frequently used standards.
      - Outcome standard—judged as capable based on the outcome of decision. Patients are less likely to have their capacity questioned if they agree with the clinician. However, the standard is not what is rational to the clinician.
      - *Bartling v. Superior Court* case revolves around a 70-year-old man with inoperable lung cancer, who ended up with mechanical ventilation in an intensive care unit (ICU) following a lung biopsy. He frequently removed himself from the ventilator and was put in restraints. The Court refused to allow the clinician to discontinue the mechanical ventilation or untie Bartling's hands, and he died on the respirator 4 months later. Mr. Bartling is often referred to as the "prisoner in the ICU" case because the patient stated that he did not want to die, but did not want to live with a respirator either.
      - If the patient is in the category of mentally ill, mentally retarded, aged, an adolescent minor, or critically ill, the clinician decides whether the patient is able to participate in decision making. This standard is rejected by most.
      - Functional standard—most widely used standard. Does the patient have (1) the ability to

communicate choices, (2) the ability to understand relevant information, (3) the ability to appreciate the situation and its consequences, and (4) the ability to reach conclusions rationally?

   2. **Determining Capacity**
      - Capacity should be based on the importance of the decision at hand (i.e., taking an aspirin vs. a cardiac transplant).
      - When there is doubt because of the patient's clinical situation, the significance of the decision, or dispute among care providers, a psychiatric or neurologic consultation is important.
      - No international clinical, legal, or ethical consensus about competence criteria exists because competence determinations are not essentially objective matters.
      - Instruments that measure traits of mental status, but not specifically decision-making capacity are the following: Mini-Mental Status Examination, Mattis Dementia Rating Scale, Short Portable Mental Status Questionnaire, and Cognitive Capacity Screening Examination.

   3. **Depression**
      - Mild-to-moderate depression has little predictive value in determining preference toward life-sustaining treatment.
      - When severely depressed patients recover from depression, an associated increased desire exists for lifesaving medical therapy.
      - In general, life-sustaining therapy should not be withheld until efforts have been made to reverse depression.

   4. **Capacity in Older Children and Adolescents**
      - Clinician must evaluate each child and adolescent's capacity; capacity is based on functional ability, not on age.
      - Researchers have determined that children as young as 7 years have developed the capacities needed to make good decisions; although not ready for independent consent, they are capable of participation.
      - Most adolescents older than 14 years have full decisional capacity.
      - By age 12, most children have formal logical thinking and are able to think abstractly, reason deductively, consider multiple factors, and understand the future consequences.
      - Children with chronic disease have dealt with problems associated with the disease. They are obviously more prepared than the child who has just received his or her diagnosis.

   5. **Three Categories of Minors Assumed Capable**
      - Emancipated minors include minors who are married and not subject to parental control. Pregnant or parent minors, college students, and military personnel are often included in this category.

- Mature minors are adolescents who have maturity in decision making and can participate in their health care. The definition varies according to jurisdiction.
- Statutory adult is a minor who can give consent for medical and mental health services, treatment of venereal and other contagious diseases, birth control or pregnancy, substance abuse, or outpatient mental health treatment. This designation of capability varies by state.

6. **Who Makes the Decisions for an Incapacitated Patient?**
   - Designated proxies are individuals who have voluntarily assumed the role of proxy, usually as part of an advance directive.
   - Family members are usually aware of patient's values and goals. In order of priority, it is the patient's spouse, adult child of the patient, parent of the patient, an adult brother or sister, and any other relative of the patient in descending order of blood relationship.
   - Institutional committees, such as ethics committees or committees, formed specifically for the mentally ill or neonates.
   - Courts are a last resort when other modes fail to resolve a conflict. They appoint a guardian to make decisions about the patient's care.

7. **How Is the Decision Made for the Incapacitated Patient?**
   - Substituted judgment standard allows the patient's own values and definition of well-being to shape the health care decisions. The proxy focuses on what the patient would have wanted in this particular situation.
   - Research has shown that the proxy's substituted judgment is accurate approximately 62% of the time.
   - The *Quinlan*, *Cruzan*, and *Schiavo* cases were based on substituted judgment terminology.
   - The best-interest standard is applied to patients who have never been competent (retardation or children) or when the patient's opinion is unknown.
   - *Belchertown State School v. Saikewicz* was based on best interest of the patient. In this case, chemotherapy was not given for leukemia in a 76-year-old man with severe mental retardation.

D. Informed Consent
1. **Responsibility for Informed Consent**
   - The burden of ensuring informed consent lies with the clinician.
   - Shared decision making involves the patient, physician, PA, and family.
2. ***Schloendorff v. Society of New York Hospital* (1914)**
   - Justice Benjamin Cardozo wrote, "Every human being of adult years and sound mind has a right to

determine what shall be done with his own body." A woman had given consent for examination under anesthetic, but did not authorize any additional surgery. The physician removed a tumor, numerous complications ensued, and the patient suffered serious long-term morbidity.

3. **Elements of Informed Consent**
   - Preconditions include capacity to understand and decide, and voluntariness in deciding. The patient's choice implies he or she would be free from coercion, manipulation, and persuasion.
   - Information elements include disclosure of information, recommendation of a plan, and understanding of this disclosure and recommendation. This disclosure should include the purpose of the therapies, risks, consequences, benefits, probability of success, feasible alternatives, and prognosis if the therapy is not given.
   - Two standards of disclosure: (1) the professional standard, that is, the clinician discloses only what another clinician would disclose in a similar situation, and (2) reasonable-person standard, that is, what the average, reasonable person would need to know in order to decide treatment, in the presence of fully disclosed risks.
   - The clinician should confirm patients' understanding by asking them to describe in their own words the medical problem and proposed therapies.
   - Consent elements also include a decision in favor of the plan and authorization of the chosen plan.

4. **Exception to Informed Consent Requirements**
   - Emergency—life-threatening situation and patient is unable to consent.
   - Incapacity—patient is unable to consent; process must involve surrogate decision maker.
   - Patient waiver—when patients waive their right to know and tell the physician "just do what you think is best."
   - National/state waivers—when the government waives consent (i.e., vaccination programs and newborn genetic screening).

5. **Children as Decision Makers**
   - Assent by a child is agreement to treatment differentiated from a legally valid consent, which can only be given from a competent adult.
   - Assent involves telling the child what he or she can expect regarding the tests, treatments, or both, and asking for his or her willingness to accept the proposed care.

V. Clinical Issues
A. Frontiers of Medicine
1. **Stem Cells**
   - Stem cell therapy is actually a form of transplant.
   - Stem cells are pluripotent, which means they can differentiate into any other cell, except fetal cells.

- Stem cells can be collected from bone marrow, circulating blood, or cord blood and can be cultured from embryos formed through in vitro fertilization procedures or from human fetuses.
- Adult stem cells can be found among the differentiated cells of a particular tissue or organ in the body, but lack the flexibility for indefinite differentiation.
- Currently, bone marrow transplants, skin transplants for severe burns, and cornea replacements are the only forms of cell therapy done in a nonexperimental way.
- Experiments are taking place with pancreatic cells, lung tissue, brain cells, heart tissue, as well as rebuilding blood cells.
- The National Institutes of Health (NIH) was not able to find one nongovernment scientist to testify in support of President Bush's 2002 policy on stem cells. On March 9, 2009 President Obama issued an order and now NIH can support and conduct stem cell research.

2. **Cloning**
- Therapeutic cloning is not a reproductive cloning, which is intended to produce a person.
- Therapeutic cloning or somatic cell nuclear transfer involves taking genetic material from the nucleus of the donor adult cell, transferring and fusing it to an egg that has had its nucleus removed. This reconstructed egg contains the genetic material of the donor.
- This individual's DNA divides, forms a blastocyst, and then genetic material is used to give the individual an infusion of compatible new cells.
- Most scientific organizations support a ban on efforts to implant a human clone embryo for the purpose of reproduction, but support therapeutic cloning.
- Reproductive cloning is not supported by scientists because the genetic material used from adults continue to age so that a newborn could have 30-year-old genes (i.e., Dolly, the sheep, had progressive lung disease and arthritis).
- Ethical reasons to ban reproductive cloning: (1) health risks from mutation of the genes, (2) emotional risks (a child grows up knowing her mother is her sister), and (3) risk of abuse of technology.

3. **Genetic Testing**
- Genetic testing involves specific laboratory analysis of chromosomes and genes to determine whether a genetic alteration is present in an individual.
- Genetic testing may be DNA based (cystic fibrosis), chromosomal (Down syndrome), or biochemical (Tay–Sachs disease).
- The Genetic Information Nondiscrimination Act (2008) is designed to prohibit improper use of genetic information in health insurance and employment.
- Individuals have a right to this information, but they also have a right not to know.

- The clinician may be faced with an ethical dilemma—needing to safeguard the right to privacy for the patient, but also wanting to safeguard the health of family members who may be unaware of their personal risk.
- If individuals decide to know they have a genetic disease or a predisposition to a disease, they cannot lie on health insurance questionnaires; otherwise they could have committed fraud.
- HIPAA states explicitly that genetic information, in the absence of a current diagnosis of illness, shall not be considered a preexisting condition.
- Many individuals with Huntington disease choose not to have presymptomatic testing performed because this is a late-onset disorder. Individual is usually without symptoms until after the age of 35 to 40.
- A woman has the right to refuse prenatal genetic testing; however, courts have intervened and mandated prenatal testing and therapy when it is demonstrated that the health and well-being of the fetus will be affected adversely by the mother's refusal of these procedures.
- Gene therapy involves pinpointing a defective gene in a germ-line cell, replacing it with a normal version, thus preventing a disease.
- Risks of gene therapy include introducing a disease by way of a vector and a mild-to-severe immune response.

4. **Genetic Re-engineering**
- Genetic re-engineering (GM) involves technologies that alter the genetic makeup of living organisms—such as animals, plants, or bacteria by combining genes from different organisms. It is also known as recombinant DNA.
- Farmers have been selectively breeding plants and animals since the 19th century, but environmentalists have produced a significant backlash protest.
- GM offers a way to improve crop characteristics, such as yield and resistance to pests, enhance taste and quality, reduce growing time, and produce new products.
- Scientists speculate on the risk of unanticipated allergic responses, the spread of pest and herbicide resistance to unwanted plants, and the loss of flora and fauna biodiversity.

B. Reproductive Technology

1. **Abortion**
- *Roe v. Wade* (1973) protects the fundamental right to abortion.
- Debate continues: unborn child's right to life versus a woman's right to make her own decision about whether to bear a child.
- *Planned Parenthood Association of Southeastern PA v. Casey* (1992) affirmed a woman's right to terminate pregnancy until viability, and if necessary to protect her life or health. State laws regulating abortion were determined to be valid if they do

not impose an undue burden or substantial obstacle to access to abortion.

- Partial-birth Abortion Act (2003) banned these abortions in the United States and was upheld in 2007 by U.S. Supreme Court. This statute deals with a method of abortion usually used in the second trimester, from 15 to 26 weeks, some of which occur before and some of which occur after viability.
- When discussing potential outcomes of prenatal testing, it is important to include abortion.

2. In Vitro Fertilization

- Couple at risk for passing on a genetic disorder could use in vitro fertilization to create embryos, test for the condition, and discard embryos that carry the condition.
- Children can be created to be possible donors for existing siblings ("spare parts").

3. Surrogate Motherhood

- Allows infertile couple the opportunity to have a biologically related child by implanting a fertilized egg into the uterus of a surrogate.
- Sperm from man combined with egg either from a surrogate or from his wife.
- Written contract involved.
- Ethical issues: Commercial surrogacy—sperm and egg from the infertile couple, surrogate mother is essentially a "rented" womb.
- Birth mother gives custody of child to biologic father, wife adopts the child.
- Problems arise when the surrogate mother refuses to surrender custody of the baby.

4. Sterilization

- An estimated 65,000 Americans were subjected to involuntary sterilization beginning in the late 1800s through the late 1970s to prevent those considered "unfit" from passing on their traits to future generations.
- Eugenics (the study of human genetics and its application to human problems) was upheld by the U.S. Supreme Court in 1927 (*Buck v. Bell*).
- Sterilization should not occur without informed consent.

C. Mental Health

1. Professional Boundaries

- Maintain professional boundaries between the clinician and the patient in a therapeutic relationship; relationship should not be that of a friend or a family member.
- Clinicians must monitor the quality and amount of personal self-disclosure, and, as a rule, it is best to set limits.

2. Americans with Disabilities Act

- A qualified individual with a disability is defined as an individual who, with or without reasonable accommodation, can perform the essential functions of the employment position that such an individual without a disability can perform.
- Reasonable accommodations may involve job restructuring, acquisition of equipment or devices, and modification of policies or training materials.
- For health care providers recovering from substance abuse, this might include not allowing them to prescribe opioids.
- For the purposes of this Act, the phrase, *individual with a disability*, does not include an individual currently engaging in the illegal use of drugs.

3. Suicide Assessment

- Ask if patients have thoughts of killing themselves (suicidal), or have thought about ending their life. If yes, . . .
- Ask if they have a plan. If yes, . . .
- Ask if they have the means (i.e., firearms or pills). If yes, . . .
- Ask if they are willing to give you the means. If no, hospitalize.
- Also assess current level of support systems.

D. Organ Transplant

1. Ethical issues in organ transplant include (1) definitions of death; (2) maximizing the number of organs, yet demonstrating respect for donor, donor family, or both; and (3) allocation of organs.
2. Uniform Declaration of Death Act (1981) says that an individual who has sustained either (1) irreversible cessation of circulatory and respiratory functions or (2) irreversible cessation of all functions of the entire brain, including the brain stem, is dead.
3. Allocation of organs is determined by medical need, tissue matching, and length of time on a list. A tension exists between distributive justice, which would argue for the sickest candidate, and utilitarian justice, which would support giving the organ to the candidate who is likely to receive the most benefit.
   - The transplant waiting list is fair because it is maintained by a nonprofit organization, the United Network for Organ Sharing, under contract with the U.S. Department of Health and Human Services (HHS).
   - Organ donation is an act of beneficence; it is not an act of malfeasance not to choose to donate.
   - An individual can be on more than one organ procurement organization list. This double listing may be regarded as questionable, but it is legal.
4. Living donors are being used for kidney, tissue, and liver transplants. Quality of the organs is superior, with few reported long-term problems for the donors.
5. "Presumed consent" would change the US present system. The same registry process currently existing could be used. Instead of checking the list to determine whether an individual's name appeared for donation, the registry would check to see whether

individual did not wish to donate. This would remove the burden from families of making a decision while dealing with a traumatic event. Most European nations have this system with an opt-out rate of approximately 2%.

6. Arguments against legalizing the sale of human organs include (1) selling organs is disrespectful to the sanctity of life; (2) selling an organ would further disadvantage the poor in favor of the rich; (3) individuals would be vulnerable to coercion; (4) quality of the organ may be less because persons in financial need may not have access to appropriate health care.
   - Individuals who buy organs abroad are entitled to health care coverage for posttransplant care.
7. Research shows that children of transplant recipients are often premature; however, follow-up research indicates that these children are generally healthy and developing well.
8. Xenotransplantation:
   - Xenotransplantation involves transplants across species barriers; however, most have caused hyperacute rejection.
   - Potential lethal viruses could be introduced into the human body.
   - Currently banned in the United States.

E. Research on Human Subjects

1. Institutional Review Board (IRB)
- The U.S. Food and Drug Administration requires that every organization conducting research on human subjects have an IRB.
- IRBs review each study and associated documents to ensure the welfare of participants is protected.
- The IRB has the authority to approve, require modification in, or disapprove research.
- The IRB reviews the informed consent process to ensure the subjects are provided with an accurate and fair description of what the research entails, as well as the risks and benefits.
- IRB has responsibility to ensure that the subjects were not coerced in any way to participate.
- IRB assures privacy and confidentiality of participants' research records.
- IRB monitors the research to determine whether any adverse events have occurred; it has the responsibility to report these events immediately to the sponsor of the research.
- IRB conducts a continuing review at least annually until the study is closed.
- It is not uncommon for IRB members to receive financial compensation for their services. This compensation is not associated with the individual clinical trials.

2. Protection of Patients in Research
- "Protected populations" are considered to be at higher risks for undue burdens. These individuals include prisoners, economically disadvantaged persons, racial minorities, children, fetuses, pregnant women, and terminally ill individuals.
- Only individuals or organizations that are part of the clinical trial and data-monitoring process are permitted access to patients' medical records.
- If a patient does not understand the trial or procedures, the researcher or clinical trial coordinator should be notified and treatment withheld until the patient verbalizes a clearer understanding.
- Clinical trials may be terminated because of unacceptable toxicities in patients, or failure to benefit from reasonable course of the therapy.
- Collection and storage of blood and tissue samples for future research are not ethical unless full consent is obtained. Patients should be given the opportunity to refuse participation and be recontacted for informed consent as each new project is undertaken.

F. Neonates, Infants, and Children

1. Prenatal diagnosis
- Provider's own views may influence how information is presented.
- Informed consent for testing is necessary.
- Abortion could be a consequence of some types of testing, either directly (amniocentesis) or indirectly (abnormal finding leading to decision to terminate the pregnancy).
- Testing can be done to prepare for the birth of an affected child, or to make a decision about abortion.
- Should not be used to select for desirable characteristics (e.g., sex) or abortion for minor conditions.

2. Baby Doe (1982)
- The situation involved forgoing the life-sustaining treatment of an infant.
- HHS proposed regulations that prohibited discrimination against individuals with handicaps. The purpose of the regulation was to ensure that infants received all potentially effective lifesaving treatment without consideration of quality of life.
- All infants must receive appropriate nutrition, hydration, and medication, and must be given medically indicated treatment unless the infant is irreversibly comatose, the treatment would merely prolong dying, or the treatment would be futile.

3. Parent's authority to make decisions on treatment is considered part of the power that society grants parents. They have moral responsibility for their children.

4. Infants <24 weeks, or 500 g, at birth should not be resuscitated unless parents request full support and the infant is viable.

5. Infants with trisomy: Trisomy 13 or trisomy 18 have extremely poor prognosis, but infants with trisomy

21 (Down syndrome) can often function in family and work settings.

6. Parental consent is usually the only permission needed for sibling donation of bone marrow.

7. The desire to avoid emotional, financial, or other hardships cannot justify the denial of clearly beneficial care to an ill or injured child.

8. In cases of uncertainty, most err on the side of life.
   - This can ignore the suffering (i.e., suffering of infant in neonatal ICU or the suffering of chronic ventilator children).
   - Individualized prognosis, using the data of present condition and benefit–burden analysis, may be the best way to decide in cases of uncertainty.

G. HIV-AIDS

1. **Testing**
   - Many states have statutes about informed consent for testing.
   - Insurance carriers cannot legally deny insurance if an individual has HIV.
   - Carriers cannot cancel existing insurance, unless the individual lied about a preexisting condition.
   - Individuals cannot be tested for HIV without their consent, except in cases of rape, in which the victim is given the results.

2. **Reporting**
   - Tension exists between maintaining confidentiality and protecting at-risk, innocent third parties.
   - Providers have a duty to protect the public.
   - Public health model of reporting and contact tracing has not been used because of concern about discrimination of infected patients, or those perceived to be infected.
   - Now that treatment is available, the case for mandatory partner notification is stronger.
   - The patient has a right to know HIV status of the health care provider, if the provider is performing an exposure-prone procedure.

3. **Americans with Disabilities Act Protection**
   - People who are HIV-positive or have AIDS are protected under the Americans with Disabilities Act of 1990 (protects against employment discrimination based on disability) and the Rehabilitation Act of 1973 (prohibits employment discrimination of the handicapped).

4. **Autonomy of Patient to Behave Freely**
   - Someone who is HIV positive and fails to inform sexual partners may be held legally liable.
   - HIV-infected babies who receive treatment and whose mothers received treatment prenatally have 99% chance of not having HIV.
   - Without treatment, the risk of acquiring HIV is 15% to 25%.
   - Harm reduction practices, such as needle exchange and providing condoms in schools, are ethical.

H. Long-Term Care

1. **Dementia**
   - Recent research has shown that individuals with mild-to-moderate dementia can often express consistent preferences in care, and consistently name the person they wish would make decisions for them.
   - The Nursing Home Reform Act (1987) upholds the principle that residents have the right to self-determination, including the right to participate in care planning and the right to refuse treatment.

2. **Restraint-Free Environment**
   - A restraint is any device used to restrict the freedom of a person, including side-rails, belts, vests, hand mitts, and Geri chairs.
   - The Nursing Home Reform Act (1987) states that the resident has a right to be free from physical and chemical restraints imposed for the purposes of discipline or convenience.
   - Before restraining a resident, the facility must demonstrate the presence of a specific medical symptom that will require the use of restraints and how the use of restraints would (1) treat the cause of the symptom and (2) assist the resident in reaching the highest level of physical and psychosocial well-being.
   - A medication is considered a chemical restraint if administered for the primary purpose of reducing an individual's functional capacity (sedation).

3. **Residents' Bill of Rights**
   - The right to be fully informed.
   - The right to make independent decisions.
   - The right to privacy and confidentiality.
   - The right to dignity, respect, and freedom.
   - The right to security of possessions.
   - The right to be transferred or discharged.
   - The right to complain.
   - The right to visits.

4. **Residents' Council/Ombudsman**
   - Residents' Council identifies concerns that need to be addressed by the appropriate administrative person.
   - The ombudsman is a resident advocate and is often able to mediate discussions with the interdisciplinary team. The ombudsman makes sure the residents' rights and wishes are respected.
   - Residents who have swallowing difficulty and are at risk for aspiration still have a right to continue to eat foods. Nursing homes must demonstrate a discussion with family, increased supervision during eating, and informed consent of risks.
   - Resident has a right to refuse medications, as long as he or she has the capacity for decision making. Clinician must document and discuss options with family.
   - Staff has a legal obligation to report resident abuse as seen by other staff members, or from resident to resident.

I. Death and Dying

1. Cardiopulmonary Resuscitation (CPR)

- CPR was designed originally for sudden cardiac arrest caused by anesthesia, drowning, or myocardial infarctions. Instead, it is applied currently to all individuals unless they have specific orders written to the contrary.
- CPR does not need consent because it is an emergency.
- CPR is not mandated when considered futile.

2. Do Not Resuscitate (DNR)

- Patients and families must be consulted before a DNR order is written.
- However, if clinicians determine CPR would be futile, the clinicians do not need the patient's consent to not resuscitate, even though it would need to be discussed with the patient or surrogate.
- It is the patient's decision if he or she refuses CPR in advance; it is a medical decision if the patient's death is anticipated.
- DNR is suspended routinely during surgery.

3. Study to Understand Prognoses and Preferences for Outcomes and Risks of Treatment (SUPPORT)

- Population studied was 5,176 seriously ill patients in medical centers (MCs) across the country.
- Forty-seven percent of the physicians knew their patient's desire to avoid CPR; 46% of DNR orders were written in the last 2 days of life.
- Thirty-eight percent of patients who died spent at least 10 days in the ICU.
- Fifty percent of the patients who died in the hospital had family members reporting the patient was experiencing moderate-to-severe pain at least 50% of the time.
- In phase II of the study, an advanced practice nurse (APN) was used in each MC. The APNs had multiple contacts with patients, families, physicians, and hospital staff members to elicit their preferences, improve understanding of outcomes, encourage pain control, and facilitate advance-care planning. There was no significant improvement in the above statistics.

4. Persistent Vegetative State (PVS)

- Condition in which severe bilateral cerebral damage, either from an acute event or from progressive dementia, results in irreversible coma, leaving only automatic functions intact.
- Patients have no awareness, but sleep/wake cycles and other automatic responses such as eye movement, swallowing, grimacing, and papillary changes in response to light may remain functioning.
- Quinlan case (1975)—a 21-year-old woman suffered severe brain damage after an alcohol/drug overdose. She was resuscitated and was in a PVS. The father petitioned the court to allow him to remove the ventilator, and the case became the first "right to die" case in the country.
- Cruzan case (1988)—a case (similar to the Quinlan case) in which the family demanded the right to withdraw a feeding tube from this woman who was in a PVS. It was the first "right to die" case to be heard by the U.S. Supreme Court.
- This landmark Cruzan case found that it was unconstitutional to override the treatment directives of the individual and that no legal distinction existed between withdrawing and withholding of treatment.
- This case established the standard of proof to be "clear and convincing evidence," not evidence "beyond a reasonable doubt" (evidence needed to convict in criminal trials).
- Cruzan case established a constitutional right to refuse treatment based on the 14th Amendment to the U.S. Constitution, which states that "no state can deny life, liberty, or property without due process of law."
- Busalacchi case (1993)—another woman in a PVS, whose father wanted to remove the feeding tube. Nurses at the rehabilitation facility protested, stating the patient was able to express emotions, make purposeful movements, and feel pain. The U.S. Supreme Court overruled the nurses' objections, the feeding tube was removed, and the patient was allowed to die by dehydration.
- Terri Schiavo (2003)—40-year-old woman who had been in a PVS since her heart stopped at the age of 26. Mr. Schiavo wanted feeding tube removed and her parents objected, leading to the ensuing court battle. Governor Bush created "Terri's Law" to stop removal of tube in October 2003. Law violated equal protection and due process and separation of powers, not decided on privacy rights. This case was about maintaining the integrity of our constitutional system of government; no branch can encroach on the powers of another branch.

5. Withholding and Withdrawing of Treatment

- Although no ethical or legal difference exists between these two, people who participate in withdrawing of treatment report a significant emotional difference.
- Withholding treatment usually allows death before treatment is implemented. Withdrawing treatment occurs after some analysis of the case has occurred.

6. Medical Futility

- Treatment would provide insignificant benefit or improvement, not only in relation to the patient's underlying clinical condition, but also in relation to the patient's values and goals.
- Reasoning and medical experience indicate that the intervention would be highly unlikely to result in meaningful survival for patient—meaningful survival as defined by the patient.

- Treatment is ineffective more than 99% of the time.
- Treatment does not conform to accepted community standards.
- Wanglie case (1991)—woman with diagnosed PVS. Her husband and children, because of their religious beliefs, insisted that she be kept alive at all costs. Hospital petitioned the courts and courts denied the requests, affirming that Mr. Wanglie was the proper surrogate. The patient died several months after the hearing, still supported by a ventilator.

7. **Definition of Death**
   - Uniform Determination of Death Act (1981)—brain death is determined by the following:
     - Unresponsiveness to intensely painful stimuli.
     - No movement or breathing for a period of at least 1 hour, or, if on ventilator, 3 or more minutes without spontaneous breathing if the respirator is turned off.
     - No reflexes.
     - A flat electroencephalogram recorded for a minimum of 10 minutes and repeated at least 24 hours later with no change.

8. **The Principle of Double Effect**
   - Developed by Roman Catholic moral theologians in the Middle Ages, it is applied to situations in which all harmful action is impossible to avoid, and a decision must be made about whether one potentially harmful action is preferable to another.
   - The following four conditions must be present:
     - The act itself must be good (e.g., relieving pain by giving morphine).
     - The individual must sincerely intend only the good effect and not the evil (e.g., to relieve pain, not to kill the patient).
     - Bad effect cannot be the means to the good effect (e.g., respiratory depression cannot be the means to relieve pain).
     - The good effect must outweigh the bad effect (e.g., relief of pain and suffering in a dying patient even though death may be hastened).

9. **Terminal Sedation**
   - Terminal sedation is accomplished through a barbiturate or benzodiazepine infusion, and the patient ceases eating and drinking.
   - Used in rare cases at end-of-life where severe, unrelievable suffering is occurring.
   - Used to relieve physical distress to render the patient unconscious, not to intentionally end his or her life.
   - Used regularly in critical care practice to treat symptoms of suffocation in dying patients who are discontinuing mechanical ventilation.
   - Voluntary cessation of eating and drinking is, by definition, a patient's decision; the clinician's role is one of providing continued palliative care and support. Pope John II proposed in 2004 that artificial hydration and nutrition is part of care and should be provided for all patients in PVS. This continues to cause contentious debate among Catholic theologians.
   - In June 1997, the U.S. Supreme Court unequivocally supported the patient's right to refuse treatment, even if the intention is to hasten death, on the basis of the patient's right to bodily integrity.
   - Justices O'Connor and Souter wrote supporting use of medication to alleviate the pain and suffering of terminally ill patients, even to the point of causing unconsciousness or hastening death.

10. **Physician-Assisted Suicide (PAS) and Euthanasia**
    - In PAS, a physician facilitates a patient's death by providing the necessary means (e.g., phenobarbital) and/or information to enable the patient to kill himself or herself.
    - In euthanasia, a physician acts to intentionally take the life of the patient, through such means as lethal injection, thereby bringing about a death of a hopelessly ill and suffering person in a relatively quick and painless way for reasons of mercy.
    - Supporters of both focus on (1) compassion for the incurably ill who suffer and (2) respect for human dignity.
    - Opponents believe these practices undermine the trust in the patient–clinician relationship and lead to involuntary killing of handicapped, the poor, and other disenfranchised members of society.
    - *Quill v. Vacco*—the Court refused to declare that the U.S. Constitution gives terminally ill persons a fundamental right to ask for assistance in hastening their deaths by taking medications prescribed by physicians; when a person refuses life-sustaining treatment, he or she dies from underlying fatal disease or pathology; but if a patient takes a lethal medication prescribed by a physician, he or she is killed by the medication.

11. **The Right-to-Die Movement**
    - The right-to-die movement encourages engineering death, rather than facing death.
    - *Final Exit* is a book published by the Hemlock Society that gives explicit advice on how terminally ill patients can commit suicide.
    - The Oregon Death with Dignity Act was implemented in 1997 to provide PAS. In the United States, PAS is legal in the states of Oregon, Washington (2010), and Montana (2011).
    - Compassion in Dying is an organization formed in Oregon that provides support to individuals who choose to use PAS.

12. **Hospice and Palliative Care**
    - These terms were first applied to specialized care for dying patients in 1967, when Dr. Cicely

Saunders founded the first modern hospice at St. Christopher's Hospice, London, United Kingdom.

- A model for quality, compassionate care for people facing life-limiting illness. Focus is on caring, not curing.
- It is a team-oriented approach to pain management, and emotional and spiritual support for both the patient and the family.
- Hospice care is usually provided in the home, but can be provided in free-standing hospice centers, nursing homes, and hospitals.
- Bergman case (2002)—family sued physician for managing pain inadequately at end-of-life. Set a standard for adequate pain management.
- Hospice care is covered under Medicare, Medicaid, and most private insurance plans for the past 6 months of a patient's life.
- Palliative care is active, total care of patients whose disease is not responsive to curative treatment. The goal is to achieve the best possible quality of life for patients and their families through control of pain and other symptoms of psychological, social, and spiritual nature.

13. Advance Directives
- Patient Self-Determination Act of 1991—under this law, patients must be informed of their rights to accept or refuse care and make advance directives.
- Living wills are a set of instructions that indicate what individuals do or do not want when they are in a terminal condition or in a state of permanent unconsciousness.
- Health care proxy or durable power of attorney for health care indicates that a person empowered to make decisions when an individual is no longer able to make decisions for himself or herself.

J. Ethics Committees
- Joint Commission established Standards on Patient Rights and Organizational Ethics, under which all health care organizations must meet a standard of addressing ethical issues. Ethics committees have been formed to meet this standard.
- The role of the ethics committee is to improve bioethical decision making in the institution. Case consultation is a part of its role.
- Ethics consultation is indicated when differences exist among family members, interdisciplinary team members, physicians, or physician and patient/family.
- Ethics consultation is also indicated if an individual believes an ethical dilemma is not being addressed, such as when advance directives are not being followed.
- Cases brought to the ethics committee involve treatment decisions, such as withholding and withdrawing of therapy, discontinuation of life-sustaining therapy, or evaluating decision-making capacities.

- Physicians are not required to do what ethics committees recommend; however, they usually take these recommendations seriously and choose to follow some or all of them.
- Ethics committees also review policies and make recommendations for changes.

K. Managed Care and Advocacy
1. Managed care seeks to integrate the financing and delivery of health care by contracting with providers (health care professionals, clinics, and hospitals) to provide care to an enrolled patient population for a fixed premium.
   - Providers may be part of an incentive plan (i.e., their compensation may depend on their use of resources in caring for their patients).
2. Principle of justice can be in conflict with principle of patient autonomy, as providers are encouraged to make cost-effective clinical decisions (conserve scarce resources), while advocating for what is medically appropriate.
3. Issues to consider when working with or evaluating a managed care organization:
   - Quality of care—the organization has the resources, commitment, and ability to provide reasonable health care to its members.
   - Patient choice—patients are able to choose their own primary care provider and specialists, to go to the emergency room without prior approval, and make decisions concerning their own health care.
   - Advocacy—providers are able to advocate for their patients.
   - Full disclosure—patients are provided with information regarding treatment options not covered by the health care plan and provider's financial incentives that could influence treatment recommendations.
   - Internal and external appeals and grievance procedures—mechanisms are available to patients and providers to resolve disputes and disagreements about treatment.

L. Religion and Ethics/Culture and Ethics
- Patients' understanding of their illnesses may be affected by cultural or religious beliefs, which need to be taken into consideration by providers.

1. Jehovah's Witnesses
- Reject blood transfusions as a treatment modality.
- Courts have upheld the right of adult Jehovah's Witnesses to refuse blood for themselves, but have not usually upheld their right to refuse a transfusion for their children.

2. Church of Christian Science
- Advocates spiritual and natural healing. The sick are treated through prayer by the Christian Scientist healer.
- Their influence was severely curtailed in 1997 with a court decision on children's treatment. Cases

continue to make the news, as parents are tried in court.

3. **Different Cultures**
   - Cultural beliefs that could affect medical care may differ from the provider's beliefs.
   - People from some cultures rely on community elders to make decisions.
   - The patient and provider should come to an agreement on a treatment course acceptable to both.
   - Do not use family members to translate when patients do not speak English; this violates confidentiality and family members may interpret rather than translate in an effort to protect the patient.
   - Coin rubbing and cupping are traditional forms of healing in Asian cultures.
   - African Americans tend to be resistant to organ donation, advance directives, and enrollment in hospice, due to concerns about clinician premature withdrawal of life-prolonging interventions.

VI. Legal Issues

A. Civil Law
1. Law punishes wrongs against an individual.
2. The wrong is called a tort, in which parties start out unharmed then one does a wrong to the other (victim); the victim cannot be unwronged, and therefore to restore balance, a punishment is administered to the wrongdoer. The victim seeks to be "unwronged" by receiving money—financial restitution.

B. Criminal Law
1. Law punishes wrongs against the individual/group.
   - Defendants can lose their money (fine) or their lives (in jail or being executed).
   - Clinicians can also lose their licenses.

C. Laws by Representatives of Society
1. Statutes are written by the legislative branch, either federal or state.
   - Statutes are the source of most law that affects clinicians (i.e., living wills).
   - Licensure, consent to treat, Medicare and Medicaid reimbursement, and employment law are largely controlled by statutes.
2. Regulations are written by the executive branch of the government (governor of a state, president of the country).
   - The board of medicine writes the scope of care.
3. Case law is written by judges after deciding on appeals of lawsuits.
   - Case law sets a precedent and is considered written law, binding on future cases in lower courts.
   - It is referred to as common law because it is written by judges after they make a decision in a case.

D. Plaintiff and Defendant
1. Plaintiff is the wronged party, or victim, in a lawsuit.
   - Person who brings a claim or lawsuit.

2. The defendant is the perceived wrongdoer in the case.
   - Person against whom a malpractice claim is brought.

E. Elements of Malpractice
1. **Professional Misconduct**
   - Negligent care and treatment, or failure to meet the standard of care by a PA that results in harm to others.
   - Negligence is the failure to act as an ordinary prudent person or a "reasonable person" would under similar circumstances.
2. **Examples of Negligence**
   - Failure to carry out physician's orders.
   - Failure to recognize and report patient's signs and symptoms.
   - Failure to take the necessary steps in an emergency.
   - Failure to see that faulty equipment is fixed.
   - Failure to recognize dangers inherent in physician's orders.
3. **The Basis for Professional Liability**
   - Duty—PA is charged with the duty to assume the care of potential patients and act appropriately.
   - Breach of duty—PA breaches his or her duty to the patient and fails to act as a reasonable PA would in similar circumstances, based on the standard of care, statutes and regulations, or standards of professional associations.
   - Causation—Has the breach resulted in injury to the patient? To be civilly liable, the PA's failure to act in accordance with standards of care must have resulted in some harm to the patient, which the patient would have not otherwise sustained.
   - Injury or damage—actual harmful results to the patient.

F. Intentional Torts
1. **Defamation**
   - Oral or written communication to someone other than the person defamed that tends to injure the individual's reputation (diminishes esteem, respect, or confidence in the person).
2. **Assault**
   - An intentional act by one person that causes another person to fear he or she will be touched in an offensive or injurious manner.
3. **Battery**
   - An intentional act in which physical contact or touching in an offensive or injurious manner has occurred.
4. **False Imprisonment**
   - Unlawful intentional confinement of another within fixed boundaries so that the confined person is conscious of the confinement or is harmed by it.

G. Guidelines for a PA Serving as an Expert Witness

1. During litigation, the standard of care is applied to the case by the expert-witness testimony.

2. These guidelines are not meant as legal advice, but as guidance for the PA in determining whether he or she will choose to act as an expert witness.

   - Guideline 1: A PA serving as an expert witness should have current experience and knowledge in the area about which he or she is to testify.

   - Guideline 2: A PA expert must evaluate facts objectively and provide an opinion. The testimony based on a review of the medical facts should not favor either the plaintiff or the defendant, but simply the truth.

   - Guideline 3: The testimony should not attack performance that falls within acceptable standards of practice or, conversely, support obviously deficient practice.

   - Guideline 4: The PA should offer an opinion on the basis of customary practice; innovations in medical practice should be identified as such.

   - Guideline 5: The PA should testify truthfully and consistently.

   - Guide 6: The PA should not accept a contingency fee, based on the outcome of the case.

SELECTED REFERENCES

American Academy of Hospice and Palliative Medicine Web site. http://www.aahpm.org. Accessed April 4, 2012.

Beauchamp T, Childress J. *Principles of Biomedical Ethics*. 5th ed. New York, NY: Oxford University Press; 2002.

Buchanan A, Brock D, Daniels N, et al. *From Chance to Choice: Genetics and Justice*. New York, NY: Cambridge University Press; 2000.

Center for Bioethics Web Site. http://www.bioethics.net. Accessed April 4, 2012.

Chervenak FA, McCullough LB. The limits of variability. *J Perinat Med.* 1997;25(5):418–420.

Emanuel L, VonGunter C, Ferris F, eds. Education of physicians on end-of-life care (EPEC) curriculum. http://www.epec.net/EPEC/webpages/index.cfm. Accessed April 4, 2012.

Fletcher J, Spencer E, Lombardo P. *Introduction to Clinical Ethics*. 3rd ed. Hagerstown, MD: University Publishing Group; 2005.

Guidelines for ethical conduct for the physician assistant profession, policy of the American Academy of Physician Assistants, adopted May 2000, last amended May 2007. http://www.aapa.org. Accessed April 4, 2012.

Hedges R. *Contemporary Legal Issues: Bioethics, Health Care, and the Law, a Dictionary*. Santa Barbara, CA: ABC-CLIO; 1999.

Jonsen AR, Siegler M, Winslade WJ. *Clinical Ethics, a Practical Approach to Ethical Decisions in Clinical Medicine*. 5th ed. New York, NY: McGraw-Hill; 2002.

Singer P. *A Companion to Ethics*. Malden, MA: Blackwell; 2000.

Steinbock B, Arras JD, London AJ. *Ethical Issues in Modern Medicine* (2009). 6th ed. New York, NY: McGraw-Hill; 2003.

Sugarman J. *20 Common Problems: Ethics in Primary Care*. New York, NY: McGraw-Hill; 2000.

Ulrich, C, Danis, M., Ratcliffe, SJ, Garrett-Mayer, E, Koziol, D., Soeken, KL, Grady, C.

Ulrich, C, Danis, M., Ratcliffe, SJ, Garrett-Mayer, E, Koziol, D., Soeken, KL, Grady, C. Ethical conflict in nurse practitioners and physician assistants in managed care. *Nurs Res.* 2006:55(6):391–401.

Veatch R. *Transplantation Ethics*. Washington, DC: Georgetown University Press; 2000.

Environmental Emergencies

Joseph C. Krolikowski • Charles Stream

I. Venomous Bites and Stings

A. Reptile Bites

- An estimated 3 million bites and 150,000 deaths occur worldwide each year annually from venomous snakes.
- Approximately 6,000 bites each year annually, with approximately 2,000 of them from venomous snakes.
- The major venomous snakes of the world can be divided into three groups: Viperidae (vipers), Elapidae, and Hydrophiinae (sea snakes).
- Approximately 20 of the 120 snake species indigenous to North America are venomous and include pit vipers (Crotalinae subfamily of Viperidae) and coral snakes (Elapidae family). The crotaline snakes are represented by the rattlesnakes (*Crotalus* species), pygmy rattlesnakes, massauah (*Sistrurus* species), and the copperheads and water moccasins (*Agkistrodon* species).

1. Crotaline (Pit Viper) Bites

- The crotaline snakes are called pit vipers because of depressions or pits located midway between and below the level of the eye and nostril that function as a heat receptor that guides strikes at warm-blooded prey or predators.

PATHOPHYSIOLOGY

- Crotaline venom is a complex enzyme mixture that causes local tissue injury, systemic vascular damage, hemolysis, fibrinolysis, and neuromuscular dysfunction.
- Hypovolemia, coagulopathy, cranial nerve weakness, respiratory failure, and altered mental status.

CLINICAL FEATURES

- Fang marks, localized pain, and progressive edema, nausea and vomiting, weakness, oral numbness or tingling of tongue and mouth, tachycardia, dizziness, and muscle fasciculation.
- Systemic effects with tachypnea, tachycardia, hypotension, and altered level of consciousness. In general, local swelling at the bite site becomes apparent within 15 to 30 minutes, but in some cases, it may not start for several hours.
- Edema may progress to involve an entire limb within an hour. Edema near an airway or in a muscle compartment may threaten life or limb without the presence of systemic effects.

DIAGNOSIS

- Presence of fang marks and a history consistent with exposure to a snake plus evidence of tissue injury.
- Clinically, the injury may be manifested in three ways: local injury, coagulopathy, or systemically.
- The absence of any of these manifestations for a period of 8 to 12 hours after the bite indicates a dry bite.

TREATMENT

- Immediate transport to the emergency department.
- Tourniquets are contraindicated.
- Constriction bands may be of some use: an elastic bandage or Penrose drain, rope, or a piece of clothing wrapped circumferentially above the bite, applied with enough tension to restrict superficial venous and lymphatic flow while maintaining distal pulses.
- Advanced life support as indicated.
- Rapid intravenous isotonic fluid infusion for hypotension.
- Supplemental oxygen.
- Limb immobilization continued during transport to reduce further venom absorption.
- Cleanse the wound area.
- Tetanus prophylaxis.
- Antivenom is the mainstay of therapy.

2. Coral Snake (Elapid) Bite

- North American coral snakes include the eastern coral snake (*Micrurus fulvius fulvius*), the Texas coral snake (*Micrurus fulvius tener*), and the Arizona (Sonoran) coral snake (*Micruroides euryoxanthus*).
- The eastern coral snake is found primarily in the southeast United States.
- The Texas and Arizona coral snakes are found primarily in the states that bear their names.
- Venom is primarily composed of neurotoxic components.

CLINICAL FEATURES

- Primary neurologic effects: salivation, dysarthria, diplopia, bulbar paralysis with ptosis, fixed and contracted pupils, dysphagia, dyspnea, and tremors and seizures.
- Cause of death is paralysis of respiratory muscles. Signs and symptoms may be delayed up to 12 hours.

DIAGNOSIS

- Presence of fang marks and a history consistent with exposure to a snake.

TREATMENT

- Hospital admission for observation.
- Antivenin (*Micrurus fulvius*), administered to patients who have definitely been bitten because it may not be possible to prevent further effects or reverse effects that have already developed.
- Respiratory monitoring.
- Bites by the Sonoran coral snake are mild, and antivenom is not usually needed.

B. Spider Bites

1. Brown Recluse Spider Bites

ETIOLOGY

- The brown recluse spider (*Loxosceles reclusa*) is one of the most common species found in the United States, with an endemic range in the south-central United States, from Texas to Georgia and Iowa to Louisiana.
- Approximately 1-cm body, a tan to brown coloration, and a violin-shaped mark on its dorsal cephalothorax.
- Prefers warm, dry areas such as abandoned buildings, woodpiles, and cellars.

PATHOPHYSIOLOGY

- The venom of the brown recluse has multiple enzymes (hyaluronidase, alkaline phosphate, 5′-ribonucleotide phosphohydrolase, and sphingomyelinase D).
- Sphingomyelinase D is the major enzyme responsible for necrosis.
- Necrotic wounds are possible through neutrophil activation, platelet aggregation, and intravascular thrombosis.

CLINICAL FEATURES

- Initial bite is painless, usually prohibiting definitive identification of the spider.
- Most common manifestation is mild erythematous lesion that will become firm and heal over several days to weeks.
- Occasionally, a more serve local reaction occurs, starting with mild to severe pain for several hours with discoloration within the first 24 hours.
- This lesion may become necrotic over the next 3 to 4 days, with eschar formation by the end of the first week.

MANAGEMENT

- Tetanus prophylaxis.
- Analgesics.
- Antibiotics when appropriate.
- Surgery consult for lesions >2 cm.
- Dapsone and hyperbaric treatment controversial.
- Hospitalization for system reactions.

2. Black Widow Spider Bites

ETIOLOGY

- The black widow spider (*Latrodectus mactans*) is found in woodpiles, basements, garages, and sheds.
- Classic orange-red hourglass-shaped marking.
- Female spiders range in body size up to 1.5 cm in length with leg spans of 4 to 5 cm.
- Female spider will aggressively defend her web, particularly when guarding her eggs.
- Most bites occur between April and October and are usually seen on the hands and forearm.
- Male spider is approximately one-third the size of the female, lighter in color, and bite cannot penetrate human skin.

PATHOPHYSIOLOGY

- Active component of the venom is α-latrotoxin, acting through a calcium-mediated mechanism leading predominately to the release of acetylcholine and norepinephrine from nerve terminals.

CLINICAL FEATURES

- Initial bite is felt as a pinprick sensation at the bite site, followed by increasing local pain that may spread quickly to include the entire bitten extremity.
- Erythema appears 20 to 60 minutes after the bite.
- In two-thirds of bites, a small <5-mm erythematous macule develops.
- In one-third of bites, initial erythema evolves into a larger "target lesion" with blanched center and surrounding erythema.
- Patients may complain of cramping of the larger muscle groups (trunk, back, and abdomen), which becomes generalized and may be mistaken for a surgical abdomen.
- Confirmatory testing is not available; however, the presence of the characteristic lesion in association with severe pain and muscle spasms is pathognomonic.
- Patients may develop hypertension, and symptoms such as headache, nausea, diarrhea, diaphoresis, photophobia, and dyspnea.

MANAGEMENT

- Supportive care of airway, breathing, and circulation.
- Cleanse the bite site.
- Pain and muscle spasm can be controlled with opioids and benzodiazepines.
- Serve envenomation admission is required for continued analgesia.
- Administration of *Latrodectus* antivenin often causes rapid resolution of symptoms and can shorten the course of illness.
- *Lactrodectus* antivenin is administered by intramuscular injection. It is derived from horse serum and hypersensitivity reactions are possible.

C. Bee Stings (Hymenoptera)

ETIOLOGY
- Most allergic reactions occur from wasp, hornet, and yellow jacket stings.

PATHOPHYSIOLOGY
- Venom composed of many substances.
- Histamine.
- Melitin, causes degranulation of basophils and mast cells.

CLINICAL FEATURES
- **Local reaction:**
  - Urticaria.
  - Pain.
  - Erythema.
  - Edema.
  - Pruritus.
- **Systemic/anaphylactic reaction:**
  - Urticaria.
  - Itchy eyes.
  - Cough.
  - Bronchospasm.
  - As the reaction progresses, patients may experience respiratory and cardiovascular failure.

MANAGEMENT
- Oral antihistamines.
- Analgesics.
- Steroids.
- Bronchospasm responds to inhaled albuterol.
- Hypotension should be treated with crystalloids; may require dopamine and epinephrine.
- Severe reactions require treatment with 1:1,000 epinephrine subcutaneously; 0.3 to 0.5 mL for an adult and 0.01 mL per kg for a child (0.3 mL maximum).
- Patients who experience hymenoptera reactions should be referred to an allergist and prescribed an EpiPen.

D. Marine Fauna Stings, Trauma, and Envenomation

EPIDEMIOLOGY
- There is little information known on the epidemiology of marine injuries and envenomation.
- The most common envenomation incidents occurred with jellyfish stings.
- In the United States, thousands of cases of minor jelly fish stings occur yearly from *Physalia* (Portuguese man-of-war) and *Chrysaora* species.
- Of the 373 species of shark, 32 have been described in attacks on humans.
- Minor trauma is most frequently caused by coral cuts sustained underwater, usually involving the extremities.

CLINICAL FEATURES
- Abrasions, puncture wounds, lacerations, and crush injuries.
- Shark bites are associated with substantial tissue loss, hemorrhagic shock, hypothermia, and near-drowning fatalities.
- Coral cuts are associated with local stinging, erythema, pruritus, and urticaria, which may progress to cellulitis secondary to potentially pathogenic bacteria.

TREATMENT
- Copious irrigation of the affected area and exploration and debridement of tissue.
- Supportive care for hemorrhagic shock, hypothermia, and anaphylaxis.
- Soft-tissue X-rays should be ordered to identify foreign bodies.
- Tetanus prophylaxis.
- Aerobic and anaerobic cultures should be obtained.
- Patients with grossly contaminated soft-tissue injuries should be started on antibiotic therapy that covers *Staphylococcus* and *Streptococcus* species; *Vibrio* species should be covered with a third-generation cephalosporin.

II. Near-Drowning

DEFINITION
- Near-drowning is defined as survival longer than 24 hours after a submersion event.

EPIDEMIOLOGY
- In the United States, drowning is the fourth leading cause of accidental death overall and is the second leading cause of death in those under 15 years of age.
- There are an estimated over 500,000 submersion events per year in the United States.
- Near-drowning events also occur in pools, open bodies of water, toilets, buckets, and bathtubs.

PATHOPHYSIOLOGY
- "Dry-drowning," occurs when there is laryngospasm, followed by hypoxia leading to loss of consciousness.
- "Wet-drowning," occurs more commonly, in which there is aspiration of water into the lungs causing washout of pulmonary surfactant resulting in diminished gas transfer across the alveoli, atelectasis, and ventilation perfusion mismatch. Resulting in hypoxemia and metabolic acidosis.

PREHOSPITAL TREATMENT
- Rapid, cautious rescue.
- C-spine immobilization.
- Cardiopulmonary resuscitation.
- Supplemental oxygen.

EMERGENCY DEPARTMENT
- Secure the airway, provide oxygen, and assist ventilation as necessary.
- Administer warmed isotonic intravenous fluids.

- Warming adjuncts (e.g., blankets, overhead warmers, and warming devices) should be used.
- If after 4 to 6 hours the patient still requires oxygen, has an abnormal pulmonary examination (rales, rhonci, rhonchi, wheeze retractions, etc.), or deteriorates in the emergency department, reassessment and admission or transfer to a monitored bed is needed.
- All near-drowning victims who require emergency department resuscitation should be admitted to an intensive care unit for continuous cardiopulmonary and frequent neurologic monitoring.

III. Lightning Injuries

EPIDEMIOLOGY

- Approximately 300 lightning injuries occur each year in the United States, of which there are about 100 deaths; the US locations with the greatest numbers of incidents include Arizona, Arkansas, Florida, Mississippi, New Mexico, and Wyoming.

PATHOPHYSIOLOGY

- Lightning is a high-voltage direct current (DC) discharge of energy.
- Mechanisms of lightning strikes: direct strike, side flash—when a nearby object is struck and current through the air; contact strike—when an object the person is carrying is struck; ground current—when lightning hits the ground and is transferred to a person.
- Cardiac arrest from DC depolarization of the myocardium causing asystole and respiratory arrest secondary to depolarization of the medullary respiratory center.

CLINICAL FEATURES

- Varying level of mental status.
- Dysrhythmias.
- Burns.
- Cataracts, retinal detachment, corneal lesions, macular degeneration.
- Myoglobinuria.
- Fetal death, placental abruption.

TREATMENT

- Advanced cardiac life support (ACLS) resuscitation for cardiac and respiratory arrest and cardiac dysrhythmias.
- C-spine immobilization.
- IV access.
- Tetanus prophylaxis.
- Hospital admission for close cardiac and neurologic monitoring.

IV. Carbon Monoxide Poisoning

EPIDEMIOLOGY

- Carbon monoxide (CO) poisoning is responsible for greater morbidity and mortality than any other toxin.

- CO is formed from the incomplete combustion of any fossil fuel.
- Exposure is more common in northern climates during colder months.

PATHOPHYSIOLOGY

- CO is an odorless, colorless, nonirritating gas.
- Clinical manifestations can develop with levels as low as 200 parts per million.
- CO binds to hemoglobin about 240 times greater than oxygen.
- Poisoning of the myocardial myoglobin causes decrease in contractility, cardiac output, and oxygen delivery.

CLINICAL FEATURES

- Fatigue.
- Malaise.
- Flulike symptoms; nausea, vomiting.
- Altering variances of level of consciousness.
- Seizures.
- Hypotension.
- Respiratory arrest.
- Myocardial ischemia/arrest.

DIAGNOSIS

- Elevated COHb levels.
- Pulse oximetry.
- Chest radiographs.

EMERGENCY DEPARTMENT TREATMENT

- Attention to airway, breathing, and circulation.
- High-flow 100% oxygen with a tight-fitting mask and reservoir.
- Hyperbaric oxygen therapy is indicated for severe poisoning.

V. Burns

A. Thermal Burns

EPIDEMIOLOGY

- There are more than 1 million burn injuries each year in the United States.
- Burn injuries account for:
  - 700,000 emergency department visits.
  - 45,000 hospitalizations.
  - 4,500 deaths.

PATHOPHYSIOLOGY

- Severity of burn injury is related to the rate at which heat is transferred to the skin, resulting in varying degrees of coagulation, stasis, and hyperemia.

CLINICAL FEATURES

- Burn size is calculated as the percentage of body surface area, either with the "rule of nines," or the Lund and Browder burn diagram.
- Burn depth is described in degrees: first, second, third, and fourth.
- Clinically, burns are classified as superficial partial-thickness, deep partial-thickness, and full-thickness.

- Superficial partial-thickness burns develop blisters and are painful; capillary refill is intact.
- Deep partial-thickness burns are white to yellow in color; two-point discrimination is diminished; capillary refill and pain sensation are absent.
- Full-thickness burns are charred, pale, and leathery in appearance.
- Smoke inhalation can develop into upper airway edema indicated by singed nasal hair, soot in the nose or mouth, carbonaceous sputum, and wheezing.
- CO poisoning should be suspected in all patients.

DIAGNOSIS
- Chest radiograph for smoke inhalation-related injuries; may need to perform flexible fiber-optic bronchoscopy to confirm the diagnosis.
- COHb levels should be obtained.

TREATMENT
- Secure airway, breathing, and circulation.
- High-flow oxygen should be administered.
- Endotracheal intubation should be performed for patients who present with perioral burns, stridor, circumferential neck burns, altered mental status, or respiratory distress.
- Two large-bore intravenous lines.
- Fluid resuscitation directed by the Parkland formula.
- Foley catheter.
- Narcotic analgesia.
- Burns should be cooled either with cold water or with application of cool compresses.
- Escharatomy may need to be performed to circumferential burns.
- Hyperbaric oxygen therapy for those patients who have suffered smoke inhalation.
- Tetanus toxoid prophylaxis.

B. Chemical Burns

EPIDEMIOLOGY
- It is estimated that 5% to 10% of all US burn center admissions are related to chemical burns.
- Common household offending agents are lye, disinfectants, paint removers, bleach, and sulfuric acid.

PATHOPHYSIOLOGY
- Acid burns cause a coagulation necrosis with formation of a leathery eschar.
- Alkali burns result in a liquefaction necrosis that creates passage of hydroxyl ions into deep tissues.

CLINICAL FEATURES
- Skin damage is dependent on the type of agent.
- Pain and tissue destruction.
- Acid burns produce dark brown or black skin discoloration.
- Alkali burns produce soft, gelatinous, brownish eschars; may progress to full-thickness burns.
- Chemical burns of the eye cause redness, pain, and tearing and are considered a medical emergency.

DIAGNOSIS
- pH paper can help differentiate the difference between acid and alkali exposure to the eye.

TREATMENT
- Copious irrigation to the involved area.
- Ocular irrigation with 1 to 2 L of normal saline for a minimum of 1 hour, and a return of the pH to neutral (pH 7.4).
- Gluconate gel applied topically to skin.
- IV fluid resuscitation.
- Analgesia.
- Tetanus toxoid prophylaxis.

C. Electrical Burns

EPIDEMIOLOGY
- Electrocution is the fifth leading cause of fatal occupation injuries in the United States.
- Responsible for approximately 800 deaths annually.
- Household accidents are most common in children.

PATHOPHYSIOLOGY
- Electricity causes damage by direct effects of current on cells, and thermal damage from the heat generated by the resistance of tissues.

CLINICAL FEATURES
- Thermal burns.
- Cardiac arrest, ventricular fibrillation, arrhythmias.
- Hemorrhage, arterial and venous thrombosis, ischemia.
- Loss of consciousness, suppression of respiratory center, seizures, paralysis.
- Rhabdomyolysis.
- Myoglobinuria, renal failure.
- Cataracts.

DIAGNOSIS
- Diagnosis is based on history of event and exposure.
- Elevated creatine kinase due to myocardial damage.
- CT scan of the head for those patients with severe head injury, coma, or varying altered mental status changes.
- ECG to rule cardiac abnormalities.

EMERGENCY DEPARTMENT TREATMENT
- Secure airway, breathing, and circulation.
- High-flow oxygen through air mask.
- Continuous cardiac monitoring.
- Blood pressure monitoring.
- Two large-bore IV lines; IV crystalloid fluid.
- ACLS as needed.
- Tetanus prophylaxis.
- Seizures are treated with standard therapy.
- General surgery consult for evidence of deep tissue injury.

VI. Mushroom and Plant Poisoning

EPIDEMIOLOGY
- Children account for 80% of all plant-related exposures, and mushroom poisonings are the most common.

- Ninety-five percent of fatalities associated with mushrooms in the United States are due to the *Amanita* species.

PATHOPHYSIOLOGY
- The toxins in plants and mushrooms produce physiologic ranging from gastrointestinal and neurologic to organ failure and death.
  - Toxins:
    - Psilocybin and psilocin:
    - Neuroactive chemicals producing hallucinogenic effects similar to lysergic acid diethylamide.
  - Ricin:
    - Cytotoxin causing multiple organ failure.
  - Gyromitrin:
    - Causes hepatic necrosis and inhibits the cytochrome P450 system.
  - Amatoxins:
    - Bind to hepatocytes and inhibit messenger RNA.
  - Amygdalin:
    - Metabolized to hydrocyanic acid leading to acute cyanide poisoning.

CLINICAL FEATURES
- Toxicity from mushroom poisoning occurring within 1 hour of ingestion usually indicates a benign course.
- Toxicity caused by mushroom poisoning >6 hours following ingestion indicates a more severe prognosis.
- Gastrointestinal:
  - Abdominal pain, nausea, vomiting, hematemesis, chemical burns to the oropharynx.
- Neurologic:
  - Seizures, delirium, hallucinations, and death.
- Cardiovascular:
  - Dysrhythmias, hypotension, and conduction defects.
- Dermatologic:
  - Contact dermatitis.
- Muscarinic and cholinergic effects.
- SLUDGE syndrome (*s*alivation, *l*acrimation, *u*rination, *d*efecation, *g*astrointestinal *h*ypermotility, and *e*mesis).

DIAGNOSIS
- On the basis of history of ingestion and symptom onset.
- Cholinergic, anticholinergic involvement should be assessed on physical examination.
- Laboratory analysis should include electrolytes, creatinine, blood urea nitrogen, liver enzymes, and coagulation studies if poisoning is suspected.

TREATMENT
- Supportive care with attention to airway, breathing, and circulation.
- Activated charcoal to decontaminate the gastrointestinal tract.
- High-dose penicillin or cimetidine therapy to block amatoxin uptake into the liver.
  - Penicillin G: 0.3 to 1.0 million units/kg/day.
- Cimetidine: 10 g per day.
- Bowel irrigation.
- Liver transplant when aspartate aminotransferase is >2,000 IU, prothrombin time >50 seconds, or grade 2 hepatic encephalopathy.
- High-dose pyridoxine (25 mg per kg) with neurologic symptoms associated with exposure to gyromitrin.
- Atropine for severe muscarinic effects.
- Orellanine toxicity requires fluid and electrolyte replacement and hemodialysis.
- Amatoxin, gyromitrin, or orellanine exposure requires admission for at least 48 hours; otherwise if asymptomatic after 4 to 6 hours of treatment, can be discharged.

VII. Cold Emergencies

A. Hypothermia

EPIDEMIOLOGY
- Defined as a core temperature of <35° C (95° F).
- More than 700 people die each year in the United States as a result of hypothermia.

PATHOPHYSIOLOGY
- Hypothermia is a result of heat loss by conduction, convection, radiation, or evaporation.
- Exposure to cold environments, slowed metabolic rate, sepsis, depressed CNS, and drug use can predispose hypothermia.

ETIOLOGY
- Environmental.
- Metabolic.
- Hypothalamic and CNS dysfunction.
- Drug induced.
- Sepsis.

CLINICAL FEATURES
- Abnormally low body temperature.
- Drowsiness that may progress to confusion, lethargy, and coma.
- Bradycardia.
- Bradypnea.
- Shivering.
- Weakness.
- Discolored (purple) fingers and toes.
- ECG changes in hypothermia:
  - T-wave inversions.
  - PR, QRS, QT prolongation.
  - Osborn (J) wave.
- Dysrhythmias: sinus bradycardia, atrial fibrillation or flutter, nodal rhythms, AV block, PVCs, ventricular fibrillation, asystole.

TREATMENT
- Gentle rewarming techniques.
- Aggressive handling can precipitate ventricular fibrillation.
- Airway and cardiac support as necessary.
- Warmed intravenous fluids.
- Thiamine-depleted patients (alcoholics) should be administered intravenous thiamine 50 mg.
- Respiratory and cardiac monitoring.

B. Frostbite

EPIDEMIOLOGY
- Elderly, alcoholic abuse, homeless, and the psychiatric populations are at an increased risk.

PATHOPHYSIOLOGY
- Hypothermia causes increased blood viscosity, extracellular ice formation, intracellular dehydration, and lysis leading to progressive tissue loss.

CLINICAL FEATURES
- Early symptoms: shivering, weakness, fatigue, drowsiness, lethargy, and impaired coordination.
- Later findings: bradycardia, hypotension, and hypoventilation.
- Rhabdomyolysis, acute renal failure.
- ECG may show PR, QRS, and QT interval prolongations and Osborn J waves.
- First-degree frostbite—edema, burning, erythema, stinging, and burning.
- Second-degree frostbite—same as above plus blistering.
- Third-degree frostbite—involves deeper layers of skin; hemorrhagic blisters, necrosis, and blue-gray discoloration.
- Fourth-degree frostbite—involves deep tissue injuries of the subcutaneous tissue, muscle, and bone.

DIAGNOSIS
- Hypothermia is diagnosed when the core body temperature is below 35° C or 95° F.

EMERGENCY DEPARTMENT TREATMENT
- Rapid rewarming with water at 107° F.
- Narcotic pain control.
- Penicillin G 500,000 units every 6 hours for 48 to 72 hours.
- Clear blisters can be debrided; hemorrhagic blisters should be left intact.
- Airway, breathing, and circulation.
- ECG.
- Suspected thiamine depletion should receive thiamine 100 mg IV or IM.
- Suspected hypothyroidism should receive IV thyroxine and hydrocortisone 100 mg.
- More aggressive rewarming may need to be performed through gastric, bladder, peritoneal, and pleural lavage.
- Hospital admission for any patient suffering more than superficial frostbite and hypothermia.

VIII. Heat Emergencies

EPIDEMIOLOGY
- Four hundred deaths annually in the United States.
- Children and elderly individuals are at an increased risk.

PATHOPHYSIOLOGY
- Evaporation is the primary mechanism for heat dissipation in a hot environment.
- Exposure to heat stress augments cardiac output, circulation is shifted to the peripheral circulation, vasodilatation occurs, and sweating is enhanced.
- Heat stroke causes endothelial injury, coagulation disorders, circulatory failure, and ultimately multiorgan failure.

CLINICAL FEATURES
- Core temperature ranges from 40° to 47° C.
- Neurologic abnormalities—ataxia, confusion, agitation, seizures, coma.
- Anhidrosis may be present.
- Lactic acidosis.

DIAGNOSIS
- Diagnosis should be considered in the setting of heat stress, hyperthermia, and altered mental status.

EMERGENCY DEPARTMENT TREATMENT
- Airway, breathing, and circulation.
- High-flow supplemental oxygen.
- Monitor core temperature.
- Rehydrate with normal saline or lactated Ringer's.
- Cooling of the patient with fans and spraying the body with tepid water.
- Benzodiazepines for seizures.
- Check electrolytes every few hours.
- Hospital admission.

A. Heat Cramps
- Painful spontaneous contraction of the skeletal muscles.
- Occur during physical activity or after vigorous activity.
- Treatment includes oral or intravenous fluid and salt replacement in a cool location.

B. Heat Exhaustion
- Can occur by two different means, but is often a combination of water depletion and sodium depletion.
- Water depletion occurs when it is hot and there is insufficient water intake or supply.
- Sodium depletion occurs when fluid losses are replaced with significant amounts of isotonic fluids.

CLINICAL FEATURES
- Core body temperature is normal or below 40° C.
- Nausea, vomiting, lightheadedness, headache, tachycardia, and orthostatic hypotension.

- Neurologically intact.
- Electrolyte and hematologic findings are variable depending on the degree of fluid and electrolyte losses.

EMERGENCY DEPARTMENT TREATMENT

- Fluid and electrolyte replacement either orally or intravenously.
- Admission is recommended when critical electrolyte imbalances exist or in patients with congestive heart failure secondary to the time needed to amend the electrolyte and/or fluid deficiencies.
- May progress to heat stroke, therefore if symptoms do not improve after 30 minutes of treatment, core temperature should be cooled to 39° C.

C. Heat Stroke

- Mortality rates as high as 80%.
- Fatal if untreated.
- Differentiation between exertional and nonexertional heat stroke is not necessary because treatment is identical and urgent.

CLINICAL FEATURES

- Core body temperature >40° C.
- Include those seen in heat exhaustion along with confusion, inappropriate behaviors, hallucinations, seizures, hemiplegia, decorticate and decerebrate posture and coma.
- Laboratory studies including, CBC, comprehensive metabolic panel, CPK, arterial blood gas, coagulation profile, ECG, urinalysis chest radiographs, and head CT can assist in identifying end organ damage and ruling out other causes of the altered mental status.

EMERGENCY DEPARTMENT TREATMENT

- Resuscitation including airway, breathing, and circulation. High-flow oxygen and rehydration with normal saline or lactated Ringer's.
- Cooling of the patient with fans and spraying the body with tepid water.
- Hospital admission.

IX. Infectious Diseases

A. American Trypanosomiasis (Chagas Disease)

ETIOLOGY

- Protozoan *T. cruzi*.
- Prevalent in Latin America northward to Texas.
- Vector is the assassin bug that is active in the evening hours.
- Leading cause of congestive heart failure in Latin America.

CLINICAL FEATURES

- Acute illness last for 3 weeks to 3 months with fever, unilateral periorbital edema, lymphadenopathy, edema at the site of the bite, hepatosplenomegaly.
- Latent phase with destruction of nerve cell ganglia causing cardiomyopathy, congestive heart failure, arrhythmias, decreased gastrointestinal performance.
- Peripheral blood smear or culture identifies the parasite in acute illness.
- Serology or muscle biopsy in the latent phase.

TREATMENT

- Nifurtimox orally four times daily for 90 to 120 days depending on age.

B. Human African Trypanosomiasis (African Sleeping Sickness)

ETIOLOGY

- Protozoan *T. brucei gambiense* and *T. brucei rhodesiense*.
- Prevalent in South/Central America and sub-Sahara Africa.
- Vector is the tsetse fly.

CLINICAL FEATURES

- Painless chancre 2 to 3 days after bite that increases in size and resolves after 2 to 3 weeks.
- Fever, fatigue, wasting, changes in behavior, encephalitis, anemia, pancarditis, coma, and death.
- Diagnosis is completed with peripheral blood smears, aspiration of lymph nodes, bone marrow and cerebral spinal fluid examination.

TREATMENT

- Infectious disease consult.

C. Leishmaniasis

ETIOLOGY

- Protozoan.
- Prevalent in Central/South America, Africa, Asia, and the Mediterranean.
- Vector is the sand fly.

CLINICAL FEATURES

- Chronic, systemic disease including fever, wasting, pancytopenia, hepatosplenomegaly, hypergammaglogulnemia.
- High fatality due to secondary infections including pneumonia, dysentery, and tuberculosis.

TREATMENT

- Infectious disease consult.

SELECTED REFERENCES

Tintinalli JE, Stapczynski JS, Cline DM, et al, eds. *Tintinalli's Emergency Medicine, A Comprehensive Study Guide*. 7th ed. Singapore: McGraw Hill Medical; 2011.

21

Preventive Medicine

Parmjeet S. Saini • Patrick C. Auth

I. Primary Prevention

FAMILY VIOLENCE OR DOMESTIC VIOLENCE

1. **Definition**
   - Willful intimidation, battery, sexual assault, or other abusive behavior perpetrated by a family or household member or intimate partner against another with the goal of establishing and maintaining power and control.

2. **Epidemiology**
   - Approximately 1 million children are identified as physically abused in the United States each year.
   - In the United States, approximately 1 to 4 million women are physically, sexually, or emotionally abused by their intimate partners each year.
   - Women are 7 to 14 times more likely to suffer severe physical injuries from an assault by an intimate partner.
   - In 90% of abuse cases, the perpetrator is a family member, usually an adult child or spouse.

3. **Screening**
   - Family Violence Prevention Funds and Health and Human Services (HHS) recommend routine screening as opposed to indicator-based screening for all female patients older than 14 at primary care settings, emergency departments, pediatrics, and mental health clinics.
   - Confidential documentation will increase outcomes and opportunities for identification and intervention and document and report abuse and/or neglect, such as burns, bruises, and repeated suspicious traumatic injury.
   - Screening for child abuse in the primary care setting can include physical examination as well as screening questionnaires.
   - Consider using *Hawaii Risk Indicators Screening Tool* followed by the *Kempe Family Stress Inventory*.
   - The Domestic Violence Survivor Assessment (DVSA) tool can help health care providers and abused women identify issues and feelings created by domestic violence and helps guide counseling.
   - More research is needed to develop screening tools that are effective in the general population.

4. **Recommendation**
   - Reporting child and elder abuse to protective services is mandatory in most states, and several states have laws requiring mandatory reporting of intimate partner violence.
   - The American Academy of Pediatrics (AAP) and the American Medical Association (AMA) recommend that physicians remain alert for the signs and symptoms of children's physical and sexual abuse in the routine examination.
   - The AMA encourages physicians to inquire routinely about their patients' domestic violence histories and refer those patients with violence-related problems for medical and/or community-based services.
   - The Centers for Disease Control (CDC) and U.S. Preventive Services Task Force (USPTF) on Community Preventive Services found that home visitation programs aimed at children with a high risk of maltreatment (e.g., single or young mothers, low-income households, families with low birth-weight infants) were effective in decreasing maltreatment episodes.
   - The American College of Obstetricians and Gynecologists (ACOG) guidelines on domestic violence recommend that physicians routinely ask women direct, specific questions about abuse.
   - The American Academy of Family Physicians (AAFP) notes that family physicians can provide early intervention in family violence through routine screening and the identification of abuse, and recommends that physicians be alert to the presence of family violence in virtually every patient encounter.

UNINTENTIONAL HOUSEHOLD INJURIES AMONG PERSONS 0 TO 19 YEARS OLD

1. **Definition**
   - Public health-related unintentional accidental injury.
   - Unintentional injuries are the leading cause of morbidity and mortality among children in the United States.

2. **Epidemiology**
   - In the United States, on average 12,175 children and adolescents (0 to 19 years) die each year from an unintentional injury. The death rate for males was almost twice the rate for females.
   - *Injuries due to transportation were the leading cause of death for children.* Combining all unintentional injury

deaths among those between 0 and 19 years, motor vehicle traffic-related deaths were the leading cause.

- *The leading causes of injury death differed by age group.* For children younger than 1 year, two-thirds of injury deaths were due to suffocation. Drowning was the leading cause of injury death for those 1 to 4 years of age. For children and adolescents (5 to 19 years), the most injury-related deaths were due to being an occupant in a motor vehicle traffic crash.

- Poisoning death rate for those older than 15 years is at least five times the rate for the younger age group.

- *Risk of injury death varied by race.* An injury death rate was highest for American Indians and Alaska Natives and was lowest for Asian or Pacific Islanders. Overall death rates for Whites and African Americans were approximately the same.

- *Injury death rates varied by state, depending upon the cause of death.* Overall, NE states have the lowest injury-related death rates. Fire, burn, and transportation-related injuries death rates were highest in some of the SE states.

- Approximately 21.8 million persons aged ≥15 years sustained nonfatal, unintentional injuries, resulting in approximately $67.3 billion in lifetime medical costs (2008).

3. Screening

- Injury Center suggests screening for Child Maltreatment Prevention, Motor Vehicle Safety, and Older Adult Falls. Screening should be an ongoing process at primary care and community-based settings.

4. Recommendation

- The CDC's Community Guide "recommends child safety seat use laws, community-wide information and enhanced enforcement campaigns, and distribution or incentive programs plus education, enforcement programs to increase safety seat use in infants and children."

- The CDC recommends 0.08 blood alcohol concentration laws, lower blood alcohol concentration laws for young drivers, minimum legal drinking age laws, sobriety checkpoints, mass media campaigns, school-based programs, and alcohol server intervention training programs.

- AAFP, AAP, and AMA support primary enforcement of occupant restraint system legislation and counseling of all parents and patients older than 2 years about accidental injury prevention, and document the use of occupant restraint systems. In addition, providers should provide up-to-date, appropriate information for parents on car safety seat choices and proper use. Motor vehicle occupant injuries (MVOI) between physicians and their patients and the use of active, approved restraints for both adults and children should also be discussed.

- The ACOG recommends that clinicians counsel all women on the use of seat belts and that pregnant women be counseled on proper seat belt use during pregnancy and driving while intoxicated (DWI) alert for riding with the DWI drivers.

PREVENTION OF FALLS IN OLDER ADULTS—FALL AND GAIT DISORDERS (ALSO SEE PAGE 419)

1. Definition

- An unexpected event in which the participant falls and comes to rest on the ground, floor, or lower level.

2. Epidemiology

- Each year, one in every three adults aged 65 and older falls, which can lead to moderate to severe injuries, such as hip fractures and head traumas, and can even increase the risk of early death.

- Common occurrence among older adults, affecting approximately 30% of persons older than 65 years each year.

- Most common cause of nonfatal injuries and hospital admissions for trauma.

- The highest rates were for injuries that occurred in or around the tub or shower (65.8 per 100,000) and injuries that happened on or near the toilet (22.5 per 100,000).

- Hip fracture is common after fall; over 90% of hip fractures are caused by falling; women sustain three-quarters of all hip fractures.

- The most common are fractures of the spine, hip, forearm, leg, ankle, pelvis, upper arm, and hand.

- White women are much more likely to sustain hip fractures than are African American or Asian women; people 85 years and older are 10 to 15 times more likely to sustain hip fractures than are those aged 60 to 65.

3. Screening

- During routine visits, a provider should ask elderly patients about history of falls; observe any change in mental status, change in vision, and difficulty in transferring from bed to chair/bathroom; and observe patients' gait.

4. Recommendation

- Exercising regularly, focus on increasing leg strength and improving balance. Tai Chi programs are effective.

- Reviewing medicines—both prescription and over-the-counter—to reduce side effects and interactions that may cause dizziness or drowsiness.

- Eye examination/vision check once a year.

- Making home safety improvements by reducing tripping hazards, adding grab bars and railings, and improving lighting.

- Getting adequate calcium and vitamin D in your diet, undertaking a program of weight-bearing exercise, and getting screened and treated for osteoporosis.

MOTOR VEHICLE OCCUPANT RESTRAINTS

1. **Definition**
   - MVOI are related to motor vehicle accidents (MVA) when the seat belt and *child safety seats* are not used by the motor vehicle occupants (passengers).

2. **Epidemiology**
   - Each year, MVA take the lives of more than 40,000 people in the United States and result in 2.7 million emergency department visits.
   - Leading cause of death among individuals between 3 and 33 years of age in the United States and cause morbidity for the nearly 3 million people who sustain nonfatal injuries annually.
   - Proper use of seat belt or motor vehicle occupant restraints (child safety seats, booster seats, and lap-and-shoulder belts) is associated with a 45% to 70% reduction of fatality risk. Improper use reduces the efficacy of restraints substantially.
   - All 50 states currently have laws requiring child safety seats for infants and children, and 49 states and the District of Columbia have adult seat belt laws.
   - All 50 states, the District of Columbia, and Puerto Rico have laws that make it illegal to drive with a blood alcohol concentration of 0.08 g per dL or higher, and rates of alcohol involvement among fatal crashes have decreased during the past two decades.
   - Despite widespread regulation and overall increases in safer motor vehicle-related behaviors, recent crash data show that more than 50% of fatalities were among unrestrained occupants and nearly 40% involved alcohol.

3. **Screening**
   - Increasing the correct use of occupant restraint devices and decreasing alcohol-related driving (i.e., driving while under the influence of alcohol or riding with drivers who are under the influence of alcohol) are among the most important strategies to effectively reduce MVA-related fatalities.

4. **Recommendation**
   - Counseling in primary care setting to increase the proper use of child safety seats, increase the use of safety belts, and reduce alcohol-impaired driving.

CHEMOPROPHYLAXIS

A. Pertussis (Also see page 374, Section G-Whooping Cough and page 361 Immunization Schedule)

1. **Definition**
   - A cough illness lasting at least 2 weeks with one of the following: paroxysms of coughing, inspiratory "whoop," or post tussive vomiting, without any other apparent cause (as reported by a health professional).

2. **Epidemiology**
   - Pertussis is an endemic (common) disease in the United States, with periodic epidemics every 3 to 5 years and frequent outbreaks.
   - Since the 1980s, there has been an increase in the number of reported cases of pertussis in the United States, especially among 10- to 19-year-olds and infants younger than 6 months.
   - The primary goal of pertussis outbreak control efforts is to decrease morbidity (amount of disease) and mortality (death) among infants; a secondary goal is to decrease morbidity among persons of all ages.
   - Polymerase chain reaction (PCR) tests vary in specificity, so obtaining culture confirmation of pertussis for at least one suspicious case is recommended any time there is suspicion of a pertussis outbreak.
   - Institutional outbreaks of pertussis are common. Outbreaks at middle and high schools can occur as protection from childhood vaccines fades. In school outbreaks, prophylaxis is recommended for close classroom and team contacts—and the pertussis booster vaccine (Tdap), depending on age. Pertussis outbreaks in hospitals and other clinical settings can put infants and other patients at risk (Figure 21-1).

3. **Screening**
   - Infants younger than 6 months, who are at greatest risk for severe disease and death, continue to have the highest reported rate of pertussis, with a 60% increase in incidence observed between 2008 and 2009.
   - PCR tests of nasopharyngeal swabs or aspirates can be a rapid, sensitive, and specific test for pertussis. Preferably, it should be used in addition to bacterial cultures, not as a replacement for culture tests.
   - Clinical case and positive PCR tests are considered confirmed cases by the health department. Patients who have not been coughing for at least

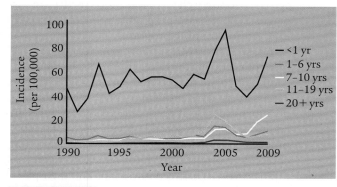

FIGURE 21–1. Reported pertussis incidence of age group 1990 to 2009. (Courtesy of the CDC, National Notifiable Diseases Surveillance System, 2009.)

14 days are considered probable cases unless the cough continues for 14 days.

- Isolation of *Bordetella pertussis* by culture is considered to be definitive for pertussis. The *B. pertussis* bacteria are fastidious; therefore, culturing may be difficult.

4. **Recommendation**
- Vaccination of susceptible persons is the most important preventive strategy against pertussis. Universal childhood pertussis vaccine recommendations have been implemented since the mid-1940s.
- Postexposure prophylaxis. A macrolide can be administered as prophylaxis for close contacts of a person with pertussis if the person has no contraindication to its use: azithromycin, erythromycin, clarithromycin, alternate agent (TMP–SMZ).

METABOLIC DISORDERS, NUTRITIONAL AND ENDOCRINE DISORDERS (ALSO SEE PAGE 228–229)

A. Obesity (Adult)
1. **Definition**
- Obesity ranges are determined by using weight and height to calculate the "body mass index (BMI)."
- An adult who has a BMI between 25 and 29.9 is considered overweight.
- An adult who has a BMI of 30 or higher is considered obese.

2. **Epidemiology**
- It is estimated that more than 34% of adults aged 20 and older in the United States are obese (defined as having a BMI of 30 or higher) and therefore at increased risk for cancer, diabetes, and coronary heart disease (CHD).
- Approximately 65% of obese adults aged 20 and older reported being told by their health care provider that they were overweight.
- Poor, near-poor, and middle-income obese adults were less likely than high-income obese adults to report being told by their health care provider that they were overweight.
- Obese adults with less than a high school education and those with a high school education were less likely than obese with at least some college to report being told by their health care that they were overweight.
- Obese women aged 20 and older were more likely than men to report being told by a doctor or health professional that they were overweight.

3. **Screening**
- The U.S. Preventive Services Task Force (USPTF) recommends that clinicians screen all adult patients for obesity and offer intensive counseling and behavioral interventions to promote sustained weight loss for obese adults.

- The AAFP recommends that intensive counseling involve more than one session per month for at least 3 months (2003).

4. **Recommendation**
- The CDC recommends counting calories and not eating more calories than the body is using, reducing time spent watching television and other sedentary behaviors, building physical activity into regular routines, creating opportunities for physical activity at work sites and in communities.
- The Agency for Healthcare Research and Quality (AHRQ) recommends physician-based exercise and diet counseling as an effective strategy for a weight loss intervention and regular exercise and a health aid in maintaining normal blood cholesterol levels, weight, and blood pressure, reducing the risk of heart disease, stroke, and diabetes.

PHYSICAL ACTIVITY
1. **Definition**
   The CDC defines physical activity as follows:
- Recommend physical activity—moderate-intensity activities in a usual week (i.e., brisk walking, vacuuming, or anything that results in small increases in breathing or heart rate) for ≥30 minutes per day, ≥5 days per week; or vigorous-intensity activities in usual week (i.e., running, heavy hard work or anything else that causes large increases in breathing or heart rate) for ≥20 minutes per day, ≥3 days per week, or both.
- Insufficient physical activity—doing more than 10 minutes per week of moderate or vigorous-intensity lifestyle activities (i.e., household, transportation, or lifestyle activities), but less than the recommended level of activity.
- Inactivity—less than 10 minutes per week of moderate or vigorous-intensity lifestyle activities (i.e., household, transportation, or leisure-time activity).
- Leisure-time inactivity—no reported physical activities (i.e., any physical activities or exercise such as running, calisthenics, golf, gardening, or walking) in the previous month.

2. **Epidemiology**
- According to CDC and USPSTF, 36 States reported (2008) that 25% of their population reported no leisure-time physical activity.
- According to the 2007 Youth Risk Behavior Surveillance System, 17% of high school youths are physically active.

3. **Screening**
- The AAFP recognizes that regular physical activity is desirable.

4. **Recommendation**
- The USDHHS (Healthy People 2020), CDC, AAFP, AAP, The American Heart of Association, and ACOG recommend that healthcare providers

counsel individuals physical activity based on the health benefits of physical activity.

- The *2008 Physical Activity Guidelines for Activity* recommends adults should do at least 150 minutes of moderate intensity (e.g., brisk walking) or 75 minutes of vigorous-intensity physical activity (e.g., jogging, running) per week or an equivalent combination of the two.
- For additional health benefits, adults should do more than 300 minutes of moderate intensity or 150 minutes of vigorous-intensity activity per week or an equivalent combination of the two.
- Older adults should engage in muscle-strengthening activities on at least 2 days of the week to improve.

HORMONE REPLACEMENT THERAPY

1. **Definition**
   - There is controversy around the risks and benefits of the use of hormone replacement therapy (HRT) in women going through menopause and having decrease in estrogen levels.

2. **Epidemiology**
   - White women are more likely to receive HRT counseling than black or Hispanic women with the same level of education; women with higher levels of education were more likely to receive counseling than women with less education, regardless of race or ethnicity.
   - Women who had received recent preventive health services such as mammograms, Pap smears, and general examinations were much more likely to have received HRT counseling than those who had not. The more recent the services, the greater the likelihood the women had received HRT counseling.

3. **Screening**
   - The American College of Physicians recommended that heathcare providers discuss HRT with all women around the time of menopause (40 to 60 years of age, the years when menopause is most likely to occur).

4. **Recommendation**
   - The USPSTF recommends against the routine use of combined estrogen and progestin for the prevention of chronic conditions in postmenopausal women.
   - The USPSTF found evidence that the use of combined estrogen and progestin results in the reduced risk of fracture and colorectal cancer.
   - The USPSTF found that combined estrogen and progestin has no beneficial effect on CHD and may even pose an increased risk. Other harms included an increased risk for breast cancer, venous thromboembolism, stroke, cholecystitis, dementia, and lower global cognitive function.
   - The USPSTF could not assess the effects of combined estrogen and progestin on the incidence of ovarian cancer, mortality from breast cancer or CHD, or all-cause mortality. The USPSTF concluded that the harmful effects of combined estrogen and progestin are likely to exceed the chronic disease prevention benefits in most women.
   - The USPSTF recommends against the routine use of unopposed estrogen for the prevention of chronic conditions in postmenopausal women who have had a hysterectomy.

II. Child and Adolescents

DENTAL CARIES IN PRESCHOOL CHILDREN (ALSO SEE PAGE 22–23)

1. **Definition**
   - Dental caries (i.e., tooth decay) is an infectious, multifactorial, communicable disease caused by demineralization of tooth enamel in the presence of a sugar substrate and cariogenic bacteria found in plaque.
   - *Streptococcus mutans* is considered to be the primary strain of bacteria causing tooth decay.
   - When plaque is not regularly removed, it may calcify to form calculus (tartar) and dental caries.
   - Fluoride reduces the incidence of dental caries and slows or prevents cavities.

2. **Screening**
   - Health care providers are encouraged to screen for dental caries and identify risk factors for childhood dental caries during routine visits: frequent consumption of foods and beverages containing sugars and sticky foods, frequent bottle- and breast-feeding on demand, maternal or sibling caries, repetitive use of "sippy cup," poor oral hygiene, inadequate fluoridation, and lack of dental visits.

3. **Epidemiology**
   - According to the CDC, dental caries affects more than one-fourth of US children aged 2 to 5 years, and half of those aged 12 to 15 years, half of all children and two-thirds of adolescents aged 12 to 19 years from lower-income families have decay.
   - Less than one of three children enrolled in Medicaid received at least one preventive dental screening.
   - Children and adolescents from some racial and ethnic groups have more untreated tooth decay—40% of Mexican American children aged 6 to 8 years have untreated decay, compared with 25% of non-Hispanic white.

4. **Recommendation**
   - The USPSTAF and AAFP recommend that health care providers prescribe oral fluoride supplementation to prevent dental caries based on age and fluoride concentration of patient's water supply for infants and children aged 6 months through 16 years residing in areas with inadequate fluoride in the water supply (<0.6 pm).

EXERCISE (PHYSICAL ACTIVITY)

1. **Definition**
   - Physical activity is any bodily movement that results in the expenditure of energy and includes aerobic, muscle strengthening, and bone strengthening activities.
   - According to the CDC, physical activity for children and adolescents is measured on a scale of 0 to 10, where sitting is a 0 and the highest level of activity is a 10, moderate-intensity activity is a 5 or 6 and vigorous-intensity activity is a level 7 to 8.
   - Aerobic activity moderate-intensity includes brisk walking, and vigorous-intensity includes running; muscle strengthening includes gymnastics or push-ups; and bone strengthening activities include jumping rope or running.

2. **Epidemiology**
   - According to Healthy People 2020, the following factors have a positive association with physical activity:
     - Children aged 4 to 12; gender (boys), belief in ability to be active (self-efficacy) and parental support.
     - Adolescents aged 13 to 18; parental education, gender (boys) and personal goals, physical education/school sports, belief in ability to be active (self-efficacy and support of friends and family).
     - Environmental influences positively associated with physical activity among children and adolescents include presence of sidewalks, having a destination/walking to a particular place, access to public transportation, low traffic density, access to neighborhood or school play area and/or recreational equipment.

3. **Screening**
   - The AAFP *recognizes that regular physical activity is desirable*. The effectiveness of physician's advice and counseling in this area is uncertain (2002).

4. **Recommendation**
   - The *2008 Physical Activity Guidelines for Activity* recommends that children should be active at least 60 minutes daily and that most of this time should be spent in either moderate (i.e., brisk walking) or vigorous-intensity physical activity (i.e., running) on at least 3 days per week, to include aerobic, muscle strengthening, and bone strengthening activities.
   - The AAFP recommends that prolonged periods of physical inactivity should be discouraged in both the home and the school.
   - Adults should do at least 150 minutes a week of moderate intensity (e.g., brisk walking) or 75 minutes a week of vigorous-intensity aerobic physical activity. Aerobic activity should be performed in episodes of at least 10 minutes and should be spread throughout the week.
   - The AAFP recommends that parents encourage their children to be physically active as part of their daily routine. The benefits of physical activity include increased cardiovascular endurance, improved large muscle strength and endurance, increased flexibility, maintenance of proper body weight, and reduction of stress.

HEALTHY DIET (NUTRITION)

1. **Definition**
   - The *Dietary Guidelines for Americans, 2010* emphasizes the following goals for a healthy diet:
     - Balance calories with physical activity to manage weight.
     - Consume more of certain foods and nutrients such as fruits, vegetables, whole grains, fat-free and low-fat dairy products, and seafood.
     - Consume fewer foods with sodium (salt), saturated fats, *trans* fats, cholesterol, added sugars and refined grains.

2. **Epidemiology**
   - According to the CDC, most youths in the United States do not meet the recommendations for eating fruits and vegetables and whole grains each day, and exceed the recommended maximum daily intake of sodium (1,500 to 2,300 mg each day).
   - Children and adolescents between the ages of 2 and 18 years consume 40% of their daily calories from empty calories from soda, fruit drinks, dairy desserts, grain desserts, pizza, and whole milk.
   - Adolescents drink more full-calorie soda per day than milk. Males aged 12 to 19 years drink an average of 22 oz of full-calorie soda per day, more than twice their intake of fluid milk (10 oz), and females drink an average of 14 oz of full-calorie soda and only 6 of fluid milk.

3. **Screening**
   - Health care providers are encouraged to screen for healthy eating to reduce the risk of heart disease, cancer, stroke, and diabetes in children and adolescents; in addition, it is important for proper growth and development and can prevent health problems such as obesity, dental caries, and iron deficiency.

4. **Recommendation**
   - The Dietary Guidelines for Americans recommends a diet rich in fruits and vegetables, whole grains, and fat-free and low-fat dairy products for persons aged 2 years and older.
   - The guidelines also recommend that children, adolescents, and adults limit the intake of solid fats (major sources of saturated and trans fatty acids), cholesterol, sodium, added sugars, and refined grains.

LEAD LEVELS IN CHILDREN AND ADOLESCENTS (ALSO SEE PAGE 303–304)

1. **Definition**
   - Lead is an element found in flaking lead paint, artist's paints, fruit tree sprays, solder, brass alloys, home-glazed pottery, and fumes from burning batteries.
   - Repetitive ingestion of small amounts of lead is more serious than a single massive exposure.
   - Toxic effects are more likely to occur if more than 0.5 mg of lead per day is absorbed.
   - Lead poison causes symptoms including weakness, irritability, weight loss, vomiting, ataxia, headache, colicky abdominal pain, decreased growth in height, delayed sexual maturation, increased dental caries, and impaired neurologic development (e.g., behavioral changes, mental impairment, seizures, and coma).

2. **Epidemiology**
   - The incidence and prevalence of lead poisoning in children has decreased since the removal of lead from paint and gasoline in the 1970s; however, there are approximately 310,000 US children younger than 5 years that have elevated blood lead levels.

3. **Screening**
   - Health care providers are encouraged to identify children at risk, eliminate exposure to known sources, and ensure adequate nutrition, including preventing and correcting iron deficiency, as key strategies in the care of all children.
   - Healthcare providers should perform targeted screening for lead poisoning in children who are Medicaid-enrolled or –eligible, foreign born, or identified as high-risk by the CDC.

4. **Recommendation**
   - The CDC recommends a blood lead level of 10 μg per dL (0.48 μmol per L) or higher as abnormal and requiring follow-up and intervention; lead levels lower than 10 μg per dL can affect cognitive development.
   - Recommendations for treatment of elevated blood levels include a thorough environmental investigation, laboratory testing when appropriate, iron supplementation for iron-deficient children, and chelation therapy for blood lead levels of 45 μg per dL or more. Prevention consists of education and avoidance of lead-contaminated products.

III. Cancer

BREAST CANCER (ALSO SEE PAGE 400–401)

1. **Definition**
   - Cancer that forms in tissues of the breast, usually the ducts and lobules.

2. **Epidemiology**
   - Most common cancer in pregnant and postpartum women, occurring in about 1 in 3,000 pregnant women.
   - Average patient is between 32 and 38 years, many women choosing to delay childbearing; it is likely that the incidence of breast cancer during pregnancy will increase.
   - Estimated new cases and deaths from breast cancer in the United States (2011): new cases—230,480 (females), 2,140 (males); and deaths—39,520 (females), 450 (males).
   - Decline in cancer deaths among white women in this country, but survival has decreased among black women, with 28% more likely to die from the disease.

3. **Screening**
   - The USPSTF recommends screening mammography (Grade B), with or without clinical breast examination (CBE), every 1 to 2 years for women aged 40 and older. (Grade B net benefit is moderate to substantial.)

4. **Recommendations**
   - CDC makes the following recommendations: have a regular breast examination, control weight and exercise, know your family history, find out the risks and benefits of HRT, and limit the amount of alcoholic drinks.

COLORECTAL CANCER (PAGE 399)

1. **Definition**
   - Most common type is adenocarcinomas.

2. **Epidemiology**
   - Estimated new cases and deaths from colon cancer in the United States (2011): new cases—101,340 (colon), 39,870 (rectal); and deaths—49,380 (colon and rectal combined).
   - Third most common type of cancer and the second leading cause of cancer death in the United States.
   - Prevention of colorectal cancer includes modifying risk factors such as weight, physical activity, smoking, and alcohol use, as well as screening for early disease.

3. **Screening**
   - Screening is important because early stages of colorectal cancer may not present any symptoms, and also because abnormal growths can be detected before they develop into cancer.
   - Early detection increases treatment options and the chances for survival. The USPSTF recommends colorectal cancer screening for men and women aged 50 years and continuation until age 75.
   - The screening tests include fecal occult blood test (FOBT), flexible sigmoidoscopy, colonoscopy, proctoscopy, and barium enema.
   - Insufficient evidence to assess the benefits and harms of CT colonography and fecal DNA testing as screening modalities for colorectal cancer.

4. **Recommendations**
   - High-sensitivity FOBT or fecal immunochemical-testing annually, flexible sigmoidoscopy every 5 years, double-contrast barium enema every 5 years,
   - CT colonography (virtual colonoscopy) every 5 years, colonoscopy every 10 years, fecal DNA at an unspecified interval.
   - Adults aged 50 to 75 years—screen with high sensitivity FOBT, sigmoidoscopy, or colonoscopy.

LUNG

1. **Definition**
   - Cancer of air passages, small cell lung cancer(SCLC) and non-small cell lung cancer (NSCLC).
2. **Epidemiology**
   - In the United States, the estimated cases of lung cancer (SCLC and NSCLC)—new cases: 221,130 and deaths: 156,940 (2011).
   - The most common types of NSCLC are squamous and of SCLC, adenocarcinoma.
   - Leading cause of death accounting for one of every four deaths both in men and in women.
   - NSCLCs are associated with cigarette smoke, whereas adenocarcinomas may be found in patients who have never smoked.
   - As a class, NSCLCs are relatively insensitive to chemotherapy and radiation therapy compared with SCLCs.
   - SCLC accounts for approximately 15% of bronchogenic carcinomas; at the time of diagnosis, approximately 30% of patients will have tumors confined to the hemithorax of origin, the mediastinum, or the supraclavicular lymph nodes.
   - Five-year survival rates were higher for whites (52.7 %) than for blacks (47.5 %) with stage I or II disease. For stages III and IV disease, 5-year survival rates were 17.7% for whites and 19.6% for blacks.
3. **Screening**
   - In patients considered to be at high risk for developing lung cancer, no screening modality for early detection has been shown to alter mortality.
4. **Recommendations**
   - The USPSTF concludes that the evidence is insufficient to recommend for or against screening asymptomatic persons for lung cancer with either low-dose computerized tomography (LDCT), chest X-ray (CXR), sputum cytology, or a combination of these tests.
   - CDC makes the following recommendations: stop smoking, control weight and exercise, know your family history, and limit the amount of alcohol drinks.

ORAL

1. **Definition**
   - Cancer of oral cavity.
2. **Epidemiology**
   - In the United States, new cases were estimated to be 39,400 and deaths, 7,900 (2011).
   - Tobacco (cigarettes, cigars, pipes, betel or mixed tobacco and smokeless tobacco) users or alcohol users are at elevated risk for oral cancer; and they are at particularly high risk if they use both tobacco and alcohol.
   - Persistent oral infection by carcinogenic strains of human papillomavirus (HPV), and chronic sun exposure of lips are also at increased risk.
3. **Screening**
   - USPSTF concludes insufficient evidence to recommend routine screening of adults for oral cancer. Recommend oral examination during routine health care visits.
4. **Recommendations**
   - Encouraged not to use tobacco and to limit alcohol use to decrease their risk of oral cancer as well as heart disease, stroke, lung cancer, and cirrhosis.

OVARIAN

1. **Definition**
   - Mostly epithelial carcinomas.
2. **Epidemiology**
   - Estimated new cases and deaths from ovarian cancer in the United States in 2011—new cases, 21,990 and deaths, 15,460.
3. **Screening**
   - CA 125 levels, transvaginal ultrasound, and pelvic examinations.
4. **Recommendations**
   - Genetic testing for *BRCA1/2* mutation that can increase chances for breast/ovarian cancer.
   - Most breast and ovarian cancer is *not* caused by mutations in these genes; *BRCA1/2* genetic testing will be helpful only for a small number of women.
   - CDC recommends general cancer prevention, such as control weight; more fruit and vegetables; exercise; know your family history; and limit the amount of alcohol drinks.

PROSTATE (ALSO SEE PAGE 399)

1. **Definition**
   - Cancer of prostate common in older men.
2. **Epidemiology**
   - The American Cancer Society estimates about 240,890 new cases and 33,720 deaths in the United States (2011).
3. **Screening**
   - Prostate-specific antigen (PSA) and rectal examination.
4. **Recommendations**
   - CDC recommends general cancer prevention, such as control weight; more fruit and vegetables; exercise; know your family history; and limit the amount of alcohol drinks.

SKIN

1. **Definition**
   - Skin cancer; it could be melanoma, basal cell, squamous cell, and neuroendocrine carcinoma of skin.
2. **Epidemiology**
   - The American Cancer Society estimates that in 2011, there were 1,000,000 new cases and fewer-than 1,000 deaths.
3. **Screening**
   - The only widely proposed screening procedure for skin cancer is visual examination of the skin, including both self-examination and clinical examination.
4. **Recommendations**
   - The USPSTF concludes that the current evidence is insufficient to assess the balance of the risk and benefits of using a whole-body skin examination by a primary care clinician or patient skin self-examination for the early detection of cutaneous melanoma, basal cell cancer, or squamous cell skin cancer in the adult general population.
   - The USPSTF concludes that the evidence is insufficient to recommend for or against routine counseling by primary care clinicians to prevent skin cancer.

TESTICULAR (ALSO SEE PAGE 398)

1. **Definition**
   - Testicular cancer common in young or middle-aged men, or germ cell cancer.
2. **Epidemiology**
   - The American Cancer Society estimates 8,290 new cases and 350 deaths (2011).
3. **Screening**
   - α-Fetoprotein (AFP), beta-human chronic gonadotropin (β-hCG), and lactase dehydrogenase (LDH) should be measured before removing the involved testicle.
4. **Recommendations**
   - The USPSTF, AAFP, and AAP recommend against screening for testicular cancer in adolescent or adult males. The American Cancer Society does not recommend testicular self-examination. Most testicular cancers are discovered accidentally by the patient or their partner. Potential harm associated with screening testicular cancer includes false-positives, anxiety, and harms from diagnostic tests or procedures.

TOBACCO CESSATION

1. **Epidemiology**
   - Tobacco use is the leading preventable cause of death, disease, and disability in the United States. Each year, around 443,000 people die from smoking or exposure to secondhand smoke, and another 8.6 million suffer from a serious illness from smoking.
   - CDC reports about 46.6 million adults in the United States smoke, and 88 million nonsmokers are exposed to secondhand smoke.
   - Adult smoking rates vary across the United States, but the states with the most smokers are in the Midwest and Southeast regions.
   - Smokers are two to four times more likely to develop heart disease, double the risk for stroke.
2. **Screening and Recommendations**
   - To increase tobacco use cessation, the United States Public Health States (USPHS) on Community Preventive Services recommends increasing the unit price of tobacco products, conducting mass media education campaigns with community interventions, and providing telephone-based cessation counseling.
   - USPHS recommends that brief advice by medical providers to quit smoking is an effective intervention.
   - HHS provides single toll-free number 1-800-QUIT NOW.
   - All 50 states offer some degree of telephone-based tobacco cessation services.

CARDIOVASCULAR

AAA—Abdominal Aortic Aneurysm.

1. **Epidemiology**
   - AAA is more common in men and in individuals aged 65 years and older. AAA is less common in women and with black race/ ethnicity.
   - AAA (from 2.9 to 4.9-cm diameter) are present in 1.3% of men (0% of women) aged 45 to 54 years and 2.5% (5.2% of women) of men aged 75 to 84 years.
2. **Screening**
   - USPSTF recommends one-time screening for AAA by ultrasound in men aged 65 to 75 years who have ever smoked and do not recommend ultrasound for those who have never smoked.
3. **Recommendations**
   - Less than 3.0 cm, no further screening; 3.0 to 3.9 cm, periodic re-screening with abdominal ultrasound until age 75 and expert opinion.
   - 4.0 to 5.4 cm, rescreening with ultrasound and one expert opinion, at 6 months following first screening; every year until age 75.
   - Greater than or equal to 5.5 cm, refer to vascular surgery for AAA repair 2. Grade A periodic surveillance offers comparable mortality benefit to routine elective surgery.

HTN

1. Definition
According to CDC

Blood Pressure Levels	
Normal	Systolic: <120 mm Hg
	Diastolic: <80mm Hg
At risk (prehypertension)	Systolic: 120–139 mm Hg
	Diastolic: 80–89 mm Hg
High	Systolic: 140 mm Hg or higher
	Diastolic: 90 mm Hg or higher

2. Epidemiology
- About one out of three US adults—31.3%—has high blood pressure (nearly 68 million), a major risk factor for heart disease, stroke, congestive heart failure, and kidney disease.
- In 2010, high blood pressure will cost the United States $76.6 billion in health care services, medications, and missed days of work.
- About 70% of those with high blood pressure and who took medication had their high blood pressure controlled. The control rate was 46.6% among all hypertensive patients.
- Twenty-five percent of American adults have pre-hypertension—blood pressure numbers that are higher than normal, but not yet in the high blood pressure range. Prehypertension raises your risk for high blood pressure.
- High blood pressure increases the risk for heart disease and stroke, the first and third leading causes of death.

3. Screening
- The USPSTF recommends screening for high blood pressure in adults aged 18 years and older.

4. Recommendations
- The National Guideline Clearinghouse (NGC) and the American Dietetic Association (ADA) recommend dietary interventions, including Dietary Approaches to Stop Hypertension (DASH), dietary pattern and weight management, physical activity interventions, behavioral interventions, and pharmacotherapy.

CORONARY HEART DISEASE

1. Epidemiology
- Leading cause of death in most Northern European, North American, and other industrialized Caucasian societies.
- Leading cause of death among African Americans, Native Americans, or Alaska Natives, Hispanics, and Whites. One-third of all deaths over age 35 are related to CHD.
- By the age of 60, 1 in 5 men and 1 in 17 women have some form of CHD. One in 15 men and women will eventually have a stroke.
- Every year about 785,000 Americans have a first heart attack. Another 470,000 who have already had one or more heart attack have another attack.
- In 2011, heart disease will cost the United States $444 billion (in health care services, medications, and lost productivity).

2. Screening and Recommendations
- The USPSTF found insufficient evidence to recommend for or against routine screening with electrocardiogram (ECG), exercise treadmill (ETT), or electron-beam computerized tomography (EBCT) scanning for coronary calcium for either the presence of severe coronary artery stenosis (CAS) or the prediction of CHD events in adults at low or high risk for CHD events.

EYE

A. Glaucoma (Also See Pages 9–10)

1. Definition
- There are four major types of glaucoma: open-angle (chronic) glaucoma, angle-closure (acute) glaucoma, congenital glaucoma, and secondary glaucoma. In the United States, it is the second most common cause of blindness, and it is a leading cause of blindness worldwide.

2. Epidemiology
- An estimated 2.2 million Americans have glaucoma, and a similar number may have the disease without knowing it. 120,000 are blind as a result of glaucoma.
- Risk factors include African Americans older than 40 years, everyone older than 60 years, Mexican Americans, and those with a family history of glaucoma.
- Primary open-angle glaucoma is the most common type of glaucoma.

3. Screening
- The USPSTF found insufficient evidence to recommend for or against screening adults for glaucoma.

4. Recommendation
- Complete eye examination before age 40, or sooner if you have the above-mentioned risk factors for glaucoma or other eye problems.
- Laser eye surgery for high risk of acute glaucoma.

CATARACT

1. Definition
- Clouding eye lens.

2. Epidemiology
- An estimated 20.5 million Americans aged 40 or older have cataract in either eye.
- One of the leading treatable causes of blindness in the world.
- By age 80, more than half of all people in the United States either have a cataract or have had cataract surgery.

3. Screening
- Visual acuity, dilated eye examination test, and tonometry.

4. **Recommendation**
   - Complete eye examination before age 40, or sooner if you have above-mentioned risk factors for cataract or other eye problems.

AGE-RELATED MACULAR DEGENERATION

1. **Definition**
   - Associated with aging, which gradually destroys sharp, central vision.
2. **Epidemiology**
   - More than 1.6 million Americans older than 60 years have advanced age-related macular degeneration (AMD).
   - Common among people aged 50 and older.
   - Most common cause of blindness and vision impairment in Americans aged 60 and older.
3. **Screening and Recommendation**
   - Recommendations for preventionand screening of AMD include the following: do not smoke; prevent overexposure to the sunlight by wearing sunglasses and a hat; eat a variety and nutritious diet that includes leafy green vegetables, fruit, fish, and foods containing vitamins D, E, and C and ω-3 fatty acids; maintain a healthy weight; keep blood pressure at a normal level; follow a regular exercise routine; regularly visit an eye doctor for comprehensive eye examinations; and perform Amsler grid tests at home.

MUSCULOSKELETAL DISORDERS

A. Osteoporosis (Pages 220–275)

1. **Definition**
   - A condition characterized by decreased bone strength and microarchitectural deterioration of bone tissue that increases bone fragility and risk of fractures.
2. **Epidemiology**
   - In the United States, 8 million women and 2 million men have osteoporosis; it is estimated that 50% of Americans older than 50 years will be at risk for osteoporotic fractures during their lifetime.
   - Occurs more frequently with increasing age as bone tissue is progressively lost.
   - Prevalence rates are higher in women than in men; rates vary by race, with the highest in whites; and rates for all demographic groups increase with age.
   - In women, the loss of ovarian function (typically at about age 50) precipitates rapid bone loss; occurs in men and women with underlying conditions (see Chapter 9, section IV.A.) or major risk factors associated with bone demineralization.
   - Causes approximately 1.5 million fractures annually in the United States, mainly of the spine and hip.
3. **Screening**
   - The dual energy X-ray absorptiometry (DXA) is used to predict fractures, to diagnose osteoporosis, and to select patients for treatment.
   - DXA of the hip is the strongest predictor of hip fracture, and most DXA testing includes measurements of the hip and lumbar spine (central DXA).
   - The most commonly used non-DXA test in the United States is quantitative ultrasound (QUS) of the calcaneus.
   - QUS avoids ionizing radiation, and is inexpensive, portable, and feasible for primary care settings.
4. **Recommendation**
   - The USPSTF recommends screening for osteoporosis in women aged 65 years or older and in younger women whose fracture risk is equal to that of a 65-year-old woman who has no additional risk factors.
   - The USPSTF concludes that the current evidence is insufficient to assess the balance of benefits and harms of screening for osteoporosis in men.
   - Osteoporosis Screening Recommendations of Other Organizations (Table 21-1).

TERTIARY PREVENTION AND DISEASE MANAGEMENT

A. Antimicrobial Resistance (AMR) (Also see pages 338–339 and 345–347)

1. **Definition**
   - According to the World Health Organization, AMR is the resistance of a microorganism to an antimicrobial medicine to which it was previously sensitive. AMR is a consequence of the use, particularly the misuse, of antimicrobial medicines and develops when a microorganism mutates or acquires a resistance gene.
2. **Epidemiology**
   - According to the CDC, there are 440,000 new cases of multidrug-resistant tuberculosis (MDR-TB) emerging annually, resulting in at least 150,000 deaths.
   - A high percentage of hospital-acquired infections are caused by highly resistant bacteria such as methicillin-resistant *Staphylococcus aureus* (MRSA).
3. **Screening**
   - Healthcare provides can prevent the spread of antibiotic resistance by prescribing antibiotic therapy when it will most likely be beneficial to the patient, using antibiotics that target likely pathogens and using antibiotics for the appropriate dose and duration.
4. **Recommendations**
   - Veiw CDC's adult and pediatric academic detail sheets for recommended prescribing guidelines for providers http://www.cdc.gov/getsmart/campaign-materials/info-sheets/adult-approp-summary.html and http://www.cdc.gov/getsmart/campaign-materials/info-sheets/child-practice-tips.html.
   - Pediatric treatment guidelines for upper respiratory infections: http://www.cdc.gov/getsmart/campaign-materials/pediatric-treatment.html.

TABLE 21-1.	Osteoporosis Screening Recommendations of Other Organizations	
Organization	**Recommendations**	
	Women	**Men**
National Osteoporosis Foundation	BMD testing for all women ≥65 y and postmenopausal women <65 y, based on risk factor profile	BMD testing for all men ≥70 y and men aged 50–69 y, based on risk factor profile
World Health Organization	Indirect evidence supports screening women ≥65 y, but no direct evidence supports widespread screening programs using BMD testing	–
American College of Physicians	–	Clinicians should assess older men for osteoporosis risk factors and use DXA to screen men at increased risk who are candidates for drug therapy for osteoporosis
American Congress of Obstetricians and Gynecologists	BMD testing for all women ≥65 y and postmenopausal women <65 y who have one or more risk factors	–

BMD, bone mineral density; DXA, dual energy X-ray absorptiometry.

SELECTED REFERENCES

Agency for Healthcare Research and Quality (AHRQ). http://www.ahrq.gov/CLINIC/uspstfix.htm.

American Academy of Family Physicians. http://www.aafp.org/online/en/home/clinical/exam/physicalactivity.html.

A-Z topics from CDC.http://www.cdc.gov/az/.

Cancer. http://www.cancer.gov/cancertopics/types/colon-and-rectal.

Clinical Preventive Services resources for PA (AAPA). http://www.aapa.org/advocacy-and-practice-resources/clinical-issues/clinical-topics/clinical-preventive-services.

Evidence Review literature review for fall prevention.http://www.uspreventiveservicestaskforce.org/uspstf11/fallsprevention/fallsprevart.pdf.

Fall prevention brochureand literature. http://www.cdc.gov/Homeand RecreationalSafety/Falls/fallsmaterial.html.

Grading for Recommendations. http://www.uspreventiveservicestaskforce.org/uspstf/gradespre.htm#drec.

Injury prevention and control. http://www.cdc.gov/injury/overview/data.html.

MMWR Fatalities and Injuries from Falls Among Older Adults—United States, 1993–2003 and 2001–2005. http://www.cdc.gov/mmwr/preview/mmwrhtml/mm5545a1.htm.

Multiple interventions in these areas have been recommended. Recommendations can be accessed at: http://www.thecommunityguide.org/mvoi/.

My plate.gov: http://www.choosemyplate.gov.

National Center for Victim of Crime. http://www.ncvc.org/ncvc/main.aspx?dbName=DocumentViewer&DocumentID=32347.

National Institute of Aging. http://www.nia.nih.gov/HealthInformation/Publications/falls.htm.

Other resources for Preventive Medicine. http://www.uspreventiveservicestaskforce.org/resources.htm.

Preventive medicine recommendations, screening and counseling by topic. http://epss.ahrq.gov/ePSS/Topics.do?ttid=1.

Recommendations for Adults. http://www.uspreventiveservicestaskforce.org/adultrec.htm.

Recommendations for Children. http://www.uspreventiveservicestaskforce.org/tfchildcat.htm.

State Indicator Report on Physical Activity, 2010 National Action Guide. http://www.cdc.gov/physicalactivity/downloads/PA_State_Indicator_Report_2010_Action_Guide.pdf.

The National Highway Traffic Safety Administration. http://www.nhtsa.gov.

Three priority areas for prevention. http://www.cdc.gov/injury/about/priorities.html.

US Preventive Task Force: A-Z topics http://www.uspreventiveservicestaskforce.org/uspstopics.htm.

US Preventive Task Force. http://www.uspreventiveservicestaskforce.org/.

22

Study and Test-Taking Strategies

Jeffrey Bonfield

How to Study

This section will detail some test preparation techniques that can help you learn more in less time. Although there is no single test preparation technique that is ideal for everyone, there are some things that all good techniques have in common.

Being actively engaged with the material is a fundamental characteristic of the best study techniques. One of the most common ways to stay active with material is to organize information, so that it makes sense to you. A couple of common organization structures are outlines and mind maps. The process of rationally organizing information helps turn information into knowledge. Another important step for physician assistants is to consider how you would apply the information in practice. If you are asking yourself how you would use each piece of information as a PA, you are more likely to retain the information and be able to apply it on the test. The final and arguably most important way to stay actively engaged with the material is to test yourself.

One way to test your memory is the flashcard method. Few people have time to create and use flashcards for the quantity of material on the PANCE/PANRE, but we can gain most of the benefits of flashcards in far less time by understanding what it is about flashcards—beyond repetition—that aids in memorization. The essentials of using flashcards are to have a cue phrase on one side of the card and everything you need to know about that topic on the other side, then to look at the cue phrase and try to remember everything that is on the other side of the card. Even if you remember very little of the information, the act of making an effort to remember and then reading the information makes it more likely that you will retain the information. By analogy, the effort to remember creates a folder in your mind, so that when you read the information, you will file it in the correct place. This makes the information easier to recall during the exam.

As it is time-consuming to make flashcards, you can simply use the information in this text by reading the main headers in bold—your cue phrases—while covering the information below until you have made an effort to recall it. The header serves as the front of the flashcard and the covered information below serves as the back. If you use the text this way, you will find that you retain information far more efficiently than if you had simply read the information passively, like you are reading a novel.

As stated earlier, organizing information is another important way to learn faster and more thoroughly. All review books and textbooks try to organize information logically. This is helpful, but you can take it further. One method is to organize information based on similarities and—more importantly—distinctions. When answering multiple choice questions such as those on the PANCE/PANRE, being clear on the characteristics that distinguish one thing from another is extremely important. You can expect that the test makers will give you two answers that look right, but there is always some distinguishing characteristic that makes one answer better than the other. That distinction could be a single symptom or contraindication. If you look for those distinctions while you are studying, you will be ready for the questions. As you answer the practice questions on the Web site that accompanies this book, you will see how important knowing distinctions can be.

Although memorization is important, doing well on the PANCE/PANRE is not simply a matter of memorizing information. You must understand that information and be able to apply it to the test questions. To better understand the material, you will benefit from referring to other sources, such as textbooks. As with all studying, it is important to be active while reading. One way to encourage active reading is to read a paragraph and then stop and try to put what you read into your own words. It is important to be honest with yourself by asking questions like "Is this information mine or do I just understand it while I'm reading it?" Simply understanding what you read without being able to put it into practice is not enough for the PANCE/PANRE.

One way to ensure that you are ready to put the information you are reading into practice is to imagine you are treating a real patient and ask yourself "What would I see?" and "What would I do?" Asking yourself these two questions can help make the information you are reading more real for yourself. Some people like to visualize situations. Others prefer to verbalize them. Whatever method works for you, if you are able to make the material real for yourself while you are studying, it will be easier to remember and apply later.

Using the Web Site

Whether you take a complete practice PANCE/PANRE or shorter practice exams, the Web site that accompanies this text will identify your strengths and weaknesses. Use the diagnostic information to identify the content and clinical skills that you need to strengthen. In addition, as you review your incorrect answers and those correct answers about which you were not confident, make note of the areas you need to study. If you did not know one detail about a subject, it is likely you also lack some information surrounding that specific detail. It is usually worthwhile to cast a wide net when trying to fill gaps in knowledge.

Preparing for the Exam

In addition to reviewing specific material, there are more general ways to prepare yourself for the PANCE/PANRE. Simply knowing information and how to apply it is not always enough to ensure success on the exam; you must maintain your energy and focus throughout the exam. One of the factors that affect many students is the length of the PANCE/PANRE. The exam can be compared to a marathon, and similar to the way one prepares for such a long race, it is useful to prepare for a long exam.

Just as marathon runners familiarize themselves with the route of a race, it is helpful to familiarize yourself with the testing site at which you will take your exam. The fewer uncertainties and distractions you have on the day of the exam, the easier it will be to concentrate all your energy on the questions themselves. Similarly, it is helpful to know exactly what you will eat the night before, the morning of, and during breaks in the exam. Food might seem like an inconsequential element, but your hunger or blood sugar level could severely affect how well you concentrate as the exam progresses. Plan your meals ahead of time and bring snacks to the exam, whether you think you will need them or not.

You may have been given suggestions like, "Don't drink coffee the morning of the exam." This might seem like reasonable advice because the stimulant effect of the caffeine will wear off during the exam. Still, if you are a coffee drinker and you drink a specific amount of coffee every morning, it makes sense to drink that same amount of coffee on the morning of the exam. Similarly, some students wonder if they should take medication for anxiety or attention deficit disorder. For this and similar questions, the answer is the same: do not try anything new on the day of the exam. If you take medication for anxiety before every exam, it makes sense to take it before the PANCE/PANRE. If, on the other hand, you have never tested the effects of a medication on yourself, it is very risky to try it for the first time on the PANCE/PANRE. Simply put, you know what works for you. If you do not know about something, it is safest *not* to try it for the PANCE/PANRE.

Overcoming Test Anxiety

Most people suffer to some degree from test anxiety. Test anxiety can take many forms: some people "draw a blank" or their minds race; others try to finish exams as quickly as possible. In extreme cases, some people even fall asleep during an exam or express physical manifestations of their anxiety. All reactions arise in part from the activation of the sympathetic nervous system.

We usually think of the sympathetic nervous system as being activated when we are in mortal danger, but it reacts to subtler stimuli as well. Anything that is perceived as a challenge can activate the sympathetic nervous system. That is a good thing because, correctly interpreted, the system helps us perform our best in challenging situations. The problem comes when the system is not correctly interpreted by our minds. Most often, misinterpretation takes place when a "fight" response is appropriate, but our minds react with "flight." That is what happens when, during a test, we are not as focused as we want to be.

It is easy to image having the correct response to our sympathetic nervous system if, for instance, we wake up and our house is on fire. We would probably run out of the house, and we would run better and faster than we would run in a normal situation. That is flight mode working for us. If, on the other hand, a loved one were trapped under a 150 kg section of wall that had fallen on him or her in the fire, we would be able to lift the wall and carry the person out of the house. That is fight mode working for us.

An exam, however, does not look like a house on fire. Everyone is sitting. Everyone is quiet. It does not look like a situation in which we should fight, but it is. Fight mode will help us focus and bring all of our energy to beating the exam.

It may sound funny to say "beat the exam," but that is exactly the attitude that will best prepare you for success. Imagine for a moment that you are a football player and an opponent is coming down the field with the ball. That opponent is trying to beat you. In order to beat your opponent, it is best to be in fight mode. The fight response will focus your mind and actions. Similar to the football player, the exam is challenging you. Each question is testing your knowledge and ability. If you are not energized to beat the exam, it has a better chance of beating you. If we are not in fight mode, our minds might misinterpret the situation and slip us into flight mode. Flight mode causes those negative responses: a racing or wandering mind, the urge to finish the exam quickly, or negative physical manifestations of anxiety.

Now it should be clear why "fight" is the optimal attitude, but how do we get into fight mode? The first thing to remember is that logic and reason are not enough. It is not enough to say to yourself, "I've studied the material and know I can do well on the exam." Those are good things to know and tell yourself, but they are not enough to create and sustain fight mode. Just as athletes motivate themselves by exercising and yelling just before a match, you should find a way to motivate yourself before an exam. Some people use music to motivate themselves to fight; others exercise. Dancers and runners tend to use quieter, more internal ways of getting focused. Figure out what works for you and use it.

During the exam, if you find that you are not thinking as clearly as you would like, stop and take a few deep breaths. Your respiration is the only physical manifestation of an activated sympathetic nervous system that is in your control. Deep breaths will help convince your mind that despite your activated sympathetic nervous system, you are really okay. After assuring yourself physically that you are okay, go back to the exam and fight! Remember that this is your exam. Just as a football player "owns" the field, own your exam.

Taking the Exam

The difference between people who consider themselves good test takers and those who consider themselves bad test takers is usually one simple strategy. Bad test takers look for the correct answer, whereas good test takers look for the wrong ones. It is true that you must choose the single best answer, but that is not what the creators of the exam do. Good test takers capitalize on the fact that the exam makers write a question and then they have to come up with answers that are not as good as the answer they have in mind. If you look for the reason why each answer is wrong, you will see more clearly why one answer is better than another. Eliminating one or two answers will probably be easy. Then, when you have narrowed your choices down to two or three, cast doubt on each. Think, "How did they make this answer wrong?" Remember, the test makers have to make all but one answer wrong, so look for what's wrong with each answer. When you find something wrong with all but one answer, you've found your choice.

INDEX

Note: Page numbers followed by *f* indicate figures; those followed by *t* indicate tables.